# Comprehensive
# Handbook of
# Cognitive Therapy

# Comprehensive Handbook of Cognitive Therapy

Edited by

**ARTHUR FREEMAN**
*University of Pennsylvania*
*Philadelphia, Pennsylvania*

**KAREN M. SIMON**
*University of Pennsylvania*
*Philadelphia, Pennsylvania*

**LARRY E. BEUTLER**
*Arizona Health Sciences Center*
*Tucson, Arizona*

and

**HAL ARKOWITZ**
*University of Arizona*
*Tucson, Arizona*

Plenum Press • New York and London

Library of Congress Cataloging in Publication Data

Comprehensive handbook of cognitive therapy / edited by Arthur Freeman . . .
[et al.].
    p.    cm.
  Includes bibliographies and index.
  ISBN 0-306-43052-5
  1. Cognitive therapy—Handbooks, manuals, etc. I. Freeman, Arthur M.
  [DNLM: 1. Behavior Therapy. 2. Cognition. WM 425 C737]
RC489.C63C66   1989
616.89′142—dc19
DNL/DLC                                                                    89-3880
for Library of Congress                                                    CIP

10 9 8 7 6 5 4

© 1989 Plenum Press, New York
A Division of Plenum Publishing Corporation
233 Spring Street, New York, N.Y. 10013

Printed in the United States of America

# Contributors

HAL ARKOWITZ, Department of Psychology, University of Arizona, Tucson, Arizona

DONALD H. BAUCOM, Department of Psychology, University of North Carolina at Chapel Hill, Chapel Hill, North Carolina

AARON T. BECK, Center for Cognitive Therapy, Department of Psychiatry, University of Pennsylvania, Philadelphia, Pennsylvania

E. EDWARD BECKHAM, University of Oklahoma Health Sciences Center, Oklahoma City, Oklahoma

LARRY E. BEUTLER, Department of Psychiatry, College of Medicine, University of Arizona, Tucson, Arizona

MICHAEL D. BOLTWOOD, Counseling Psychology Program, School of Education, Stanford University, Stanford, California

WAYNE A. BOWERS, Department of Psychiatry, University of Iowa, Iowa City, Iowa

JAMES C. COYNE, University of Michigan Medical School, Ann Arbor, Michigan

DENISE DAVIS, Department of Psychiatry, Vanderbilt University, Nashville, Tennessee

RAYMOND DiGIUSEPPE, Institute for Rational-Emotive Therapy, New York, New York

E. THOMAS DOWD, Department of Educational Psychology, Kent State University, Kent, Ohio

JANET SASSON EDGETTE, Department of Mental Health Sciences, Hahnemann University, Philadelphia, Pennsylvania

DAVID J. A. EDWARDS, Department of Psychology, Rhodes University, Grahamstown, South Africa

BRUCE N. EIMER, Departments of Psychiatry and Rehabilitation Medicine, Abington Memorial Hospital, Abington, Pennsylvania

ALBERT ELLIS, Institute for Rational-Emotive Therapy, New York, New York

NORMAN EPSTEIN, Department of Family and Community Development, University of Maryland, College Park, Maryland

ARTHUR FREEMAN, Center for Cognitive Therapy, Department of Psychiatry, University of Pennsylvania, Philadelphia, Pennsylvania

MEYER D. GLANTZ, Division of Clinical Research, National Institute of Drug Abuse, Rockville, Maryland

JOEL O. GOLDBERG, Department of Psychiatry, University of Toronto, Toronto, Ontario, Canada

LESLIE S. GREENBERG, Department of Psychology, York University, Downsview, Ontario, Canada

PAUL D. GUEST, Program 3, Patton State Hospital, Patton, California

SHEENAH HANKIN-WESSLER, Cognitive Therapy Associates, 103 East 86th Street, and Pace University, New York, New York

MO THERESE HANNAH, Department of Psychology, University of Arizona, Tucson, Arizona

W. J. JACOBS, Department of Psychology, University of Lethbridge, Lethbridge, Alberta, Canada

F. MATTHEW KRAMER, Behavioral Sciences Division, U.S. Army Natick Research, Development, and Engineering Center, Natick, Massachusetts

RICHARD S. LAZARUS, Department of Psychology, University of California, Berkeley, California

RUSSELL C. LEAF, Department of Psychology, Rutgers University, New Brunswick, New Jersey; and Institute for Rational-Emotive Therapy, New York, New York

BARRY McCARTHY, Department of Psychology, American University, and Washington Psychological Center, Washington, DC

THOMAS V. MERLUZZI, Department of Psychology, University of Notre Dame, Notre Dame, Indiana

L. NADEL, Department of Psychology, University of Arizona, Tucson, Arizona

TERRY M. PACE, Department of Educational Psychology, University of Nebraska, Lincoln, Nebraska

CHRISTINE PADESKY, Center for Cognitive Therapy, Newport Beach, California

CARLO PERRIS, Department of Psychiatry, University of Umea, Umea, Sweden

MAURICE F. PROUT, Institute for Graduate Clinical Psychology, Widener University, Chester, Pennsylvania

LAURA RICE, Department of Psychology, York University, Downsview, Ontario, Canada

HUGH ROSEN, Department of Mental Health Sciences, Hahnemann University, Philadelphia, Pennsylvania

JEREMY SAFRAN, Clarke Institute of Psychiatry, Toronto, Ontario, Canada

G. RANDOLPH SCHRODT, JR., Department of Psychiatry and Behavioral Sciences, University of Louisville School of Medicine, and Norton Psychiatric Clinic, Louisville, Kentucky

BRIAN F. SHAW, Department of Psychiatry, University of Toronto, Toronto, Ontario, Canada

KAREN M. SIMON, Center for Cognitive Therapy, Department of Psychiatry, University of Pennsylvania, Philadelphia, Pennsylvania

LAURIE A. STALKER, Department of Psychiatry, University of Pennsylvania, Philadelphia, Pennsylvania.

D. J. TATARYN, Department of Psychology, University of Arizona, Tucson, Arizona

JOHN T. WATKINS, University of Oklahoma Health Sciences Center, Oklahoma City, Oklahoma

MARJORIE WEISHAAR, Department of Psychiatry and Human Behavior, Brown University, Providence, Rhode Island

RICHARD L. WESSLER, Cognitive Therapy Associates, 103 East 86th Street, and Pace University, New York, New York

DAVID M. WHITE, Department of Mental Health Sciences, Hahnemann University, Philadelphia, Pennsylvania

JESSE H. WRIGHT, Department of Psychiatry and Behavioral Sciences, University of Louisville School of Medicine, and Norton Psychiatric Clinic, Louisville, Kentucky

# Foreword

In reviewing the Contents of this *Handbook* edited by Freeman, Simon, Beutler, and Arkowitz, I am both impressed and gratified with the enormous strides made by cognitive-behavior therapy since the late 1960s. A perusal of the Contents reveals that it is used with adults, children, couples, and families; it is clinically appropriate for such problems as anxiety, depression, sexual dysfunctions, and addictions; and it is employed in conjunction with psychopharmacological and other psychotherapeutic interventions.

It was in the mid-1960s when Breger and McGaugh published an article in the *Psychological Bulletin,* taking behavior therapists to task for using only classical and operant principles in devising their therapeutic interventions. Breger and McGaugh argued that the field of learning was undergoing a major revolution, paying considerably more attention to cognitive processes than had previously been the case. In short, they criticized the growing behavioral orientation for being limited in its exclusively peripheralistic orientation.

At the time, behavior therapists were initially somewhat resistant to any allusion to cognitive metaphors. Indeed, my own initial reactions to the Breger and McGaugh article was quite negative. Yet, in rereading their critique, many of their suggestions now seem most appealing. No doubt, I and my behavior colleagues lacked the appropriate "cognitive set" for incorporating such contradictory information. Nonetheless, the clinical evidence for the relevance of cognitive factors in the behavior change process was simply too compelling to ignore. An increasing number of behavior therapists started to question whether the array of techniques available to them might be too narrowly comprised and began to consider the possibility that the addition of cognitive conceptualizations might help in expanding upon available behavioral procedures.

At the 1968 meeting of the American Psychological Association, I had the honor of chairing a symposium entitled "Cognitive Processes in Behavior Modification." The participants included Louis Breger, Gerald Davison, Thomas D'Zurilla, Gordon Paul, and Stuart Valins. The abstract for the symposium read as follows:

> This symposium discusses the important direct influence of such processes as expectation, attribution, reasoning, and planning on behavior change and independent functioning. The predominant conceptualization of the "behavior therapies" as conditioning techniques involving little or no cognitive influence on behavior is questioned. It is suggested that current procedures should be modified and new procedures developed to capitalize more on the human organism's unique capacity for cognitive control.

Unlike the earlier behavioral procedures that were made available to the field, cognitive techniques grew more out of a clinical need than an extrapolation from experimental findings.

ix

It was noticed by clinical behavior therapists that patients/clients often engaged in internal dialogues that could have a significant impact on their lives. By changing what clients/patients told themselves, it was argued, changes in emotion and behavior might ensue.

With increased experience in using cognitive procedures, it has become evident that the assessment and modification of what clients/patients "tell themselves" within any particular situation is not always as straightforward as it originally seemed. What is more often of interest is determining not so much what they are deliberately thinking but rather the more elusive *meaning* that they may be assigning to a given event. Thus, although clients/patients might not always be able to directly report certain cognitions, they will nonetheless acknowledge that they were reacting emotionally or behaviorally "as if" they were saying certain things to themselves.

To explain this phenomenon, an increasing number of cognitive-behavior therapists have recently adopted an information-processing model as a useful paradigm. This model, which has been popular in experimental cognitive psychology for a number of years, postulates several nonconscious cognitive processes that operate both on incoming and stored information. Thus, when individuals interact with their environment, potential distortions may occur by virtue of selective attention, inappropriate classification of events, idiosyncratic storage of information, and/or inaccurate retrieval from memory.

In making a move from an early associationistic premise to a more constructivistic viewpoint, the concept of "schema" has been suggested as being particularly useful in understanding this distortion process. In the most general sense, a schema refers to a cognitive representation of one's past experiences with situations or people, which eventually serves to assist individuals in constructing their perception of events within that domain. Although there are varying definitions of a schema, most reflect three basic assumptions: First, a schema is said to involve an organization of conceptually related elements, representing a prototypical abstraction of a complex concept. From a clinical vantage point, these complex concepts are likely to consist of types of situations (e.g., being criticized) and/or types of persons (e.g., authority figures). Specific examples are said to be stored in a schema as well as the relationship among these exemplars. Second, a schema is induced from the "bottom up," based on repeated past experiences involving many examples of the complex concept it represents. Finally, a schema is seen as guiding the organization of new information, much like a template or computer format allows for attending to or processing some information but not others.

Among the advantages of a schema is that it can facilitate learning and the recognition, recall, and comprehension of information that is schema-relevant. It allows us to chunk information into larger, more meaningful units—so called "knowledge structures"—giving a sense of meaning to the world around us. It also helps us to fill in the gaps when there are missing observations and provides us with greater confidence in making predictions about our world. At the same time, those advantages can serve as liabilities, particularly if a schema is no longer relevant to one's current life situation. In essence, our past interactions with the world have provided us with the propensities to view the world—or ourselves—in given ways, even though these perceptions may no longer be valid.

In depicting a model of human cognition that has important implications for the therapeutic change process, George Kelly suggested in the 1950s that there exist certain core assumptions that individuals have about themselves and others. Contemporary cognitive-behavior therapists refer to these as "silent assumptions" or "core organizing principles." Kelly hypothesized that under such core assumptions may be found more peripheral ones, hierarchically arranged according to the types of situations in which they manifest themselves. At the very bottom of this hierarchical organization, there exists specific life events.

In addressing the issue of how people change, the crucial question becomes whether therapists should proceed by facilitating "top-down" or "bottom-up" changes. That is, should the emphasis be on cognitive change, in the hope that it will result in behavior change, or is specific behavior change required in order to bring about change in one's core cognitions? This is most reminiscent of the psychodynamic and behavioral opposing emphases on "insight" versus "action." The essence of a cognitive-behavioral intervention is that it needs to make use of *both* top-down and bottom-up interventions. Top-down interventions, reflecting the deductive component of the change process, provide clients/patients with the conceptual categories essential for the recognition, classification, storage, and retrieval of relevant life events. Bottom-up methods, facilitating the inductive element in change, are needed to transform pure hypothetical categories into experience-based schemata.

These are but some of the issues with which this *Handbook* attempts to grapple. And in doing so, it provides the therapist and researcher with clinical and conceptual guidelines that are essential for functioning within a cognitive-behavioral orientation.

MARVIN R. GOLDFRIED

*Stony Brook, New York*

# Preface

The compilation of a handbook on any subject necessarily involves bringing together a large number of diverse people addressing a common theme. However, the compilation of this handbook has brought together collaborators with even more diverse backgrounds than is usually the case. We find, even among the editors, that the entire spectrum of psychological orientations is represented: Freeman was originally trained in a psychoanalytic model and at the Adlerian Institute in New York; Simon was originally a radical behaviorist who became a social-learning theorist while working with Albert Bandura at Stanford University; Arkowitz's background was originally behavioral, and he has more recently moved toward an integrated behavioral-psychodynamic approach; and Beutler evolved from a client-centered tradition and now considers himself an eclectic therapist who is committed to integrating many treatment models.

Furthermore, all of these orientations—as well as several others—are represented by the other contributors. Among our contributors we have individuals with backgrounds that are behavioral, psychodynamic, family systems, gestalt, psychopharmacological, eclectic, as well as cognitive. This volume is representative of the fact that cognitive-behavioral therapy (CBT), in general, has become a meeting place for all theorists. All of the contributors are now working from a broad cognitive perspective in the psychotherapy or research that they conduct. The contributors represent those who teach psychotherapy, those who research psychotherapy outcomes, those who practice psychotherapy, and those who represent combinations of the above.

We believe that this diversity is not a coincidence, but represents a real difference between cognitive therapy and many other forms of therapy. Given the relative youth of what has been termed the *cognitive revolution* the contributors were, of necessity, trained in the older, more established schools of therapy. Although the roots of a cognitive-behavioral focus in therapy can be traced back to the early writings of Freud, Adler, Horney, Sullivan, Frankl, and others, it was not until the mid-twentieth century that CBT emerged as a discrete entity. (There are those who still insist that CBT come "back into the fold." The fold is in some cases more narrowly focused behavior therapy, and in other cases more orthodox psychoanalytic therapy.)

What has led to the increasing interest in CBT? First, experimental research has shown cognitive therapy to be an effective treatment of various psychological disorders. Therapists who desire to be effective in their treatment of their patients should be drawn to cognitive therapy. Cognitive therapy does not prohibit addressing any form of clinical phenomena—it avoids neither the past nor present; neither the cognitive, the behavioral, nor emotional; neither the situational nor the characterological. Therefore, it is a congenial approach for therapists with diverging interests and original orientations who are open to the idea of reconceptualizing their clinical observations.

Second, cognitive therapy is a powerful example of therapeutic eclecticism. It gathers and uses techniques from a variety of approaches, but insists that interventions have a theoretical rationale, offer testable hypotheses, and be based on the case conceptualization. With an overriding orientation and conceptualization, the therapist is in a position to generate novel interventions that are tailor-made for the particular patient. This is also very appealing for many therapists.

Furthermore, cognitive therapy is new enough, on the one hand, not to be rigidly entrenched in terms of "correct" background, while on the other hand not having experienced intense enough prejudice to have closed ranks against "outsiders." Thus, cognitive therapy appeals to—and is open to—a wide variety of therapists and researchers.

This is good for cognitive therapy and for this handbook. It is good for cognitive therapy because once a therapeutic approach has reified its boundaries, it has stopped growing. However, rather than becoming static, cognitive therapy is continually being infused with new ideas for conceptualization and application from these various sources. It is good for this handbook because there is the creativity of many different perspectives, brought to bear on clinical problems within the CBT focus. As a result, we are able to bring readers innovative treatment packages for problematic clinical syndromes and populations. More than this, we hope that through the examples provided by others, the reader will be inspired to expand the horizons of cognitive therapy even further. Thus, an increasing number of clinicians will seek to apply it to more and new populations and an increasing number of researchers will seek to test its effectiveness and the validity of its assumptions and conceptualizations. If cognitive therapy lives up to its promise to be as an effective model of treatment for a broad range of symptoms and populations as we think it will, then a truly comprehensive treatment of psychopathology will eventually be achieved.

The editors would like to thank a number of people: first and foremost are the contributors to this volume. Each has contributed his or her theoretical and personal perspectives openly and in great detail. The excellence of their material has made editing this volume an exciting experience, and has given us the opportunity to meet and work with colleagues from throughout the United States, Canada, South Africa, and Sweden.

Eliot Werner, senior editor for Medical and Behavioral Sciences at Plenum, has been involved with this project since its inception. Eliot's good humor, friendship, professionalism, and perseverance have been very helpful in seeing this book to completion.

Each of the editors have specific people to thank. Arthur Freeman and Karen Simon would like to thank Joanne Muñiz and Donna Battisto for their expert secretarial and logistical assistance. Hal Arkowitz would like to thank Imogene Flett for her secretarial assistance and general helpfulness through all aspects of this project. Larry Beutler would like to thank Linda Fowler for her secretarial assistance and his colleagues in the Department of Psychiatry (University of Arizona) for their patience. His contribution was also partially supported by NIMH Grant MH 39859.

# Contents

# I

# Theory and Research

From its inception, there has been a close interaction of theory, research, and practice in cognitive therapy. This interplay is rather unusual among the psychotherapies, most of which have emphasized one or another of these areas at the expense of the others. For example, psychoanalytic psychotherapy rests on an elaborate theoretical substrate but has been lacking both in empirical research and in the development of practical guidelines. By contrast, behavior therapy has contributed a great deal to clinical technique and empirical research but encompasses only a rudimentary theory of psychopathology and behavior change. In concert with our view that cognitive therapy has made significant contributions to theory, research, and practice, the first part of this volume will examine the theoretical foundations and empirical status of cognitive therapy. These chapters will provide a basis for the clinical applications that will be presented in the second part.

It is only fitting that a *Comprehensive Handbook of Cognitive Therapy* should open with chapters from two pioneers and leaders of cognitive therapy: Albert Ellis and Aaron T. Beck. The chapters by these two important cognitive therapists provide us with a background in the history and current status of theory in cognitive therapy.

Ellis chronicles the long history and contemporary growth of cognitive therapy in Chapter 1. He traces the origins of a broadly defined cognitive theory to such early religious thinkers as Lao-tse, Confucius, and Buddha. The important influence of the early Stoic philosophers is nicely illustrated in Ellis's description of the forces that shaped his own development as a cognitive therapist. In his chapter, we can see the evolution of cognitive therapy from a purely cognitive approach to a cognitive-behavioral one and, finally, to one that incorporates both the role of affective arousal and relevant features of other psychotherapies.

Aaron Beck and Marjorie Weishaar present a comprehensive and updated version of the cognitive therapy of psychopathology and psychotherapy in Chapter 2. Beck and Weishaar provide us with a major statement of the theory underlying psychopathology and address the role of both cognitive change and affective arousal in the change process. According to Beck and Weishaar, the cognitive bases of psychopathology can be found in schema-relevant vulnerabilities. These vulnerabilities result in what they call "cognitive profiles," which represent the particular distortions and systematic biases that characterize each of the major disorders. The description of these profiles should stimulate further research and thinking in the area, all the more so because the authors extend their thinking far beyond the familiar clinical problems usually addressed by cognitive therapy, and take us into lesser understood problem areas such as anorexia, obsessions, compulsions, suicide, and paranoid states.

Cognitive therapy has been impressive in its ability to stimulate empirical research in assessment, as well as in treatment process and outcome. Chapters 3 and 4 provide a state-of-the-art review of research in each of these areas. In Chapter 3, Goldberg and Shaw describe significant technological and methodological issues confronting the measurement of cognition. Their discussion underlines issues in the measurement of cognition within a wide variety of clinical problems (e.g., depression, anxiety, medical and psychosomatic disorders, smoking, alcohol and substance abuse, and even schizophrenia). In each case, they review the empirical status of cognitive measurement and suggest directions for future research and applications.

In a complementary way, Beckham and Watkins take a careful look at clinically meaningful research on outcome and process in cognitive therapy in Chapter 4. The effectiveness of cognitive therapy for depression has been clearly demonstrated, although comparative studies with other therapists have raised many unresolved issues. In spite of some promising outcome data on other clinical disorders, the clear efficacy of cognitive therapy for them has yet to be firmly established. With this literature clearly in mind, the authors turn their attention to the uncertain role of cognitive change in behavioral and affective change. They provide an elucidating discussion of the relationship of process and outcome in cognitive therapy and discuss how future research might profit by understanding more about this relationship.

The next set of chapters turns our attention to basic theoretical issues in cognitive therapy. In 1977, Gordon Bower, an eminent cognitive scientist, explored the possible points of contact between cognitive sciences and social learning theory. Chapters 5, 6, and 7 explore the results of 10 years of effort to find and develop the linkages that could lead to cross-fertilization.

In Chapter 5, Tataryn, Nadel, and Jacobs point out that an interest in cognitive factors in psychotherapy leads naturally to the need for the scientific understanding of cognition itself, and it is in this domain that the cognitive scientist can have major input. They argue that cognitive science has demonstrated that much of what we call "cognitive" occurs outside of conscious awareness, and they review the implications of nonconscious mental processing for understanding cognition in cognitive therapy. The authors conclude with a stimulating discussion of repression, that is, the "means by which certain controlling features of a person's cognitive makeup become unconscious." Two new ways of thinking about repression are presented, both emerging from recent advances in the cognitive and biological sciences. These are areas that they believe provide a rich opportunity for contact between cognitive sciences and cognitive therapy.

The theoretical and empirical work of Richard Lazarus on emotion and coping has been highly influential in the field of personality and clinical psychology for many years. In Chapter 6, Lazarus argues that cognition is the key to functioning and change, providing motivational direction, emotional significance, and connecting action to its environmental context. He further argues that cognitive change alone is not capable of producing integrated functioning without coordinated changes in motivation and emotion as well. Finally, he argues that an understanding of human behavior and functioning is incomplete without incorporating the influence of environmental factors. In the concluding section of this chapter, Lazarus discusses the relevance of his theoretical arguments for the application of cognitive therapy and psychotherapy.

In Chapter 7, Beutler and Guest focus their attention on one of the most critical issues in cognitive therapy—the role of cognitive change. Their chapter takes a broad and scholarly look at identifying and explicating the role of cognitive change in cognitive therapy and psychotherapy. This chapter presents us with a descriptive comparison of the roles assigned to cognitive change by cognitive scientists and by different schools of psychotherapy as well. The last section of this chapter presents an integrative perspective on the issues, by bringing the theoretical and empirical perspectives into an integrative language system and theory of change.

From rather different perspectives, then, these three chapters on basic theoretical issues provide some new looks at old issues and raise new ideas that may well influence the future course of cognitive therapy and research.

What relationship does cognitive therapy and theory have to other major therapies and theories? This broad question is addressed in Chapters 8 through 11. Convergences and divergences among cognitive, behavioral, and psychodynamic therapies are considered by Arkowitz and Hannah in Chapter 8. They compare these approaches along such applied dimensions as patient selection, the role of assessment, the nature of the therapy relationship, and the role of technique. In addition, they examine the visions of human nature embodied in these three approaches as well as exploring how the three theories conceptualize change in psychotherapy. Although there is considerable variation among the specific dimensions, the authors conclude that cognitive therapy falls somewhere between behavioral and psychodynamic therapies, sharing more in common with each of these than they, in turn, do with one another. Using their comparative analysis as a basis, the authors conclude their chapter by abstracting what they believe are a set of common factors that may, at least in part, underly the effectiveness of the three therapies. They present a model of change centering on the concept of *behavioral enactments*. In this view, behavioral enactments mediate change and involve elements of staging, enactment with affective arousal, self-observation, disconfirmation of expectancies, and cognitive restructuring.

Recently, there has been an increased interest in experiential theories in the research literature on psychotherapy, and this has been largely due to the work of the authors of Chapter 9—Greenberg, Safran, and Rice. Comparisons between experiential therapy and cognitive therapy are made with reference to targets for change, relationship stances, and change processes. The authors argue that some of the general similarities that they abstract become more differentiated when the specific therapeutic tasks in experiential therapy are considered. The authors examine how each therapy works with cognition and affect and argue that cognitive therapy can learn much about affect from experiential therapy, whereas experiential therapy can learn much about cognition from cognitive therapy. They discuss the importance of a common information-processing language to facilitate real interchange between these two important therapy approaches.

In Chapter 10, Rosen has attempted to build a bridge between the theoretical work of Piaget and cognitive therapy. In the first part of this chapter, he provides us with an informative and succinct summary of Piaget's thinking. In the second part, the author argues that there are some unique and intimate connections that can be made between these two ways of thinking. His goal is to make explicit the implied connections that he believes exist, the knowledge of which may maximize their utility. Rosen applies Piagetian concepts to such important issues as the change process in psychotherapy and strategies of applied therapy. The developmental stages in therapy, the roles of cognitive structures in maintenance generalization, of change, and the concept of equilibration are presented as linking principles between the two approaches. Because Piaget himself did not extend his thinking to the area of psychotherapy, Rosen's task is a major one and will hopefully stimulate further thinking in this area.

Dowd and Pace also draw heavily from constructivist approaches in their attempt to apply such thinking to cognitive therapy in Chapter 11. They develop the argument that constructionist viewpoints share the assumption that we develop our own reality through our self-schemata and tacit rules. The authors discuss the implications of this assumption for change in psychotherapy and cognitive therapy. In addition, they discuss the interesting concepts of first- and second-order change. First-order change involves a change in specific behavior, whereas second-order change refers to a shift in the levels of meaning that govern behavior. The importance of the concept of second-order change is exemplified by the use of paradoxical techniques in cognitive therapy and psychotherapy.

Taken as a group, these four chapters place cognitive therapy into the context of other major therapies and theories that have preceded it.

In Chapter 12, the final chapter of this section, Coyne invites us to "think postcognitively" about depression. He points to a number of serious problems with the traditional cognitive theory of psychopathology in general and depression in particular. He argues that many cognitive therapy constructs are ambiguous and circular. In Coyne's view, a basic problem with the cognitive therapy perspective is that it arbitrarily ". . . separates what people say they think from the circumstances in which it is said, the conditions of their lives, and how they and those around them cope." Coyne argues for a postcognitive perspective that places greater emphasis on contextual and transactual factors than does the current cognitive therapy approach. Although critical of cognitive perspectives, Coyne acknowledges the efficacy of cognitive therapy for depression. He attempts to reconcile this apparent paradox by arguing that cognitive therapy works not so much by changing cognitions but by encouraging new transactions between the client and his or her environment. The editors of this volume believe that cognitive therapy can only develop in a healthy way in the face of constructive criticisms from both within the cognitive approach and from those outside of it. Coyne's chapter presents significant challenges to the cognitive perspective and one that cognitive theorists and reactionists will do well to consider.

It is our hope that this part on theory and research in cognitive therapy will give the interested reader a picture of the current state of affairs as well as directions that need to be addressed in the future. The strengths as well as the limitations of the cognitive approach emerge rather clearly from this section of the book, and we hope that it will provide a foundation for the reader before turning to the second part of this book on clinical applications.

# 1

# The History of Cognition in Psychotherapy

ALBERT ELLIS

## EARLY BEGINNINGS

The history of cognition in psychotherapy starts with the history of cognition in self-help philosophy. For although the early philosophers concentrated on explaining nature, the world, and—incidentally—the nature of humans in the world, some of the most outstanding Eastern and Western philosophers focused on the nature of humans and how they could help themselves by understanding the cognitions that led them to become "emotionally" disturbed and how they could use this understanding to overcome their disturbances. Significantly enough, the earliest major philosophers that we now remember and who still have a rather profound influence over us were greatly concerned with these problems—and not merely with those of comprehending nature and the world.

Take the influential Eastern philosophers, for example. In the sixth century B.C., Lao-tse founded Taoism, preaching right conduct of the external spirit of righteousness and holding that forms and ceremonies are entirely useless. Around the same time, Confucius set forth precepts dealing with morals and the family system; and his *Maxims* was a work that is still taught as a guide for people's daily life and espoused a practical, utilitarian philosophy. Another famous sixth-century B.C. philosopher was Gautama Buddha, who presumably abandoned the ascetic life, which he practiced for a while and found that emancipation of spirit came to him under a pipal tree (the Sacred Bo tree) at Buddh Gaya (from which came his title, Buddha, or Enlightened One). Although all these individuals were philosophers (and founders of religions), they were basically cognitive (or cognitive-behavioral) therapists; and their followers were, in a sense, clients.

It is similar with several of the early Greek and Roman philosophers. Socrates, in the fifth century B.C., particularly emphasized self-understanding and often preached what was, for his day, an unconventional method of life—so much so, in fact, that he was accused of corrupting the youth of Athens and was forced to drink hemlock in prison to atone, as it were, for his

ALBERT ELLIS • Institute for Rational-Emotive Therapy, New York, New York 10021.

"sins." Plato, Socrates's most outstanding student and writer of his views, carried on his self-help views. Epicurus, in the fourth century B.C., emphasized that pleasure is the main good and end of morality and of life but he largely preached long-range instead of short-range hedonism and held that genuine pleasure was a life of prudence and honor.

Zeno of Cytium, another Greek philosopher, founded the Stoic school in the late fourth and early third centuries B.C. and taught its principles in Athens for more than 50 years. He was followed by Chrisippus and by Panaetius of Rhodes, who introduced Stoicism into Rhodes. We do not have much of the writings of speeches of the early Stoics, nor do we even have the actual writings of the popular Stoic, Epictetus, but we do have those of Epictetus's pupil, Flavius Arrian, who wrote down his lectures, when he gave them during the first century A.D. in Rome and who has thereby given us his main works, the *Discourses* and his *Enchiridion* (*Manual*), which have been in print since 1890 (Epictetus). We also have the Stoic writings of Cicero (106–43 B.C.) and Seneca (54 B.C.?—A.D. 39).

Epictetus was a particularly influential Stoic, who in the first century A.D. wrote that "people are disturbed not by things, but by the views which they take of them." The Roman Emperor, Marcus Aurelius (1890), was raised with the Stoic philosophy of Epictetus and incorporated it into his famous book, *Meditations,* which again is one of the oldest self-help books still in print. The Stoic philosophy has a good deal of rationality about it, but it also has its weak points because it has fatalism as its basis. Thus, Marcus Aurelius (1890, p. 15) advised:

> Accept everything which happens, even if it seems disagreeable, because it leads to this, to the health of the universe and to the prosperity and felicity of Zeus. For he would not have brought on any man what he has brought, if it were not useful for the whole.

This is not exactly the sanest philosophy in the world, but it obviously is designed to help people be reasonably happy and accepting even when faced with severe adversity. The same can be said about much of the philosophy of the Old and the New Testament, the Jewish and the Christian Bibles. Many of the books of the Bible—particularly the Book of Job, Proverbs, and several parts of the New Testament—include a great deal of advice to troubled people and really consist of self-help material. As I said in one of my talks to the American Psychological Association some years ago, if we look at it from a cognitive-behavioral standpoint, the Bible is (as it has been for centuries) probably the most widely sold and read of the vast number of self-help books that have existed for the last thousand years (Ellis, 1978).

Following the early philosophers and religionists, innumerable other thinkers throughout the ages have presented ideas and practical suggestions for people to follow when they feel emotionally disturbed and behave in a self-defeating manner. To list the ones who were most profound and influential in this respect would take a chapter in its own right. Let me merely mention, in this respect, Thomas Aquinas, Thomas À Kempis, Baruch Spinoza, Immanuel Kant, Arthur Schopenhauer, Ralph Waldo Emerson, Henry David Thoreau, and Bertrand Russell. Kant, in particular, was highly influential in glorifying ideas, intellect, and reasoning and greatly affected the rise of Adlerian psychotherapy and of rational-emotive therapy (Ansbacher & Ansbacher, 1956; Ellis, 1981). Schopenhauer wrote a persuasive book called *The World as Will and Idea,* as well as many practical essays on the supposedly good life. Emerson's *Essays,* particularly his famous essay on self-reliance, started the fashion for an emormous number of self-help books. Bertrand Russell's *Marriage and Morals* (1929) and *Conquest of Happiness* (1950) have for many years been bibles to less religious and more liberal intellectuals.

Finally, if we are still to remain in the philosophic area, Kierkegaard started the existential revolution when the nineteenth century was under way, and Martin Heidegger (1962) and Paul Tillich (1953), along with many other influential existentialists, carried on their kind of thinking and made it one of the bulwarks of self-help writings in the last half century. Although all the writers and thinkers I have named in the last few paragraphs were quite concerned with human feelings and with self-defeating behaviors, they have in common a set of beliefs that hold that emotional upsetness largely originates in illogical, unrealistic, and irrational thinking and that humans have the distinct ability to monitor this kind of thinking, to reflect on it, and to change it, so that they significantly help themselves solve their everyday problems and their fairly severe disturbances.

This brings us, a little belatedly, to the fields of psychology, psychiatry, and social work. In the second part of the nineteenth and the early part of the twentieth centuries, psychologists were mainly academic rather than clinical, and psychotherapy was mainly done by psychiatrists. But these psychiatrists were largely philosophically and cognitively oriented, and because many of them were engaged in hypnotism, they emphasized suggestion (after Bernheim (1886/1947)) and autosuggestion (after Coué (1923).

They were also clearly cognitive in several other important respects. Thus—as Raimy (1975) has noted—Paul Dubois (1904/1907) strongly insisted that "incorrect ideas" produced psychological distress and wrote a well-known book advocating persuasion, *The Psychic Treatment of Nervous Disorders,* which was unknown to me when I originated rational-emotive therapy (RET) in 1955 but was in many ways as direct, active, and argumentative as rational-emotive therapy often is. Déjerine and Gaukler (1913) also advocated active-directive persuasion and their book was popular in the early 1900s.

Pierre Janet (1893) believed that hysterics had "fixed ideas" or idées fixe and that these ideas had to be changed in the course of treating these "neurotics." Joseph Breuer (Breuer & Freud, 1895/1965) agreed with Janet but used the term *unconscious pathogenic ideas* to describe severe disturbance. And Freud, going along with Breuer, also used the term *ideogenic* to show the main causation of many neurotic problems.

Unfortunately (I would personally say), Freud (1965) and his followers (Fenichel, 1945) later began to emphasize—and probably overemphasize—the role of emotion and transference in human disturbance (not realizing that "transference" is really overgeneralization and therefore still largely ideogenic). So classical psychoanalysis began to diverge far from the cognitive track. But many less classical analysts—including Adler, Fromm, Sullivan, Horney, Rado, and Arieti—were more philosophic and less emotive (not to mention less archaeological!) than Freud and began to emphasize cognition in their work far more heavily than the old master was wont to do.

For a discussion of strong cognitive influences in the works of leading neo-Adlerians and neo-Freudians, see several relevant chapters in Mahoney and Freeman (1985). Remember, too, in this connection that, although Freud often wrote as if psychoanalysis almost entirely consisted of working through transference and countertransference feelings, especially during the first few months of psychoanalytic therapy, his main final and ultimate tool consisted of interpretation—which is as cognitive as any therapist could possibly be. He also resorted at times to behavioral methods and to unusually short-term treatment and frequently was much more active-directive than he often cared to admit (Wortis, 1954).

In any event, before the Freudian revolution, psychotherapy was profoundly cognitive and at times even clearly cognitive-behavioral (Wick, 1983), even when it was practiced almost exclusively by physicians and psychiatrists. Then, in the later nineteenth century, psychologists began to get into the act. William James (1914), taking off from Emerson and some religious thinkers, began to write in a hardheaded fashion about the role of ideas and beliefs in therapy; and a host of other psychological therapists, such as Munsterberg (1919), followed in his tracks. Freudianism, however, still ruled the roost up until the 1940s—despite the efforts of Adler (1927, 1929) and several neo-Adlerians to revise it.

Then came a somewhat dramatic breakthrough. Following up some of the ideas of Gordon Allport (1937), Prescott Lecky (1943) insisted that people with low self-concept *defined* themselves that way and that they invariably had the ability to *re*define their self-images. Andrew Salter (1949) started the assertion training movement by taking some of the behavioral theories of Pavlov, Watson, and Skinner and directing people to recondition themselves. He was mainly behavioral, but he also stated and implied that people could imagine themselves doing differently and could cognitively retrain themselves when they were shy and unassertive. Snygg and Combs (1949) noted that "inadequate differentiations" of the phenomenal field led to psychological disturbances. Julian Rotter (1954), emphasizing expectancy theory, came up with the first major social learning theory of emotional upsetness and its treatment. George Kelly (1955) published a brilliant theory of cognition and disturbance that he significantly entitled, *The Psychology of Personal Constructs*. This was by far the most comprehensive explanation of the role of ideas in the creation of emotional problems that had been written up to that time; and it is still a classic.

## RATIONAL-EMOTIVE THERAPY (RET) AND COGNITIVE-BEHAVIORAL THERAPY (CBT)

Spurred on by the writings of some of these psychologists—but not, oddly enough, by those of George Kelly, whom I had not yet read—I created rational-emotive therapy (RET) during the first few months of 1955. I had previously been a practicing psychoanalyst, but after 6 years of doing classical analysis and analytically oriented psychotherapy, I became thoroughly disillusioned with their inefficiencies by 1953 and began exploring other, more effective avenues of therapy. My widespread library researches culminated in two monographs: *New Approaches to Psychotherapy Techniques* (Ellis, 1955a) and "Psychotherapy Techniques for Use with Psychotics" (Ellis, 1955b).

As I abandoned psychoanalysis, I returned to my early love, with which I had been involved since the age of 16 and in which I had done voluminous reading—the field of philosophy. And I also went back to behavior therapy—which I had used on myself in my late adolescence and early adulthood to overcome my severe fears of public speaking and my social anxiety about encountering young females whom I wished to date (Ellis, 1972b). So I became the first major cognitive-behavioral therapist by actively practicing RET, by doing a pioneering outcome study of it (Ellis, 1957a), and by forcefully promoting it in talks, workshops, articles, and books (Ellis, 1957b, 1958a,b, 1962).

Although I did not realize it at that time, without yet reading Paul Dubois (whose main book I read in 1957, two years after originating RET), I reinvented some of his very active-persuasive therapeutic procedures. I also, right from the start, went beyond Eysenck (1960) and Wolpe (1958) by often employing *in vivo* (rather than imaginal) desensitization and also by preceding Stampfl (Stampfl & Levis, 1967) in the advocacy of implosive rather than gradual desensitization. From the beginning, I also included some highly emotive exercises and practices in RET.

Although, therefore, I did not by any means wholly invent cognitive-emotive-behavioral methodology, I think I can safely say that I was the first modern therapist to give it heavy emphasis and considerable publicity. Because of this, I am often acknowledged as the father of RET and the grandfather of cognitive-behavioral therapy.

Moreover, whereas George Kelly (1955) was mainly a cognitive behaviorist—because his main treatment method was fixed role playing and by no means consisted (as one might think it would) of cognitive persuasion or disputing—I have always been a behavioral cognitivist. Most of my actual treatment process in RET consists of active-directive cognitive debating—with emotive and behavioral homework always integrally included but with a strong emphasis on helping clients achieve a profound—and preferably quite conscious—philosophic or attitudinal change.

As I have indicated before, there were two main factors that strongly influenced me to substitute RET for psychoanalytic and psychoanalytically oriented psychotherapy: the early history (and effectiveness over the centuries) of philosophical cognitive therapy and the recent history (and, again, effectiveness) of behavioral therapy. When I first formulated RET, behavior therapy was in its real infancy because the early experiments of John B. Watson and his students (Jones, 1924a,b; Watson & Rayner, 1920) had been effective but had not led to notable success when used with adults. Pavlov (1927) was also honored in theory but not used, except in the Soviet Union, in practice. Wolpe had done some early experimental work with animals but not applied it, as he did later (Wolpe, 1958) to humans. Followers of Skinner (1953) were beginning to get somewhere in applying his principles, but there was (as there still often is) a great deal of opposition to their "conditioning" experiments. Moreover, virtually all the behaviorists, especially Skinner and Wolpe and their students, were almost pathologically allergic to words like *thinking* and *cognition* (as some of them still stubbornly are!).

By a fortunate accident, however, my early psychotherapeutic efforts were importantly tied up with a special school of therapy that has always been cognitive-behavioral, although when I began to practice in 1943 it was an exceptionally little-known school. That field was sex therapy, in which I started to do somewhat pioneering work during the early 1940s. For sex therapy has always, almost by necessity, been cognitive-behavioral. As was the case with general psychotherapy, it got fairly well under way in the mid-nineteenth century and was almost entirely the province of physicians. Richard von Krafft-Ebing (1886/1922) investigated the processes of sexual pathology and had some distinct ideas on what to do about curing afflicted individuals. Havelock Ellis (1897/1936) went much further into the nuances of normal, as well as "abnormal," sexuality and also wrote voluminously on some practical solutions to sex problems. They were followed by a host of other fairly well-known sex therapists, virtually all of them physicians—such as Iwan Bloch (1907), August Forel (1908/1922), William J. Robinson (1915), W. F. Robie (1920/1925), and H. W. Long (1922).

These sex therapists, without knowing too much about the art and science of formal psychotherapy, did two main things with their patients: First, they gave them information about effective sex functioning and relieved them of their guilt and shame about "wrong" or "abnormal" acts that they were doing; and, second, they gave them activity homework assignments—to have more or less intercourse, to engage in noncoital relations, to use certain kinds of sex positions instead of other kinds, and to think about nonsexual things (when they came to orgasm too quickly) and about sexual fantasies (when they came to orgasm too slowly or did not reach it at all). In a word, they were quite cognitive-behavioral.

When, therefore, I practiced sex therapy in the 1940s I not only derived much of my information from these pioneering other therapists but I also realized that teaching people new ways of thinking and behaving and getting them to practice *in vivo* homework assignments were just about the only good ways to help them overcome their sexual problems. Without exactly consciously thinking of myself as such, I thereby became a cognitive-behavioral therapist with my sex, marriage, and family cases. Consequently, when I abandoned psychoanalysis—with which I particularly became disillusioned because it did *not* help my clients who had severe sex problems but often seemed to exacerbate such problems—I easily fell into cognitive-behavioral therapy for virtually all my clients, including most of them who had regular problems of anxiety, depression, rage, and self-pity without having any serious sexual correlates of these problems.

In any event, I most probably would never have created rational-emotive therapy had I not been, prior to my psychoanalytic training and practice, a fairly effective sex therapist. And the entire field of general psychotherapy today would probably not be as cognitive-behaviorally oriented had not Masters and Johnson (1970) followed a similar path to mine, in which they, too, read the early sexologists (and my own early writings on sex treatment [Ellis, 1953, 1954]) and led the field of sex therapy in the cognitive-behavioral direction. Seeing that their procedures worked, other outstanding sex therapists—such as Annon (1974, 1975), Hartman and Fithian (1972), and Kaplan (1974)—soon followed suit; so that cognition and behavioral methodology has today become the supreme method of choice in dealing with most serious sex problems.

## THE GROWTH OF RET AND CBT

Cognitive-behavioral sex therapy, however, only became truly popular in the early 1970s. Before that time, it was practiced by physicians—especially, by urologists and gynecologists—and to some extent by psychologists, psychiatrists, and social workers. But it was recognized as a special kind of "sex therapy" and not particularly as psychotherapy. Wolpe (1958) and Lazarus (Wolpe & Lazarus, 1966) pioneered in placing it as a normal part of behavior therapy, but it was not recognized as being particularly cognitive except by a few practitioners (Ellis, 1953, 1954, 1958b, 1960, 1962).

In the meantime, modern cognitive and cognitive-behavioral therapy began to develop and become more and more popular in its own right. After I presented my first major paper on rational-emotive therapy at the American Psychological Association convention in Chicago in 1956 (Ellis, 1958a), Aaron Beck began to do intensive research on thinking and depression in the late 1950s and published his first major article on the subject in the *Archives of General Psychiatry* in 1963. Meanwhile, I had collected most of my early articles on RET, published from 1956 onward, and incorporated them in revised form in *Reason and Emotion in Psychotherapy* (Ellis, 1962). In 1966, Richard Lazarus brought out his influential book, *Psychological Stress and the Coping Process*; in 1965 William Glasser published his popular book, *Reality Therapy*; and in 1967, Beck published his first book on cognitive therapy, *Depression: Clinical, Experimental, and Theoretical Aspects*. The modern revolution in cognitive-behavioral psychotherapy was by now under way!

Developments in the field of cognitive-behavior therapy have been so many and so profound since it began to get really going in 1955 that it would be next to impossible to list even all the major events that had transpired since that time. Let me, therefore, give a reasonably brief summary that will tend to show how things have been going and how they are still tending to proceed in this important area of psychotherapy.

### 1955 TO 1959

Rational-emotive therapy (RET) and cognitive-behavioral therapy (CBT) at first grew slowly, largely through my own talks, seminars, and writings; and they often aroused more opposition than acceptance because they were strongly opposed by leading psychoanalysts, client-centered therapists, and experiential therapists. However, the first popular book on cognitive therapy—*How to Live with a Neurotic* (Ellis, 1957b)—was published, as well as the first book applying RET specifically to sex problems and sex therapy—*Sex without Guilt* (Ellis, 1958b). The writings of George Kelly (1955) and of Viktor Frankl (1959) began to have some real impact. The nonprofit Institute for Rational Living (later to become the Institute for Rational-Emotive Therapy) was organized and began to train therapists in cognitive therapy and to sponsor public presentations as well as workshops for the profession. Whereas RET had begun as a form of individual therapy in 1955, it was expanded into the practice of group therapy in 1959; and it also began to make a name for itself in the field of marital and family therapy (Ellis & Harper, 1961a). Aaron Beck began to work, with his associates, on a reliable inventory for measuring depression and included in this instrument a good many cognitive questions (Beck, Ward, Mendelson, Mock, & Erbaugh, 1961, 1962).

Beck (1961) continued his systematic investigations of the cognitive elements in depression and published his seminal paper, "Thinking and Depression" (Beck, 1963). Eric Berne (1961, 1964) began to publish immensely popular writings on transactional analysis. RET started to gain significant support, first from my professional writings, particularly *Reason and Emotion in Psychotherapy* (Ellis, 1962); and then it began to gain wide popular recognition from my popular writings, especially from the first edition of the *Guide to Rational Living* (Ellis & Harper, 1961b) and from *A Guide to Successful Marriage* (originally entitled, *Creative Marriage*) (Ellis & Harper, 1961a). My sex books, which incorporated a good deal of RET material, not only sold well in their original hardcover editions but became best-sellers in paperback form—especially, *The Art and Science of Love* (Ellis, 1960), *Sex and the Single Man* (Ellis, 1963a), and *The Intelligent Woman's Guide to Manhunting* (Ellis, 1963b).

## 1960 TO 1964

RET began to gain significant support, largely because of my books, workshops, and writings. Aaron Beck published his first articles on cognitive therapy (1961, 1963). Eric Berne (1961, 1964) began to publish immensely popular writings on transactional analysis, particularly *Games People Play*. Eysenck (1964) introduced RET and cognitive therapy to the behavior therapy movement in his book, *Experiments in Behaviour Therapy*. Frank (1963) came out with the first edition of *Persuasion and Healing* that included a section on RET and strongly promoted the thesis that all effective psychotherapy largely is ideological and persuasive. Jay Haley (1963), influenced by the work of Milton Erickson, published his first book, *Strategies of Psychotherapy*, which had some significant cognitive-behavioral interventions and techniques included in it.

## 1965 TO 1969

The Institute for Rational-Emotive Therapy was chartered as a training institute by the Regents of the State of New York, began its fellowship and associate fellowship training programs, and began to publish its journal, *Rational Living*. Several doctoral theses and other outcome studies began to be published on RET and CBT, as well as some books and writings by myself and other authors on RET (Ard & Ard, 1969; Ellis, 1965a,b). Albert Bandura (1969) brought out an extremely influential book on behavior therapy that had an unusually cognitive emphasis, *Principles of Behavior Modification*. Other important and highly popular books on cognitive therapy were published by Eric Berne (1966), Milton Erickson (1967), William Glasser (1965), Richard Lazarus (1966), Thomas Harris (1969), and Watzlawick, Bevan, and Jackson (1967).

A number of tests of irrational beliefs, based on the 12 major ones that I outlined in *Reason and Emotion in Psychotherapy*, began to be published and to lead to many empirical studies of their reliability and validity. Most notable and most used in this respect was the Irrational Beliefs Tests of Jones (1968). Going further than incooporating RET into group therapy procedures, I originated and began to train other RET practitioners to lead rational-emotive encounter marathon groups (Ellis, 1969). In these marathon procedures, a good many experiential and emotive exercises were incooporated with the usual cognitive-behavioral procedures that were generally used in RET.

## 1970 TO 1974

Many research studies and theses on the efficacy of RET and CBT began to be done in the psychological laboratories of Albert Bandura, Donald Meichenbaum, Marvin Goldfried,

Gerald Davison, Michael Mahoney, and other psychologists who specialized in these two forms of therapy. Masters and Johnson (1970) brought out *Human Sexual Inadequacy,* which sparked the publication of scores of other books and hundreds of articles on cognitive-behavioral sex therapy. Michael Mahoney (1974) published a highly influential work that reviewed the history and the practice of cognition and behavior modification. Mahoney's work, in addition to Bandura's earlier book, gave considerable respectability to CBT and began to place it in the forefront of the psychotherapy movement. A large number of other significant books on RET and CBT were published, including those by Alberti and Emmons (1970), Berne (1972), Ellis (1971, 1972a,b, 1973), Goldfried and Merbaum (1973), Haley (1973), Hauck (1973, 1974), Knaus (1974), A. Lazarus (1971), Masters and Rimm (1974), Maultsby (1975), Spivak and Shure (1974), Tosi (1974), Watzlawick, Weakland, and Fisch (1974), and Young (1974).

By this time, in the early 1970s, RET and CBT were truly coming of age and were beginning to become the new kid on the block, and in some ways the most influential kid on the block, in the entire realm of psychotherapy. Moreover, where previously only the field of behavior therapy significantly produced a great many outcome studies of a technical nature, cognitive-behavioral therapy now started to do likewise; and from the 1970s onward began to produce literally scores of controlled experimental studies, the great majority of which showed that when CBT was tested against a group of subjects having no therapy or having some other form of therapy, it tended to bring forth more successful results.

## 1975 TO 1979

The cognitive-behavioral revolution in psychotherapy erupted into full bloom, with additional scores of confirming outcome studies being published and innumerable therapists beginning to favor RET and CBT (DiGiuseppe, Miller, & Trexler, 1979; Ellis, 1979; Miller & Berman, 1983; Smith & Glass, 1977). So many significant texts on RET and CBT were also published that it is difficult to list even the most outstanding ones. Some of the influential ones included those by Bandler and Grinder (1978), Bandura (1977), Beck (1976), Beck, Rush, Emery, and Shaw (1979), Diekstra and Dassen (1977a,b), Ellis and Abrahms (1978), Ellis and Grieger (1977), Ellis and Whiteley (1979), Erickson and Rossi (1979), Goulding and Goulding (1979), Goldfried and Davison (1976), Kanfer and Goldstein (1975), Guerney (1977), Haley (1976), Janis and Mann (1977), Kendall and Hollon (1979), Lange and Jakubowski (1976), A. Lazarus (1976), Meichenbaum (1977), Morris and Kanitz (1975), Raimy (1975), Seligman (1975), Singer and Pope (1978), and Spivack, Platt and Shure (1976).

At the same time, many best-selling self-help books using RET and CBT appeared, including Dyer's (1976) fabulously successful *Your Erroneous Zones* and my own highly successful *How to Live with a Neurotic* (revised edition) (Ellis, 1975), *Sex and the Liberated Man* (Ellis, 1976), *Anger—How to Live with and without It* (Ellis, 1977), and *A New Guide to Rational Living* (Ellis & Harper, 1975). Other popular RET and CBT books for the public included *Overcoming Procrastination* (Ellis & Knaus, 1977), *I Can if I Want To* (A. Lazarus & A. Fay, 1975), *Help Yourself to Happiness* (Maultsby, 1975), and *Fully Human, Fully Alive* (Powell, 1976).

During this period of time, the distinguished journal, *Cognitive Therapy and Research,* was founded under the editorship of Michael Mahoney and the *Cognitive Behaviorist* was founded and edited by Thomas Dowd. Aaron Beck founded the Center for Cognitive Therapy in Philadelphia; and a number of RET and CBT institutes were developed in the United States and Europe.

## 1980 TO 1986

The cognitive-behavioral revolution continued. Not without criticism, because a number of prominent and hard-headed psychologists began to take issue with it. Thus, Zajonc (1980) insisted that the role of cognition in emotion was distinctly overplayed. Schwartz (1982), Beidel and Turner (1986), and T. Smith (1982) wrote critical reviews of cognitive-behavioral theories and therapy. Wolpe (1980) kept taking potshots at any form of therapy that cavalierly talked about cognitions and underplayed behavioral conditioning of a noncognitive nature.

Nonetheless, RET and CBT forged ahead in regard to their influence on professionals and members of the public. Darrell Smith (1982) published an article in the *American Psychologist* showing that the 10 most influential psychotherapists, according to a survey of 800 clinical and counseling psychologists were No. 2, Albert Ellis, No. 4, Arnold Lazarus; No. 7, Aaron Beck; and No. 10, Donald Meichenbaum. He concluded that "these findings suggest quite clearly that cognitive behavior therapy is one of the major trends in counseling and psychotherapy" (1982, p. 808). Heesacker, Heppner, and Rogers (1982) analyzed approximately 14,000 references cited in three major counseling psychology journals for the last 2 complete years and discovered that, although I was No. 3 in the frequency of citations before 1957, after 1957 I was easily the most frequently cited author in these journals. No. 6 on the list after 1957 was Meichenbaum, No. 7 was Bandura, and No. 9 was Mahoney.

To accord with this influence, scores of research studies attesting to the potential validity of CBT and RET continued; and scores of other experiments attesting to the validity of many tests of irrational beliefs were also published.

The *British Journal of Cognitive Therapy* (later to be merged with the *Behavior Therapist* into the *International Journal of Cognitive Psychotherapy*) was founded by Windy Dryden; and the *Journal of Rational-Emotive and Cognitive Behavior Therapy* replaced *Rational Living,* being initiated and edited by Paul Woods and Russell Grieger.

A large number of texts on RET and CBT continued to appear. These included books by Bard (1980), Beck and Emery (1985), Bernard and Joyce (1984), Bowers and Meichenbaum (1984), Ellis (1985a), Dryden (1984), Dryden and Golden (1986), Dryden and Trower (1986), Ellis and Bernard (1983, 1985), Ellis and Grieger (1986), Erickson (1981), Freeman (1983), Grieger (1986), Grieger and Boyd (1980), Grieger and Grieger (1982), Guidano and Liotti (1983), Janis (1983), A. Lazarus (1981), R. Lazarus and Folkman (1984), Mahoney and Freeman (1985), Maultsby (1984), McGovern and Silverman (1984), McMullin (1986), Meichenbaum and Jaremko (1983), T. Miller (1983), Reda and Mahoney (1984), Walen, DiGiuseppe, and Wessler (1980), and Wessler and Wessler (1980).

Especially notable in the 1980s was the work in cognitive behavior therapy of P. C. Kendall and S. D. Hollon, who started a series, *Advances in Cognitive Behavioral Research and Therapy* (1981) and who also took over the main editorships of *Cognitive Therapy and Research.* In addition, they published a number of outstanding books on behavioral assessment and therapy, including *Cognitive Behavioral Interventions: Theory, Research and Practice* (Kendall & Hollon, 1979); *Assessment Strategies for Cognitive-Behavioral Interventions* (Kendall & Hollon, 1980); *Cognitive Therapy and Research* (Hollon, 1983); and *Cognitive Behavioral Therapy for Impulsive Children* (Kendall & Braswell, 1984).

## SUMMARY AND CONCLUSION

The history of cognition in psychotherapy is of course not ended, as I write this chapter in September 1986. It began with philosophy and religion, was taken over for a while by psychiatry, and now seems most solidly in the hands of a large number of outstanding psychologists. It started out by being almost purely cognitive and philosophical; then it became cognitive-behavioral; and now it is becoming much more emotive as well. It is also becoming more integrative or "eclectic." Goldfried (1980) beat loudly the drum for an integration of all major therapies, as did Schwartz (1982, 1984) and a number of other leading therapists (Beutler, 1983; Bowers & Meichenbaum, 1984; Mahoney & Freeman, 1985; Meichenbaum & Jaremko, 1984; Wachtel, 1977, 1982). On the other hand, some other proponents of cognitive therapy—including A. Lazarus (1981) and myself (Ellis, 1956, 1983, 1984a,b, 1985a,b; Ellis & Dryden, 1987)—took the view that a good and comprehensive form of cognitive-behavioral therapy includes most of the best features of many other existent therapies but that it also stays within the scientific method and tends to exclude some of the unscientific aspects of psycho-analysis, transpersonal psychotherapy, and other therapies that promote inefficient and harmful (as well as beneficial) methodologies.

Many other differences also still exist in the field of cognitive therapy. Some theorists and practitioners think that it should emphasize mild or softsell methods of disputing irrational beliefs (Beck, 1976; Janis & Mann, 1977; Meichenbaum, 1977; Wessler & Hankin-Wessler, 1986). Others advocate the former, hardshell approach to talking people out of their disturbances (Ellis, 1985a, 1988; Ellis & Dryden, 1987). Some cognitivists take a highly philosophic road to minimizing illogicalities and unrealistic attitudes (Ellis, 1985a, 1988; Ellis & Dryden, 1987). Others use more behavioral methods of helping people to acquire healthy coping statements (Lazarus & Folkman, 1984; Meichenbaum, 1977; Meichenbaum & Jaremko, 1983). Some practitioners emphasize a large variety of rational, logical, and realistic arguments in helping clients to become more reasonable (Beck, 1976; Burns, 1980). Others especially emphasize teaching clients to see what their underlying absolutistic and masturbatory thinking is and, in the course of extirpating their dogmas, to reduce the unrealistic and illogical ideas that presumably are derived from their Jehovian insistences (Ellis, 1984a, 1985a, 1988; Ellis & Dryden, 1987).

Many of these important issues and differences in the field of RET and CBT are still to be resolved and require considerable more research before definitive or authoritative answers can, if ever, be given. In this respect, the whole field of cognitive-behavioral theory and methodology, in spite of its long history, still presents almost innumerable problems and questions that are not likely to be resolved by the end of this century and that will present challenges and a substantial amount of further research for, in all probability, centuries to come.

# REFERENCES

Adler, A. (1927). *Understanding human nature.* New York: Greenberg.

Adler, A. (1929). *The science of living.* New York: Greenberg.

Alberti, R. E., & Emmons, M. L. (1970). *Your perfect right.* San Luis Obispo, CA: Impact.

Allport, G. (1937). *Personality: A psychological interpretation.* New York: Holt.

Annon, J. S. (1974). *The behavioral treatment of sexual problems* (Vol. 1). New York: Harper & Row.

Annon, J. S. (1975). *The behavioral treatment of sexual problems* (Vol. 2), Honolulu: Enabling Systems.

Ansbacher, H. L., & Ansbacher, R. (1956). *The individual psychology of Alfred Adler.* New York: Basic Books.

Ard, B. N., Jr., & Ard, C. (Eds.). (1969). *Handbook of marriage counseling.* Palo Alto, CA: Science and Behavior Books.

Bandler, R., & Grinder, J. (1978). *The structure of magic* (2 vols.). Palo Alto: Science and Behavior Books.

Bandura, A. (1969). *Principles of behavior modification.* New York: Holt, Rinehart & Winston.

Bandura, A. (1977). *Social learning theory.* Englewood Cliffs, NJ: Prentice-Hall.

Bard, J. (1980). *Rational-emotive therapy in practice.* Champaign, IL: Research Press.

Beck, A. T. (1961). A systematic investigation of depression. *Comprehensive Psychiatry, 2,* 162–170.

Beck, A. T. (1963). Thinking and depression. *Archives of General Psychiatry, 9,* 324–333 (reprinted in New York by the Institute for Rational-Emotive Therapy).

Beck, A. T. (1967). *Depression.* New York: Hoeber-Harper.

Beck, A. T. (1976). *Cognitive therapy and the emotional disorders.* New York: International Universities Press.

Beck, A. T., & Emery, G. (1985). *Anxiety disorders and phobias.* New York: Basic Books.

Beck, A. T., Rush, A. J., Shaw, B. F., & Emery, G. (1979). *Cognitive therapy of depression.* New York: Guilford.

Beck, A. T., Ward, C. H., Mendelson, M., Mock, J., & Erbaugh, J. R. (1962). Reliability of psychiatric diagnosis. *American Journal of Psychiatry, 119,* 351–357.

Beidel, D. C., & Turner, S. M. (1986). A critique of the theoretical bases of cognitive-behavioral theories and therapy. *Clinical Psychology Review, 6,* 177–197.

Bernard, M. E., & Joyce, M. R. (1984). *Rational-emotive therapy with children and adolescents.* New York: Wiley.

Berne, E. (1961). *Transactional analysis in psychotherapy.* New York: Grove.

Berne, E. (1964). *Games people play.* New York: Grove.

Berne, E. (1966). *Principles of group treatment.* New York: Oxford.

Berne, E. (1972). *What do you say after you say hello?* New York: Grove.

Bernheim, H. (1947). *Suggestive therapeutics.* New York: London Book Company. (Originally published 1886)

Beutler, L. E. (1983). *Eclectic psychotherapy: A systematic approach.* New York: Pergamon.

Bloch, I. (1907). *The sexual life of our time.* New York: Rebman.

Bowers, K. S., & Meichenbaum, D. (1984). *Cognition and the unconscious.* New York: Plenum Press.

Breuer, J., & Freud, S. (1965). *Studies in hysteria.* Vol. 2 of *The Standard Edition of the Complete Psychological Works of Sigmund Freud.* New York: Basic Books. (Originally published 1895)

Burns, D. D. (1980). *Feeling good: The new mood therapy.* New York: Morrow.

Coué, E. (1923). *My method.* New York: Doubleday, Page.

Derine, J., & Gaukler, E. (1913). *Psychoneurosis and psychotherapy.* Philadelphia: Lippincott.

Diekstra, R., & Dassen, W. (1976). *Rationale therapie.* Amsterdam: Swets & Zeitlinger.

Diekstra, R., & Dassen, W. (1977). *Inlieding tot de rationele therapie.* Ambsterdam: Swets & Zeitlinger.

DiGiuseppe, R. A., Miller, N. J., & Trexler, L. D. (1979). A review of rational-emotive psychotherapy outcome studies. In A. Ellis & J. M. Whiteley (Eds.), *Theoretical and empirical foundations of rational-emotive therapy* (pp. 218–235). Monterey, CA: Brooks/Cole.

Dryden, W. (1984). *Rational-emotive therapy: Fundamentals and innovations.* Beckenham, Kent: Croom-Helm.

Dryden, W., & Ellis, A. (1986). Rational-emotive therapy (RET). In W. Dryden & W. Golden (Eds.), *Cognitive-behavioural approaches to psychotherapy* (pp. 129–168). London: Harper & Row.

Dryden, W., & Golden, W. (Eds.). (1986). *Cognitive-behavioural approaches to psychotherapy.* London: Harper & Row.

Dryden, W., & Trower, P. (Eds.). (1986). *Rational-emotive therapy: Recent developments in theory and practice.* Bristol, England: Institute for RET (UK).

Dubios, P. (1907). *The psychic treatment of nervous disorders.* New York: Funk & Wagnell. (Originally published 1904.)

Dyer, W. (1976). *Your erroneous zones.* New York: Funk and Wagnalls.

Ellis, A. (1953). Is the vaginal orgasm a myth? In A. P. Pillay & A. Ellis (Eds.), *Sex, society and the individual* (pp. 155–162). Bombay: International Journal of Sexology Press.

Ellis, A. (1954). *The American sexual tragedy.* New York: Twayne and Grove Press (Rev. ed., New York: Lyle Stuart and Grove, 1962)

Ellis, A. (1955a). New approaches to psychotherapy techniques. Brandon, VT: *Journal of Clinical Psychology Monograph Supplement,* Vol. 11.

Ellis, A. (1955b). Psychotherapy techniques for use with psychotics. *American Journal of Psychotherapy, 9,* 452–476.

Ellis, A. (1957a). Outcome of employing three techniques of psychotherapy. *Journal of Clinical Psychology, 13,* 344–350.

Ellis, A. (1957b). *How to live with a neurotic: At home and at work.* New York: Crown. (Rev. ed., Hollywood, CA: Wilshire Books, 1975.)

Ellis, A. (1958a). Rational psychotherapy. *Journal of General Psychology, 59,* 35–49. (Reprinted: New York: Institute for Rational-Emotive Therapy.)

Ellis, A. (1958b). *Sex without guilt.* New York: Lyle Stuart (Rev. ed., New York: Lyle Stuart, 1965.)

Ellis, A. (1960). *The art and science of love.* Secaucus, NJ: Lyle Stuart.

Ellis, A. (1962). *Reason and emotion in psychotherapy.* Secaucus, NJ: Lyle Stuart.

Ellis, A. (1963a). *Sex and the single man.* Secaucus, NJ: Lyle Stuart.

Ellis, A. (1963b). *The intelligent woman's guide to manhunting.* New York: Lyle Stuart. (Rev. ed.: *The intelligent woman's guide to dating and mating.* Secaucus, NJ: Lyle Stuart, 1979.)

Ellis, A. (1965a). *Homosexuality.* Secaucus, NJ: Lyle Stuart.

Ellis, A. (1965b). *Suppressed: Seven key essays publishers dared not print.* Chicago: New Classics House.

Ellis, A. (1969). A weekend of rational encounter. *Rational Living, 4*(2), 1–8.

Ellis, A. (1971). *Growth through reason.* North Hollywood, CA: Wilshire Books.

Ellis, A. (1972a). Psychotherapy without tears. In A. Burton (Ed.), *Twelve therapists* (pp. 103–126). San Francisco: Jossey-Bass.

Ellis, A. (1972b). *Psychotherapy and the value of a human being.* New York: Institute for Rational-Emotive Therapy.

Ellis, A. (1973). *Humanistic psychotherapy: The rational-emotive approach.* New York: McGraw-Hill.

Ellis, A. (1975). *How to live with a neurotic* (Rev. ed.). North Hollywood, CA: Wilshire Books.

Ellis, A. (1976). *Sex and the liberated man.* Secaucus, NJ: Lyle Stuart.

Ellis, A. (1977). *Anger—How to live with and without it.* Secaucus, NJ: Citadel Press.

Ellis, A. (1978). Rational-emotive therapy and self-help therapy. *Rational Living, 13*(1), 2–9.

Ellis, A. (1979). Rational-emotive therapy: Research data that support the clinical and personality hypotheses of RET and other modes of cognitive-behavior therapy. In A. Ellis & J. M. Whiteley (Eds.), *Theoretical and empirical foundations of rational-emotive therapy* (pp. 101–173). Monterey, CA: Brooks/Cole.

Ellis, A. (1981). The place of Immanuel Kant in cognitive psychotherapy. *Rational Living, 16*(2), 13–16.

Ellis, A. (1983). *The case against religiosity.* New York: Institute for Rational-Emotive Therapy.

Ellis, A. (1984a). The essence of RET—1984. *Journal of Rational-Emotive Therapy, 2*(1), 19–25.

Ellis, A. (1984b). Is the unified-interaction approach to cognitive-behavior modification a reinvention of the wheel? *Clinical Psychology Review, 4,* 215–218.

Ellis, A. (1985a). *Overcoming resistance: Rational-emotive therapy with difficult clients.* New York: Springer.

Ellis, A. (1985b). Two forms of humanistic psychology: Rational-emotive therapy vs. transpersonal psychology. *Free Inquiry, 15*(4), 14–21.

Ellis, A. (1987). A sadly neglected cognitive element in depression. *Cognition Therapy and Research, 11,* 121–146.

Ellis, A. (1988). *How to stubbornly refuse to make yourself miserable about anything–yes, anything!* Secaucus, N.J.: Lyle Stuart.

Ellis, A., & Abrahms, E. (1978). *Brief psychotherapy in medical and health practice.* New York: Springer.

Ellis, A., & Bernard, M. E. (Eds.). (1983). *Rational-emotive approaches to the problems of childhood.* New York: Plenum Press.

Ellis, A., & Bernard, M. E. (Eds.). (1985). *Clinical applications of rational-emotive therapy.* New York: Plenum Press.

Ellis, A., & Dryden, W. (1987). *The practice of rational-emotive therapy.* New York: Springer.

Ellis, A., & Grieger, R. (Eds.). (1977). *Handbook of rational-emotive therapy* (Vol. 1). New York: Springer.

Ellis, A., & Grieger, R. (1986). *Handbook of rational-emotive therapy* (Vol. 2). New York: Springer.

Ellis, A., & Harper, R. A. (1961a). *A guide to successful marriage.* North Hollywood, CA: Wilshire Books.

Ellis, A., & Harper, R. A. (1961b). *A guide to rational living.* Englewood Cliffs, NJ: Prentice-Hall.

Ellis, A., & Harper, R. A. (1975). *A new guide to rational living.* North Hollywood, CA: Wilshire Books.

Ellis, A., & Knaus, W. (1977). *Overcoming procrastination.* New York: New American Library.

Ellis, A., & Whiteley, J. M. (1979). *Theoretical and empirical foundations of rational-emotive therapy.* Monterey, CA: Brooks/Cole.

Ellis, H. (1936). *Studies in the psychology of sex* (2 vols.). New York: Random House. (Originally published 1897.)

Epictetus. (1890). *The collected works of Epictetus.* Boston: Little, Brown.

Erickson, M. H. (1967). *Advanced techniques of hypnosis and therapy: Selected papers of Milton H. Erickson.* Edited by Jay Haley. New York: Grune & Stratton.

Erickson, M. H. (1981). *A teaching seminar with Milton H. Erickson.* Edited with commentary by J. K. Zeig. New York: Brunner/Mazel.

Eysenck, H. J. (1960). *Handbook of abnormal psychology: An experimental approach.* New York: Basic Books.

Eysenck, H. J. (Ed.) (1964). *Experiments in behavior therapy.* New York: Macmillan.

Fenichel, D. (1945). *The psychoanalytic theory of neurosis.* New York: Norton.

Forel, A. (1922). *The sexual question.* New York: Physician's and Surgeon's Book Company. (Originally published 1908.)

Frank, J. (1963). *Persuasion and healing.* Baltimore, MD: Johns Hopkins.

Frankl, V. (1959). *Man's search for meaning.* New York: Pocket Books.

Freeman, A. (Ed.). (1983). *Marital and family therapy.* New York: Guilford.

Freeman, A., & Greenwood, V. (1986). *Cognitive therapy.* New York: Human Sciences Press.

Freud, S. (1965). *Standard edition of the complete psychological works of Sigmund Freud.* London: Hogarth.

Glasser, W. (1965). *Reality therapy.* New York: Harper & Row.

Goldfried, M. R. (1980). Toward the delineation of therapeutic change principles. *American Psychologist, 35,* 991–999.

Goldfried, M. R., & Davision, G. (1976). *Clinical behavior therapy.* New York: Holt, Rinehart & Winston.

Goldfried, M. R., & Merbaum, M. (Eds.). (1973). Behavior change through self-control. New York: Holt, Rinehart & Winston.

Goulding, M. M., & Goulding, R. L. (1979). *Changing lives through redecision therapy.* New York: Brunner/Mazel.

Grieger, R. M. (Ed.). (1986). *Rational-emotive couples therapy.* A special issue of *Journal of Rational-Emotive Therapy.* New York: Human Sciences Press.

Grieger, R., & Boyd, J. (1980). *Rational-emotive therapy: A skills-based approach.* New York: Van Nostrand Reinhold.

Grieger, R., & Grieger, I. (Eds.). (1982). *Cognition and emotional disturbance.* New York: Human Sciences Press.

Guerney, B. G., Jr., (1977). *Relationship enhancement: Skill-training programs for therapy, problem-prevention and enrichment.* San Francisco: Jossey-Bass.

Guidano, V. F., & Liotti, G. (1983). *Cognitive processes and emotional disorders.* New York: Guilford.

Haley, J. (1963). *Strategies of psychotherapy.* New York: Grune & Stratton.

Haley, J. (1973). *Uncommon therapy: The psychiatric techniques of Milton H. Erickson.* New York: Norton.

Haley, J. (1976). *Problem-solving therapy.* San Francisco: Jossey-Bass.

Harris, T. (1969). *I'm OK, you're OK.* New York: Harper & Row.

Hartman, W., & Fithian, M. (1972). *Treatment of sexual dysfunction.* Long Beach, CA: Center for Marital and Sexual Studies.

Hauck, P. A. (1973). *Overcoming depression.* Philadelphia, PA: Westminster.

Hauck, P. A. (1974). *Overcoming frustration and anger.* Philadelphia, PA: Westminster.

Heesacker, M., Heppner, P. P., & Rogers, M. E. (1982). Classics and emerging classics in psychology. *Journal of Counseling Psychology, 29,* 400–405.

Heidegger, M. (1962). *Being and time.* New York: Harper & Row.

Hollon, S. D. (1983). *Cognitive therapy and research.* New York: Plenum Press.

James, W. (1914). *Varieties of religious experience.* London: Longmans Green.

Janet, P. (1898). *Nevroses et idée fixes* (2 vols.). Paris: Alcan.

Janis, I. L. (1983). *Short-term counseling.* New Haven, CT: Yale University Press.

Janis, I. L., & Mann, L. (1977). *Decision-making.* NewYork: Free Press.

Jones, M. C. (1924a). The elimination of children's fears. *Journal of Experimental Psychology, 7,* 383–390.

Jones, M. C. (1924b). A laboratory study of fear: The case of Peter. *Journal of Genetic Psychology, 31,* 308–315.

Jones, R. (1968). *A factored measure of Ellis' irrational belief systems with personality and maladjustment correlates.* Unpublished doctoral dissertation, Texas Tech College.

Kanfer, F. H., & Goldstein, A. P. (Eds.). (1975). *Helping people change.* New York: Pergamon.

Kaplan, H. S. (1974). *The new sex therapy.* New York: Brunner/Mazel.

Kelly, G. (1955). *The psychology of personal constructs* (2 vols). New York: Norton.

Kendall, P. C., & Hollon, S. D. (Eds.) (1981). *Advances in cognitive behavior research and therapy* (Vol. 1). New York: Academic.

Kendall, P. C. (Ed.). (1983). *Advances in cognitive behavioral research and therapy* (Vol. 2). New York: Academic Press.

Kendall, P. C., & Braswell, L. (1984). *Cognitive behavioral therapy for impulsive children.* New York: Guilford.

Kendall, P. C., & Hollon, S. (Eds.). (1979). *Cognitive behavioral interventions: Theory, research and procedures.* New York: Academic Press.

Kendall, P. C., & Hollon, S. D. (1980). *Assessment strategies for cognitive-behavioral interventions.* New York: Academic Press.

Kanus, W. (1974). *Rational emotive education.* New York: Institute for Rational-Emotive Therapy.

Krafft-Ebing, R. von. (1922). *Psychopathia Sexualis.* Brooklyn: Physician's and Surgeon's Book Company. (Original publication, 1886)

Lange, A., & Jakubowski, P. (1976). *Responsible assertive behavior.* Champaign, IL: Research Press.

Lazarus, A. A. (1971). *Behavior therapy and beyond.* New York: McGraw-Hill.

Lazarus, A. A. (1976). *Multimodal therapy.* New York: Springer.

Lazarus, A. A. (1981). *The practice of multimodal therapy.* New York: McGraw-Hill.

Lazarus, A. F., & Fay, A. (1975). *I can if I want to.* New York: Morrow.

Lazarus, R. S. (1966). *Psychological stress and the coping process.* New York: McGraw-Hill.

Lazarus, R. S., & Folkman, S. (1984). *Stress, appraisal, and coping.* New York: Springer.

Lecky, P. (1943). *Self-consistency.* New York: Doubleday/Anchor.

Long, H. W. (1922). *Sane sex life and sane sex living.* New York: Eugenics.

Mahoney, M. J. (1974). *Cognition and behavior modification.* Cambridge, MA: Ballinger.

Mahoney, M. J., & Freeman, A. (Eds.). (1985). *Cognition and psychotherapy.* New York: Plenum Press.

Marcus Aurelius (1890). *Meditations.* Boston: Little, Brown.

Masters, W., & Johnson, V. A. (1970). *Human sexual inadequacy.* Boston: Little, Brown.

Masters, J., & Rimm, D. C. (1974). *Behavior therapy.* New York: Academic Press.

Maultsby, M. C., Jr. (1971). *Handbook of rational self-counseling.* Lexington, KY: Rational Self Help Books.

Maultsby, M. C., Jr. (1975). *Help yourself to happiness: Through rational self-counseling.* New York: Institute for Rational-Emotive Therapy.

Maultsby, M. C., Jr. (1984). *Rational behavior therapy.* Englewood Cliffs, NJ: Prentice-Hall.

McGovern, T. E., & Silverman, M. S. (1984). A review of outcome studies of rational-emotive therapy from 1977 to 1982. *Journal of Rational-Emotive Therapy, 2*(1), 7–18.

McMullin, R. (1986). *Handbook of cognitive therapy techniques.* New York: Norton.

Meichenbaum, D. (1977). *Cognitive-behavior modification.* New York: Plenum.

Meichenbaum, D., & Jaremko, M. E. (Eds.). (1984). *Stress reduction and prevention.* New York: Plenum Press.

Miller, R. C., & Berman, J. S. (1983). The efficacy of cognitive behavior therapies: A quantitative review of the research evidence. *Psychological Bulletin, 94,* 39–53.

Miller, T. (1983). *So you secretly suspect you're worthless, well . . .* Manlius, NY: Tom Miller.

Morris, K. T., & Kanitz, J. M. (1975). *Rational-emotive therapy.* Boston: Houghton Mifflin.

Munsterberg, H. (1919). *Technique of psychotherapy.* Boston: Houghton Mifflin.

Pavlov, I. (1927). *Conditioned reflexes.* New York: Liveright.

Powell, J. (1976). *Fully human, fully alive.* Niles, IL: Argus.

Raimy, V. (1975). *Misunderstandings of the self.* San Francisco: Jossey-Bass.

Reda, M. A., & Mahoney, M. J. (Eds.). (1984). *Cognitive psychotherapies.* Cambridge, MA: Ballinger.

Robie, W. F. (1925). *The art of love.* Ithaca, NY: Rational Life Press. (Originally published 1920.)

Robinson, W. J. (1915). *Treatment of sexual impotence.* New York: Critic and Guide.

Russell, B. (1929). *Marriage and morals.* New York: Liveright.

Russell, B. (1950). *The conquest of happiness.* New York: New American Library.

Salter, A. (1949). *Conditioned reflex therapy.* New York: Creative Age.

Schwartz, R. M. (1982). Cognitive-behavior modification: A conceptual review. *Clinical Psychology Review, 2,* 267–293.

Schwartz, R. M. (1984). Is rational-emotive therapy a truly unified interactive approach?: A reply to Ellis. *Clinical Psychology Review, 4,* 219–226.

Seligman, M. E. P. (1975). *Helplessness.* San Francisco: Freeman.

Singer, J. L., & Pope, K. S. (Eds.). (1978). *The power of human imagination.* New York: Plenum Press.

Skinner, B. F. (1953). *Science and human behavior.* New York: Macmillan.

Smith, D. (1982). Trends in counseling and psychotherapy. *American Psychologist, 37,* 802–809.

Smith, M. L., & Glass, G. V. (1977). Meta analysis of psychotherapy outcome studies. *American Psychologist, 32,* 752–760.

Smith, T. W. (1982). Irrational beliefs in the cause and treatment of emotional distress: A critical review of the rational emotive model. *Clinical Psychology Review, 2,* 505–522.

Snygg, D., & Combs, A. W. (1959). *Individual behavior.* New York: Harper.

Spivack, G., & Shure, M. (1974). *Social adjustment in young children.* San Francisco: Jossey-Bass.

Spivack, G., Platt, J., & Shure, M. (1976). *The problem-solving approach to adjustment.* San Francisco: Jossey-Bass.

Stampfl, T. G., & Levis, D. J. (1967). Essentials of implosive therapy. *Journal of Abnormal Psychology, 72,* 496–503.

Tillich, P. (1953). *The courage to be.* New Haven: Yale University Press.

Tosi, D. J. (1974). *Youth: Toward personal growth, a rational-emotive approach.* Columbus, OH: Merrill.

Wachtel, P. L. (1977). *Psychoanalysis and behavior therapy: Toward an integration.* New York: Basic Books.

Wachtel, P. L. (1982). *Resistance.* New York: Plenum Press.

Walen, S. R., DiGiuseppe, R., & Wessler, R. L. (1980). *A practitioner's guide to rational-emotive therapy.* New York: Oxford.

Watson, J. B., & Rayner, R. (1920). Conditioned emotional reactions. *Journal of Experimental Psychology, 3,* 1–14.

Watzlawick, P., Bevan, A., & Jackson, D. (1967). *Pragmatics of human communication.* New York: Norton.

Watzlawick, P., Weakland, J., & Fisch, R. (1974). *Change.* New York: Norton.

Wessler, R. A., & Wessler, R. L. (1980). *The principles and practice of rational-emotive therapy*. San Francisco, CA: Jossey-Bass.

Wessler, R. A., & Hankin-Wessler, S. W. R. (1986). Cognitive appraisal therapy. In W. Dryden & W. Golden (Eds.), *Cognitive-behavioural approaches to psychotherapy* (pp. 196–223). London: Harper Row.

Wick, E. (1983). Psychotherapy focus: Old and new. *Voices, 18*(4), 34–38.

Wolpe, J. (1958). *Psychotherapy by reciprocal inhibition*. Stanford, CA: Stanford University Press.

Wolpe, J. (1980). Cognitive behavior: A reply to three commentaries. *American Psychologist, 35,* 112–114.

Wolpe, J., & Lazarus, A. A. (1966). *Behavior therapy techniques*. New York: Pergamon.

Wortis, J. (1954). *Fragments of an analysis with Freud*. New York: Simon & Schuster.

Young, H. (1974). *Rational counseling primer*. New York: Institute for Rational Emotive Therapy.

Zajonc, R. B. (1980). Feeling and thinking: Preferences need no inferences. *American Psychologist, 35,* 151–175.

# 2

# Cognitive Therapy

## AARON T. BECK AND MARJORIE WEISHAAR

## HISTORY

### PRECURSORS

Cognitive therapy has been influenced by a variety of theories of psychopathology and the process of therapy. At the theoretical level, it has been primarily influenced by three sources: (1) the phenomenological approach to psychology, (2) structural theory and depth psychology, and (3) cognitive psychology. The "phenomenological" approach to psychology is rooted in Greek Stoic philosophy. It maintains that one's view of self and one's personal world largely determine behavior. This concept appears in Kant's (1798) emphasis on conscious subjective experience and in the more contemporary writings of Adler (1936), Alexander (1950), Horney (1950), and Sullivan (1953).

The second major influence on cognitive therapy was structural theory, particularly Freud's conceptualization of cognitions being hierarchically arranged into primary and secondary processes. Primary-process thinking is analogous to the rigid, primitive cognitive processing that goes on during psychological distress. Secondary-process thinking, with its greater flexibility and finer discrimination, is what cognitive therapy regards as the "normal" coding system.

The third influence on cognitive therapy has been cognitive psychology, from Kelly's (1955) formulations of "personal constructs" and elucidation of the role of beliefs in behavior change to the current work of Richard Lazarus (1984), which gives primacy to the role of cognition in emotional and behavioral change.

### DEVELOPMENT

Cognitive Therapy developed out of Beck's early research on depression (Beck 1963, 1964, 1967). Trained in psychoanalysis, Beck tried to substantiate Freud's theory of depres-

---

AARON T. BECK • Center for Cognitive Therapy, Department of Psychiatry, University of Pennsylvania, Philadelphia, Pennsylvania 19104.     MARJORIE WEISHAAR • Department of Psychiatry and Human Behavior, Brown University, Providence, Rhode Island 02912.

sion as having at its core "anger turned on the self." By examining the thoughts and dreams of depressed patients, he noted themes not of anger but of defeat. Further experimental testing and clinical observation revealed a consistent negative bias in the cognitive processing of depressed patients. The cognitive theory of emotional disorders was developed to describe the shifts in information processing that occur in psychopathology.

Concurrent with Beck's research was the work of Albert Ellis (1962), which similarly focused on patients' thoughts and beliefs. Both Ellis and Beck believe that people can consciously adopt reason, and both view the patient's underlying assumptions as targets of intervention. Similarly, both advocate active dialogues with patients, rather than passive listening. Despite conceptual and stylistic differences between Rational Emotive Therapy and Cognitive Therapy, they provided considerable foundation and impetus for what has become a range of cognitive-behavior therapies.

The work of a number of contemporary behaviorists influenced the development of cognitive therapy. Bandura's social learning theory and concepts of expectancy of reinforcement, self- and outcome efficacies, interaction between person and environment, modeling, and vicarious learning (Bandura 1977a,b) catalyzed the shift in behavior therapy to the cognitive domain. Similarly, Mahoney (1974, 1977) outlined the cognitive mediation of human learning. The paradigm shift in behavior therapy from a conditioning model to one that includes cognitive processing allowed for a proliferation in research into the nature of cognitive processing in emotional disorders and into treatment interventions aimed at cognitions.

## THEORY OF PSYCHOPATHOLOGY

Cognitive therapy can be thought of as a system of psychotherapy: (1) a theory of personality and psychopathology, (2) a body of knowledge, and (3) an integrated program of strategies and techniques.

The theory is based on the conception that an organism needs to process information in an adaptive way in order to survive. If we did not utilize a functional apparatus for taking in relevant data, synthesizing it, and formulating a plan of action on the basis of that synthesis, we would soon be killed or starve to death. Much of this processing is automatic and outside of awareness. Further, the process is not necessarily rational, logical, or veridical. It is usually functional in the sense that it serves to promote the basic requirements of the organism— specifically, survival and reproduction. In some cases, as in mate selection, it may be advantageous or adaptive to process information in an overly optimistic way. This would encourage bonding and reproductive success. However, in certain risk situations, it is more beneficial to exaggerate the probability of harm, thus allowing the organism to escape and continue to contribute to the gene pool.

The information-processing apparatus can be construed as containing several related coding systems. These systems are designed by evolutionary and developmental (learning) processes to select specific data, integrate them, interpret them, and store a selected sample. The systems also draw on a specific memory residue to match with present experiences. The memory thus serves as a guide to interpreting current events.

The specific coding elements are composed of rules (assumptions, attitudes) that translate experiences into usable information. An example of a rule is "strangers may be dangerous." The rules are formed by learning: by interaction between experiences and the primodial coding system.

In psychopathology, a specific, more primitive coding system is activated and may assume precedence over the "normal" coding systems. Thus in anxiety, the relevant coding system consists of the following parts: (1) attention—hypervigilance for data relevant to danger; (2) selection of data relevant to danger; (3) overinterpretation of danger; and (4) increased access to danger themes in memory.

The intrusion of the more primitive coding system produces a skewing of information processing. This "cognitive shift" introduces a systematic bias into the interpretations and inferences in various psychopathological conditions such as anxiety disorders, depressive disorders, mania, paranoid states, obsessive-compulsive neurosis, and others. The specific bias can also account for the symptomatology of the various psychological disturbances. Thus, an individual whose processing has shifted to a fixation of attention and interpretation of themes of loss or defeat is likely to be depressed. Similarly, the anxiety patient experiences a systematic bias toward themes of danger; in paranoid conditions, the skewing is in the direction of indiscriminate attribution of abuse or interference. The manic patient shows a skewing toward exaggerated interpretations of personal gain.

People are predisposed to experience the cognitive shift as a result of the interaction of certain dysfunctional attitudes and life situations. For example, a person who has an attitude that a loss of status represents a major reduction of his or her worth may, under the stress of many minor losses or even a single major loss, shift into the mode of interpreting most experiences as a serious defeat. A person who believes that she or he is vulnerable to sudden death may, after exposure to a life-threatening disorder in him- or herself or another person, begin to interpret normal body sensations as a sign of an impending catastrophe and experience a panic attack. Other specific sets of beliefs can predispose people to other psychiatric disorders.

## THEORY OF CAUSALITY

Psychological distress is the ultimate consequence of the interaction of innate, biological, developmental, and environmental factors. There is no single "cause" of psychopathology. Depression, for example, has a number of predisposing factors such as hereditary susceptibility, physical disease leading to neurochemical abnormalities, developmental traumata leading to cognitive vulnerabilities, inadequate personal experiences or identifications to provide coping mechanisms, and maladaptive cognitive patterns such as unrealistic goals, assumptions, or imperatives. Precipitating factors include physical disease, chronic stress, or severe and acute stress. *Cognitions do not "cause" depression or any other psychopathological disorder* but are an intrinsic part of the disorder.

In terms of cognitive processing, individuals experience psychological distress when they perceive a situation as threatening to their vital interests. At such times, there is a functional impairment in normal cognitive processing: Perceptions and interpretations of events become highly selective, egocentric, and rigid. The person has a decreased ability to "turn off" distorted thinking or self-correct perceptions, to concentrate, recall, or reason. Corrective functions, which allow reality testing and refinement of global conceptualizations, are weakened.

## COGNITIVE DISTORTIONS

During psychological distress, the shift to a more primitive information-processing system is apparent in systematic errors in reasoning, called cognitive distortions (see Beck, 1967). These include the following.

*Arbitrary inference*—drawing a particular conclusion in the absence of substantiating evidence or even in the face of contradictory evidence. An example of this is the working mother who concludes after a busy workday, "I'm a terrible mother."

*Selective abstraction*—conceptualizing a situation on the basis of a detail taken out of context, ignoring other relevant information. An honoree at a banquet was not asked to speak before her admirers. She concluded, "They don't really think I'm that great because they didn't ask for a speech."

*Overgeneralization*—formulating a general rule based on one or a few isolated incidents and applying the rule broadly to other situations. An example of this is the man who concluded after a brief affair, "I'll never get close to anyone because I can't."

*Magnification and minimization*—viewing something as far more or far less significant than it actually is. Upon putting a minor dent in her car, a young woman concluded that she was a terrible driver who had had a major collision.

*Personalization*—attributing external events to oneself in the absence of any causal connection. After being treated brusquely by a supervisor, a man concluded, "I must have written a bad quarterly report."

*Dichotomous thinking*—categorizing experiences in one of two extremes; for example, a complete success or a total failure. A doctoral candidate said, "I must be the best student in this department, or I've failed."

## COGNITIVE VULNERABILITY

The shift to the primitive information-processing system is triggered by the interaction of personal and environmental factors. Each individual has a set of idiosyncratic vulnerabilities that predispose one to psychological distress. These vulnerabilities appear related to personality structure, to one's fundamental beliefs about the self and the world. These fundamental cognitive structures are called schemata. Schemata develop early in life from personal experiences and identification with significant others. Early conceptualizations are reinforced by further learning experiences and, in turn, influence the formation of other beliefs, values, and attitudes.

As enduring cognitive structures, schemas may be positive, thereby providing coping mechanisms, or they may be negative and dysfunctional. They may be general or highly specific. A person may even have competing schemas. Schemas are usually latent but become activated and hypervalent when triggered by stimuli, such as life events.

The basic nature of schemas and the notion of cognitive vulnerability are illustrated in the following conceptualization of the borderline personality disorder, which, according to cognitive therapist Jeffrey Young (1983), is characterized by intense emotional reactions to events, abrupt shifts in mood particularly to anxious agitation or anger, impulsive and counterproductive acts, and unstable interpersonal relationships. The predominant cognitive distortions operating are dichotomous thinking (particularly seeing oneself or others as all good or all bad) and "subjective reasoning" (equating feelings with facts).

Young conceptualizes the borderline patient as having early negative schemas that are central to his or her psychological functioning. Typical schemas are, "There's something fundamentally wrong with me"; "People should support me and should not criticize, abandon, disagree with or misunderstand me;" and "I am my feelings." With such schemas about the self and others, the delicate emotional balance of the borderline patient is easily upset by any perceived abandonment or transgression. The behavioral and emotional patterns that one would label *personality* are derived from these rules about life and the self. Other disorders may be characterized by similar core beliefs, but they are less strong or rigidly held.

Schemas are also present as "conditional assumptions," attitudes that have an implicit "if–then" format. An example frequently found among depression-prone individuals is, "If I don't succeed at everything I do, nobody will respect me" or "If a person doesn't like me, it means I'm unlovable." Such individuals may function without difficulty until they experience a defeat or rejection. At that point, their underlying assumptions become relevant, and they may begin to believe that no one respects them or they are unloveable. Usually, such beliefs can be corrected in brief therapy. However, if they constitute core beliefs, extended treatment is necessary.

## SYSTEMATIC BIAS IN PSYCHIATRIC DISORDERS

A systematic bias in information processing is characteristic in psychiatric disorders. It distorts both "external" information, such as communication from other people, and "internal" information, such as bodily sensations during a panic attack. The kind of bias found in some disorders appears in Table 1.

In the next sections, the cognitive profiles of several disorders are presented in order to demonstrate biased cognitive processing in psychopathology.

# COGNITIVE PROFILES

## DEPRESSION

Depression is characterized by the cognitive triad, reflecting the depressed individual's negative view of the self, the world, and the future. This person perceives himself or herself as inadequate, deserted, and worthless. The negative view of the world is reflected in beliefs that unreasonable demands are present and that immense barriers prevent the person from obtaining goals. The world holds no pleasure or gratification. The depressed individual's view of the future is pessimistic: Current problems will persist and perhaps get worse. The person often sees no way out of his or her difficulties. This hopelessness may lead to suicidal ideation.

The motivational, behavioral and physical manifestations of depression are rooted in these cognitive constellations. The motivational problems observed in depression, often referred to as the "paralysis of will," stem from expectations of failure, a low sense of self-efficacy, and a perceived inability to cope with the consequences of failure.

Similarly, increased dependency on others reflects the negative view of the self as incompetent, a magnification of the difficulty of everyday tasks, and the desire for someone more competent to take over. Indecisiveness also reflects the belief that one is incapable of making the right decision.

Physical symptoms of depression such as low energy, fatigue, and inertia also stem from negative expectations. Initiating activity, paradoxically, tends to reduce retardation and fa-

TABLE 1. The Cognitive Profile of Psychological Disorders

| Disorder | Systematic bias |
| --- | --- |
| Depression | Negative view of self, experience, and future |
| Hypomania | Positive view of self, experience, and future |
| Anxiety disorder | Physical or psychological threat |
| Panic disorder | Catastrophic misinterpretation of bodily or mental experiences |
| Phobia | Threat in specific, avoidable situations |
| Paranoid state | Attribution of negative bias to others |
| Hysteria | Belief in motor or sensory abnormality |
| Obsession | Repetitive warning or doubting about safety |
| Compulsion | Rituals to ward off doubts or threat |
| Suicidal behavior | Hopelessness |
| Anorexia nervosa | Fear of appearing fat (to self or others) |
| Hypochondriasis | Belief in serious medical disorder |

tigue. This is due, in part, to the refutation of negative expectations and the demonstration of motor ability.

## ANXIETY

Anxiety disorders are conceptualized as the excessive functioning of normal survival mechanisms. The same responses that protect an organism from external threat become maladaptive when excessively or incorrectly activated in psychosocial situations. These basic responses consist of a cognitive set that makes decisions quickly and tends to be overinclusive in its discrimination of threatening stimuli and physiological reactions that are automatic and do not distinguish between physical danger and psychosocial threat.

Anxious individuals tend to overestimate the risk and magnitude of perceived danger. "Normal" individuals make more accurate assessments of harm and are also able to correct their misperceptions using logic and evidence. Anxious individuals have difficulty recognizing cues of safety and other evidence that would reduce the threat of danger, including their own ability to cope.

## HYPOMANIA

The cognitive bias in hypomania or mania is opposite that in depression. The hypomanic or manic patient selectively perceives gains in each life experience, ignores negative experiences or reinterprets them as positive, and unrealistically expects favorable outcomes in the future.

The exaggerated perceptions of worth, abilities, and accomplishments lead to feelings of euphoria. The continued stimulation from inflated self-evaluations and overly optimistic expectations provide vast amounts of energy and drive the manic individual into continuous goal-seeking activity.

## PANIC DISORDER

Patients with panic disorder tend to interpret any unexplained symptom or sensation as a sign or impending physical or mental disaster. Their information-processing system focuses on physical or psychological experiences and interprets these as sources of internal information that some catastrophe is about to occur. Symptoms are interpreted in idiosyncratic ways: For one person, rapid heartbeat signals a heart attack; for another, shortness of breath means he or she will stop breathing; yet another person will interpret lightheadedness as a sign of imminent fainting. The key characteristic of panic attacks is the patients' interpretations that one of their vital systems (cardiovascular, respiratory, or central nervous system) will collapse and, as a result, they will die or go crazy. This fear makes them hypervigilant toward any internal sensations, thereby magnifying any sensations that would go unnoticed in other people.

In addition to errors in perceptions and interpretation, individuals who experience panic attacks show a specific "cognitive deficit" during the attack: the inability to use logic and evidence to calm themselves or to view their symptoms realistically.

## AGORAPHOBIA

Patients who have had one or more panic attacks in certain locations or situations will avoid that situation because they associate it with extreme discomfort and catastrophic predictions. Even the anticipation of being in that situation may increase vigilance to sensations and may trigger a variety of symptoms. Agoraphobic patients may eventually become housebound or so restricted in their activities that they cannot travel far from home and rely on a companion if they are to travel any distance.

In phobias, the cognitive bias is the anticipation of physical or psychological harm in circumscribed situations. As long as that situation is avoided, the patient may feel comfortable. When they are in that situation, however, they experience the autonomic arousal typical of anxiety disorders. As a result of this unpleasant reaction, their avoidance is reinforced.

In "evaluation phobias," there is fear of disparagement or failure in social or performance situations. The behavioral and physiological reactions to the potential threat (rejection, devaluation, failure) may actually interfere with the patient's functioning and cause what the patient fears will happen.

## PARANOID STATE

The information-processing system in the paranoid person is biased toward attributing prejudice to others in their interactions with him or her. The paranoid patient assumes that others are unjustly and deliberately malicious, abusive, interfering, or critical. In contrast to the depressed individual who suffers a loss of self-esteem when he or she perceives criticism, the paranoid individual gets angry over the injustice of the presumed attacks.

## OBSESSIONS AND COMPULSIONS

The information processing of persons with obsessions is biased in the direction of emphasizing uncertainty in situations that ordinary prudence would deem as safe. The uncertainty is usually assigned to some situation that has some risk involved, but the degree of doubt and worry is inordinate and excessive for the degree of actual risk. The person experiences continual doubts when there is no evidence of danger and even in the face of reassurances.

Patients may continually doubt whether they have performed an act necessary to guarantee safety (e.g., turning off a gas oven, locking the doors at night, washing germs from one's hands). A key characteristic in obsessive disorder is this sense of responsibility that patients are accountable for having taking an action or failed to take an action that could be harmful to them or their families.

Compulsions consist of attempts to reduce excessive doubts or worries by performing a ritual that will prevent the anticipated disaster. A handwashing compulsion, for example, is based on the person's belief that he or she remains contaminated by dirt and germs and must remove it from his or her body. Dirt may signify a source of physical disease to the person or may be seen as a source of odors that would offend other people.

## SUICIDAL BEHAVIOR

Suicidal behavior has been found to have specific associated cognitive characteristics that warrant its inclusion as a separate cognitive profile. The cognitive processing in suicidal individuals has two features. First, suicidal individuals have a high degree of hopelessness; the greater the hopelessness, the more likely they are to commit suicide (Beck, Steer, Kovacs, & Garrison, 1985). Second, suicidal individuals have poor problem-solving skills, often apparent in their interpersonal relationships at work or school. Although poor problem-solving skill interacts with hopelessness to increase suicidal risk, it is a factor, in itself, in suicide potential.

## ANOREXIA NERVOSA

Both anorexia nervosa and bulimia are behavioral manifestations of a constellation of maladaptive beliefs. The beliefs center around the assumption, "My weight and shape determine my worth and/or my social acceptability." Contiguous to this assumption are beliefs such as, "I will look ugly if I gain much more weight," "The only thing in my life that I can control is my weight," and "If I let go and eat, there will be no stopping and I will become obese."

Patients with anorexia show the following distortions in information processing: They misinterpret feelings of fullness after eating as signs they are getting fat, and they interpret their image in a photograph or mirror as heavier than it is.

## THEORY OF PSYCHOTHERAPY

The goals of cognitive therapy are to correct faulty information processing and to modify dysfunctional beliefs and assumptions that maintain maladaptive behaviors and emotions. Cognitive therapy is a collaborative process between patient and therapist that employs both behavioral and verbal techniques to examine the patient's beliefs, challenge the dysfunctional ones, and provide skills and experience that promote more adaptive cognitive processing.

Cognitive therapy initially focuses on symptom relief, including distortions in logic and problem behaviors. Ultimately, it aims at modifying underlying assumptions and correcting the patient's systematic bias in thinking. In order to cause these changes, the patient's beliefs are treated as hypotheses to be tested. Then they are logically examined and tested through behavioral experiments, jointly determined by therapist and patient. Structural change occurs with the modification of these assumptions to fit more closely with the reality of the situation and with the practice of behaviors congruent with new, more adaptive assumptions.

Therapeutic change occurs along several channels: cognitive, behavioral, and affective. Cognitive change promotes behavioral change by allowing the patient to adopt a perspective that allows risk taking. In turn, the practice of new behaviors serves to validate the new perspective. Emotions can be moderated by considering evidence and facts and by expanding one's perspective to allow for alternative interpretations of events. Emotions play a role in cognitive change, for learning is more salient when emotions are triggered. Thus the cognitive, behavioral, and affective channels interact in therapeutic change. Cognitive therapy emphasizes the primacy of cognition in initiating and maintaining therapeutic change.

Cognitive change occurs at several levels: in voluntary thoughts, in continuous or "automatic" thoughts, and in assumptions. These levels of cognition are hierarchically arranged according to the degree of accessibility and stability. Thus the most accessible and least stable type of cognition is voluntary thought, for voluntary thoughts can be activated at will and are temporary.

Automatic thoughts come to mind spontaneously and are the thoughts that intercede between a stimulus event and one's emotional and behavioral reactions to it. They are more stable and less accessible than voluntary thoughts. Patients often need to be trained to recognize automatic thoughts. Yet, automatic thoughts are generally quite powerful. They are accompanied by affect and, at the time they are experienced, are plausible, highly salient, and consistent with that person's logic. Despite the cognitive distortions present in automatic thoughts, they are familiar and, therefore, accurate or veridical to that person. Because of their mediating role between stimuli and responses and because of the presence of cognitive distortions, much attention is given to automatic thoughts in the early stages of therapy.

Automatic thoughts not only reveal distortions in information processing but represent the patient's beliefs and underlying assumptions. When an underlying assumption is triggered by a situation or circumstance, automatic thoughts are generated. Thus automatic thoughts are often the therapist's access to the patient's underlying assumptions. For example, a patient with the belief, "Unless I am loved, I am nothing," would have a proliferation of negative automatic thoughts following the breakup of a relationship. Assumptions generally concern how one conceptualizes oneself and the world. They are rules learned from one's own experience or from others. They shape perceptions into cognitions, formulate goals and values, provide interpretations, and assign meanings to events. Assumptions may be quite stable and out of the patient's awareness.

Core beliefs, called schemata, are the most stable cognitive structures and are generally reached by a process of inference. Therapy aims at identifying schemata and counteracting their negative effects. If these core beliefs or assumptions themselves can be changed, the patient is less vulnerable to future distress.

## MECHANISM OF CHANGE IN COGNITIVE THERAPY

Several mechanisms appear to underlie successful forms of psychotherapies: (1) a framework that is comprehensible to the patients and compatible with their belief systems, (2) the patients' affective engagement in applying the framework in the problematic situations, and (3) reality testing in the problematic situations.

The framework or rationale of Wolpe's systematic desensitization is that successive approximations to a threatening scene, when accompanied by muscle relaxation, result in neutralizing a conditioned fear. One of the rationales of psychoanalysis is that uncovering early memories or unconscious material allows them to be assimilated by the conscious ego. The framework of cognitive therapy is that the modification of dysfunctional cognitions and assumptions leads to affective and behavioral change.

Change can only occur if the patient is engaged in the problematic situation and *experiences affective arousal*. According to cognitive therapy, cognitive constellations underlie affect and become accessible and modifiable only with *affective arousal*. In the language of cognitive therapy, these are "hot cognitions." The importance of engagement may be illustrated by contrasting depressed and phobic patients. Because depression is so pervasive, the "hot cognitions" are present and available for examination in the therapist's office. In contrast, phobic or panic disorder patients generally have little distress in the presence of the therapist and may have little anxiety anywhere outside the phobic or stimulus situation. In order to produce change among phobics and panic patients, anxiety has to be induced, either through *in vivo* exposure, imagery, or provocative techniques such as hyperventilation. Consequently, anxiety-related cognitions become highly salient, accessible, and open to testing and modification.

Simply arousing affect and the accompanying cognitions is usually not sufficient to cause *lasting* change. Individuals may go through catharses or abreactions continuously through their lives without receiving any benefit. The therapeutic situation in cognitive therapy allows the patient to experience emotional and cognitive arousal simultaneously and to reality-test the cognitions. In cognitive therapy, reality testing is highly organized: The examination of the evidence and logic supporting dysfunctional cognitions allows the patient to recognize that a particular situation has been misconstrued. It prompts the recognition of thinking deviations as well as the disconfirmation of specific beliefs held by that individual.

# PROCESS OF PSYCHOTHERAPY

## THE THERAPEUTIC RELATIONSHIP

Cognitive therapy is founded on a collaborative relationship between therapist and patient. The patient thus assumes the role of an active co-investigator, providing the cognitive "data" to be examined: the thoughts and images that occur in various situations. Together the patient and therapist set the goals for therapy as well as the agenda for each session.

The therapist acts as a guide to understanding how cognitions influence affect the behav-

AARON T. BECK and
MARJORIE
WEISHAAR

ior. As needed, the therapist also provides skills training and designs behavioral experiments that serve as corrective experiences. In cases of severe depression or anxiety, the therapist may take a very directive role in order to help the patient organize his or her thoughts and wishes. Later in therapy or in cases of less severe distress, the patient may take the lead in determining homework assignments, setting new goals, and the like.

The patient assumes responsibility for therapy by helping to set goals for therapy, by self-observing and monitoring thoughts and images, and by completing homework assignments that may include both behavioral and cognitive endeavors. The patient also provides feedback to the therapist on progress in therapy, including problems with the therapy or therapist.

Thus, cognitive therapy uses a learning model of psychotherapy. The therapist uses well-developed and efficacious cognitive and behavioral techniques specific to targeted symptoms. The therapist provides a rationale for each technique used. This demystifies therapy, increases the patient's understanding of and participation in therapy, and reinforces the learning paradigm with patients gradually assuming more responsibility for therapy.

### STRATEGIES

The overall strategies of Cognitive Therapy center around a collaborative enterprise designed to explore the dysfunctional interpretations and distorted meanings attached to the patient's experiences and to modify them when they are found to be unrealistic or unreasonable. Collaborative empiricism engages the patient as a practical scientist who ordinarily interprets stimuli in a functional way but who has been temporarily thwarted by the shift or bias in gathering and integrating information. The therapist and patient work together in gathering evidence and testing hypotheses based on the patient's operating beliefs.

The second strategy, labeled *guided discovery,* is directed toward unraveling the various facets of the patient's present experiences and past history to discover what themes may be running through his or her misperceptions and beliefs.

### INITIAL GOALS OF THERAPY

The therapist works with the patient to produce a shift back to the functional level of information processing. In theoretical terms, the process is initiated by disconfirmation of the patient's faulty interpretations and conclusions regarding experiences that he or she considers personally relevant. Two aspects of information processing are exploited in this process. First, the therapist and patient draw on reality testing by refocusing the patient's attention to the evidence that is contradictory to his or her conclusions. Second, the patient's ability to admit different data into informative processing is enhanced by pushing the patient to make observations of all the relevant data in a situation, not simply the data that are consistent with the patient's dysfunctional beliefs. Similarly, setting up experiments to test beliefs broadens one's focus of attention and introduces alternative explanations.

Thus by allowing new information that is discrepant with previous beliefs to enter the information-processing system and by expanding the patient's discriminating and evaluative functions, there is a return to the normal coding system.

## TREATMENT OF SPECIFIC DISORDERS

The treatment of each of the psychiatric disorders is guided by the "cognitive profile" for each of these disorders. Depending upon the specific cognitive profile of a disorder, techniques are applied to reverse or neutralize the particular cognitive distortions and dysfunctions characteristic of a particular disorder. It should be emphasized that the cognitive profile simply presents a kind of map for synthesizing the information and other data relevant to the patient. Thus, within the outlines of the cognitive map, the specific details of an individual case are organized. This "detailed map" then serves as the guide for the therapy.

## Depression

In the mild to moderate depressions, it is possible to begin immediately to deal with individuals' misinterpretations and negative beliefs about themselves, their personal world, and the future. Oftentimes, the patient's negative reactions to therapy and expectations of rejection from the therapist can be immediately elicited and evaluated in the therapy session.

In the more severe cases of depression, it is important to start off with behavioral tasks. Thus a daily activity schedule is set up with the patient. This would include such items as getting out of bed when not sleeping, tending to essential hygienic details, and attempting to be more active generally. Specific tasks may be agreed upon and worked into the graded task assignment, the rationale of which is to start with easily mastered tasks and then work up to the more difficult ones. The more retarded, and particularly the hospitalized patients, may have a wide variety of negative thoughts regarding the activities such as, "I won't be able to do it," "I would feel silly," or "It won't do any good." These cognitions in themselves can be set up as hypotheses that the patient can then test as part of the graded task assignment.

When the patient is already active, then the more purely cognitive procedures may be used. The patients track their automatic thoughts, particularly when they precede or accompany a negative feeling. They are asked to full out the Daily Record of Dysfunctional Thoughts and are trained to give reasonable or rational responses to their negative automatic thoughts. As therapy progresses, the patients' underlying beliefs such as, "If I'm not successful, then I am a failure" or "If somebody doesn't like me, it means I'm socially undesirable," are examined in the same way as automatic thoughts; namely in terms of the evidence supporting them, the logical basis on which they rest, and empirical testing.

## Anxiety Disorders

With patients who have intense anxiety, it is often important to delay any of the behavioral tasks until a certain cognitive groundwork has been laid. These patients have to be given a framework for them to integrate the experiences that would correct their exaggerated expectations. Thus a patient who has strong fears and inhibitions relevant to asserting herself would be encouraged to explore all of the presumed catastrophic occurrences that would eventuate from unsuccessful self-assertion. She could then weigh the magnitude of pain resulting from a reversal and compare it with the potential gain from self-assertion. Further, the patient would be encouraged to reexamine the importance attached to certain specific situations. It often turns out that, on examination, the person realizes that one of the reasons a specific "failure" seemed so devastating is that the individual attaches too much importance to that particular situation. In the early stages, various imagery techniques are extremely helpful. Patients can be encouraged to "live through" a situation by imagining that it is occurring right in the therapist's office. The patient can then be asked to imagine the worst possible outcome and the best possible outcome. This type of imaging technique helps to give the patient greater perspective of the feared situation and constitutes a learning experience in itself.

After the patient has undergone some preliminary cognitive restructuring as a result of the use of Socratic questioning, reevaluation of anticipated catastrophes, and imagery techniques, then he or she is encouraged to try out what he or she has learned in a threatening situation. Here again, the tasks are assigned in a graded way so that the person is only gradually exposed to the threatening situation. In this situation, the patient does continue to monitor automatic thoughts and, when possible, to reevaluate them.

In depression, the main thrust is toward disconfirming a strong belief such as, "I can't do anything" or "Nothing brings me pleasure." A single disconfirming episode (in which the patient is able to do something that he or she did not expect to be able to do or get some unexpected pleasure) can significantly undermine this strongly belief. In anxiety, on the other hand, a series of positive outcomes do not in themselves prove that a negative outcome might not occur (even though one sees a whole flock of white swans, this does not prove that all swans are white; the next one might be a black one). Thus the initial work is done in terms of reducing the catastrophizing regarding the importance of a negative outcome and also teaching the patient coping techniques; that is, how to cope with a situation in order to improve the chances of a positive outcome and also how to deal with a negative outcome that might occur.

## PANIC DISORDER

In panic disorders, the treatment is focused on the tendency of the patient to make "catastrophic misinterpretations" about bodily sensations or mental experiences. The first one or two sessions are devoted to determining the precise nature of the patient's symptoms and how she or he misinterprets them. Careful attention is paid to the specific automatic thought that occurs during the panic attack, the situation in which the panic attack is likely to occur, and the prodromal symptoms of the attack. By the third session, the therapist and patient are generally ready to give the patient a different interpretation of the symptoms leading to the panic attack (reattribution). In most cases, it is possible to produce a "mini-panic attack" through hyperventilation, exercise, use of imagery, or other stimuli. The particular techniques depend upon the specific demands of a specific case. The patient is also taught distraction techniques as a way of showing that the panic attack is controllable. Following this, the patient is encouraged to go into the situations in which panic attacks can occur and to apply the techniques of rational restructuring based on what she or he has learned in her or his prior interviews. It is often desirable for a patient to go through at least one more panic attack after the preliminary cognitive restructuring, but without using rational responses in order to demonstrate to the patient that the panic attack in itself does not constitute a serious danger.

## PARANOID STATE

In treating paranoid states, it is crucial to establish a good collaborative relationship with the patient. Above all, it is essential that the patient trust the therapist. In applying the cognitive profile, it is important for the therapist to realize that some areas of the patient's belief may be "so hot" that they could be better left explored to a later date.

The initial interventions can consist of having the patient monitor his or her automatic thoughts regarding other people's presumed bias toward him or her and then encouraging him or her to look for alternative explanations for their presumed noxious behavior. Next, certain basic beliefs such as "I can't trust anybody" or "everybody is out to get me" can be subjected to a logical and empirical analysis. The therapist should be alert to find at least a single episode that can disconfirm an absolute statement (such as, "everybody mistreats me") because a single disconfirmation if accepted by the patient can undermine the absolutistic thinking.

## OBSESSIONS AND COMPULSIONS

These patients can be treated initially by encouraging them to notice the automatic thoughts and images that they have at the time there is an urge to carry out a compulsive act. These images often portray the full magnitude of the patients' fears that propel them to carry on such redundant activities such as handwashing and the like. It would become apparent in a good number of cases that the individual responds to the catastrophic ideation or images as though there is a high probability of this occurring. Thus, the catastrophizing methods are important. It is also crucial to steer the patient to recognize the overresponsibilitizing thoughts such as ''If I don't do these compulsions and something bad happens, it would be awful'' or ''It is my responsibility to protect my own life and those of my family.''

In treating compulsions, typical behavioral methods may be used. The most common ones are ''response prevention,'' in which the patient is prevented from engaging in compulsive rituals such as handwashing. The other method is ''exposure,'' in which the patient is exposed to a mass of the threatening material, such as a pile of dirty towels. This method is akin to the ''flooding'' techniques often used by behavior therapists. In using these behavioral methods, it is important to elicit the patient's thinking and images. By testing the reality of these thoughts and images, the patient is able to cognitively restructure the fears of contamination and the like.

### SUICIDAL BEHAVIOR

In treating the suicidal patient, it is important to promote a good relationship with him or her from the beginning and to establish bridges from one therapy session to the next so as to discourage the patient from making a suicide attempt between sessions. The therapist immediately starts to explore the patient's hopelessness in using a variety of cognitive techniques to try to get the patient to view her or his problems more objectively. The therapist teaches the patient to cope with particularly with the type of ''dichotomous'' (all-or-nothing) thinking characteristic of many suicidal patients.

Suicidal patients seem to operate according to certain beliefs such as ''If my boyfriend doesn't respond to me, it means he doesn't like me and I will always be alone.'' By attacking the hopelessness and the self-defeating beliefs, the therapist is able to get the patient to recognize that there are important solutions to life's problems and that she or he does not need to turn to suicide in order to escape from them.

Another problem that is typical of the cognitive profile of suicidal patients is their ''cognitive deficit.'' In contrast to other patients, they seem to have a peculiarly lacking ability in solving highly charged problems in relationship to other people or to their job or carrer. When they are thwarted in one of these endeavors, they seem to be unable to generate alternative solutions to the problem. If their accustomed way of dealing with a situation suddenly does not work, they do not seem to be able to think of other ways of dealing with this situation. Thus a good part of the therapy has to be devoted to ''problem-solving'' techniques such as defining the problem, generating alternative ways of solving the problem, and implementation of the solution.

### ANOREXIA NERVOSA

A number of investigators, such as Christopher Cooper, in Edinburgh, David Garner, in Toronto, and Christopher Fairburn, in Oxford, have developed techniques for dealing with patients with anorexia nervosa and bulimia. For the most part, the therapists work initially with giving the patients a kind of graded task assignment in terms of attempting to increase their food intake. Fairly rapidly, however, the therapist starts to discuss with the patient specific faulty beliefs regarding eating and its effect on body weight; the importance of appearance; and the patient's insistence on self-control. As therapy progresses, the cognitive analysis may spread out to include various beliefs not relevant immediately to the weight disorder.

### HYPOCHONDRIASIS

The most important work on the cognitive approaches to hypochondriasis has been done by Salkovskis and Clark in Oxford and together with Warwick in London. The working formulation with this type of patient is that he or she cannot tolerate any type of fear regarding a possible medical disorder and continuously seeks reassurance from the doctors. Going to the doctors thus becomes a way of life that in no way neutralizes his or her fears but on a temporary basis does make him or her feel more comfortable. One of the unique features of the treatment is to set up the following hypothesis: "Because you have been seeing doctors for the past 5 years, you tell me that your complaints have not gotten any better and indeed have gotten worse." The therapist then tries to induce the patient to test the following hypothesis: "Going to doctors does not make me feel better." The therapist then proposes a different hypothesis that the patient is encouraged and usually agrees to test out, that is, not to go to the doctor for any of the typical physical symptoms for an extended period of time, for example, 3 months, to see what happens.

Aside from this particular type of intervention, various other techniques that have been described in terms of the decatastrophizing for panic and the evaluation of cognitions, such as in depressive disorder, may be utilized.

# CURRENT STATUS

## EMPIRICAL AND TREATMENT OUTCOME STUDIES

Cognitive therapy gained its preeminence as a treatment for unipolar depression. The cognitive model of depression is the most comprehensive model of the psychological processes of depression (Beck, 1967; Beck, Rush, Shaw & Emery, 1979). Research has provided empirical support for this model (summarized by Beck & Rush, 1978) as studies demonstrating the efficacy of cognitive therapy continue to accumulate. An unpublished study by Don Ernst reports that 86 (86%) of 99 studies support specific hypotheses of the cognitive model of depression. Thirty (88%) of 34 studies support hypotheses of bias in information processing.

Recently, a meta-analysis of cognitive therapy for depression found a greater degree of change, as measured on the Beck Inventory, for cognitive therapy patients than those on a waiting-list control, and those receiving pharmacotherapy, behavior therapy, interpersonal therapy, or other forms of psychotherapy (Dobson, in press).

Two controlled studies support the efficacy of cognitive therapy in the treatment of anxiety (Durham & Turvey, 1987; Lindsay, Gamsu, McLaughlin, Hood, & Espie, 1987). Other outcome studies reflect the application of cognitive techniques to other clinical problems, including dysthymic disorder, drug abuse, alcoholism, panic disorder, anorexia, and bulimia.

## SUICIDE RESEARCH

Cognitive therapy has also focused research efforts on the study of suicide, developing assessment scales for suicide risk, key theoretical concepts, and treatment interventions. The Scale for Suicide Ideation (Beck, Kovacs, & Weissman, 1979), the Suicide Intent Scale (Beck, Schuyler, & Herman, 1974) and the Hopelessness Scale (Beck, Weissman, Lester, & Trexler, 1974) are all used clinically in assessing the dimensions of suicidality. Recently, the Hopelessness Scale has been indicated as having some predictive validity for suicide completion. A 10-year longitudinal study of 207 depressed, suicidal patients found that 90% of patients with a score of 9 or more on the Hopelessness Scale eventually killed themselves. Only one patient with a score less than 9 completed suicide (Beck, Steer, Kovacs, & Garrison, 1985). Hopelessness as a predictor of ultimate suicide has been supported in two subsequent studies (Drake & Cotton, 1986; Fawcett, Scheftner, Clark, Hedeker, Gibbons, & Coryell, 1987).

Research into cognitive processing in anxiety disorders identifies four major types of distortions: (1) overestimating the probability of the feared event; (2) overestimating the severity of the feared event; (3) underestimating one's coping resources; and (4) underestimating rescue factors (Beck, 1976). Clark and Beck (1988) found that the main cognitions in anxiety concern unrealistic perceptions of danger or threat and/or catastrophic thinking about the loss of control, illness, or changes in relationships. The cognitive model of anxiety and specific treatment interventions appear in *Anxiety Disorders and Phobias: A Cognitive Perspective* (Beck & Emery, 1985).

## CONCLUSIONS

Cognitive therapy is a system of psychotherapy based on a theory of personality and psychopathology that gives primacy to cognitive processing in the development of psychological distress. How a person structures his or her experience strongly influences how that person feels and behaves. Cognitive therapy has been influenced by a number of forms of psychotherapy, most notably psychodynamic therapy and behavior therapy. In terms of behavior therapy, the paradigm shift from behavior modification to cognitive-behavior therapies coincided with the development of cognitive therapy. The interaction between them yielded empirically validated treatment interventions and a more comprehensive understanding of the interconnections among cognition, affect, and behavior.

Cognitive therapy offers a comprehensive theory of psychopathology, well-defined therapeutic strategies, and a wide variety of efficacious and integrated techniques. Cognitive therapy is not only testable but readily teachable. To achieve proficiency in cognitive therapy requires a combination of the basic qualities of the "good" psychotherapist (warmth, acceptance, and regard), a good conceptualization of the patient's problems, and the appropriate application of cognitive strategies and techniques.

## REFERENCES

Adler, A. (1936). The neurotic's picture of the world. *International Journal of Individual Psychology, 2,* 3–10.

Alexander, F. (1950). *Psychosomatic medicine: Its principles and applications.* New York: Norton.

Bandura, A. (1977a). *Social learning theory.* Englewood Cliffs, NJ: Prentice-Hall.

Bandura, A. (1977b). Self-efficacy: Toward a unifying theory of behavior change. *Psychological Review, 84,* 191–215.

Beck, A. T. (1963). Thinking and depression: 1. Idiosyncratic content and cognitive distortions. *Archives of General Psychiatry, 9,* 324–333.

Beck, A. T. (1964). Thinking and depression: 2. Theory and therapy. *Archives of General Psychiatry, 10,* 561–571.

Beck, A. T. (1967). *Depression: Clinical, experimental, and theoretical aspects.* New York: Hoeber. (Republished as *Depression: Causes and treatment.* Philadelphia: University of Pennsylvania Press, 1972).

Beck, A. T. (1976). *Cognitive therapy and the emotional disorders.* New York: International Universities Press.

Beck, A. T., & Rush, A. J. (1978). Cognitive approaches to depression and suicide. In G. Serban (Ed.), *Cognitive defects in the development of mental illness* (published under the auspices of the Kittay Scientific Foundation). New York: Bruner/Mazel.

Beck, A. T., Schuyler, D., & Herman, I. (1974). Development of the suicidal intent scales. In A. T. Beck, H. L. P. Resnik, & D. J. Lettieri (Eds.), *The prediction of suicide* (pp. 45–56). Bowie, MD: Charles Press.

Beck, A. T., Weissman, A., Lester, D., & Trexler, L. (1974). The measurement of pessimism: The Hopelessness Scale. *Journal of Consulting and Clinical Psychology, 42,* 861–865.

Beck, A. T., Kovacs, M., & Weissman, A. (1979). Assessment of suicidal intention: The Scale for Suicidal Ideation. *Journal of Consulting and Clinical Psychology, 47,* 343–352.

Beck, A. T., Rush, A. J., Shaw, B. F., & Emery, G. (1979). *Cognitive therapy of depression*. New York: Guilford Press.

Beck, A. T., & Emery, G. (1985). *Anxiety and phobias: A cognitive approach*. New York: Basic Books.

Beck, A. T., Steer, R. A., Kovacs, M., & Garrison, B. (1985). Hopelessness and eventual suicide: A 10 year study of patients hospitalized with suicidal ideation. *American Journal of Psychiatry, 142*, 559–563.

Clark, D. M., & Beck, A. T. (1988). Cognitive approaches. In C. G. Last, & M. Hersen (Eds.), *Handbook of anxiety disorders* (pp. 362–385). New York: Pergamon.

Dobson, K. S. (in press). A meta-analysis of the efficacy of cognitive therapy for depression. *Journal of Consulting and Clinical Psychology*.

Drake, R. E., & Cotton, P. G. (1986). Depression, hopelessness, and suicide in chronic schizophrenics. *British Journal of Psychiatry, 148*, 554–559.

Durham, R. C., & Turvey, A. A. (1988). Cognitive therapy versus behavioral therapy in the treatment of chronic and general anxiety: Outcome at discharge and at six-month follow-up. *Behavior Therapy and Research*, pp. 229–234.

Ellis, A. (1962). *Reason and emotion in psychotherapy*. New York: Lyle Stuart.

Ernst, D. (1987). *A review of systematic studies of the cognitive model of depression*. Unpublished manuscript, Center for Cognitive Therapy, Philadelphia.

Fawcett, J., Scheftner, W., Clark, D., Hedeker, D., Gibbons, R., & Coryell, W. (1987). Clinical predictors of suicide in patients with major affective disorder: A controlled prospective study. *American Journal of Psychiatry, 144*, 35–40.

Horney, K. (1950). *Neurosis and human growth: The struggle toward self-realization*. New York: Norton.

Kant, I. (1798). *The classification of mental disorders*. Konigsberg, Germany: Nicholovius.

Kelly, G. (1955). *The psychology of personal constructs*. New York: Norton.

Lazarus, R. (1984). On the primacy of cognition. *American Psychologist, 39*(2), 124–129.

Lindsay, W. R., Gamsu, C. V., McLaughlin, E., Hood, E. M., & Espie, C. A. (1987). A controlled trial of treatment for generalized anxiety. *British Journal of Clinical Psychology, 26*, 3–15.

Mahoney, M. J. (1974). *Cognition and behavior modification*. Cambridge, MA: Ballinger.

Mahoney, M. J. (1977). Reflections on the cognitive-learning trend in psychotherapy. *American Psychologist, 32*, 5–13.

Rush, A. J., Beck, A. T., Kovacs, M., & Hollon, S. (1977). Comparative efficacy of cognitive therapy and imipramine in the treatment of depressed outpatients. *Cognitive Therapy and Research, 1*, 17–37.

Sullivan, H. S. (1953). *The interpersonal theory of psychiatry*. New York: Norton.

Young, J. E. (1983, August). *Borderline personality: Cognitive theory and treatment*. Paper presented at the Annual Meeting of the American Psychological Association.

# 3

# The Measurement of Cognition in Psychopathology

## Clinical and Research Applications

Joel O. Goldberg and Brian F. Shaw

## INTRODUCTION

With the increasing growth and success of cognitive treatments for a variety of psychopathological conditions, there has been an accompanying need to identify the cognitions associated with dysfunction, to quantify the changes in therapy, and to evaluate beliefs that predict treatment responsiveness. The cognitive measurement field has harvested a diverse range of assessment techniques and instruments. However, the research and development of cognitive assessment methods tends to neglect important principles in test and measurement construction that has made it more difficult for interesting techniques to find their way from the laboratory into clinical practice.

In the chapter that follows, we will describe significant technological and methodological issues facing cognitive assessment developers and then suggest what appear to be promising research prospects in the area of measurement. An emphasis will be placed on research techniques that have special relevance to the practitioner, rather than attempting a comprehensive review of the field. Practical and theoretical issues in assessment methodology are outlined to provide background for the administration and interpretation of popular, currently available techniques. Both the clinician and investigator want measures (1) that will predict certain outcomes such as treatment responses or relapse potential, (2) that will measure the changes in areas hypothesized to be important contributors to suffering and, (3) that will facilitate understanding of the psychopathological condition (either as part of a functional assessment or a theoretical formulation).

To assist in the examination of a variety of measures, a description will be made of important techniques in the psychopathological domains of most interest to cognitive thera-

Joel O. Goldberg and Brian F. Shaw • Department of Psychiatry, University of Toronto, Toronto, Ontario M5T 1R8, Canada.

pists. In the most heavily studied area of affective disorders, specific recommendations are offered for the development of a battery of cognitive measures. In this way, we hope that it will allow some practical and reasoned suggestions for clinical assessment strategies.

## METHODOLOGICAL ISSUES

There are several conceptual and methodological issues that face developers and users of cognitive assessment devices, including: (1) the desire for theory to guide the construction and use of instruments (Korchin & Schuldberg, 1981), (2) concern for psychometric purity (adequate reliability and validity), and (3) the need for standardization of techniques.

One problem is the extent to which a diverse variety of internal processes can be made available for examination by the clinician or researcher. For example, Beck's (1976) theory postulates a host of cognitive variables such as self-schema, cognitive distortions, dysfunctional attitudes, and automatic thoughts. Beidel and Turner (1986) criticized cognitive theories because cognitive variables have not been organized adequately using traditional information-processing models, although there have been previous descriptions of levels of categorization (Arnkoff & Glass, 1982). One typology proposed by Hollon and Kriss (1984) suggests that cognitive "structures" like self-schema are essential organizing principles that guide behavior. Cognitive "processes" are seen as patterns of thinking, reflecting styles or modes of operation, whereas cognitive "products" represent the resultant expressed thoughts or conscious verbalizations.

An interesting parallel exists in the traditional psychological assessment literature. Sundberg and Tyler (1962) referred to three ways of conceptualizing assessment data: (1) as "signs" of an underlying, theoretical structure, (2) as "correlates" of related characteristics, and (3) as "samples" of an individual's behavior. Just as the three levels of data analysis require decreasing need for extrapolation in order to interpret the assessment findings, so the tripartite levels of cognitive variables (structures, processes, products) can be viewed as increasingly closer to observable behavior.

Traditional behavior therapists have argued strongly that assessment techniques should require few inferential assumptions and instead remain close to observables (Goldfried & Kent, 1972). Cognitive theorists and clinicians, however, have now become more interested in "going beyond the information given" (Bruner, 1973) in order to examine constructs such as self-schema by making use of imagery, fantasies, and personal meaning inquiries. From a methodological viewpoint, cognitive "products" would appear to be most easily available for the kinds of measurement that could be interpreted at the "sample" level. Techniques such as thought sampling, thought listing, and some endorsement methods such as the Automatic Thoughts Questionnaire (ATQ; Hollon & Kendall, 1980) were developed to examine easily accessible cognitions. As one considers how to evaluate variables such as cognitive "processes" and cognitive "structures," the object of measurement is farther removed from direct observation. Some theorists (Sobel, 1981) have suggested that to understand personal concerns and idiosyncratic processing requires the use of unstructured materials such as projective methods that offer an opportunity to make interpretations at the "correlate" and "sign" levels. In fact, specialized projective methods, such as TAT-like cards, have been described by cognitive researchers (Meichenbaum, 1977; Sobel, 1981).

One fundamental concern with tools that purport to measure cognitive variables is the question of whether a particular test measures a hypothesized inner process, essentially an issue of construct validity (Cronbach & Meehl, 1955). To establish the construct validity of a measurement device does not involve simply collecting a single set of observations. Rather, the validation process depends on a gradual accumulation of evidence from diverse research studies that provide stepwise gains in confidence. Such incremental validity is a long process designed to prove the value of an instrument (Campbell & Fiske, 1959). As an example, validation research in the cognitive assessment area might include the examination of the relationship of cognitive measures to classic information-processing variables such as selective attention and different aspects of memory functioning.

Several issues are pertinent to the content validity of cognitive measures. The most clinically useful instruments and the ones that have generated the most empirical activity have been composed of item content derived from theoretical models (e.g., Beck, Bandura, Seligman, Bruch). Thus the Dysfunctional Attitude Scale (DAS; Weissman, 1980) has been employed in a wide range of diverse studies encompassing a variety of biopsychosocial contexts in large part because of the relevance of the items to testing the cognitive theory of depression (see Beck, Rush, Shaw, & Emery, 1979).

Second, the ''content'' of measurement devices can vary in the degree to which the method is most appropriate for specific versus general psychopathological groups. Some tests, such as the Smoking Self-Efficacy Scale, fall into a ''narrow band'' in the sense that the content is only relevant to the select group of tobacco-dependent individuals. Other methods, such as ''think-aloud'' procedures, are more generic. Problems in interpretation can arise when a narrow-band test is employed with populations for which the measure was not designed. For example, low scores on the Sexual Self-Efficacy Scale may be suggestive of beliefs about sexual inadequacy in erectile dysfunction patients but could reflect depressive libido disturbance in affective disordered individuals.

The psychometric tradition has emphasized the importance of publishing normative information about measures that have been developed (APA Standards, 1974). Within the cognitive assessment literature, however, there has been a virtual absence of typical conversion-scoring methods such as standard scores, T-scores, and percentile scores in order to permit comparison of a individual's performance relative to normative groups. Instead, ''cutoff'' scores are described, based on deviation from the group mean. Confusion results when investigators offer different cutoff criteria, usually due to differences in group mean findings or different stringency in definition of deviation (one standard deviation or two standard deviations). Because many of the measures described in this chapter have been employed primarily in a research context, some consideration should be made regarding how the normative data might best be used to allow clinicians to make interpretations based on an individual's responses.

It is necessary to establish the level of dysfunction found by the instrument in samples of individuals who are known to be symptomatic. A problem arises with many instruments that have relied exclusively on undergraduate samples to derive normative data because they have questionable generalizability (though this may not be as serious a problem for psychopathological disorders that are found commonly in student groups, such as test anxiety). In some cases, different norms for inpatient and outpatients may be required to obtain appropriate severity-level comparison groups. Finally, if the measure is hypothesized to evaluate cognitive dysfunction in a particular psychopathological group, then the level of performance of other psychopathologically disturbed samples should be investigated.

The developers of cognitive assessment inventories consistently neglect to report three essential test construction indices, namely ''sensitivity,'' ''specificity,'' and ''accuracy.'' Sensitivity concerns the extent to which a test correctly identifies actual instances of the attribute being measured (''true hits''). Specificity refers to whether a test can correctly identify noninstances of the attribute (''true misses''). Accuracy establishes the extent to which a test classifies both the correct cases and correct noninstances in their appropriate categories. As an example, a study that examines a proposed cutoff score for the DAS test in samples of depressives and nondepressed psychiatric controls would involve the following calculations: (1) Sensitivity would be determined by the number of depressives with DAS scores above the proposed cutoff compared to the total number of depressives; (2) specificity would be determined by the number of controls below the proposed cutoff compared to the total number of controls; and (3) accuracy would be determined by the number of depressives above the cutoff and the number of controls below the cutoff compared to the total number of cases. Using this methodology enables researchers to establish the most suitable cutoff scores to maximize psychometrically determined accuracy.

Related to the issue of content validity, a number of endorsement measure attitude scales fail to report factor analytic and internal consistency studies of the test items. Inspection of individual items may reveal that the content is not homogeneous. The problem is especially critical for attitude measures because theoretical models typically do not make predictions based on the severity or number of maladaptive beliefs but rather make postulates about the nature or content of dysfunction. As such, the establishment of theoretically relevant factor dimensions can be useful in distinguishing the kind of cognitive dysfunction (i.e., factor analytic studies of the Dysfunctional Attitude Scale, DAS; Weissman, 1980, and the Eating Disorder Inventory, EDI; Garner, Olmstead, & Polivy, 1983).

Predictive validity is the extent to which a measure can determine characteristics or behaviors that emerge at a later time. One important issue is whether it is possible to predict which individuals eventually develop symptoms. The establishment of predictive validity is essential for instruments that measure cognitive processes hypothesized to be causes of clinical disturbance. Such processes must be shown to be evident prior to symptom onset (cf. vulnerability studies using the EDI and the DAS). A second issue, of clinical concern, is whether an assessment measure is able to predict which individuals respond to therapy. For example, self-efficacy scales attempt to specify cognitions thought to be associated with successful treatment outcome.

Consideration of important individual difference variables has been neglected when applying a particular measure to a person or special population. Although the readability of some tests has been examined empirically (Berndt, 1983), instruments such as belief scales were developed originally using undergraduate samples and so, clinicians should examine whether the item content is meaningful for their clinical populations, particularly those with varied educational backgrounds. Another individual difference attribute concerns the empirical finding that persons differ in their ability to report and make use of imagery (Strosahl, Ascough, & Rojas, 1986); the cognitions of some individuals may be less amenable to measurement using methods that rely upon imaginal processes. Further, some techniques such as "think aloud" and "videotape reconstruction" are rather unusual methods that require individuals to verbalize their ongoing thinking, planning, and problem solving. Being able to think aloud or reconstruct thoughts involves varying amounts of "training" in order to allow individuals to perform such skills; the length of time is usually unspecified in studies. The effects of differing amounts of such "practice" in acquiring the skill to permit the use of such methods can be considered as reactive "instrumentation" effects. These effects are a potentially significant source of individual difference variability. In fact, the acquisition of skills such as articulating a problem-solving strategy or describing an attributional pattern may be therapeutic and have potential benefit to the individual, yet the question is raised about determining when research involving training in a technique becomes a quasi-intervention study.

The issue of individual differences is relevant in another way for endorsement methods. A problem arises in that it is possible for individuals to derive idiosyncratic meanings in responding to a test item. As an illustration, concerns exist about the Hopelessness Scale (HS; Beck, Weissman, Lester, & Trexler, 1974) because of observed inverse relationship between HS scores and social desirability found in normals (Linehan & Nielson, 1981) and also with suicidal patients (Mendonca, Holden, Mazmanian, & Dolan, 1983). It has been suggested that some suicidal individuals may choose to check off every item because of an idiosyncratic negative self-presentation response sct, rather than because they have hopeless beliefs (Linehan & Nielsen, 1983). Meaning checks or inquires are rarely conducted in conjunction with the administration of endorsement inventories (Arnkoff & Glass, 1982; Kendall, 1982). Thus one approach to the problem of idiosyncratic meanings is to ask for additional ratings that provide information beyond the presence or absence of a belief by further inquiring about the degree to which the statement is important (for example, see the ATQ).

## TECHNIQUES OF COGNITIVE ASSESSMENT

Several attempts have been made to categorize the methods available to measure cognitions and cognitive processes. Kendall and Hollon (1981), for example, assigned the techniques into four descriptive categories: recording, endorsement, production, and sampling methods. Glass and Arnkoff (1982) have suggested that assessment instruments could be viewed in terms of their degree of structure and temporal occurrence in the evaluation process. Some techniques, such as endorsement via questionnaires are structured and are administered following performance, whereas other methods, such as "think aloud," are relatively unstructured and accompany performance. The main kinds of assessment methods used by cognitive therapists and researchers consist of think-aloud procedures, recording of spontaneous speech, self-monitoring, thought listing, thought reconstruction, random sampling, and endorsement inventories containing statements regarding attributions, attitudes, and self-efficacy beliefs.

The use of *"think-aloud" procedures* has been described in detail by Genest and Turk (1981). Essentially, an individual is asked to provide a continuous monologue while performing a task. Thus, in the case of an individual with anxiety about doing mathematics, the person is given a problem to solve and is requested to "say everything which comes to your mind" (Blackwell, Galassi, Galassi, & Watson, 1985). In practice, individuals find the technique unusual and often quite difficult to maintain, and so, prompts are usually given after an extended silence ("remember to say out loud what comes to your mind"). Ericsson and Simon (1984) have noted criticisms of the method, especially the potential lack of veridicality between expressed speech and thinking processes. For example, one cannot equate silence with cessation of cognitive activity. Nevertheless, a main advantage of the method is that it formalizes the traditional assessment practice of recording an individual's spontaneous speech emitted during task performance. As an example, a delusional patient was assessed recently, and he began adding circles to copy-drawing designs, saying out loud "this looks like a first World War tank." The content of speech accompanying performance can be quite revealing of the nature of the problem-solving difficulty in this case, psychotic elaborations. The main disadvantage with think-aloud procedures is their reactivity, such that instruction to verbalize thoughts can inhibit or distract from actual task performance (Blackwell, Galassi, Galassi, & Watson, 1985). As well, a standardized instruction set or coding and scoring procedures have not been established. These are essential for the techniques to be considered an assessment method, capable of replication across research studies.

*Self-monitoring* has been described in the behavioral assessment literature (e.g. Nelson, 1977) as a technique in which smokers, alcoholics, obese individuals, and others are asked to record antecedent and consequent events surrounding their maladaptive behaviors. Beck, Rush, Shaw, and Emery (1979) extended this behavioral technique to self-monitoring of dysfunctional thoughts that accompany depressive mood. Similarly, a study by Sewitch and Kirsch (1984) asked individuals to use small booklets to record anxiety-related thoughts. Ciminero, Nelson, and Lipinski (1977) suggest that the main weakness of the method is inaccurate, biased, and falsified records.

*Random sampling of thoughts* (Hurlburt, 1979) is an interesting variation of self-monitoring. Typically, individuals are given a paper that gives off a "beep" signal, according to designated variable interval schedules and then asked to write down self-reports, a technique that has been used in experimental studies of introspection (Klinger, 1977). A main advantage of the method is the opportunity to examine information acquired in the natural environment without specifying any necessary conditions for writing down reports. Csikszentmihalyi and Larson (1984) used the technique, which they labeled the *Experience Sampling Method* (ESM), to permit the examination of cognitions of adolescents during their daily activities.

The ESM instructions were, "As you were beeped, what were you thinking about?" The technique makes minimal retrospective memory demands (cf. Ericsson & Simon, 1984) because the request is for immediate recall. The adolescents were quite productive in responding to the ESM, which elicited thoughts during periods of conflict ("thinking about the bullshit exiting my sister's mouth"), periods while alone ("what it would be like to be a model in Paris"), and periods during classroom activity ("the guy next to me is drawing the neatest airplane"). Clearly, the technique was intrusive ("how much I hate explaining this survey over and over and over") and may not be acceptable to individuals in clinical practice who wish to maintain discretion. However, thought sampling has been used successfully in populations where the goal is to increase skills in the natural environment, such as Williams and Rappoport's (1983) study of cognitive reports of agoraphobics.

*Thought reconstruction* is a technique that typically requires individuals to think out loud while viewing a videotape of their performance or viewing their role playing of a situation. A popular use of the method is with couples experiencing marital distress (Fichten, 1984) as a way of eliciting the distorted attributions and self-serving biases that often fuel marital conflict (Wright & Fichten, 1976). A problem noted by Genest and Turk (1981), who used the technique to examine cognition associated with laboratory-induced pain, is that the reports may reflect *post hoc* rationalizations and explanations (cf. Meichenbaum, 1977) and thus is highly susceptible to retrospective memory distortion (Ericsson & Simon, 1984).

A variant of videotape thought reconstruction is *thought listing* (Cacioppo & Petty, 1981) where individuals are asked to write down their thoughts immediately after experiencing a problem situation. Blackwell *et al.* (1985) recently compared thought listing and think-aloud procedures with math-anxious students. They found that thought listing was less intrusive and so did not inhibit performance, yet far fewer cognitions were recorded compared to think aloud. The few reports that were listed, however, seemed quite relevant to strategic plans and so tended to be revealing of the nature of the interference with solving the math problems.

*Imagery techniques* have been used as a main ingredient in some forms of behavioral therapy, such as systematic desensitization and as an adjunctive method in cognitive therapy (Meichenbaum, 1977; Singer, 1974). As a tool for assessment, individual differences in imagery ability may be a relevant dimension in predicting good therapy outcome, especially in treatments that rely considerably on use of imaginal processes. Although some problems have been noted with imagery self-report measures (McLemore, 1976), Strosahl and Ascough (1981) suggest that behavioral and physiological methods are inadequate alternatives for discriminating good from poor imagers. The currently available individual difference measures attempt to evaluate the ability to make effective use of imagery (Anderson, 1981) as well as try to quantify imaginal processes using instruments such as the Short Imaginal Processes Inventory (Huba & Tanaka, 1983).

*Endorsement scales* comprise the most common methods employed by cognitive researchers and clinicians. The tendency for investigators to construct a new instrument for each attempted outcome study has led to a proliferation of measures, which are often lacking in adequate psychometric "qualifications" to be considered a test in the traditional sense. The main advantage of endorsement scales is their potential ability to sample many domains through specifying particular item content (i.e., anxiety, depression, eating problems) relevant to a theoretical model (i.e., Beck, Bandura, Seligman, Bruch). A key problem is that an individual may choose to endorse a particular item without ever having experienced that thought, because his or her response (either true/false or agree/disagree) is directed toward item content provided by the test.

In the cognitive-behavior therapies, investigators and clinicians have been left to their own preferences and interpretive experience to custom-design an assessment battery depending on the patients' presenting problems. In fact, it is hoped that this chapter may be of value to increase awareness about important measures and assessment strategies as well as their advantages and limitations. As this endeavor is not a new one in the field, our aspiration was for breadth of survey, and to a degree, novelty of topic in reviewing significant clinical domains.

# CLINICAL DOMAINS

### AFFECTIVE DISORDERS

Spurred on by many advances in cognitive-behavioral theories and therapies, the affective disorders have received a significant amount of clinical and research attention in the past 15 years. Diagnostically, the affective disorders refer to several categories of depression (for example, major depression, dysthymia, and mania). The review that follows will be limited to measures of depression because there has been no empirical work evaluating specific cognitions associated with mania, although depression instruments have been applied to that population.

The cognitive assessment of depression has been previously described by several reviewers (for example, Shaw & Dobson, 1981; Segal & Shaw, 1987; Hammen & Krantz, 1985; Rush, 1984). In an attempt to distill the most important methods, a summary will be provided for the main measures, particularly those that in our view have special clinical relevance. The reader interested in greater detail should consult these other chapters.

In pursuit of the goals of clinical description, evaluation of change, and prediction of outcome, the clinician has available a number of instruments for the purpose of the cognitive assessment of depression. The methods include (1) descriptive measures of cognition associated with depression; (2) measures of change that are useful in documenting therapeutic gains; and (3) measures with predictive relevance to the roblem of relapse.

Many measures are available to describe the specific cognitive changes associated with depression. Most of these involve endorsement scales to detect cognitions such as negative ideation (Automatic Thoughts Questionnaire; Hollon & Kendall, 1980), hopelessness (Hopelessness Scale; Beck *et al.*, 1974), distorted thinking (Cognitive Bias Questionnaire; Krantz & Hammen 1979; Cognitive Response Test; Watkins & Rush, 1983; Cognitive Error Questionnaire; Lefebvre, 1981), biased attributional style (Attributional Style Questionnaire; ASQ; Peterson, Semmel, von Baeyer, Abramson, Metalsky, & Seligman, 1982), and dysfunctional attitudes (Dysfunctional Attitude Scale; Weissman, 1980; Irrational Beliefs Test; Jones, 1969). These instruments do a reasonable job within the constraints of endorsement report methodology in documenting cognitive change. Most of these measures reflect the patient's state at a point in time when he or she is depressed. The instruments correlate reasonably well with depression severity scales. Some like the ATQ are highly correlated (i.e., $r$'s in the range of .80) with depression severity measures (the Beck Depression Inventory, BDI: Beck *et al.*, 1979; Hamilton Rating Scale for Depression, HRSD: Hamilton, 1960), whereas others such as the DAS or the ASQ have only moderate correlations.

Typically, therapists assess their patients prior to the treatment and again at the end of treatment. During cognitive therapy, the patient will be encouraged to complete several homework assignments employing the Daily Record of Dysfunctional Thoughts, DRDT; Beck *et al.*, 1979), thereby providing another source of information. Furthermore, some thought listing or even think-aloud procedures may also be employed during treatment. The reader should also note that some cognitive items are available in the BDI, the 24-item HRSD and other depression measures (see Shaw, Vallis, & McCabe, 1985).

Assuming that a therapist wants a thorough sampling of cognitions associated with depression, what measures could the practitioner be advised to select? Keeping in mind three central functions of cognitive assessment (description, measurement of change, prediction of treatment response or relapse), a selection of instruments will be offered based upon clinical experience with the measures, significant empirical findings and admittedly, our subjective preferences. The suggested battery, would include the Hopelessness Scale, the Dysfunctional Attitude Scale, the Automatic Thoughts Questionnaire, and the Self-Control Schedule.

It is distressing that all of these measures involve self-report, but, at present, other assessments based on experimental methods (i.e., self-schema measures such as self-referent encoding: Kuiper, Olinger, MacDonald, & Shaw, 1985; Dobson & Shaw, 1987) are not sufficiently well developed to be used in the clinic.

The Hopelessness Scale (HS: Beck *et al.*, 1974) measures the person's negative expectations about future events based upon a 20-item scale. (''I never get what I want so it's foolish to want anything''). The value of the HS lies in its ability to predict suicidal behavior (Beck, Steer, Kovacs, & Garrison, 1985). Practically, it may also be relevant in identifying a negative response set that may interfere with the patient's commitment to therapy. There have been reports that the HS is confounded by a bias toward social undesirability (e.g., in suicidal patients: Mendonca *et al.*, 1983). This confound is particularly apparent in survey studies of a normal population (Linehan & Nielson, 1981). Nevertheless, the reader should recognize that some depressed/anxious patients will have high scores not because they have a suicidal orientation (Kowalchuk, 1986) but because they see themselves as personally undesirable. These latter issues can be pursued in clinical interviews with the patient.

The DAS (Weissman, 1980) is one of the most controversial scales in the field (see Shaw, 1988). Two 40-item scales (Form A and Form B) are available, and considerable psychometric work has been conducted in order to establish its reliability and validity (Weissman, 1980). The DAS appears to be more sensitive to nonendogenous depressions compared with endogenous depressions (Giles & Rush, 1982; Zimmerman & Coryell, 1986). Knowing the DAS score is useful to predict treatment outcome because patients with higher scores tend to respond *less* well to therapy (Keller, 1983; Sotsky, Glass, & Shea, 1986). High scores on the DAS have also been shown to identify some patients who will relapse, regardless of the type of treatment they received (Rush, Weissenburger, & Eaves, 1986; Simons, Murphy, Levine, & Wetzel, 1986). Individuals with many dysfunctional attitudes may experience increased life stress (Olinger, Kuiper & Shaw, 1987; Wise & Barnes, 1986), leading to depressive symptoms. Finally, the DAS has been factor-analyzed (Cane, Olinger, Gotlib, & Kuiper, 1986) with two main factors, Approval by Others and Performance Evaluation, emerging. Future research will examine the extent to which the two DAS factors correspond to Beck's (1983) proposal of two depressive personality predispositions called sociotropic and autonomous types (Segal, Goldberg, & Vella, 1987).

On balance the DAS is worthy of being in our basic battery for its usefulness in describing possible cognitive vulnerabilities associated with depression. It also has value in the prediction of posttreatment and follow-up status. It is not particularly specific to major depression (see Dobson & Shaw, 1986; Hollon, Kendall & Lumry, 1986) but has a fairly high sensitivity to the disorder.

The Automatic Thoughts Questionnaire (ATQ) is included because of its usefulness in eliciting common self-verbalizations in depression. The instrument is easily administered, has good face validity, and includes an evaluation of the degree of belief in the ideation as well as the estimated frequency of occurrence. The ATQ is highly state-dependent and thus has some value in measuring change over the course of treatment (Harrell & Ryan, 1983). The ATQ is relatively sensitive to depressed states (Blackburn & Smyth, 1985), although like many of these endorsement instruments, it is not specific to major depression. In therapy, it is sometimes useful to relate the patients' responses on the ATQ to their written homework assignments using the Daily Record of Dysfunctional Thoughts. The DRDT is used extensively in the treatment and yet is difficult to employ as an outcome measure because of lack of adequate psychometric properties (see Persons & Burns, 1985). Future research on the relationship between these sources of information about the patient's thinking would be instructive. For now we include the ATQ in our battery because of its sensitivity to change.

The Self-Control Schedule (SCS: Rosenbaum, 1980) is included because it informs the clinician about the patient's use of certain problem-solving strategies to control their emotional responses. One aspect tapped by the SCS may be the patient's self-efficacy (Bandura, 1977). We included it because Simons, Lustman, Wetzel, & Murphy (1985) found it to be a predictor of response to cognitive therapy with the group of high scorers (presumably reflecting those individuals with the strongest beliefs about their own role in effecting personal change) showing the best outcome.

The cognitive assessment of depression continues to be a problematic area. A number of difficulties exist with the reliability and validity of many instruments. Many are new scales in the early stages of development and have not been given the proper scientific study after their first introduction. For example, Beckham, Leber, Watkins, Boyer, and Cook (1986) introduced the Cognitive Triad Inventory, a measure designed to assess the three aspects of Beck's (1976) theory, negative view of the self, world, and future. This instrument consists of 30 items, 10 in each subscale. Some of the items overlap with items from the BDI. Only further research will determine the value of this scale, including the stability of the subscales.

Of course, for specific assessment, the clinician will want to select an assessment method that best fits the situation. In this regard the dictionary of behavioral assessment (Hersen & Bellack, 1988) may be of considerable value. New methods are being developed on a regular basis. Some like the unprompted causal attribution method (Peterson, Bettes, & Seligman, 1985) or the Cognitive Distortion Questionnaire (Burns, Shaw, & Croker, 1987) involve a more open-ended format than the endorsement scales. These methods require trained judges but are of value in investigating the patient's unforced responses.

## ANXIETY DISORDERS

Clearly, anxiety has a significant cognitive component. Some theorists have maintained that cognitive factors such as appraisals of threat (Lazarus & Folkman, 1984) and maladaptive beliefs (Beck & Emery, 1985; Ellis, 1962) play an important etiological role. As the anxiety construct is an extremely diverse one, some scales have been developed for specific situations or conditions (Endler & Hunt, 1966). It is generally accepted that cognitive variables reflecting anxiety must be understood in the context of other response modes, specifically psychophysiological and behavioral modes (see Nietzel & Bernstein, 1981). In this section, a number of measures pertinent to social anxiety and lack of assertiveness, test anxiety, agoraphobia, dental anxiety, and obsessional worry will be introduced.

As indicated in Segal and Shaw (1987), the cognitive assessment of anxiety, in contrast to depression, has seen the use of a wider range of methodologies. Thus investigators have constructed measures that tap specific concerns (e.g., self-efficacy ratings about approach behavior to a feared object) and have developed techniques that tap a broad base (e.g., articulated thoughts during a stimulated interaction). With anxiety, then, there is a better opportunity to assess specific situation–person interaction.

Social anxiety or social phobia in the DSM-III framework includes phobic disorders (e.g., agoraphobia, social phobia, simple phobia) and anxiety states (e.g., panic disorder, generalized anxiety disorder, and obsessive-compulsive disorder). If clinicians want to assess their anxious patients from a cognitive perspective, they are advised to consider some of the following tests. The Social Interaction Self-Statement Test (Glass, Merluzzi, Biever, & Larsen, 1982) may be used to identify a sample of positive and negative ideation associated with heterosexual social anxiety. As assertiveness difficulties are likely related to social evaluative anxiety, the Subjective Probability of Consequences Inventory (SPCI; Fiedler & Beach, 1978) is often useful. The SPCI elicits the types of consequences individuals anticipate following refusal behavior. Of course, two commonly used tests in this field are the Fear of Negative Evaluation Scale (FNE; Watson & Friend, 1969) and the Social Avoidance and Distress Scale (SAD; Watson & Friend, 1969). These scales will help to evaluate the person's degree of apprehension about disapproval and the individual's experience of discomfort in social situations.

Clinicians who deal with social anxiety often prefer to use real or simulated social interactions as one context for observation. Thus, procedures such as thought listing are particularly relevant (for example, see Davison, Robins, & Johnston, 1983; Halford & Foddy, 1982; Segal & Marshall, 1985). Performance anxiety or test anxiety has received considerable empirical attention (see Arnkoff, 1986). Typically, the main cognitive assessment of performance anxiety is a thought-listing procedure such as the measure proposed by Cacioppo, Glass, and Merluzzi (1979). This procedure basically identifies the valence (positive, negative, or neutral) of the thoughts within an idiographic format.

The cognitive assessment of specific phobias tends to be dealt with on an *ad hoc* basis. Dental phobia is a notable exception, mostly because of the work by Kent (1985a) and Wardle (1984). Building on the research of Butler and Mathews (1983) who asked generalized anxiety patients to estimate the probability that certain events would occur and to rate how bad or costly it would be if the negative events did occur, Kent (1985a) found that highly anxious dental patients perceived a higher likelihood of negative events (e.g., "the next time you have a filling you will find the drilling extremely painful"). Women were found to perceive the cost of negative events as being greater. In general, anxious patients recall more pain than they actually experienced during previous appointments (Kent, 1985b).

Agoraphobia or alternatively, panic disorder with phobic avoidance, is one of the most actively researched anxiety disorder. From a cognitive perspective, the Agoraphobic Cognitions Questionnaire (ACQ; Chambless, Caputo, Bright, & Gallagher, 1984) assesses the frequency of self-statements. By combining the ACQ with its companion scale, the Body Sensation Questionnaire (BSQ; Chambless *et al.*, 1984), the clinician will obtain a reasonably base of information of the cognitions in agoraphobia. Of course, it bears remembering that agoraphobia is a condition involving many feared situations (Williams, 1985), and the clinician would do well to detect commonalities among the various threats. Furthermore, Clark (1986) emphasized that the catastrophic interpretation of normal bodily sensations is an important aspect of the assessment of panic disorder. The reader is advised to combine the cognitive assessment measures with other instruments to evaluate phobic avoidance and the expected consequences of a panic or anxiety attack.

Clark and Hemsley (1985) introduced the Distressing Thoughts Questionnaire (DTQ), a self-report inventory that measures six anxious and six depressive thoughts/images across five parameters (frequency, sadness, worry, dismissal, and disapproval). Like the ATQ, this instrument taps several parameters. It does not, however, provide the clinician with the specific cognitive content but instead addresses thematic issues (e.g., thoughts or images of personally unacceptable sexual acts). Like most scales in this area, more work on the validity of the DTQ is needed.

Salkovskis (1985) presented an interesting paper on obsessive-compulsive problems from a cognitive-behavioral perspective. Although he did not identify specific cognitive assessment procedures, he differentiated the intrusive thoughts associated with an obsessional disorder and the negative automatic thoughts (Beck *et al.*, 1979) associated with anxiety and/or depression. Clinically, the importance of this distinction emerges when the therapist considers an intervention. With intrusive thoughts, the demand (from the patient) is to neutralize the ideation with reassurance or positive statements. Automatic thoughts, on the other hand, are dealt with with specific interventions (e.g., examining evidence, pursuing consequences, exploring meaning), including behavioral challenges of this ideation. It will be instructive when assessments of this condition are designed to differentiate the range of negative automatic thoughts that have been described clinically.

In summary, the cognitive assessment of anxiety has been reasonably well developed. Most of the currently used instruments utilize the self-endorsement format, but there are several thought-listing paradigms available. In parallel with the development of the depression literature, more recent efforts have focused on the experimental study of anxiety using schema-related evaluations or other laboratory methodologies (e.g., Foa & McNally, 1986; Mathews & MacLeod, 1985).

## MEDICAL AND PSYCHOSOMATIC DISORDERS

There has been a burgeoning growth of cognitive treatments for a variety of medical problems and conditions (DSM-III, AXIS III Disorders), including acute and chronic pain (Turk, Meichenbaum, & Genest, 1983), headaches (Bakal, Demjen, & Kaganov, 1981), coping with arthritis (Bradley, 1983), coping with cancer and cancer treatment side effects (Morrow, 1986; Taylor, Lichtman, & Wood, 1984), preparation for surgery (Kendall *et al.,* 1979; MacDonald & Kuiper, 1983) and cardiac-proneness behavior (Levenkron, Cohen, Mueller, & Fisher, 1983). However, very few studies have attempted to develop measures specifically designed to evaluate the cognitive changes associated with improvements. In fact, the serious neglect of cognitive assessments was a main failure cited in a recent review of behavioral medicine (Bradley & Kay, 1985). Several investigations have provided evidence for cognitive mediators in laboratory analysis (e.g., Neufeld & Thomas, 1977), yet there has been a paucity of studies demonstrating effects in clinical situations.

One exception is the self-report Cognitive Error Questionnaire that was designed to assess the distorted cognitive styles of catastrophizing, overgeneralization, personalization, and selective abstraction found in 48 situations associated with chronic low-back pain (Lefebvre, 1981). A study by Smith, Pollick, Ahern, and Adams (1986) found that overgeneralization was particularly related to disability symptoms in a sample of 138 outpatients. A number of investigations have attempted to measure cognitive variables associated with cardiac proneness, essential hypertension, and Type A behavior. Baer, Collins, Bourianoff, and Ketchell (1979) developed a 16-item self-report Brief Hypertension Instrument containing anxiety-producing and anger-related attitudes (e.g., "I sometimes try and get even rather than forgive and forget") that was cross-validated in samples of 332 hypertensive and 335 controls. Because several theorists have implicated hostility as a major factor in Type A behavior (Shekelle, Gale, Ostfeld, & Oglesby, 1983; Williams *et al.,* 1980) future work might consider applying measures related to anger beliefs (Novaco, 1977). In addition, there is some evidence that perceived self-efficacy is related to lower heart rate, blood pressure, and other physiological measures (Bandura, Reese, & Adams, 1982; Bandura, *et al.,* 1985) that has led to suggestions to evaluate self-efficacy beliefs in cardiac patients (Ewart, Taylor, Reese, & Debusk, 1984).

Several studies have examined the impact of cognitive therapeutic techniques designed to alleviate distress related to surgery (MacDonald & Kuiper, 1983); however, there has been a neglect of actual measurement of associated cognitive changes. Neufeld and Kuiper (1983) proposed that high Dysfunctional Attitude Scale scorers may be most vulnerable to postoperative depressions. The importance of developing adequate cognitive measurement is underscored by evidence supporting Cohen and Lazarus's (1973) theory that information-based preparation improves recovery for "copers" but actually hinders recovery for "avoiders" (MacDonald & Kuiper, 1983). In addition, there is evidence that suggests that negative thoughts are inversely related to clinician's ratings of postcardiac catheterization surgical adjustment as measured by Kendall *et al.*'s (1979) 20-item self-report Self-Statement Inventory.

Investigations with cancer patients have highlighted the role of cognitive factors such as beliefs about problems with coping (Meyerowitz, Heinrich, & Schag, 1983). Preliminary studies have evaluated coping attitudes (Silverman 1986; Weisman & Sobel, 1979) and attributions of blame (Taylor *et al.*, 1984; Burish *et al.*, 1984). Hopeful beliefs that control over cancer symptoms is possible were associated with better adjustment. However, future work might consider the hypothesis of Cohen and Lazarus (1973) and attempt to develop individual difference measures to distinguish "copers" from "avoiders" before applying information-based cancer education programs.

## SMOKING

Tobacco dependence is considered psychopathological by the DSM-III classification scheme. Smoking-cessation programs have made use of a variety of psychotherapeutic methods from hypnotherapy to behavioral techniques in order to help individuals stop smoking.

Research has attempted to measure the contribution of self-efficacy cognitions as a predictor of success in smoking-cessation programs (Condiotte & Lichtenstein, 1981; DiClemente, 1981; Godding & Glaslow, 1985). Typically, investigators have developed their own self-efficacy questionnaires (Colletti, Supnick, & Payne, 1985; Condiotte & Lichtenstein, 1981) to measure smoking-related beliefs. In addition, because the psychological and physiological effects of cessation are quite idiosyncratic with unknown causes (Murray & Lawrence, 1984), some attention has been given to measuring the relationship between self-efficacy cognitions and withdrawal symptoms (Killen, Maccoby, & Taylor, 1984). From a different perspective, earlier attempts to measure cognitive factors in smoking treatments were conducted by Keutzer (1968). She constructed an 18-item Effective Cognitive Dissonance (ECD) scale to measure smoker's beliefs posited to maintain dependence ("the pleasure I get, which is certain, outweighs the health hazard, which is uncertain"; "I personally know of at least one very old person who has smoked most of his life yet who continued to be in fine health"). Several investigations found a significant relationship between ECD scores and smoking treatment outcome (Best & Steffy, 1971; Best, 1975; Keutzer, 1968) however, the psychometric properties of the cognitive dissonance index have not been adequately examined.

## ALCOHOLISM AND SUBSTANCE ABUSE

The role of cognitive factors in maintaining problem drinking has led to self-control therapies (Carey & Maisto, 1985) and cognitive behavioral treatment (Sanchez-Craig, Annis, Bornet, & MacDonald, 1984). As well, experimental studies have examined cognitive factors in maintaining alcohol abuse, including alcohol-related expectancies (Annis & Davis, 1986; Brown, Goldman, & Christiansen, 1985).

One issue, noted by several authors, is that the cognitive distortions, biases, and misperceptions of alcoholic caseworkers (Bailey, 1970), nurses (Harlow & Goby, 1980), family practice residents (Fisher, Fisher, & Mason, 1976), and therapists (Emery & Fox, 1981) mitigate against effective treatment. Kilty (1975) developed a 40-item Attitudes Towards Alcoholism (ATA) scale using a demographically stratified community sample of 205 people, a group of 119 graduate social work students, as well as cross-validation samples of 17 professionals who attended alcoholism workshops, and 32 alcohol caseworkers. The ATA items pertain mainly to beliefs about alcoholism ("When alcohol is used in moderation, it can produce creative and original thinking"). However, an inspection of the item content suggests that the scale is actually multivariate with at least four distinct factors, only two of which pertain directly to alcohol beliefs. Other items are more related to general self-esteem issues ("I certainly feel useless at times"). If further work in developing the scale were being considered, then one might attempt to integrate the observations of Emery and Fox (1981) who noted some therapist's misconceptions, such as "all alcoholics are weak, dependent individuals." The development of a therapist's attitude scale is relevant because of the suggestion that attitudinal shifts in counselors improves the treatment of alcoholics (Fisher *et al.,* 1976).

Other investigators have attempted to develop belief measures for alcoholics themselves. One measure of alcohol-related beliefs has been described by Brown *et al.* (1985). The Alcohol Expectancy Questionnaire consists of 90 items pertaining to expectations about the beneficial effects of alcohol ("after a few drinks, I'm in a better mood," or "alcohol enables me to fall asleep more easily"). The scale was validated using 171 alcoholics, 344 college students, and 64 medical patient controls. In addition, Annis and Davis (1986) describe a Situational Confidence Questionnaire, a 100-item self-report instrument (42-item short form) designed to measure self-efficacy beliefs for alcohol-related situations ("If I wanted to heighten my sexual enjoyment, I would be able to resist the urge to drink").

In the area of substance abuse, Gossop (1978) has examined cognitive and other mediators of dependency, including heroin, amphetamine, and barbiturate addiction. Using a validation sample of 40 primarily abusers, Eiser and Gossop (1979) constructed a 15-item Perceptions about Addiction Scale with items such as "getting stoned is one of the things that gives me the most pleasure in life." Some of the items pertain to attitudes toward treatment ("I've never made a serious effort to give up drugs on my own") and beliefs about others ("I don't think I could ever turn down drugs if someone offered them to me"). Considerable psychometric work in obtaining reliability and validity data as well as conducting factor-analytic studies is required in order to refine the scale. One suspects that the attitudinal dimensions combine cognitive distortions, self-efficacy beliefs, and attitudes toward others in this atheoretically constructed instrument.

## SCHIZOPHRENIA AND PSYCHOTIC DISORDERS

Cognitive impairment is a hallmark symptom of schizophrenia (Winters & Neale, 1983) with clinical and experimental evidence pointing to information-processing deficits in schizophrenics (Saccuzzo & Braff, 1986) and children at high risk (Asarnow, Steffy, MacCrimmon, & Cleghorn, 1978). Direct management of psychotic thought disorder typically involves pharmacological interventions (Andreason, 1984), though some attempts have been made to modify the content and extent of delusional thinking using self-instruction and behavioral techniques (Meichenbaum, 1969; Nydegger, 1972). Bellack (1986) has argued that diminished research and clinical interest in schizophrenia by behaviorally oriented investigators has encouraged the exclusive medication management of psychotic behavior despite the utility of psychotherapeutic techniques such as social skills training and aftercare programs.

One exception to the virtual absence of belief and attributional measures for this population consists of work conducted by Soskis and Bowers (1969) that seems to parallel current self-efficacy belief investigations. The Soskis Attitudes Towards Illness Questionnaire (SA-TIQ) is a 55-item self-report scale that measures 11 dimensions about beliefs about responsibility for the psychosis ("I can find the real cause of my illness in myself") and attitudes about dealing with the problems ("I think that I am up to solving problems"). Some attempts have been made to examine the relationship between SATIQ scores and posthospital adjustment (Soskis & Bowers, 1969) and more recently between SATIQ scores and schizophrenia psychotherapy outcome (Gunderson *et al.,* 1984). The psychometric properties of the scale however, remain unexplored, including lack of factor-analytic verification for the validity of the multivariate subscales. There does appear to be some promise in attempting to develop attitudinal and attributional measures that relate to posthospital adjustment and rehospitalization rates, even in these more chronically disturbed populations.

A major source of difficulty facing schizophrenics upon discharge is the biased attitudes of the public as well as hospital and institutional workers (Mayo & Havelock, 1970), who hold misconceptions that may also have been adopted by investigators where interest has shifted away from the disorder (Bellack, 1986). Future studies could explore shifts toward more positive attitudes by caregivers in improving treatment outcome, similar to studies of alcohol caseworkers.

Finally, Haynes (1986) has proposed a cognitive-behavioral model for nonschizophrenic paranoid disorders. His view attempts to understand the rigid hypervigilant beliefs of paranoid individuals (Heilbrun, 1975); however, there have been no reported attempts to develop cognitive-behavioral measures of paranoid cognitions.

## MARITAL PROBLEMS AND SEXUAL DYSFUNCTIONS

Marital therapy has been influenced by experimental evidence that has linked marital dysfunction to a number of cognitive factors such as distorted perceptions of spouse behavior (Fichten, 1984; Wright & Fichten, 1976), blaming attributions (Fincham, 1985; Fincham & O'Leary, 1983), rigid cognitive style (Tyndall & Lichtenberg, 1985), poor decision making (Olson & Ryder, 1970; Weiss, 1984), problems in perceived controllability of the relationship (Miller, Lefcourt, & Ware, 1983), and unrealistic beliefs about the marriage (Epstein & Eidelson, 1981). In fact, beginning attempts have been made to integrate cognitive techniques into marital therapy (Berley & Jacobsen, 1984; Epstein, 1982; Johnson & Greenberg, 1985).

Fichten (1984) has used videotape reconstruction of marital disagreements to elicit self-serving biases and distorted attributions, whereas Weiss (1984) has employed videotapes to obtain problem-solving orientation ratings.

Miller *et al.* (1983) developed a 44-item self-report Marital Locus of Control Scale that examines perceptions of controllability in a marriage ("It seems to me that maintaining a smooth functioning marriage is simply a skill; things like luck don't come unto it"). Internal consistency analyses and validation using marital satisfaction ratings are reported for a sample of 230 married students, but the applicability to maritally distressed couples seeking counselling remains to be demonstrated. Cognitive therapy has been applied to treatment of sexual dysfunction (Fox & Emery, 1981), and cognitive techniques such as distraction and attentional focus have been used in traditional sex therapy (Beck & Barlow, 1984). A number of attitude measures have been developed to assess sex-related beliefs including an Attitudes Towards Homosexuality Scale (MacDonald, Huggins, Young, & Swanson, 1973), Attitudes of Heterosexuals to Homosexuality (Cerny & Polyson, 1984; Larsen, Reed, & Hoffman, 1980), Sex Role Inventory (Bem, 1974, 1975), Negative Attitudes Toward Masturbation (Abramson & Mosher, 1975; Mosher & Abramson, 1977), and the Sexual Attitudes and Experiences Questionnaire (Zuckerman, Tushup, & Finner, 1976). As well, a study developed a measure of sexual self-efficacy using a sample of 56 individuals with erectile dysfunction (Libman, Rothenberg, Fichten, & Amsel, 1985).

## EATING DISORDERS

Accompanying the development of cognitive therapy for anorexic and bulimic patients (Cooper & Fairburn, 1984; Rossiter & Wilson, 1985) have been attempts to construct measures of dysfunctional attitudes towards food, weight, and body image. Early work in evaluating the cognitions of anorexics was flawed because of inadequate methodology that used informal interviews (Crisp, 1965) or unvalidated questionnaires (Bhanji and Thompson, 1974; Browning & Miller, 1968). More recently theorists have suggested that the evaluation of dysfunctional attitudes is especially important because anorexics may be troubled by distorted cognitions that persist even after clinical improvements in weight normalization have been achieved.

Garner *et al.* (1983) developed a 64-item self-report measure, The Eating Disorder Inventory (EDI). The EDI consists of statements such as "If I gain a pound, I worry that I will keep gaining". Eight subscales pertaining to various aspects of anorexia and bulimia were validated using factor-analytic methods to establish internal consistency in a sample of 113 anorexics. A study by Cooper, Cooper, & Fairburn (1985) found that mean subscale scores for those anorexics were significantly higher compared to a psychiatric outpatient sample on all but one dimension. Because the scale is multivariate, including attitudinal, interpersonal, behavioral, and affective aspects, one might argue that the EDI is not a pure cognitive instrument. Nevertheless, the EDI is clearly a theory-based assessment device with dimensions such as the Perfectionism subscale and Drive for Thinness subscale that were developed to reflect constructs proposed by Bruch's (1973) etiological model of high-achievement expectations.

In contrast, an earlier instrument developed by Garner and Garfinkel (1979) called the Eating Attitudes Test (EAT) is mainly a symptom scale ("I feel bloated after meals") rather than a belief measure. The EAT measure has been validated in large samples of anorexic women (Garner, Olmstead, Bohr, & Garfinkel, 1982) and female normals attending a family planning clinic (Cooper, Waterman, & Fairburn, 1984). The EDI and EAT measure show some correlation between relevant subscales (EDI Drive for Thinness with EAT Dieting, $r$ = .80; EDI Bulimia with EAT Bulimia, $r$ = .85), according to Garner *et al.* (1983), yet factor-analytic work shows that a substantial amount of the variance is not shared.

A study by Clinton and McKinlay (1986) compared EAT scores of anorexics, recovered anorexics, psychiatric controls, and normals. Their investigation found that recovered eating-disordered patients were similar to symptomatic anorexics because they continue to show elevated EAT scores that were significantly higher than both control groups despite evidence of improved clinical functioning. The remission finding supports the theory that distorted cognitions about food, eating, weight, and body image persist despite symptom alleviation. However, the EAT data were not replicated in an investigation by Toner, Garfinkel, and Garner (1987), who found that symptomatic anorexics had significantly higher scores compared to the three comparison groups. On the other hand, both symptomatic and remitted anorexics showed elevations on several EDI factors compared to controls in the Toner *et al.* (1987) investigation. The EAT scale has been used as an outcome measure in cognitive therapy in anorexics (Cooper & Fairburn, 1984) and bulimics (Ordman & Kirschenbaum, 1985), and both the EAT and EDI have been employed in long-term follow-ups (Toner, Garfinkel, & Garner, 1986). According to the typology of Hollon and Kriss (1984), one suspects that the EAT is a measure that can be best described as a "cognitive product," whereas the EDI taps dimensions more closely linked to the cognitive "schemata" and "processes" of eating-disordered individuals.

Several other investigations have attempted to evaluate cognitive variables related to eating disorders. O'Leary (1985) cites self-efficacy studies that have evaluated the hypothesis that beliefs about the ability to regulate one's weight while obtaining nourishment contribute to eventual recovery in a sample of bulimics (Schneider & Agras, 1985). Another line of research constructed a measure of anorexic's beliefs about themselves and their treatment (Goldberg, Halmi, Eckert, Casper, Davis, & Roper, 1980) using a 63-item self-report scale that has been found to be related to recovery from inpatient therapy (Steinhausen, 1986). Because the first factor is significantly loaded with items pertinent to powerlessness in effecting changes

("Frankly, the treatment I am getting here seems confused and inconsistent"; "The medical staff often blame me for their own goofups"), the scale may, in fact, be strongly associated with self-efficacy.

Other work that has applied Bandura's (1977) self-efficacy theory to eating problems has focused on obese individuals. Glynn and Ruderman (1986) developed an Eating Self-Efficacy Scale (ESES) using a normative sample of 618 undergraduates and 32 weight-loss-clinic attenders. They found a low but significant relationship between ESES scores and weight loss in the clinic sample.

Finally, Ruderman (1985) has examined a variety of cognitive variables related to eating and dieting in a college student sample. She found that students who were especially concerned about dieting according to Herman, Polivy, Pliner, Threlkeld, and Munic's (1978) Revised Restraint Scale showed rigid, distorted beliefs as measured by the Rational Beliefs Inventory (Shorkey & Whiteman, 1977) but not depressive cognitions as assessed by the Cognitive Bias Questionnaire (Krantz & Hammen, 1979).

# CONCLUSION

It is becoming increasingly difficult to write a chapter on the cognitive assessment of psychopathology and health-related problems. The number of assessment instruments is staggering, and yet there is a significant difficulty in finding a consensus on the value of these measures especially because many tests have been used primarily in research contexts. Clinical practice being what it is places demands that assessments be useful for individual interpretations rather than for group means analysis and that methods be cost-effective for the patients and the clinician. As a result, paper-and-pencil endorsement measures rather than more cumbersome procedures tend to be used. On the other hand, it is important for the practitioner to recognize that this complicated assessment field has been quick to construct new measures but slow to expand its clinical applicability with an empirical base.

# REFERENCES

American Psychological Association. (1974). *Standards for educational and psychological tests and manuals.* Washington, DC: Author.

Anderson, M. P. (1981). Assessment of imaginal processes: Approaches and Issues. In T. V. Merluzzi, C. R. Glass, & M. Genest (Eds.), *Cognitive assessment* (pp. 149–187). New York: Guilford.

Andreason, N. C. (1984). *The broken brain: The biological revolution in psychiatry.* New York: Harper & Row.

Annis, H. M., & Davis, C. S. (1986). Assessment of expectancies in alcohol dependent clients. In A. Marlatt & D. Donovan (Eds.), *Assessment of addictive behaviors.* New York: Guilford.

Arnkoff, D. B. (1986). A comparison of the coping and restructuring components of cognitive restructuring. *Cognitive Therapy and Research, 10,* 147–158.

Arnkoff, D. B., & Glass, C. R. (1982). Clinical cognitive constructs: Examination, evaluation and elaboration. *Advances in cognitive behavioral research and therapy* (Vol. 1, pp. 2–35). New York: Academic Press.

Asarnow, R. F., Steffy, R. A., MacCrimmon, D. J., & Cleghorn, J. M. (1978). An attentional assessment of foster children at risk for schizophrenia. In L. C. Wynne, R. C. Cromwell, & S. Matthysse (Eds.), *The nature of schizophrenia* (pp. 339–358). New York: Wiley.

Baer, P. E., Collins, F. H., Bourianoff, G. G., & Ketchell, M. F. (1979). Assessing personality factors in essential hypertension with a brief self-report instrument. *Psychosomatic Medicine, 41,* 321–330.

Bailey, M. B. (1970). Attitudes toward alcoholism before and after a training program for social caseworkers. *Quarterly Journal of Studies on Alcohol, 31,* 669–683.

Bakal, D. A., Demjen, S., & Kaganov, J. A. (1981). Cognitive behavioral treatment of chronic headache. *Headache, 21,* 81–86.

Bandura, A. (1977). Self-efficacy: Toward a unifying theory of behavioral change. *Psychological Review, 84,* 191–215.

Bandura, A., Reese, L. B., & Adams, N. E. (1982). Microanalysis of action and fear arousal as a function of differential levels of perceived self-efficacy. *Journal of Personality and Social Psychology, 43,* 5–21.

Bandura, A., Taylor, C. B., Williams, S. L., Mefford, I. N., & Barchas, J. D. (1985). Catecholamine secretion as a function of perceived self-efficacy. *Journal of Consulting and Clinical Psychology, 53,* 406–414.

Beck, A. T. (1976). *Cognitive therapy and the emotional disorders.* New York: International Universities Press.

Beck, A. T. (1983). Cognitive therapy of depression: New perspectives. In P. J. Clayton & J. E. Barrett (Eds.), *Treatment of depression: Old controversies and new approaches* (pp. 265–290). New York: Raven Press.

Beck, A. T., & Emery, G. (1985). *Anxiety disorders and phobias.* New York: Basic Books.

Beck, A. T., Weissman, A., Lester, D., & Trexler, L. (1974). The measurement of pessimism: The Hopelessness Scale. *Journal of Consulting and Clinical Psychology, 42,* 861–865.

Beck, A. T., Rush, A. J., Shaw, B. F., & Emery, G. (1979). *Cognitive therapy of depression.* New York: Guilford.

Beck, A. T., Steer, R. A., Kovacs, M., & Garrson, B. S. (1985). Hopelessness and eventual suicide: A 10-year prospectus study of patients hospitalized with suicidal ideation. *American Journal of Psychiatry, 142,* 559–563.

Beck, J. G., & Barlow, D. H. (1984). Current conceptualization of sexual dysfunction: A review and an alternative perspective. *Clinical Psychology Review, 4,* 363–378.

Beckham, E. E., Leber, W. R., Watkins, J. T., Boyer, J. L., & Cook, J. B. (1986). Development of instrument to measure Beck's cognitive triad: The Cognitive Triad Inventory. *Journal of Consulting and Clinical Psychology, 54,* 566–567.

Beidel, D. C., & Turner, S. M. (1986). A critique of the theoretical bases of cognitive-behavioral theories and therapy. *Clinical Psychology Review, 6,* 177–197.

Bellack, A. S. (1986). Schizophrenia: Behaviour therapy's forgotten child. *Behaviour Therapy, 17,* 199–214.

Bem, S. (1974). The measurement of psychological androgyny. *Journal of Consulting and Clinical Psychology, 42,* 155–158.

Bem, S. (1975). Sex-role adaptability: One consequence of psychological androgyny. *Journal of Personality and Social Psychology, 31,* 634–639.

Berley, R. A., & Jacobson, N. S. (1984). Causal attributions in intimate relationships: Toward a model of cognitive-behavioral marital therapy. In P. Kendall (Ed.), *Advances in cognitive-behavioral research and therapy* (Vol. 3, pp. 1–90). New York: Academic Press.

Berndt, D. S. (1983). Readability of self-report depression inventories. *Journal of Consulting and Clinical Psychology, 51,* 627–628.

Best, J. A. (1975). Tailoring smoking withdrawal procedures to personality and motivational differences. *Journal of Consulting and Clinical Psychology, 43,* 1–8.

Best, J. A., & Steffy, R. A. (1971). Smoking modification procedures tailored to subject characteristics. *Behaviour Therapy, 2,* 177–191.

Bhanji, S., & Thompson, J. (1974). Operant conditioning in the treatment of anorexia nervosa: A review and retrospective study of 11 cases. *British Journal of Psychiatry, 124,* 166–172.

Blackwell, R. T., Galassi, J. P., Galassi, M. D., & Watson, T. E. (1985). Are cognitive assessments equal? A comparison of think aloud and thought listing. *Cognitive Therapy and Research, 9,* 399–413.

Blackburn, I. M., & Smyth, P. (1985). A test of cognitive vulnerability in individuals prone to depression. *British Journal of Clinical Psychology, 24,* 61–62.

Bradley, L. A. (1983). Coping with chronic pain. In T. G. Burish & L. A. Bradley (Eds.), *Coping with chronic disease: Research and application.* New York: Academic Press.

Bradley, L. A., & Kay, R. (1985). The role of cognition in behavioral medicine. In P. Kendall (Ed.), *Advances in cognitive behavioral research and therapy* (Vol. 4, pp. 137–209). New York: Academic Press.

Brown, S. A., Goldman, M. S., & Christiansen, B. A. (1985). Do alcohol expectancies mediate drinking patterns of adults? *Journal of Consulting and Clinical Psychology, 53,* 512–519.

Browning, C. H., & Miller, S. I. (1968). Anorexia nervosa: A study in prognosis and management. *American Journal of Psychiatry, 124,* 1128–1132.

Bruch, H. (1973). *Eating disorders.* New York: Basic Books.

Bruner, J. S. (1973). *Beyond the information given: Studies in the psychology of knowing.* New York: Norton.

Burish, T. G., Carey, M. P., Wallston, K. A., Stein, M. J., Jamison, R. N., & Lyles, J. N. (1984). Health locus of control and chronic disease: An external orientation may be advantageous. *Journal of Social and Clinical Psychology, 2,* 326–332.

Burns, D. D., Shaw, B. F., & Croker, W. (1987). Thinking styles and coping strategies of depressed women: An empirical investigation. *Behaviour Research and Therapy, 25,* 223–225.

Butler, G., & Mathews, A. (1983). Cognitive processes in anxiety. *Advances in Behavior Research and Therapy, 5,* 51–62.

Cacioppo, J. T., & Petty, R. E. (1981). Social psychological procedures for cognitive response assessment: The thought-listing technique. In T. V. Merluzzi, C. R. Glass, & M. Genest (Eds.), *Cognitive assessment* (pp. 308–342). New York: Guilford.

Cacioppo, J. T., Glass, C. R., & Merluzzi, T. V. (1979). Self-statements and self-evaluations: A cognitive response analysis of heterosexual anxiety. *Cognitive Therapy and Research, 3,* 249–262.

Campbell, D. T., & Fiske, D. W. (1959). Convergent and discrimant validation by the multitrait-multimethod matrix. *Psychological Bulletin, 56,* 81–105.

Cane, D. B., Olinger, L. J., Gotlib, I. H., & Kuiper, N. A. (1986). Factor structure of the Dysfunctional Attitude Scale in a student population. *Journal of Clinical Psychology, 42,* 307–309.

Carey, K. B., & Maisto, S. A. (1985). A review of the use of self-control techniques in the treatment of alcohol abuse. *Cognitive Therapy and Research, 9,* 235–251.

Cerny, J. A., & Polyson, J. (1984). Changing homonegative attitudes. *Journal of Social and Clinical Psychology, 3,* 366–371.

Chambless, D. L., Caputo, C., Bright, P., & Gallagher, R. (1984). Assessment of fear in agoraphobics: The Body Sensations Questionnaire and the Agoraphobic Cognition Questionnaire. *Journal of Consulting and Clinical Psychology, 52,* 1090–1097.

Ciminero, A. R., Nelson, R. O., & Lipinski, D. P. (1977). Self-monitoring procedures. In A. R. Ciminero, K. S. Calhoun, & H. E. Adams (Eds.), *Handbook of behavioral assessment.* New York: Wiley.

Clark, D. M. (1986). A cognitive approach to panic. *Behaviour Research and Therapy, 24,* 461–470.

Clark, D. A., & Hemsley, D. (1985). Individual differences in the epxerience of depressive and anxious, intrinsic thoughts. *Behaviour Research and Therapy, 23,* 625–633.

Clinton, D. N., & McKinlay, W. W. (1986). Attitudes to food, eating and weight in acutely ill and recovered anorexics. *British Journal of Clinical Psychology, 25,* 61–67.

Cohen, F., & Lazarus, R. S. (1973). Active coping processes, coping dispositions and recovery from surgery. *Psychosomatic Medicine, 35,* 375–389.

Colletti, G., Supnick, J. A., & Payne, J. J. (1985). The Smoking Self-Efficacy Questionnaire (SSEQ): Preliminary scale development and validation. *Behavioral Assessment, 7,* 249–260.

Condiotte, M. M., & Lichtenstein, E. (1981). Self-efficacy and relapse in smoking cessation programs. *Journal of Consulting and Clinical Psychology, 49,* 648–658.

Cooper, P. J., & Fairburn, C. G. (1984). Cognitive behavior therapy for anorexia nervosa: Some preliminary findings. *Journal of Psychosomatic Research, 28,* 493–499.

Cooper, P. J., Waterman, G. C., & Fairburn, C. G. (1984). Women with eating problems: A community survey. *British Journal of Clinical Psychology, 23,* 45–52.

Cooper, Z., Cooper, P. J., & Fairburn, C. G. (1985). The specificity of the Eating Disorder Inventory. *British Journal of Clinical Psychology, 24,* 129–130.

Crisp, A. H. (1965). Clinical and therapeutic aspects of anorexia nervosa: A study of 30 cases. *Journal of Psychosomatic Research, 9,* 67–78.

Cronbach, L. J., & Meehl, P. E. (1955). Construct validity in psychological tests. *Psychological Bulletin, 52,* 281–302.

Csikszentmihalyi, M., & Larson, R. (1984). *Being adolescent: Conflict and growth in the teenage years.* New York: Basic Books.

Davison, G. C., Robins, C., & Johnston, M. K. (1983). Articulated thoughts during simulated situations: A paradigm for studying cognition in emotion and behavior. *Cognitive Therapy and Research, 7,* 17–40.

DiClemente, C. C. (1981). Self-efficacy and smoking cessation maintenance: A preliminary report. *Cognitive Therapy and Research, 5,* 175–187.

Dobson, K. S., & Shaw, B. F. (1986). Cognitive assessment with major depressive disorders. *Cognitive Therapy and Research, 10,* 13–29.

Dobson, K. S., & Shaw, B. F. (1987). Specificity and stability of self-referent encoding in clinical depression. *Journal of Abnormal Psychology, 96,* 34–40.

Eiser, J. R., & Gossop, M. R. (1979). Hooked or sick: Addicts' perceptions of their addiction. *Addictive Behaviors, 4,* 185–191.

Ellis, A. (1962). *Reason and emotion in psychotherapy.* New York: Lyle & Stuart.

Emery, G., & Fox, S. (1981). Cognitive therapy of alcohol dependency. In G. Emery, S. D. Hollon, & R. C. Bedrosian (Eds.), *New directions in cognitive therapy* (pp. 181–200). New York: Guildford Press.

Endler, N. S., & Hunt, J. McV. (1966). Sources of behavioral variance as measured by the S-R inventories of anxiousness. *Psychological Bulletin, 65,* 336–346.

Epstein, N. (1982). Cognitive therapy with couples. *American Journal of Family Therapy, 10,* 5–16.

Epstein, N., & Eidelson, R. J. (1981). Unrealistic beliefs of clinical couples: Their relationship to expectations, goals and satisfaction. *American Journal of Family Therapy, 9,* 13–22.

Ericsson, K. A., & Simon, H. A. (1984). *Protocol analysis*. Cambridge: M.I.T. Press.

Ewart, C. K., Taylor, C. B., Reese, L. B., & Debusk, R. F. (1984). Effects of early myocardial infarction exercise testing on self-perception and subsequent physical activity. *American Journal of Cardiology, 51,* 1076–1080.

Fichten, C. S. (1984). See it from my point of view: Videotape and attribution in happy and distressed couples. *Journal of Social and Clinical Psychology, 2,* 125–142.

Fiedler, R., & Beach, L. R. (1978). On the decision to be assertive. *Journal of Counsuling and Clinical Psychology, 46,* 537–546.

Fincham, F. D. (1985). Attribution processes in distressed and nondistressed couples: 2. Responsibility for marital problems. *Journal of Abnormal Psychology, 94,* 183–190.

Fisher, J. V., Fisher, J. C., & Mason, R. L. (1976). Physicians and alcoholics: Modifying behavior and attitudes of family-practice residents. *Journal of Studies on Alcohol, 11,* 1686–1693.

Foa, E. B., & McNally, R. J. (1986). Sensitivity to feared stimuli in obsessive-compulsives: A dichotic listening analysis. *Cognitive Therapy and Research, 10,* 477–485.

Fox, S., & Emery, G. (1981). Cognitive therapy of sexual dysfunctions: A case study. In G. Emery, S. D. Hollon, & R. C. Bedrosian (Eds.), *New directions in cognitive therapy* (pp. 160–180). New York: Guilford.

Garner, D. M., & Garfinkel, P. E. (1979). The eating attitudes test: An index of symptoms of anorexia nervosa. *Psychological Medicine, 9,* 273–279.

Garner, D. M., Olmstead, M. P., Bohr, Y., & Garfinkel, P. (1982). The Eating Attitudes Test: Psychometric features and clinical correlates. *Psychological Medicine, 12,* 871–878.

Garner, D. M., Olmstead, M. P., & Polivy, J. (1983). Development and validation of a multidimensional eating disorder inventory for anorexia nervosa and bulimia. *International Journal of Eating Disorders, 2,* 15–34.

Genest, M., & Turk, D. C. (1981). Think aloud approaches to cognitive assessment. In T. V. Merluzzi, C. R. Glass, & M. Genest (Eds.), *Cognitive assessment* (pp. 233–269). New York: Guilford.

Giles, D. E., & Rush, A. J. (1982). Relationship of dysfunctional attitude and dexamethasone response in endogenous and nonendogenous depression. *Biological Psychiatry, 17,* 1303–1314.

Glass, C. R., & Arnkoff, D. B. (1982). Think cognitively—Selected devices in cognitive assessment and therapy. In P. C. Kendall (Ed.). *Advances in Cognitive Behavioral Research and Therapy* (Vol. 1). New York: Academic.

Glass, C. R., Merluzzi, T. V., Biever, J. L., & Larsen, K. H. (1982). Cognitive assessment of social anxiety: Development and validation of a self-statement questionnaire. *Cognitive Therapy and Research, 6,* 37–55.

Glynn, S. M., & Ruderman, A. J. (1986). The development and validation of an eating self-efficacy scale. *Cognitive Therapy and Research, 10,* 403–420.

Godding, P. R., & Glasgow, R. E. (1985). Self-efficacy and outcome expectations as predictors of controlled smoking status. *Cognitive Therapy and Research, 9,* 583–590.

Goldberg, S. C., Halmi, K. A., Eckert, E. D., Casper, R. C., Davis, J. M., & Roper, M. (1980). Attitudinal dimensions in anorexia nervosa. *Journal of Psychiatric Research, 15,* 239–251.

Goldfried, M. R., & Kent, R. N. (1972). Traditional vs. behavioral personality assessment: A comparison of methodological and theoretical assumptions. *Psychological Bulletin, 77,* 409–420.

Gossop, M. (1978). Drug dependence: A study of the relationship between motivation, cognitive, social and historical factors, and treatment variables. *Journal of Nervous and Mental Disease, 166,* 44–50.

Gunderson, J. G., Frank, A. F., Katz, H. M., Vannicelli, M. L., Frosch, J. P., & Knapp, P. H. (1984). Effects of psychotherapy in schizophrenia: II. Comparative outcome of two forms of treatment. *Schizophrenia Bulletin, 10,* 564–598.

Halford, K., & Foddy, M. (1982). Cognitive and social skills correlates of social anxiety. *British Journal of Clinical Psychology, 21,* 17–28.

Hamilton, M. (1960). A rating scale for depression. *Journal of Neurology, Neurosurgery and Psychiatry, 12,* 56–62.

Hammen, C. L., & Krantz, S. E. (1985). Measures of psychological processes in depression. In E. E. Beckham & W. R. Leber (Eds.), *Handbook of depression: Treatment, assessment and research* (pp. 408–444). Homewood, IL: Dorsey.

Harlow, P. E., & Goby, M. J. (1980). Changing nursing students' attitudes toward alcoholic patients: Examining effects of a clinical procticum. *Nursing Research, 29,* 59–60.

Harrell, T. H., & Ryon, N. B. (1983). Cognitive-behavioral assessment of depression: Clinical validation of the Automatic Thoughts Questionnaire. *Journal of Consulting and Clinical Psychology, 51,* 721–725.

Haynes, S. N. (1986). A behavioral model of paranoid behaviours. *Behaviour Therapy, 17,* 266–287.

Heilbrun, A. B. (1975). A proposed basis for delusional formulation within an information-processing model of paranoid development. *British Journal of Social and Clinical Psychology, 14,* 63–71.

JOEL O. GOLDBERG
and BRIAN F. SHAW

Herman, C. P., Polivy, J., Pliner, P., Threlkeld, J., & Munic, D. (1978). Distractibility in dieters and non-dieters: An alternative view of externality. *Journal of Personality and Social Psychology, 36,* 536–548.

Hersen, M., & Bellack, A. S. (1988). *Dictionary of behavioral assessment techniques.* London: Pergamon.

Hollon, S. D., & Kendall, P. C. (1980). Cognitive self statements in depression: Development of an automatic thoughts questionnaire. *Cognitive Therapy and Research, 4,* 383–396.

Hollon, S. D., & Kriss, M. R. (1984). Cognitive factors in clinical research and practice. *Clinical Psychology Review, 4,* 35–76.

Hollon, S. D., Kendall, P. C., & Lumry, A. (1986). A specificity of depressotypic cognitions in clinical depression. *Journal of Abnormal Psychology, 95,* 52–59.

Huba, G. J., & Tanaka, J. S. (1983). Confirmatory evidence for three daydreaming factors in the Short Imaginal Processes Inventory. *Imagination, Cognition and Personality, 3,* 139–147.

Hurlburt, R. T. (1979). Random sampling of cognitions and behaviour. *Journal of Research in Personality, 13,* 103–111.

Johnson, S. M., & Greenberg, L. S. (1985). Differential effects of experiential and problem-solving interventions in resolving marital conflict. *Journal of Consulting and Clinical Psychology, 53,* 175–184.

Jones, R. G. (1969). A factored measure of Ellis' irrational belief system. Doctoral dissertation, Texas Technological College, *Dissertation Abstracts International, 29,* 4379B–4380B.

Keller, K. E. (1983). Dysfunctional attitude and the cognitive therapy for depression. *Cognitive Therapy and Research, 7,* 437–444.

Kendall, P. C. (1982). Behavioral assessment and methodology. In C. M. Franks, G. T. Wilson, P. C. Kendall, & K. D. Brownell (Eds.), *Annual review of behavior therapy* (Vol. 8, pp. 39–81). New York: Guilford.

Kendall, P. C., Williams, L., Pechacek, T. F., Graham, L. G., Shisslak, C. S., & Herzoff, N. (1979). Cognitive-behavioral and patient education interventions in cardiac catheterization procedures: The Palo Alto medical psychology project. *Journal of Consulting and Clinical Psychology, 47,* 49–58.

Kendall, P. C., & Hollon, S. D. (1981). Assessing self-referent speech: Methods in the measurement of self-statements. In P. C. Kendall & S. D. Hollon (Eds.), *Assessment strategies for cognitive-behavioral interventions* (pp. 85–118). New York: Academic Press.

Kent, G. (1985a). Cognitive processes in dental anxiety. *British Journal of Clinical Psychology, 24,* 259–264.

Kent, G. (1985b). Memory for dental pain. *Pain, 21,* 187–197.

Keutzer, C. S. (1968). A measure of cognitive dissonance as a predictor of smoking treatment outcome. *Psychological Reports, 22,* 655–658.

Killen, J. D., Maccoby, N., & Taylor, C. B. (1984). Nicotine gum and self-regulation training in smoking relapse prevention. *Behavior Therapy, 15,* 234–248.

Kilty, K. M. (1975). Attitudes toward alcohol and alcoholism among professionals and nonprofessionals. *Journal of Studies on Alcohol, 36,* 327–347.

Klinger, E. (1977). *Meaning and void: Inner experience and the incentives in peoples' lives.* Minneapolis: University of Minnesota Press.

Korchin, S. J., & Schuldberg, D. (1981). The future of clinical assessment. *American Psychologist, 36,* 1147–1158.

Kowalchuk, B. (1986). *Suicidal orientation as a belief system: Preliminary findings with psychiatric patients.* Unpublished doctoral dissertation, York University, Toronto, Canada.

Krantz, S., & Hammen, C. L. (1979). Assessment of cognitive bias in depression. *Journal of Abnormal Psychology, 88,* 611–619.

Kuiper, N. A., Olinger, L. G., MacDonald, M. R., & Shaw, B. F. (1985). Self-schema processing of depressed and nondepressed content. The effects of vulnerability to depression. *Social Cognition, 3,* 77–93.

Larsen, K. S., Reed, M., & Hoffman, S. (1980). Attitudes of heterosexuals toward homosexuality: A Likert-type scale and construct validity. *Journal of Sex Research, 16,* 245–257.

Lazarus, R. S., & Folkman, S. (1984). *Stress, appraisal, and coping.* New York: Springer.

Lefebvre, M. F. (1981). Cognitive distortion and cognitive errors in depressed psychiatric and low back pain patients. *Journal of Consulting and Clinical Psychology, 49,* 517–525.

Levenkron, J. C., Cohen, J. D., Mueller, H. S., & Fisher, E. B. (1983). Modifying the Type A coronary-prone behavior pattern. *Journal of Consulting and Clinical Psychology, 51,* 192–204.

Libman, E., Rothenberg, I., Fichten, C. S., & Amsel, R. (1985). The SSES-E: A measure of sexual self-efficacy in erectile functioning. *Journal of Sex and Marital Therapy, 11,* 233–247.

Linehan, M. M., & Nielsen, S. L. (1981). Assessment of suicide ideation and parasuicide & hopelessness and social desirability. *Journal of Consulting and Clinical Psychology, 49,* 773–775.

Linehan, M. M., & Nielsen, S. L. (1983). Social desirability: Its relevance to the measurement of hopelessness and suicidal behaviour, *Journal of Consulting and Clinical Psychology, 51,* 141–143.

MacDonald, A. P., Jr., Huggins, J., Young, S., & Swanson, R. A. (1973). Attitudes toward homosexuality: Preservation of sex morality or the double standard? *Journal of Consulting and Clinical Psychology, 40*, 161–164.

MacDonald, M. R., & Kuiper, N. A. (1983). Cognitive-behavioral preparations for surgery. *Clinical Psychology Review, 3*, 27–39.

Mathews, S. A., & MacLeod, C. (1985). Selective processing of threat cues to anxiety states. *Behavior Research and Therapy, 23*, 563–569.

Mayo, C., & Havelock, R. G. (1970). Attitudes toward mental illness among mental hospital personnel and patients. *Journal of Psychiatric Research, 7*, 291–298.

McLemore, C. (1976). Factorial validity of imagery measures. *Behavior Research and therapy, 14*, 399–408.

Meichenbaum, D. (1969). The effects of instructions and reinforcement on thinking and language behaviour in schizophrenics. *Behavior Research and Therapy, 7*, 101–114.

Meichenbaum, D. (1977). *Cognitive behavior modification: An integrative approach.* New York: Plenum Press.

Mendonca, J. D., Holden, R. R., Mazmanian, D., & Dolan, J. (1983). The influence of response style on the Beck Hopelessness Scale. *Canadian Journal of Behavioural Science, 15*, 237–247.

Meyerowitz, B. E., Heinrich, R. L., & Schag, C. C. (1983). A competency-based approach to coping with cancer. In T. G. Burish & L. A. Bradley (Eds.), *Coping with chronic disease: Research and applications.* New York: Academic Press.

Miller, P. C., Lefcourt, H. M., & Ware, E. E. (1983). The construction and development of the Miller Marital Locus of Control Scale. *Canadian Journal of Behavioral Science, 15*, 266–279.

Mosher, D. L., & Abramson, P. R. (1977). Subjective sexual arousal to films of masturbation. *Journal of Consulting and Clinical Psychology, 45*, 796–799.

Morrow, G. R. (1986). Effect of the cognitive heirarchy in the systematic desensitization treatment of anticipatory nausea in cancer patients: A component comparison with relaxation only, counseling and no treatment. *Cognitive Therapy and Research, 10*, 421–446.

Murray, A. L., & Lawrence, P. S. (1984). Sequelae to smoking cessation: A review. *Clinical Psychology Review, 4*, 143–157.

Nelson, R. O. (1977). Methodological issues in assessment and self-monitoring. In J. D. Cone & R. P. Hawkins (Eds.), *Behavioral assessment: new directions in clinical psychology.* New York: Bruner/Mazel.

Neufeld, R. W. J., & Kuiper, N. A. (1983). Stress-relevant deviance and sources of stress negotiation difficulties in the medical setting. *Canadian Journal of Behavioral Science, 15*, 334–350.

Neufeld, R. W. J., & Thomas, P. (1977). Effects of perceived efficacy of a prophylactic controlling mechanism on self-control under pain stimulation. *Canadian Journal of Behavioral Science, 9*, 224–232.

Nietzel, M. T., & Bernstein, D. A. (1981). Assessment of anxiety and fear. In M. Hersen & A. S. Bellack (Eds.), *Behavioral assessment: A practical handbook* (pp. 215–245). New York: Pergamon.

Novaco, R. W. (1977). Stress innoculation: A cognitive therapy for anger and its application to a case of depression. *Journal of Consulting and Clinical Psychology, 45*, 600–608.

Nydegger, R. V. (1972). The elimination of hallucinatory and delusional behaviour by verbal conditioning and assertive training: A case study. *Journal of Behavior Therapy and Experimental Psychiatry, 3*, 225–227.

O'Leary, A. (1985). Self-efficacy and health. *Behavior Research and Therapy, 23*, 437–451.

Olinger, L. J., Kuiper, N. A., & Shaw, B. F. (1987). Dysfunctional attitude and stressful life events: An interactive model of depression. *Cognitive Therapy and Research, 11*, 25–40.

Olson, D. H., & Ryder, R. G. (1970). Inventory of marital conflicts: An experimental interaction procedure. *Journal of Marriage and the Family, 32*, 443–448.

Ordman, A. M., & Kirschenbaum, D. S. (1985). Cognitive-behavioral therapy for bulimia: An initial outcome study. *Journal of Consulting and Clinical Psychology, 53*, 303–313.

Persons, J. B., & Burns, D. D. (1985). Mechanisms of action of cognitive therapy: The relative contributions of technical and interpersonal interventions. *Cognitive Therapy and Research, 9*, 539–551.

Peterson, C., Semmel, A., von Baeyer, C., Abramson, L., Metalsky, G., & Seligman, M. E. P. (1982). The Attributional Style Questionnaire. *Cognitive Therapy and Research, 6*, 287–299.

Peterson, C., Bettes, B. A., & Seligman, M. E. P. (1985). Depressive symptoms and unprompted causal attributions: Content analysis. *Behavior Research and Therapy, 23*, 379–382.

Rosenbaum, M. (1980). A schedule for assessing self-control behaviors: Preliminary findings. *Behavior Therapy, 11*, 109–121.

Rossiter, E. M., & Wilson, G. T. (1985). Cognitive restructuring and response prevention in the treatment of bulimia nervosa. *Behavior Research and Therapy, 23*, 349–359.

Ruderman, A. J. (1985). Restraint and irrational cognitions. *Behavioral Research and Therapy, 23*, 557–561.

Rush, A. J. (1984). *Measurement of the cognitive aspects of depression.* Paper presented at the N.I.M.H. Workshop, The Measurement of Depression, Honolulu, Hawaii.

Rush, A. J., Weissenburger, J., & Eaves, G. (1986). Do thinking patterns predict depressive symptoms? *Cognitive Therapy and Research, 10,* 225–236.

Saccuzzo, D. P., & Braff, D. L. (1986). Information-processing abnormalities, trait- and state-dependent components. *Schizophrenia Bulletin, 12,* 447–459.

Salkovskis, P. M. (1985). Obsessive-compulsive problems: A cognitive-behavioural analysis. *Behaviour Research and Therapy, 23,* 571–583.

Sanchez-Craig, M., Annis, H. M., Bornet, H. R., & MacDonald, K. R. (1984). Random assignment to abstinence and controlled drinking: Evaluation of a cognitive behavioral program for problem drinkers. *Journal of Consulting and Clinical Psychology, 52,* 390–403.

Schneider, J. A., & Agras, W. S. (1985). A cognitive behavioral group treatment of bulimia. *British Journal of Psychiatry, 146,* 66–69.

Segal, Z. V., Goldberg, J. O., & Vella, D. D. (1987, November). *Identifying dependent and self-critical subtypes of depression.* Paper presented at the meeting of the Association for Advancement of Behavior Therapy, Boston, MA.

Segal, Z. V., & Marshall, W. L. (1985). Hetrosexual social skills in a population of rapists and child molesters. *Journal of Consulting and Clinical Psychology, 53,* 55–63.

Segal, Z. V., & Shaw, B. F. (1987). Cognitive assessment: Issues and methods. In K. S. Dobson (Ed.), *Handbook of cognitive-behavioral therapies* (pp. 361–387). New York: Guilford.

Seligman, M. E. P. (1975). *Helplessness.* San Francisco: Wilt Freeman.

Sewitch, T. S., & Kirsch, I. (1984). The cognitive content of anxiety: Naturalistic evidence for the predominance of threat-related thoughts. *Cognitive Therapy and Research, 8,* 49–58.

Shaw, B. F. (1987). The Dysfunctional Attitude Scale. In M. Hersen & A. S. Bellack (Eds.), *Dictionary of behavioral assessment techniques.* London: Pergamon.

Shaw, B. F., & Dobson, K. S. (1981). Cognitive assessment of depression. In T. V. Merluzzi, C. R. Glass, & M. Genest (Eds.), *Cognitive assessment* (pp. 361–387). New York: Guilford.

Shaw, B. F. Vallis, T. M., & McCabe, S. (1985). The assessment of the severity and symptom patterns in depression. In E. E. Beckham & W. R. Leber (Eds.), *Handbook of depression: Treatment, assessment and research* (pp. 372–407). Homewood, IL: Dorsey.

Shekelle, R. B., Gale, M., Ostfeld, A. M., & Oglesby, P. (1983). Hostility, risk of coronary heart disease, and mortality. *Psychosomatic Medicine, 45,* 109–114.

Shorkey, C. T., & Whiteman, V. L. (1977). Development of the rational behavior inventory: Initial validation and reliability. *Educational and Psychological Measurement, 37,* 527–534.

Silverman, D. C., Edbril, S., Gartrell, N., Wise, S., Botnick, L., Liao-Rosenblatt, E., & Huntley, B. (1986). A pilot study of women's attitudes towards breast-conserving surgery with primary radiation therapy for breast cancer. *International Journal of Psychiatry in Medicine, 15,* 381–391.

Simons, A. D., Lustman, P. J., Wetzel, R. D., & Murphy, G. E. (1985). Predicting response to cognitive therapy of depression: The role of learned resourcefulness. *Cognitive Therapy and Research, 9,* 79–90.

Simons, A. D., Murphy, G. E., Levine, J. L., & Wetzel, R. D. (1986). Cognitive therapy and pharmacotherapy for depression. *Archives of General Psychiatry, 43,* 43–48.

Singer, J. (1974). *Imagery and daydream methods in psychotherapy and behaviour modification.* New York: Academic Press.

Smith, T. W., Follick, M. J., Ahern, D. K., & Adams, A. (1986). Cognitive distortion and disability in chronic low back pain. *Cognitive Therapy and Research, 10,* 201–210.

Sobel, H. J. (1981). Projective methods of cognitive analysis. In T. V. Merluzzi, C. R. Glass, & M. Genest (Eds.), *Cognitive assessment* (pp. 127–148). New York: Guilford.

Soskis, D. A., & Bowers, M. B. (1969). The schizophrenic experience: A follow-up study of attitude and post-hospital adjustment. *Journal of Nervous and Mental Disease, 149,* 443–449.

Sotsky, S., Glass, D., & Shea, T. (1986). *Patient predictors of response to psychotherapy and pharmacotherapy of depression: NIMH TDCRP.* Paper presented at the meeting of the Society for Psychotherapy Research.

Steinhausen, H. C. (1986). Attitudinal dimensions in adolescent anorexic patients: An analysis of the Goldberg Anorectic Attitude Scale. *Journal of Psychiatric Research, 20,* 83–87.

Strosahl, K. D., & Ascough, J. (1981). Clinical uses of mental imagery: Experimental foundations, theoretical misconceptions and research issues. *Psychological Bulletin, 89,* 422–438.

Strosahl, K. D., Ascough, J., & Rojas, A. (1986). Imagery assessment by self-report: A multidimensional analysis of clinical imagery. *Cognitive Therapy and Research, 10,* 187–200.

Sundberg, N. D., & Tyler, L. E. (1962). *Clinical psychology*. New York: Appleton-Century-Crofts.

Taylor, S. E., Lichtman, R. R., & Wood, J. V. (1984). Attributions, beliefs about control and adjustment to breast cancer. *Journal of Personality and Social Psychology, 46,* 489–502.

Toner, B. B., Garfinkel, P. E., & Garner, D. M. (1986). Long-term follow-up of anorexia nervosa. *Psychosomatic Medicine, 48,* 520–529.

Toner, B. B., Garfinkel, P. E., & Garner, D. M. (1987). Measurement of psychometric features and their relationship to clinical outcome in the long-term course of anorexia nervosa. *International Journal of Eating Disorders, 6,* 17–27.

Turk, D., Meichenbaum, D. H., & Genest, M. (1983). *Pain and behavioral medicine: A cognitive-behavioral perspective.* New York: Guilford.

Tyndall, L. W., & Lichtenberg, J. W. (1985). Spouses' cognitive styles and marital interaction patterns. *Journal of Marital and Family Therapy, 11,* 193–202.

Wardle, J. (1984). Dental pessimism: Negative cognitions in fearful dental patients. *Behavior Therapy and Research, 22,* 553–556.

Watkins, J., & Rush, A. J. (1983). The cognitive response test. *Cognitive Therapy and Research, 7,* 425–436.

Watson, D., & Friend, R. (1969). Measurement of social-evaluative anxiety. *Journal of Consulting and Clinical Psychology, 33,* 448–457.

Weiss, R. L. (1984). Cognitive and behavioral measures of marital interaction. In K. Hahlweg & N. Jacobson (Eds.), *Marital interaction: Analysis and modification* (pp. 232–252). New York: Guilford.

Weisman, A. D., & Sobel, H. J. (1979). Coping with cancer through self-instruction: A hypothesis. *Journal of Human Stress, 5,* 3–8.

Weissman, A. N. (1980). *Assessing depressogenic attitudes: A validation study.* Paper presented at the 51st Annual meeting of The Eastern Psychological Association: Hartford, CT.

Williams, R. B., Haney, T. L., Lee, K. L., Kong, Y., Blumenthal, J. A., & Whalen, R. (1980). Type A behavior, hostility and coronary atherosclerosis. *Psychosomatic Medicine, 42,* 539–549.

Williams, S. L. (1985). On the nature and measurement of agoraphobia. In M. Hersen, R. M. Eisler & P. M. Miller (Eds.) *Progress in Behavior Modification* (Vol. 19, pp. 109–144). New York: Academic Press.

Williams, S. L., & Rappoport, A. (1983). Cognitive treatment in the natural environment for agoraphobics. *Behavior Therapy, 14,* 299–313.

Winters, K. C., & Neale, J. M. (1983). Delusions and delusional thinking in psychotics: A review of the literature. *Clinical Psychology Review, 3,* 227–253.

Wise, E. H., & Barnes, D. R. (1986). The relationship among life events, dysfunctional attitudes, and depression. *Cognitive Therapy and Research, 10,* 257–266.

Wright, J., & Fichten, C. S. (1976). Denial of responsibility, videotape feedback and attribution theory: Relevance for behavioral marital therapy. *Canadian Psychological Review, 17,* 219–230.

Zimmerman, M., & Coryell, W. (1986). Dysfunctional attitudes in endogenous and nonendogenous depressed in-patients. *Cognitive Therapy and Research, 10,* 339–346.

Zuckerman, M., Tushup, R., & Finner, F. (1976). Sexual attitudes and experiences: Attitudes and personality correlates and changes produced by a course in human sexuality. *Journal of Consulting and Clinical Psychology, 44,* 7–13.

# 4

# Process and Outcome in Cognitive Therapy

## E. Edward Beckham and John T. Watkins

In recent decades, the efficacy of psychotherapy and the process by which psychotherapy works have been increasingly scrutinized. Outcome studies have become more specific with regard to the disorder treated and the types of treatments used. With the manualization of cognitive therapy for depression (Beck, Rush, Shaw, & Emery, 1979), it has become one of the most widely researched of the psychotherapies. This chapter will describe the current status of process and outcome research in cognitive therapy. There will first be a brief review of the current state of outcome research for psychotherapy in general followed by a more detailed examination of outcome research in cognitive therapy. We will then examine the process research pertaining to cognitive therapy. Reviews of outcome studies will focus most heavily on clinically diagnosed disorders with less emphasis on analog studies.

Several reviews have found psychotherapy in general to be more helpful than no treatment (Luborsky, Singer, & Luborsky, 1975; Smith, Glass, and Miller, 1980). However, there has generally been a lack of hard evidence that one treatment is superior to another (Luborsky et al., 1975), especially over the long term (Frank, 1979). In reviewing the literature, Frank (1979) observed that there may be a short-term superiority of behavior therapy for phobias and cognitive therapy for the relief of depression. In a meta-analytic review, Smith et al., (1980) surveyed 475 studies and found that the average outcome score for all treated groups was .85 standard deviations more improved than the mean of all control groups. The effect size of cognitive therapies was considerably higher than any of the other 17 types of therapy included in the meta-analysis (Smith et al., 1980, p. 89).

In a meta-analytic review of the efficacy of cognitive behavior therapies (CBT), Miller and Berman (1983) analyzed 48 studies in which depression, anxiety, and psychophysiological disorders had been treated. Statistically, the average patient treated with CBT had an outcome .83 standard deviations more improved than the average untreated patient. CBT patients did not have significantly better outcomes than patients treated with systematic desensitization, but

E. Edward Beckham and John T. Watkins • University of Oklahoma Health Sciences Center, Oklahoma City, Oklahoma 73190.

E. EDWARD
BECKHAM and
JOHN T. WATKINS

the lack of statistical significance may have been due to the small number of comparisons (13 studies) and to the fact that the patient disorders in the studies surveyed included anxiety as well as depression. A significant difference favoring CBT over other therapies was found only on self-report measures. When effectiveness by diagnosis was examined, the effect size of CBT compared to no-treatment controls was numerically larger for depression than for treatment of anxiety and psychophysiological disorders.

Outcome studies of cognitive therapy have varied in the type of cognitive therapy tested (Beck's cognitive therapy of depression, Meichenbaum's stress innoculation training, Ellis's rational-emotive therapy), their target populations, extent of therapist training, and general methodological rigor. Most have used depressed patients, and these studies will be given the greatest amount of attention in this chapter.

## OUTCOME STUDIES OF COGNITIVE THERAPY OF DEPRESSION

Only a little over a decade ago, Shaw (1977), Taylor and Marshall (1977), and Rush, Beck, Kovacs, and Hollon (1977) provided the first empirical evidence that cognitive therapy was effective in treating depression. One methodological problem of these early studies was their lack of clearly defined diagnostic categories. More recent studies have tended to use inclusion criteria based on diagnoses by the Feighner criteria (Feighner et al., 1972), the Research Diagnostic Criteria (Spitzer, Endicott, & Robins, 1978) or the DSM-III (American Psychiatric Association, 1980). Generally, the required diagnosis has been major depression. Another trend starting with Rush et al. (1977) has been to test cognitive therapy within medical settings and to compare it with medication as a reference condition. The advantage of comparing it with tricyclic antidepressants, especially imipramine and amitriptyline, has been that they are well accepted within the medical community as effective treatments for depression. Findings of comparable or superior efficacy therefore command attention from a wide array of researchers and mental health professionals. Rush et al. (1977) compared cognitive therapy with imipramine and found the outcome with cognitive therapy to be superior at termination. Several studies followed Rush et al. (1977) in this vein and found cognitive therapy either to be more effective than tricyclic medication (Blackburn, Bishop, Glen, Whalley, & Christie, 1981, with general practice outpatients; Teasdale, Fennel, Hibbert, & Amies, 1983) or equally as effective (Beck, Hollon, Young, Bedrosian, & Budenz, 1985; Blackburn et al., 1981 with psychiatric outpatients; Elkin, Shea, Watkins, & Collins, 1986; Evans et al., 1985; Murphy, Simons, Wetzel, & Lustman, 1984). Although, on the whole, these results have been very supportive of the effectiveness of cognitive therapy for depression, medication groups do not provide a totally adequate substitute for control groups. There is, of course, a good reason for the use of medication groups because the use of control groups with severely depressed patients raises serious ethical problems. The NIMH Treatment of Depression Collaborative Research Program (TDCRP; Elkin, Parloff, Hadley, & Autrey, 1985) attempted to deal with this problem by using a pill placebo plus clinical management (minimal supportive therapy) condition. In the seven studies where control groups have been used, each has found cognitive therapy to be more effective (Comas-Diaz, 1981; Larcombe & Wilson, 1984; Reynolds & Coats, 1986; Ross & Scott, 1985; Shaw, 1977; Taylor & Marshall, 1977; Wilson, Goldin, & Charbonneau-Powis, 1983). Reporting on the TDCRP results, Elkin et al. (1986) found numerical but not statistically significant superiority for cognitive therapy over the pill–placebo treatment at termination.

Behavioral treatments for depression typically have included assertiveness training and/or training subjects to increase participation in pleasant events. Most direct comparisons of cognitive therapy with these forms of behavior therapies have failed to find a difference in efficacy (Comas-Diaz, 1981; Gallagher & Thompson, 1982; McNamara & Horan, 1986;

Rehm, Kaslow, & Rabin, 1987; Taylor & Marshall, 1977; Wilson *et al.*, 1983; Zeiss, Lewinsohn, & Munoz, 1979). Only Shaw (1977) has found cognitive therapy to be superior to behavior therapy. Reynolds and Coats (1986) made the first comparison between cognitive therapy and systematic desensitization for depression. Again they failed to find any significant difference in efficacy. Two studies (de Jong, Treiber, & Henrich, 1986; Taylor & Marshall, 1977) have reported that a combined cognitive behavioral treatment was more effective than a purely cognitive treatment. However, Taylor and Marshall also found it to be superior to a purely behavioral intervention.

The NIMH Treatment of Depression Collaborative Research Program (Elkin *et al.*, 1985) remedied many of the weaknesses of earlier CBT studies (Williams, 1984). Cognitive therapy was compared with imipramine, interpersonal psychotherapy (IPT; Klerman, Weissman, Rounsaville, & Chevron, 1984) and pill placebo plus clinical management. Patients receiving a placebo had time to talk with their pharmacotherapist about how they were feeling and to receive support (Imber *et al.*, 1986). At termination, there were no statistically significant differences between CBT and the other treatments. CBT had an outcome on depressive symptoms slightly better than placebo plus supportive therapy and slightly worse than either IPT or imipramine. CBT patients were actually worse symptomatically than placebo patients at the 4- and 8-week evaluations (Watkins, Leber, Imber, & Collins, 1986). This, of course, raises the question of why cognitive therapy was not more effective. This may perhaps be answered as process research on the TDCRP data archives is pursued.

Two groups of investigators have studied the effectiveness of cognitive therapy for geriatric depression. Thus far, it has been found to be of approximately equal efficacy with psychodynamic group therapy (Steuer *et al.*, 1984) and behavioral and relational/insight therapies (Gallagher & Thompson, 1982). Steuer *et al.* found it to be somewhat superior to the psychodynamic therapy in improving scores on cognitive items on the BDI, and Gallagher and Thompson found it to be superior to the relational/insight therapy in its effect on depressive symptoms at 1-year follow-up.

Two studies have compared the effectiveness of group versus individually administered CBT. Rush and Watkins (1981), in a pilot study contrasted individual cognitive therapy, group cognitive therapy, and individual cognitive therapy plus antidepressant medication. They found preliminary evidence that group CBT may not be as effective as individually administered CBT. There was no control group to compare with. Ross and Scott (1985) also compared group and individually administered CBT; however, they found no differences in effectiveness.

Most studies have used patients free of complications such as major physical illnesses or alcohol abuse. The treatment of depression, however, must often proceed in the context of just such complicating factors, and demonstrating efficacy for a treatment eventually means testing its utility with a wide variety of patients. Larcombe and Wilson (1984) found CBT to be superior to a waiting list in a sample of depressed patients with multiple sclerosis. Tan and Bruini (1986) found no superior effectiveness for group CBT over group supportive therapy or a wait-list control for treating depression in epileptics. However, it should be noted that depression was not the only focus of treatment in the Tan and Bruini study and that the average initial BDI score for the CBT group was less than 12. Only one study could be found that specifically addressed the issue of treating depression in alcoholics. Turner and Wehl (1984) found individual cognitive-behavioral therapy to be significantly more effective for treating depression in inpatient alcoholics than standard inpatient treatment.

The previously mentioned results regard efficacy of cognitive behavioral therapy at the time of termination from treatment. An equally important question regards whether patients treated by CBT are more immune to relapse than patients treated by medication or other psychotherapies. Cognitive theory predicts that individuals treated with cognitive therapy will be less likely to hold to dysfunctional assumptions and will possess more skills for coping with stress and depression than persons treated with pharmacotherapy or supportive therapy. For that reason, cognitive-therapy subjects would be predicted to have less depression during a follow-up period. Kovacs, Rush, Beck, and Hollon (1981) reported that patients treated with cognitive therapy in Rush *et al.* (1977) had lower levels of depression at 1-year follow-up than patients treated by pharmacotherapy. However, there was no difference in rates of relapse between the two groups. In the study of depressed elderly by Gallagher and Thompson (1982), patients treated either by cognitive or behavioral therapy maintained gains 1-year posttreatment better than patients treated by relational/insight therapy. Blackburn, Eunson, and Bishop (1986) reported a 2-year naturalistic follow-up of the earlier Blackburn *et al.* (1981) study. Patients treated by cognitive therapy or a combination of cognitive therapy and pharmacotherapy were less likely to relapse than patients treated by pharmacotherapy alone. There was no significant difference between groups, however, in average levels of symptomatology at the 6-month follow-up. The same pattern also held in the results of Simons, Murphy, Levine, and Wetzel (1986). Patients who received cognitive therapy, either alone or in combination with pharmacotherapy, were less likely to relapse than those persons receiving pharmacotherapy alone. Finally, Evans *et al.* (1985) compared follow-up results for CBT, CBT plus imipramine, imipramine alone without maintenance dosages, and imipramine with maintenance dosages. The treatment consisting of imipramine alone without maintenance resulted in higher relapse rates than the other three treatments.

In summary, the effectiveness of cognitive therapy for depression is supported by a number of studies. However, the evidence that it is more effective than other active treatments during the acute treatment phase is not conclusive. There is promising evidence that it is superior to pharmacotherapy and nonbehavioral psychotherapies in preventing relapse.

## ANXIETY DISORDERS

Much of the literature on cognitive interventions with anxiety disorders has used subclinical conditions or small numbers of subjects. For that reason, only selected studies will be reviewed here. Treatment of phobias—especially agoraphobia—has generally received the most attention. Emmelkamp and his colleagues have conducted a series of studies comparing cognitive interventions and *in vivo* exposure. Emmelkamp, Kuipers, and Eggeraat (1978) compared cognitive restructuring and prolonged *in vivo* exposure for agoraphobia and found improvement in the exposure condition to be clearly superior. The cognitive intervention consisted of: (a) learning to relabel situations and to replace irrational with rational thoughts; (b) explanation and discussion of Ellis's irrational beliefs; and (c) using coping self-statements. It apparently did not involve systematic questioning by therapists of the evidence and logic behind fear-producing thoughts, and it is not clear from the published reports that the therapists had any training in cognitive therapy. Therefore, it is not too surprising that the combined condition was not more effective than behavior therapy alone. In a further comparison of cognitive restructuring, *in vivo* exposure, and combined cognitive behavioral treatment (Emmelkamp and Mersch, 1982), the behavioral and combined treatment conditions produced greater improvement at termination. However, cognitive therapy patients improved during follow-up, and the behavioral patients relapsed so that the two groups were equivalent at follow-up, and neither group was doing as well as the combined treatment group. Emmelkamp, Brilman, Kuiper, and Mersch (1986) compared exposure *in vivo,* self-instructional training, and RET, and again found the behavioral treatment superior to the cognitive treatments in reducing agoraphobic behavior. Biran and Wilson (1981) compared guided exposure with cognitive restructuring for simple phobias (heights, elevators, darkness) and found that exposure produced superior effects on most measures. Finally, Williams and Rappoport (1983) have also found no added improvement in agoraphobics when cognitive coping procedures were added to *in vivo* exposure.

Other researchers have found more promising results for cognitive techniques. Mavissakalian, Michelson, Greenwald, Kornblith, and Greenwald (1983) used both self-instructional training and paradoxical intention for treating agoraphobia. Paradoxical intention treatment emphasized how anxious thoughts led to the feared anxiety in a self-fulfilling way and instructed subjects to reverse their thoughts regarding their fears. Both treatments were effective, with paradoxical intention being somewhat superior at posttreatment. In a later comparison of paradoxical intention, muscle relaxation, and graduated exposure for agoraphobia, all three treatments produced significant improvement, although the behavioral treatments produced effects more rapidly (Michelson, Mavissakalian, & Marchione, 1985).

Emmelkamp, Van der Helm, van Zanten, and Plochg (1980) compared the effectiveness of gradual exposure *in vivo* against *in vivo* exposure plus self-instructional training for 15 obsessive compulsive patients. The self-instructional procedures were similar to those of Meichenbaum's stress inoculation therapy. The addition of self-instructional training did not bring about greater improvement. This kind of design, however, does not yield much information about the efficacy of cognitive therapy. Studies with combination treatments for depression have often failed to find an advantage of combined over individual treatments, and the same may prove to hold true for anxiety disorders as well.

No studies using a purely cognitive treatment for panic disorder have been reported as yet. However, Clark, Salkovskis, and Chalkley (1985) tested a cognitive behavioral treatment on 18 patients with panic attacks. Therapy was based on the theory that some persons react to stress by hyperventilating, causing a drop in the partial pressure of carbon dioxide and thus resulting in physiological symptoms. Apprehensive thoughts concerning these sensations increase the hyperventilation and the symptoms. Treatment focused on educating patients about this cycle, and patients were led to reattribute their panic attacks to the hyperventilation rather than to a serious illness, such as epilepsy or heart disease. Subjects were also trained in slow breathing techniques. Frequency of panic attacks showed a sharp and significant decrease in response to this treatment package during the first 2 weeks of therapy. Further sessions employed a wider variety of standard cognitive and behavioral techniques. Treatment gains were maintained at the 6-month and 2-year follow-ups. A second study (Salkovskis, Jones, & Clark, 1986) replicated the results of the first study. It also demonstrated that the partial pressure of carbon dioxide of panic subjects was significantly below normal before treatment began and rose to normal levels by the end of treatment.

In a meta-analysis comparing cognitive therapy and desensitization for a variety of clinical and subclinical anxiety conditions (Berman, Miller, & Massman, 1985), results were found to be strongly dependent on the theoretical allegiance of the researchers. Cognitive and behavioral researchers tended to find in favor of their preferred treatments. The meta-analysis found no significant differences in outcome between the two techniques, although there was a small nonsignificant difference favoring cognitive therapy.

At the current time, there is not enough evidence to judge the value of cognitive therapy for anxiety disorders. Too much of the evidence that does exist is based on subclinical populations or on studies by behavioral researchers using selected cognitive interventions. Moreover, attempts to maintain a distinction between cognitive and behavioral procedures and thus protect internal validity may have actually caused problems with internal validity. It is not possible to fully separate cognitive and behavioral techniques. For example, cognitive therapists often encourage patients to discover negative thoughts by participating in the feared situations, noting the automatic thoughts, and testing them out.

Because there are several types of possible cognitive interventions for anxiety, it would be most fruitful for these to be compared against each other before more comparisons are done between cognitive therapy and other therapies. At the current time, there is no single cognitive therapy of anxiety that is generally accepted, as there is with depression. Beck, Emery, and Greenberg (1985) have written extensively on cognitive techniques for use with anxiety. This will hopefully lead to greater delineation and comparison of specific cognitive interventions.

Once it is determined which cognitive interventions are most effective for anxiety, comparison with other treatments will be more meaningful.

## PSYCHOSOMATIC DISORDERS

Cognitive behavior therapy has been applied to the treatment of several psychosomatic disorders, including tension and migraine headaches, duodenal ulcers, and myofascial pain. In addition, it has been used with Type A behavior. Holroyd, Andrasik, and Westbrook (1977) treated tension headaches with ''stress-coping training'' that consisted of an extensive set of cognitively oriented therapeutic procedures based upon Beck (1976), Goldfried, Decenteceo, and Weinberg (1974), and Meichenbaum (1974). The patients receiving ''stress-coping training'' showed a marked reduction in headache activity that was maintained at follow-up, whereas biofeedback patients showed more modest improvement and a waiting-list control group showed no improvement. All subjects receiving stress-coping training reported decreases in headache activity at posttreatment, with improvement ranging from 43% to 100%.

Lake, Rainey, and Papsdorf (1979) included rational-emotive therapy in a comparative study of different biofeedback procedures in the management of migraine headache. Digital temperature biofeedback alone and feedback combined with three 30-minute RET sessions were found to be no more effective than control conditions. However, three 30-minute sessions would not seem to be an adequate test of the potential effectiveness of RET with migraine headache.

Stenn, Mothersill, and Brooke (1979) successfully applied biofeedback and cognitive-behavioral modification in treating patients with myofascial pain dysfunction syndrome (MPDS), also known as temporomandibular joint pain (TMJ). Patients treated had a diagnosis of TMJ for at least 1 year with complete failure of previous conservative treatment. Eight treatment sessions were provided to all subjects. The first half hour consisted of relaxation training (half of the patients received biofeedback-assisted relaxation training) and the second half hour of one or more modules of CBT, such as examining self-statements during and prior to the occurrences of pain, developing coping skills such as assertiveness, and the use of rational-emotive therapy and stress-inoculation training. All subjects showed significant reduction in subjective-rated pain and in MPDS signs and symptoms, as rated by an independent physician blind to the treatments and treatment assignments. Because all subjects received a combination of relaxation training and CBT, it is not clear how much of the change may have been brought about by cognitive-behavior modification.

Duodenal ulcer patients were treated by Brooks and Richardson (1980) in an eight-session cognitive-behavioral protocol. The first four sessions focused on anxiety management training, which included cognitive restructuring and relaxation training. The next four sessions consisted of assertiveness training, including both cognitive and behavioral rehearsal of appropriate expression of negative emotions and correction of erroneous beliefs about asserting oneself. Treatment procedures were followed by a reduction of symptom severity, fewer days of pain, and a reduction in consumption of antacid medication. During the 3-year follow-up only one of the nine treatment patients had a recurrence of duodenal ulcer. This was a statistically significant difference from the eight control patients, five of whom required surgery and/or were victims of ulcer recurrence.

Jenni and Wollersheim (1979) compared the efficacy of stress management training, cognitive therapy, and no treatment for altering Type A personality characteristics. Stress management training consisted of visual rehearsal in which anxiety-arousing scenes were followed by adaptive responses (e.g., relaxation), whereas cognitive therapy consisted of cognitive restructuring (Ellis, 1973). Cognitive therapy was more effective than both stress-management training and no treatment in reducing self-perceived levels of Type A behavior, but neither treatment reduced subjects' cholesterol levels nor blood pressure.

Cognitive-behavior therapy would appear to be quite promising with some stress-related psychosomatic disorders, especially if one primarily considers those studies meeting basic methodological standards (treatments are not confounded, adequate control groups and amounts of treatment). Studies meeting these criteria are those by Holroyd *et al.* (1977) on tension headache and by Brooks and Richardson (1980) on duodenal ulcer.

## IMPULSE CONTROL DISORDERS

A cognitive behavioral treatment of adults with impulse control disorders has been described by Watkins (1977, 1983) and Boyer, Beckham, and Buck (1987). Boyer *et al.* reported treatment results for 154 persons for either (1) shoplifting, (2) rape or anger discontrol, (3) child molestation, or (4) exhibitionism. Only 13% of treatment completers were rearrested within 2 years of the termination, whereas 37% of treatment dropouts had been rearrested by that time. However, there was no control group to compare treatment results against. A specific goal for sexual offenders was to increase age-appropriate sexual behavior. Among sexual offenders there was a significant change away from the categories of "nonmarried, nondating," and "married, without sexual relations" to the categories of "nonmarried, dating" and "married with sexual relations". Predictors of rearrest were dropping out of treatment, being treated for pedophilia, high levels of denial, high overall MMPI elevations, and not paying for treatment (either refusing to pay or having treatment paid for by the state).

Novaco (1975, 1977a,b) has also reported success with a cognitive-behavioral approach for anger control with adults. Most studies of impulsive behavior, however, have been with children or adolescents. For instance, group anger-control training has been reported to be effective with institutionalized adolescents (Feindler, Ecton, Kingsley, & Dubey, 1986). As a result of treatment, there was an increase in self-control and appropriate verbalizations, a decrease in hostile verbalizations during conflict situations, and lower rates of fines and restrictions during treatment and follow-up. In another study of 76 aggressive boys (Lochman, Burch, Curry, & Lampron, 1984), two cognitively oriented treatments (anger coping and anger coping plus goal setting) were compared with two control treatments (goal setting minimal treatment and no treatment). Both anger-coping interventions improved aggressive and disruptive behavior to a greater degree than the two control treatments. The cognitive-behavioral treatments appeared to have their greatest impact with those boys who initially had the poorest problem-solving skills and the greatest amounts of disruptive behavior (Lochman, Lampron, Burch, & Curry, 1985).

Cognitive and relaxation treatments for anger were compared by Hazaleus and Deffenbacher (1986). Both resulted in significant anger reduction. Although some minor differences favored the cognitive intervention posttreatment, the differences disappeared by the 4-week follow-up. Compared to the control condition, both treatments led to less general and state anger, fewer physical symptoms of anger, lower daily ratings of anger, and better coping with verbal antagonism in response to provocations. A 1-year follow-up also showed a continued significant reduction in general anger for both treatment groups. However, cognitive coping skills for anger reduction appeared to generalize and assist subjects to reduce general anxiety, whereas training in relaxation coping skills surprisingly did not produce this effect. Overall, the results for the cognitive condition were said to have replicated those in the literature, but those for the relaxation condition were somewhat stronger than previously found (e.g., Novaco, 1975; Schlichter & Horan, 1981).

Combination treatments have also been examined. Kendall and Braswell (1982) randomly assigned 27 children with low self-control to either a behavioral condition, a combined cognitive-behavioral condition, or an attention control condition. Both active treatments were associated with improvements on blind ratings of hyperactivity, but only the combined cognitive-behavioral condition led to improvements in teacher ratings of self-control. The author viewed cognitive training as adding significantly to treatment effectiveness, but the behavioral component was viewed as essential. In a review of treatment studies of anger and impulse control, Kendall (1982) concluded that interventions that combine cognitive and behavioral training are superior to cognitive or behavioral training alone. There have been a number of other reports of successful use of self-control training programs involving cognitive behavioral therapy with hyperactive children (e.g., Barkley, Copeland, & Sivage, 1980; Kendall & Zupin, 1981; Neilans & Israel, 1981). Not all investigators, however, have found cognitive training to be effective with hyperactive children. Brown, Wynne, and Medenis (1985), in a comparison of cognitive therapy with methylphenidate found that only those children in the medication and the medication-plus-cognitive-therapy conditions demonstrated improvement in attentional deployment and behavioral ratings. Furthermore, the data indicated that the combined medication and cognitive-therapy condition was no more effective than that condition involving medication alone. This lack of any additive effect of cognitive therapy when combined with a stimulant has been reported elsewhere (e.g., Abikoff & Gittelman, 1985; Brown *et al.*, 1986).

## SUBSTANCE ABUSE

Although the area of substance abuse has only begun to be examined by cognitive researchers, two encouraging studies have appeared. Luborsky, McLellan, Woody, O'Brien, and Auerbach (1985) compared cognitive psychotherapy, supportive expressive psychotherapy, and drug counseling for male drug abuse clients. Patients in all three conditions improved. However, on the whole, patients receiving one of the two forms of psychotherapies had better outcomes than patients receiving drug counseling. Some differences in outcome between supportive-expressive therapy and CBT were found, in that supportive-expressive patients did better in psychological functioning and employment and CBT patients did particularly well avoiding legal problems. Oei and Jackson (1984) found encouraging results for CBT with problem drinkers on the amount of their alcohol consumption and on other other measures, such as neuroticism scores. Therapist behaviors were systematically varied, and one of the two types of cognitive treatment interventions resulted in substantial decreases in drinking and neuroticism scores (for further discussion, see the section Process Research—Experimental Manipulation). However, there was no control group, making overall interpretation of the efficacy of their treatments difficult.

## EATING DISORDERS

Several studies suggest that cognitive therapy can be an effective treatment for eating disorders. Connors, Johnson, and Stuckey (1984) used a multiple baseline approach to test a psychoeducational intervention for bulimic behavior with 20 women subjects. Cognitive restructuring was only one portion of the intervention. There was a 70% reduction in binge/purge episodes following twelve 2-hour treatment sessions. Freeman, Sinclair, Turnbull, and Annandale (1985) have reported pilot data comparing behavioral, cognitive behavioral, and group interventions with bulimia. A control group was also included. The CBT treatment involved monitoring and challenging automatic thoughts, changing maladaptive cognitions regarding weight, improving self-esteem, and increasing assertiveness. Although only initial results were available, they suggested that there were clinically significant reductions in binge frequency and eating attitudes for all three therapies compared to the control group. Ordman and Kirschenbaum (1985) compared a course of cognitive-behavioral therapy lasting an average of 15 weeks with a three-session minimal educational intervention for treating bulimia.

Full-intervention clients were taught to identify unrealistic and self-defeating cognitions regarding their eating. In addition, they received exposure with response prevention and were taught to self-monitor binging and other food-related behavior. Subjects treated with the cognitive behavioral intervention reduced their frequency of binging/vomiting, improved their psychological adjustment, and changed their food-related attitudes to a statistically greater extent than minimal intervention clients.

In an obesity study, Collins, Rothblum, and Wilson (1986) treated subjects with cognitive therapy, behavioral therapy, cognitive-behavioral therapy, or a nutrition-exercise (control) regimen. Cognitive treatment focused on thoughts regarding the role of food in subjects' lives. A wide variety of cognitive techniques were used. Behavioral techniques focused on stimulus control of eating cues, self-monitoring of calorie intake, and exercise. Although all treatments resulted in increased weight reduction compared to the control intervention, the result was statistically significant only for subjects receiving the behavioral and combined cognitive-behavioral treatments.

## THE SEARCH FOR SPECIFIC EFFECTS

The positive outcome for cognitive therapy in many of the previously mentioned studies does not establish the claim that it is cognitive change that is bringing about symptom change. It is quite possible that processes held in common with other therapies (e.g., therapeutic alliance, establishment of hope) may be the central catalytic agents. A finding that cognitive therapy produces *specific effects* (and not just greater effects) compared to other therapies would strengthen the probability that it possesses unique and effective therapy elements. Such a result was found by Rush, Beck, Kovacs, Weissenburger, and Hollon (1982) who reported differential effects of cognitive therapy and imipramine on hopelessness and self-concept in depression. Compared with imipramine, cognitive therapy resulted in significantly greater reductions in hopelessness and more generalized gains in self-concept. McNamara and Horan (1986) found evidence for greater change on cognitive measures for cognitive therapy subjects but not for greater change on behavioral measures (such as the Pleasant Events Schedule) for behavior-therapy subjects.

Apart from these two studies, however, specific effects generally have not been found for cognitive therapy. For instance, Simons, Garfield, and Murphy (1984) found that not only were cognitive therapy and pharmacotherapy equally effective in bringing about remission of clinical depression but that there was no difference in the rate of improvement on any of three cognitive measures: the Cognitive Response Test (Watkins & Rush, 1983), the Dysfunctional Attitude Scale (Weisman & Beck, 1978), or the Automatic Thoughts Questionnaire (Hollon & Kendall, 1980). Zeiss et al. (1979) compared a type of cognitive therapy with two different behavioral interventions (assertiveness training and increasing pleasant events) with moderately depressed patients. The three treatments produced equivalent symptomatic results. In addition, there were no differences on three respective target-dependent (cognitive and behavioral) measures. In a similar type of comparison, Rehm's self-control therapy was modified to be addressed toward cognitive change, behavioral change, or both (Rehm et al., 1987). The treatments not only produced similar symptomatic improvement but also equivalent improvement on cognitive and behavioral target measures. Imber, Pilkonis, Sotsky, and Elkin (1986) failed to find any difference in impact on the cognitive items of the Hamilton Rating Scale for Depression (helplessness, pessimism, worthlessness) between cognitive therapy and imipramine. In addition, Imber et al. examined the TDCRP data on other measures salient to cognitive processes, including the Dysfunctional Attitude Scale and cognitive items on the Beck Depression Inventory. Only the need for social approval factor of the DAS was found to respond preferentially to CBT over Interpersonal Psychotherapy and imipramine.

Silverman, Silverman, and Eardley (1984) treated depressed patients using a combination of pharmacotherapy and emotional support. The Dysfunctional Attitude Scale was used as a measure of depressive attitudes. Patients improved greatly on DAS scores and at posttreatment were essentially at the same average score as the normal subjects in the original validation sample for the DAS (Weissman & Beck, 1978). Similarly, Hamilton and Abramson (1983) found that depressed patients treated on an inpatient psychiatric unit were indistinguishable at discharge from control subjects on DAS and Attributional Style Questionnaire (Peterson *et al.*, 1982) scores. Neither of these studies treated patients using cognitive therapy, and yet patients attained scores on cognitive target measures in the normal range at posttreatment. This suggests that cognitive therapy is not likely to be much more effective than standard psychiatric treatment in improving dysfunctional attitudes or attributional styles during the course of a hospital stay.

In summary, the evidence for specific effects for cognitive therapy is very weak at the current time. If specific effects do occur in cognitive therapy for depression, they are likely to be limited in scope, and they have generally escaped being measured by the research instruments that have been used thus far.

## PROCESS RESEARCH

Until recently, outcome studies have usually been limited to demonstrating that a particular treatment intervention (often a treatment "package") is followed at some distant point in time by symptom alleviation and other changes. As a result, there generally has been little evidence that specific components within a treatment are related to equally specific proximal or distal changes. One role of process research is to reveal the most effective components of psychotherapy and the causal relationship between those ingredients and client change.

The identification of processes in psychotherapy and the demonstration of their relationship to change is the ultimate goal of the scientific study of psychotherapy. Kiesler (1981) has argued that scientific outcome research requires process analysis of both therapist and patient interview behaviors. Specification of exactly what these processes are has in the past often centered on broad concepts such as "combating demoralization" (Frank, 1974) and "active participation of the patient" (Gomes-Schwartz, 1978), or on relationship variables, for example, "warmth, genuineness, and empathy" (Truax & Carkuff, 1967) and "a helping relationship with a therapist" (Luborsky *et al.*, 1975). In addition, process studies have often focused on measurement of processes within therapy without attempting to relate these processes to outcome, or they have used outcome criteria that were poorly specified or overly subjective (therapist or patient self-reports).

### Significance of Demonstrated Outcome

A fruitful way for process psychotherapy research to proceed would be to examine the processes in a therapy whose efficacy has been well demonstrated. Cognitive therapy would thus seem to be an excellent choice among psychotherapies for relating process to outcome. Greenberg (1981) has commented that

> one of the most encouraging features of the cognitive behavioral approach is its combination of a focus on internal mediating events with its rigorous attempts at measuring and evaluating their change. . . . This is a domain in which research holds promise of making a major contribution to the practice of psychotherapy by illuminating some of the specific mechanisms of client change in therapy. (p. 30)

There are two basic approaches that may be taken toward process analysis. One approach, the experimental design, involves manipulating key elements of a therapy (i.e., therapist or client behaviors) and examining proximal and distal effects. Effects studied may be either symptomatic change or subsequent patient behaviors in therapy. A second approach allows the therapeutic process to unfold naturally and entails observation and measurement of key processes. Each of these approaches possesses advantages and disadvantages.

### THE NATURALISTIC APPROACH

The main advantage of the naturalistic approach is that artificial manipulations by the experimenter do not obscure the interaction between patient and therapist. Experimental designs generally impose restraints on therapist behavior that can conceal any reciprocal, unfolding interactions. A naturalistic design is likely to be more suitable than an experimental design, for example, to study the effects of patient noncompliance and resistance on therapist actions and subsequent patient actions in reaction to therapist behavior. Patient noncompliance may be followed by a variety of therapist reactions. Experimental manipulations of therapist behavior would interfere with observing how therapist behavior is typically affected by noncompliance and, in turn, how any such resulting therapist behavior then affects the client.

### Attributional Process Analysis

Naturalistic designs are useful for studying small numbers of patients intensively over long periods of time. Peterson, Luborsky, and Seligman (1983) analyzed tapes of an extended analysis of a man with chronic depression. Using the revised learned helplessness model (Abramson et al., 1978), it was predicted that global, stable, and internal attributions for bad events would lead the patient to be more depressed. Tapes of therapy sessions were monitored at places where there was an improvement or worsening of mood, and attributions of the patient before and after each mood shift were rated. Peterson et al. (1982) discovered that mood worsening tended to follow global, stable, and internal attributions by the patient.

### Path Analysis

Another way that naturalistic designs may be informative about the process of cognitive therapy is through a path analysis of symptom and behavior change. For example, it might be hypothesized that in cognitive therapy, cognitive change (C; e.g., improvement in self-esteem and hopefulness) precedes behavioral change (B; e.g., assertiveness, participation in social events), and that both have direct effects on mood (M). A path analysis model could be constructed and tested:

$$C \rightarrow B \rightarrow M$$

Of course another model could be constructed to test the opposite hypothesis: that it is behavioral change that precedes cognitive change. More elaborate models could be constructed that would include vegetative symptoms of depression, social support, environmental stressors, and so on.

### Task Analysis

Rice and Greenberg (1984) have proposed that psychotherapy research focus on patterns of change within therapy. This requires analysis of what constitutes a particular type of pattern and of "markers" that indicate the beginning of such a pattern. Such a method is interested in predictable patterns of therapist and patient behavior once such a marker occurs. Safran (1985) has suggested that one type of marker in cognitive therapy is a negative comment by a patient with no awareness of the possibility that the thought is not realistic (patient is fully immersed in the thought). A second type of marker occurs when a patient has a negative thought but knows intellectually that it is not likely to be true (divided awareness). He suggests that different therapist interventions are required depending on the type of marker.

### Other Naturalistic Studies

Persons and Burns (1985) studied one session for each of 17 depressed and anxious patients in cognitive therapy. As part of normal cognitive therapy procedure, patients were asked to describe their feelings about an upsetting event and to rate the intensity of their feelings. The degree of belief in automatic thoughts related to the events was also recorded. After the therapist and patient worked on formulating rational responses, intensity of feelings and degree of belief in automatic thoughts were again rated. Improvement in automatic thoughts and relationship with the therapist (rated after each session) were both statistically related to session outcome. Two other factors—presence of a personality disorder and high degree of belief in automatic thoughts at the beginning of a session—were negative predictors of mood change. Although the study was limited by small sample size and heterogeneity of diagnoses, it is one of the first to seriously tackle the foremost issue of process research in cognitive therapy—whether cognitive change leads to mood change. Unfortunately, its correlational nature does not rule out the possibility that it is actually mood change that is causing the cognitive change or that a third factor is causing both. Another study by Safran et al. (1987) also addresses the relationship of cognitive change and mood change within session. Cognitive change, as rated by the patient and the therapist, did not predict mood shift in the session, but it did predict degree of problem resolution between that session and the next.

Luborsky et al. (1985) studied three types of treatments for male drug abuse patients: cognitive-behavioral therapy, supportive-expressive therapy, and drug counseling. Therapist ability to develop a helping alliance as measured by the Helping Alliance Questionnaire was highly predictive of outcome. In addition, the degree to which sessions embodied CBT techniques correlated positively and significantly with improved legal status, employment status, and psychological status. The presence of supportive-expressive qualities in therapist behavior also correlated well with outcome in all three treatment groups. Purity of the CBT intervention (i.e., being free of non-CBT techniques) was significantly and positively related to better outcomes, suggesting that greater therapist adherence to the CBT manual led to better outcomes. However, it was noted by Luborsky et al. that patients' responsiveness to their therapist may have enabled the therapist to adhere to their intended technique. In fact, there is some evidence along these lines that individual differences do affect therapist adherence. Vallis and Shaw (1987) found that patient difficulty was "strongly and inversely related to therapist competency." Ratings of higher patient difficulty were associated with lower ratings of therapist competence. This relationship held both across cases and within cases. That is, not only did patient difficulty averaged across sessions covary with therapist competency averaged across sessions, but covariation was also found within series of sessions of therapist–patient dyads.

The importance of individual differences among patients in determining outcome has also been noted by Fennell and Teasdale (1987). Patients who improved rapidly in response to CBT for depression (labeled *steeps* for the gradient of change) maintained their gains and were less depressed at termination and followup than initially slow responders (*slights*). Steeps and slights were found to differ on several measures. Steeps were more likely to positively endorse the cognitive conceptualization of depression. They also received a greater positive benefit from the first homework assignment. Finally, they scored higher on a measure of depression about being depressed.

As stated before, one of the primary problems with the naturalistic approach is interpreting direction of causality. In the experimental approach, therapist behavior is protected to some degree from the influence of patient behavior, and, therefore, interpreting directionality of effect is less difficult. The experimental approach is also well suited to study low frequency or novel therapist behaviors, which would not be likely to occur in naturalistic studies.

One experimental approach to process research involves dismantling a therapy into its component parts, as has been done by Rehm *et al.* (1981) with self-control therapy. Dismantling involves a systematic variation of treatment components across groups of patients. Rehm studied four versions of self-control therapy: self-monitoring only, self-monitoring plus self-evaluation, self-monitoring plus self-reinforcement, and a combination of all three components. The self-evaluation component was similar to cognitive therapy in that it taught patients to set realistic goals and make accurate attributions for success and failure. The results were very surprising. All treatment conditions did better than the waiting-list controls. Differences among the three treatment groups were minor and tended to occur on some outcome measures but not others. In a later dismantling study (Kornblith, Rehm, O'Hara, & Lamparski, 1983), the time of treatment was lengthened from 7 to 12 weeks. Four treatments were compared: self-control principles without homework; self-monitoring plus self-evaluation; comprehensive self-control therapy; and a psychodynamic therapy group as a control. Again, no significant differences were found.

In a somewhat similar design, Jarrett and Nelson (1987) varied the sequencing of three main cognitive therapy components for depression: self-monitoring, logical analysis, and hypothesis testing. Each group received self-monitoring first, but half of the subjects were taught logical analysis before hypothesis testing, whereas the other half received hypothesis testing before logical analysis. By conducting assessments of depressive symptoms, automatic thoughts, pleasant events, and interpersonal functioning before and after each of the three components, it was possible to determine whether hypothesis testing or logical analysis was more efficacious. Self-monitoring alone was associated with reductions only in transient mood as measured by the Depression Adjective Checklist (DACL). Both logical analysis and hypothesis testing were associated with significant improvements on all measures. The interaction of time $\times$ sequence was not significant for any of the dependent measures, suggesting that hypothesis testing and logical analysis were approximately equal in effectiveness. On some measures, exposure to all components combined was associated with greater improvement than exposure to only logical analysis or hypothesis testing. However, for other measures, the combination (or more treatment) equaled the effect of logical analysis or hypothesis testing alone.

Zettle (1987) compared the efficacy of three CBT components of treating depression: distancing of thoughts, rational restructuring, and behavioral homework. Subjects receiving training in both distancing and rational restructuring improved more than subjects trained in rational restructuring only. In addition, subjects given behavioral assignments improved more than subjects who were not.

Two studies have compared the effects of thought exploration and thought challenge. Straatmeyer and Watkins (1974) and Teasdale and Fennell (1982) had one group of subjects to explore and also to challenge their negative thoughts and another group to only identify thoughts without challenging them. In both studies, the thought-challenging condition led to greater immediate improvement in mood than thought exploration. These studies and the one by Jarrett and Nelson provide very suggestive evidence that thought monitoring and exploration of negative thoughts alone are ineffective in treating depression.

Still another way of comparing component procedures of CBT has been reported by Arnkoff (1986). Students with test anxiety received either training in coping self-statements or in restructuring of irrational beliefs. Whereas the coping group showed more improvement compared to the control group, there was no significant difference in effects between the two cognitive treatments. Moreover, there were also no posttreatment differences between the two conditions on the Irrational Beliefs Test (Jones, 1969) that would logically be expected to change more in the cognitive restructuring treatment.

Oei and Jackson (1984) tested two different styles of cognitive therapy with problem drinkers. Both treatments used a combined cognitive restructuring and social skills treatment. In one group, future-oriented statements and positive self-statements were reinforced. In addition, therapists in that group used self-disclosure to demonstrate how they had dealt with their own maladaptive attitudes. In the second group, therapists avoided self-disclosure and giving opinions; they did not reinforce positive self-statements, healthy attitudes, or future-oriented statements; and they did not challenge negative self-statements. There were equal amounts of positive and aversive reinforcement given to each group, but it was given randomly to the second group. Changes in cognitions were found to precede or to parallel behavioral changes in patients. Subjects in the first group had more positive and future-oriented statements and fewer negative statements in therapy sessions. The first group also improved more on behavioral ratings of social skill and made greater decreases in alcohol consumption. Moreover, the first group maintained their decrease in drinking during a 6-month follow-up period, whereas the second group returned to pretreatment levels.

## IMPORTANT VARIABLES TO BE SCRUTINIZED IN COGNITIVE PROCESS RESEARCH

### Patient Difficulty

Cognitive therapists have recognized that there is wide variability in patient difficulty (Fennell & Teasdale, 1982). There is little empirical evidence as to the best methods of effectively overcoming noncompliance, although there have been some clinical suggestions on this topic (Burns, Adams, & Anastopoulos, 1985). This is a field that would seem to hold considerable promise for process researchers.

Presence of a personality disorder would be one variable likely to predict noncompliance (Persons & Burns, 1985), although clinical experience suggests that dependent personalities and some other types may actually be more compliant. Vallis and Shaw (1987) investigated the types of patient characteristics that were related to observer ratings of patient difficulty. Negative patient attitude toward the therapist was the strongest predictor of patient difficulty. Other variables that were significantly associated with patient difficulty were greater patient depression, lower patient activity levels, and less willingness for self-exploration. Simons, Lustman, Wetzel, and Murphy (1986) found that patients scoring high on learned resourcefulness as measured by the Self Control Schedule (Rosenbaum, 1980) were more responsive to cognitive therapy for depression, and patients scoring low on the SCS responded preferentially to a tricyclic antidepressant. Rehm *et al.* (1987) also found high scores on the Self-Control Schedule to be predictive of success for all three treatments in their study: cognitively targeted, behaviorally targeted, and combined target self-control therapy. Strength of dysfunctional assumptions may also have an effect on treatment outcome. Keller (1983) found that depressed patients who had high Dysfunctional Attitude Scale scores responded less well to cognitive therapy than those with lower scores. It is unclear how strong dysfunctional attitudes and low levels of learned resourcefulness may affect outcome—whether they affect patient behavior in therapy or inhibit symptom improvement in some other ways.

### Therapist Behavior—Purity and Competence of Cognitive Technique

The research of Luborsky *et al.* (1985) suggests that "pure" CBT interventions are more effective than interventions that blend other approaches. It would seem logical that introduction of non-CBT techniques might confuse patients and inhibit assimilation and consolidation of CBT coping skills. However, their research left unclear whether pure interventions were indeed more effective, or whether therapists were simply better able to remain true to "pure" cognitive interventions when patients were improving.

Competence is distinguished from "purity of intervention" in that it involves skillful use of all relevant aspects of cognitive therapy. For example, psychoanalytic process researchers have begun to abandon gross measures such as frequency of interpretations and have begun to investigate the "suitability" of interpretation on outcome (Silberschotz, Fretter, & Curtis, 1986). In the same way, therapist application of cognitive techniques may be skillful or unskilled in the way that it selects which negative thoughts and depressive behaviors to work on. Therapist interventions may lead toward or away from resolution of the patient's underlying cognitive schema. Little is known about relationship of competence in CBT in this sense and treatment outcome.

### Therapist and Patient Relationship

Because cognitive therapy emphasizes developing new ways of thinking, the relationship between therapist and patient is not always thought of as an important ingredient in CBT. Yet it is clearly spelled out as a necessary ingredient of cognitive therapy in Beck *et al.* (1979). Persons and Burns (1985) found relationship to relate to mood change during a single session, and Luborsky *et al.* (1985) found patient perception of the therapist's ability to form a helping relationship to correlate with outcome across all three treatments they studied, including CBT. Further work is needed to determine whether relationship provides a truly independent contribution to outcome, as suggested in the previously mentioned two studies, or whether it only potentiates the assimilation of cognitive techniques.

### Process Research in Cognitive Therapy—Conclusion

It is too early to draw any conclusions from the available process literature. Most of the methodology is quite new. Researchers are only beginning to test the primary premise of cognitive therapy—that it is cognitive change that causes symptomatic improvement. The next decade is likely to see an increasing amount of research focused on this issue, which is of the highest importance. With regard to predictors of outcome in cognitive therapy, the following constructs are promising candidates: purity and competence of CBT technique, quality of the therapist–patient relationship, cognitive style of the patient, and "patient difficulty," a broad concept that will undoubtedly prove to be very complex and heterogeneous.

### INSTRUMENTATION AVAILABLE FOR PROCESS AND OUTCOME RESEARCH

Several instruments are now available for outcome and process research in cognitive therapy. With regard to measurement of patient variables, the Beck Depression Inventory and the Hamilton Rating Scale for Depression have traditionally been the measures of choice among the multitude available to researchers for measuring depression. Because the BDI has items closely identified with the cognitive triad, a subset of BDI items can also be used to measure it specifically. The Hopelessness Scale (Beck, Weissman, Lester, & Trexler, 1974) specifically measures one aspect of the triad—view of the future. An instrument specifically designed to measure the cognitive triad—the Cognitive Triad Inventory (Beckham, Leber, Watkins, Boyer, & Cook, 1986)—is designed to measure the entire triad and to be sensitive to changes in it during a session or across the course of treatment. Other instruments measure patients' cognitive styles, for example, the Cognitive Bias Questionnaire (Krantz & Hammen, 1979); the Attributional Style Questionnaire (Peterson *et al.*, 1982); and the Self-Control Schedule (Rosenbaum, 1980). Other scales measure amounts of depressive cognitions (Automatic Thoughts Questionnaire; Hollon & Kendall, 1980), and tendency to use cognitive coping strategies (Coping Strategies Scales; Beckham & Adams, 1984). For a review of these and other instruments see Krantz and Hammen (1985) and Goldberg and Shaw (Chapter 3 in this book).

There does not appear to be a satisfactory means of measuring underlying core beliefs (dysfunctional assumptions). Two instruments have been used for this purpose, the Irrational Beliefs Test (Jones, 1969) and the Dysfunctional Attitude Scale (Weissman & Beck, 1978). However, although the DAS has been shown to have some value in predicting depressive relapse above and beyond BDI scores (Simons *et al.,* 1986), other studies suggest that the DAS simply reflects the presence or absence of depression. Two groups have suggested more idiographic approaches to assessment of core beliefs (Beckham, Boyer, Cook, Leber, & Watkins, 1984; Safran, Vallis, Segal, & Shaw, 1986), but no data on empirical validity of such methods have yet been presented.

The Cognitive Therapy Scale (Young & Beck, 1980) has been the measure primarily used thus far for scoring therapist behavior in cognitive therapy. It consists of two major sections, one measuring general interpersonal factors and a second measuring quality of application of cognitive techniques. Several studies using the CTS suggest that it can provide reliable, valid ratings of therapist competency when trained raters are used (Dobson, Shaw, & Vallis, 1985; Hollon *et al.,* 1981; Vallis, Shaw, & Dobson, 1986; Young, Shaw, Beck, & Budenz, 1981). Intraclass reliability coefficients have ranged from .54 to .96. Although the CTS was designed to assess competency, other measures have been designed to assess the degree to which therapist behaviors are consistent with the cognitive approach (DeRubeis, Hollon, Evans, & Bemis, 1982; Luborsky, Woody, McLellan, O'Brien, & Rosenzweig, 1982).

# REFERENCES

Abikoff, H., & Gittelman, R. (1985). Hyperactive children treated with stimulants: Is cognitive training a useful adjunct? *Archives of general Psychiatry, 42,* 953–961.

Abramson, L. Y., Seligman, M. E. P., & Teasdale, J. D. (1978). Learned helplessness in humans: Critique and reformulation. *Journal of Abnormal Psychology, 87,* 102–109.

American Psychiatric Association. (1980). *Diagnostic and statistical manual of mental disorders* (3rd ed.). Washington, DC: Author.

Arnkoff, D. B. (1986). A comparison of the coping and restructuring components of cognitive restructuring. *Cognitive Therapy and Research, 10,* 147–158.

Barkley, R. A., Copeland, A. P., & Sivage, C. (1980). A self-control classroom for hyperactive children. *Autism and Developmental Disorders, 10,* 75–89.

Beck, A. T. (1976). *Cognitive therapy and the emotional disorders.* New York: International Universities Press.

Beck, A. T., Weissman, A., Lester, D., & Trexler, L. (1974). The measurement of pessimism: The Hopelessness Scale. *Journal of Consulting and Clinical Psychology, 42,* 861–865.

Beck, A. T., Rush, A. J., Shaw, B. F., & Emery, G. (1979). *Cognitive therapy of depression: A treatment manual.* New York: Guilford Press.

Beck, A. T., Emery, G., & Greenberg, R. L. (1985). *Anxiety disorders and phobias: A cognitive perspective.* New York: Basic Books.

Beck, A. T., Hollon, S. D., Young, J. E., Bedrosian, R. C., & Budenz, D. (1985). Treatment of depression with cognitive therapy and amitriptyline. *Archives of General Psychiatry, 42,* 142–148.

Beckham, E. E., & Adams, R. L. (1984). Coping behavior in depression: Report on a new scale. *Behavior Research and Therapy, 22,* 71–75.

Beckham, E. E., Boyer, J. L., Cook, J. B., Leber, W. R., & Watkins, J. T. (1984, June). *Development of instrumentation for process research in cognitive therapy of depression.* Paper presented at the meeting of the Society for Psychotherapy Research, Lake Louise, Alberta, Canada.

Beckham, E. E., Leber, W. R., Watkins, J. T., Boyer, J. L., & Cook, J. B. (1986). Development of an instrument to measure Beck's cognitive triad: The Cognitive Triad Inventory. *Journal of Consulting and Clinical Psychology, 54,* 566–567.

Berman, J. S., Miller, C., & Massman, P. J. (1985). Cognitive therapy versus systematic desensitization: Is one treatment superior? *Psychological Bulletin, 97*, 451–461.

Biran, M., & Wilson, G. T. (1981). Treatment of phobic disorders using cognitive and exposure methods: A self-efficacy analysis. *Journal of Consulting and Clinical Psychology, 49*, 886–899.

Blackburn, I. M., Bishop, S., Glen, A. I. M., Whalley, L. J., & Christie, J. E. (1981). The efficacy of cognitive therapy in depression: A treatment trial using cognitive therapy and pharmacotherapy, each alone and in combination. *British Journal of Psychiatry, 139*, 181–189.

Blackburn, I. M., Eunson, K. M., & Bishop, S. (1986). A two-year naturalistic followup of depressed patients treated with cognitive therapy, pharmacotherapy and a combination of both. *Journal of Affective Disorders, 10*, 67–75.

Boyer, J. L., Beckham, E. E., & Buck, P. (1987, June). *A cognitive behavioral treatment of impulse control disorders: A naturalistic outcome study and follow-up.* Paper presented at the meeting of the Society for Psychotherapy Research, Ulm, Germany.

Brooks, G. R., & Richardson, F. C. (1980). Emotional skills training: A treatment program for duodenal ulcer. *Behavior Therapy, 11*, 198–207.

Brown, R. T., Wynne, M. E., Medenis, R. (1985). Methylphenidate and cognitive therapy: A comparison of treatment approaches in hyperactive boys. *Journal of Abnormal Child Psychology, 13*, 69–87.

Brown, R. T., Wynne, M. E., Borden, K. A., Clingerman, S., R., Geniesse, R., & Spunt, A. L. (1986). Methylphenidate and cognitive therapy in children with attention deficit disorder: A double-blind trial. *Developmental and Behavioral Pediatrics, 7*, 163–170.

Burns, D. D., Adams, R. L., & Anastopoulos, A. D. (1985). The role of self-help assignments in the treatment of depression. In E. E. Beckham & W. R. Leber (Eds.), *Handbook of depression: Treatment, assessment, and research* (pp. 634–668). Homewood, IL: Dorsey Press.

Clark, D. M., Salkovskis, P. M., & Chalkley, A. J. (1985). Respiratory control as a treatment for panic attacks. *Journal of Behavior Therapy and Experimental Psychiatry, 16*, 23–30.

Collins, R. L., Rothblum, E. D., & Wilson, G. T. (1986). The comparative efficacy of cognitive and behavioral approaches to the treatment of obesity. *Cognitive Therapy and Research, 10*, 299–318.

Comaz-Diaz, L. (1981). Effects of cognitive and behavioral group treatment on the depressive symptomatology of Puerto Rican women. *Journal of Consulting and Clinical Psychology, 49*, 627–632.

Connors, M. E., Johnson, C. L., & Stuckey, M. K. (1984). Treatment of bulimia with brief psychoeducational group therapy. *American Journal of Psychiatry, 141*, 1512–1516.

de Jong, R., Treiber, R., & Henrich, G. (1986). Effectiveness of two psychological treatments for inpatients with severe and chronic depressions. *Cognitive Therapy and Research, 10*, 645–663.

DeRubeis, R., Hollon, S., Evans, M., & Bemis, K. (1982). Can psychotherapies for depression be descriminated? A systematic investigation of cognitive therapy and interpersonal therapy. *Journal of Consulting and Clinical Psychology, 50*, 744–756.

Dobson, K. S., Shaw, B. F., & Vallis, T. M. (1985). Reliability of a measure of the quality of cognitive therapy. *British Journal of Clinical Psychology, 24*, 295–300.

Elkin, I., Parloff, M. B., Hadley, S. W., & Autrey, J. H. (1985). NIMH Treatment of Depression Collaborative Research Program: Background and research plan. *Archives of General Psychiatry, 42*, 305–316.

Elkin, I., Shea, T., Watkins, J., & Collins, J. (May, 1986). *NIMH Treatment of Depression Collaborative Research Program: Comparative treatment outcome findings.* Paper presented at the meeting of the American Psychiatric Association, Washington, DC.

Ellis, A. (1973). *Humanistic psychotherapy.* New York: Julian Press.

Emmelkamp, P. M. G., & Mersch, P. (1982). Cognition and exposure *in vivo* in the treatment of agoraphobia: Short-term and delayed effects. *Cognitive Therapy and Research, 6*, 77–88.

Emmelkamp, P. M. G., Kuipers, A. C. M., & Eggeraat, J. B. (1978). Cognitive modification versus prolonged exposure *in vivo*: A comparison with agoraphobics as subjects. *Behavior Research and Therapy, 16*, 33–41.

Emmelkamp, P. M. G., Van der Helm, M., van Zanten, B. L., & Plochg, I. (1980). Treatment of obsessive-compulsive patients: The contribution of self-instructional training to the effectiveness of exposure. *Behavior Research and Therapy, 18*, 61–66.

Emmelkamp, P. M. G., Brilman, E., Kuiper, H., & Mersch, P. (1986). The treatment of agoraphobia: A comparison of self-instructional training, Rational Emotive Therapy, and exposure in vivo. *Behavior Therapy, 10*, 37–53.

Evans, M. D., Hollon, S. D., De Rubeis, R. J., Plasecki, J. M., Quason, V. B., & Vye, C. (1985, November). *Accounting for relapse in a treatment outcome study of depression.* Paper presented at the meeting of the Association for the Advancement of Behavior Therapy.

Feighner, J. R., Robins, E., Guze, S. B., Woodruff, R. A., Winokur, G., & Munoz, R. (1972). Diagnostic criteria for use in psychiatric research. *Archives of General Psychiatry, 26,* 57–63.

Feindler, E. L., Ecton, R. B., Kingsley, D., & Dubey, D. R. (1986). Group anger-control training for institutionalized psychiatric male adolescents. *Behavior Therapy, 17,* 109–123.

Fennell, M. J. V., & Teasdale, J. D. (1982). Cognitive therapy with chronic, drug-refractory depressed outpatients: A note of caution. *Cognitive Therapy and Research, 6,* 455–460.

Fennell, M. J. V., & Teasdale, J. D. (1988). Cognitive therapy for depression: Individual differences and the process of change. *Cognitive Therapy and Research, 11,* 253–271.

Frank, J. D. (1974). Psychotherapy: The restoration of moral. *American Journal of Psychiatry, 131,* 271–274.

Frank, J. D. (1979). The present status of outcome studies. *Journal of Consulting and Clinical Psychology, 47,* 310–317.

Freeman, C., Sinclair, F., Turnbull, J., & Annandale, A. (1985). Psychotherapy for bulimia: A controlled study. *Journal of Psychiatry Research, 19,* 473–478.

Gallagher, D. E., & Thompson, L. W. (1982). Treatment of major depressive disorder in older adult outpatients with brief psychotherapies. *Psychotherapy: Theory, Research and Practice, 19,* 482–490.

Goldfried, M. R., Decenteceo, E. T., & Weinberg, L. (1974). Systematic rational restructuring as a self-control technique. *Behavior Therapy, 5,* 247–254.

Gomes-Schwartz, B. (1978). Effective ingredients in psychotherapy: Prediction of outcome from process variables. *Journal of Consulting and Clinical Psychology, 46,* 1023–1035.

Greenberg, L. S. (1981). Advances in clinical intervention research: A decade review. *Canadian Psychology, 22,* 23–37.

Hamilton, E. W., & Abramson, L. Y. (1983). Cognitive patterns and major depressive disorder: A longitudinal study in a hospital setting. *Journal of Abnormal Psychology, 92,* 173–184.

Hazaleus, S. L., & Deffenbacher, J. L. (1986). Relaxation and cognitive treatments of anger. *Journal of Consulting and Clinical Psychology, 54,* 222–226.

Hollon, S. D., & Kendall, P. C. (1980). Cognitive Self-Statements in Depression: Development of an automatic thought questionnaire. *Cognitive Therapy and Research, 4,* 383–395.

Hollon, S. D., Mandell, M., Bemis, K., DeRubeis, R., Emerson, M., Evans, M., & Kress, M. (1981). *Reliability and validity of the Young Cognitive Therapy Scale.* Unpublished manuscript, University of Minnesota.

Holroyd, K. A., Andrasik, F., & Westbrook, T. (1977). Cognitive control of tension headache. *Cognitive Therapy and Research, 1,* 121–133.

Imber, S., Glanz, L. M., Elkin, I., Sotsky, S. M., Boyer, J. L., & Leber, W. R. (1986a). Ethical issues in psychotherapy research: Problems in a collaborative clinical trials study. *American Psychologist, 41,* 137–146.

Imber, S., Pilkonis, P., Sotsky, S., & Elkin, I. (May, 1986b). *NIMH Treatment of Depression Collaborative Research Program: Differential treatment effects.* Paper presented at the meeting of the American Psychiatric Association, Washington, DC.

Jarrett, R. B., & Nelson, R. O. (1987). Mechanisms of change in cognitive therapy of depression. *Behavior Therapy, 18*(3), 227–241.

Jenni, M. A., & Wollersheim, J. P. (1979). Cognitive therapy, stress management training, and the Type A behavior pattern. *Cognitive Therapy and Research, 3,* 61–73.

Jones, R. G. (1969). A factored measure of Ellis' irrational belief system, with personality and adjustment correlates. *Dissertation Abstracts International, 29,* 4379B–4380B. (University Microfilms No. 69-6443)

Keller, K. E. (1983). Dysfunctional attitudes and the cognitive therapy for depression. *Cognitive Therapy and Research, 7,* 437–444.

Kendall, P. C. (1982). Cognitive processes and procedures in behavior therapy. *In* C. M. Franks, G. T. Wilson, P. C. Kendall, & K. Brownell (Eds.), *Annual review of behavior therapy: Theory and practice* (pp. 120–155). Gilford Press: New York.

Kendall, P. C., & Braswell, L. (1982). Cognitive-behavioral self-control therapy for children: A component analysis. *Journal of Consulting and Clinical Psychology, 50,* 672–689.

Kendall, P. C., & Zupin, V. A. (1981). Individual versus group application of cognitive-behavioral self-control procedures with children. *Behavior Therapy, 12,* 344–359.

Kiesler, D. J. (1981, June). *Process analysis: A necessary ingredient of psychotherapy outcome research.* Invited paper presented at the Society for Psychotherapy Research, Aspen, Colorado.

Klerman, G. L., Weissman, M. M., Rounsaville, B. J., & Chevron, E. S. (1984). *Interpersonal psychotherapy of depression.* New York: Basic Books.

Kornblith, S. J., Rehm, L. P., O'Hara, M. W., & Lamparski, D. M. (1983). The contribution of self-reinforcement training and behavioral assignments to the efficacy of self-control therapy for depression. *Cognitive Therapy and Research, 7,* 499–528.

Kovacs, M., Rush, A. J., Beck, A. T., & Hollon, S. D. (1981). Depressed outpatients treated with cognitive therapy or pharmacotherapy. *Archives of General Psychiatry, 38,* 33–39.

Krantz, S. E., & Hammen, C. L. (1979). The assessment of cognitive bias in depression. *Journal of Abnormal Psychology, 88,* 611–619.

Lake, A., Rainey, J., & Papsdorf, J. D. (1979). Biofeedback and Rational-Emotive Therapy in the management of migraine headache. *Journal of Applied Behavior Analysis, 12,* 127–140.

Larcombe, N. A., & Wilson, P. H. (1984). An evaluation of cognitive-behavior therapy for depression in patients with multiple sclerosis. *British Journal of Psychiatry, 145,* 366–371.

Lochman, J. E., Burch, P. R., Curry, J. F., & Lampron, L. B. (1984). Treatment and generalization effects of cognitive behavioral and goal setting interventions with aggressive boys. *Journal of Consulting and Clinical Psychology, 52,* 915–916.

Lochman, J. E., Lampron, L. B., Burch, P. R., & Curry, J. F. (1985). Client characteristics associated with behavior change for treated and untreated aggressive boys. *Journal of Abnormal Child Psychology, 13,* 527–538.

Luborsky, L., Singer, B., & Luborsky, L. (1975). Comparative studies of psychotherapies: Is it true that "Everyone has won and all must have prizes?" *Archives of General Psychiatry, 32,* 995–1004.

Luborsky, L., Woody, G., McLellan, A., O'Brien, C., & Rosenzweig, J. (1982). Can independent judges recognize different psychotherapies? An experience with manual-guided therapies. *Journal of Consulting and Clinical Psychology, 50,* 49–62.

Luborsky, L., McLellan, A. T., Woody, G. E., O'Brien, C. P., & Auerbach, A. (1985). Therapist success and its determinants. *Archives of General Psychiatry, 42,* 602–611.

Mavissakalian, M., Michelson, L., Greenwald, D., Kornblith, S., & Greenwald, M. (1983). Cognitive-behavioral treatment of agoraphobia: Paradoxical intention vs. self-statement training. *Behavior Research and Therapy, 21,* 75–86.

McNamara, K., & Horan, J. J. (1986). Experimental construct validity in the evaluation of cognitive and behavioral treatments for depression. *Journal of Counseling Psychology, 33,* 23–30.

Meichenbaum, D. (1974). *Cognitive behavior modification.* Morristown, NY: General Learning Press.

Michelson, L., Mavissakalian, M., & Marchione, K. (1985). Cognitive and behavioral treatments of agoraphobia: Clinical, behavioral, and psychophysiological outcomes. *Journal of Consulting and Clinical Psychology, 53,* 913–925.

Miller, R. C., & Berman, J. S. (1983). The efficacy of cognitive behavior therapies: A quantitative review of the research evidence. *Psychological Bulletin, 94,* 39–53.

Murphy, G. E., Simons, A. D., Wetzel, R. D., & Lustman, P. J. (1984). Cognitive therapy and pharmacotherapy: Singly and together in the treatment of depression. *Archives of General Psychiatry, 41,* 33–41.

Neilans, S. T. H., & Israel, A. C. (1981). Toward maintenance and generalization of behavior change: Teaching children of self-regulation and self-instructional skills. *Cognitive Therapy and Research, 5,* 189–195.

Novaco, R. W. (1975). *Anger control: The development and evaluation of an experimental treatment.* Lexington, MA: D. C. Heath.

Novaco, R. W. (1977a). Stress-inoculation: A cognitive therapy for anger and its application to a case of depression. *Journal of Consulting and Clinical Psychology, 45,* 600–608.

Novaco, R. W. (1977b). A stress-innoculation approach to anger management in the training of law enforcement officers. *American Journal of Community Psychology, 5,* 327–346.

Oei, T. P. S., & Jackson, P. R. (1984). Some effective therapeutic factors in group cognitive-behavioral therapy with problem drinkers. *Journal of Studies on Alcohol, 45,* 119–123.

Ordman, A. M., & Kirschenbaum, D. S. (1985). Cognitive-behavioral therapy for bulimia: An initial outcome study. *Journal of Consulting and Clinical Psychology, 53,* 305–313.

Persons, J. B., & Burns, D. D. (1985). Mechanisms of action of cognitive therapy: The relative contributions of technical and interpersonal interventions. *Cognitive Therapy and Research, 9,* 539–551.

Peterson, C., Semmel, A., von Baeyer, C., Abramson, L. Y., Metalsky, G. I., & Seligman, M. E. P. (1982). The Attributional Style Questionnaire. *Cognitive Therapy and Research, 6,* 287–300.

Peterson, C., Luborsky, L., & Seligman, M. E. P. (1983). Attributions and depressive mood shifts: A case study using the symptom-context method. *Journal of Abnormal Psychology, 92,* 96–103.

Rehm, L. P., Kornblith, S. J., O'Hara, M. W., Lamparski, D. M., Romano, J. M., & Volkin, J. I. (1981). An evaluation of major components in a self-control therapy program for depression. *Behavior Modification, 5,* 459–490.

Rehm, L. P., Kaslow, N. J., & Rabin, A. S. (1987). Cognitive and behavioral targets in a self-control therapy program for depression. *Journal of Consulting and Clinical Psychology, 55,* 60–67.

Reynolds, W. M., & Coasts, K. I. (1986). A comparison of cognitive behavioral therapy and relaxation training for the treatment of depression in adolescents. *Journal of Consulting and Clinical Psychology, 54,* 653–660.

Rice, L. N., & Greenberg, L. S. (1984). The new research paradigm. In L. N. Rice & L. S. Greenberg (Eds.), *Patterns of change: Intensive analysis of psychotherapy process* (pp. 7–25). New York: Guilford Press.

Rosenbaum, M. (1980). A schedule for assessing self-control behavior: Preliminary findings. *Behavior Therapy, 11,* 109–121.

Ross, M., & Scott, M. (1985). An evaluation of the effectiveness of individual and group cognitive therapy in the treatment of depressed patients in an inner city health centre. *Journal of the Royal College of General Practicioners, 35,* 239–242.

Rush, A. J., & Watkins, J. T. (1981). Group versus individual cognitive therapy: A pilot study. *Cognitive Therapy and Research, 5,* 95–103.

Rush, A. J., Beck, A. T., Kovacs, M., & Hollon, S. (1977). Comparative efficacy of cognitive therapy and pharmacotherapy in the treatment of depressed outpatients. *Cognitive Therapy and Research, 1,* 17–37.

Rush, A. J., Beck, A. T., Kovacs, M., Weissenburger, J., & Hollon, S. D. (1982). Comparison of the effects of cognitive therapy and pharmacotherapy on helplessness and self-concept. *American Journal of Psychiatry, 139,* 862–866.

Safran, J. (1985, June). Cognitive therapy task markers. In L. Greenberg (Chair), *Task analysis of change events.* Workshop conducted at the meeting of the Society for Psychotherapy Research, Evanston, Illinois.

Safran, J. D., Vallis, T. M., Segal, Z. V., & Shaw, B. F. (1986). Assessment of core cognitive processes in cognitive therapy. *Cognitive Therapy and Research, 10,* 509–526.

Safran, J. D., Vallis, T. M., Segal, Z. V., Shaw, B. F., Balog, W., & Epstein, L. (1987). Measuring session change in cognitive therapy. *Journal of Cognitive Psychotherapy: An International Quarterly, 1*(2), 117–128.

Salkovskis, P. M., Jones, D. R., & Clark, D. M. (1986). Respiratory control in the treatment of panic attacks: Replication and extension with concurrent measurement of behavior and $pCO_2$. *British Journal of Psychiatry, 148,* 526–532.

Schlichter, K. J., & Horan, J. J. (1981). Effects of stress inoculation on the anger and aggression management skills of institutionalized juvenile delinquents. *Cognitive Therapy and Research, 5,* 359–365.

Shaw, B. F. (1977). Comparison of cognitive therapy and behavior therapy in the treatment of depression. *Journal of Consulting and Clinical Psychology, 45,* 543–551.

Silberschatz, B., Fretter, P. B., & Curtis, J. T. (1986). How do interpretations influence the process of psychotherapy? *Journal of Consulting and Clinical Psychology, 54,* 646–652.

Silverman, J. S., Silverman, J. A., & Eardley, D. A. (1984). Do maladaptive attitudes cause depression? *Archives of General Psychiatry, 41,* 28–30.

Simons, A. D., Garfield, S. L., & Murphy, G. E. (1984). The process of change in cognitive therapy and pharmacotherapy for depression. *Archives of General Psychiatry, 41,* 45–51.

Simons, A. D., Lustman, P. J., Wetzel, R. D., & Murphy, G. E. (1985). Predicting response to cognitive therapy of depression: The role of learned resourcefulness. *Cognitive Therapy and Research, 9,* 79–89.

Simons, A. D., Murphy, G. E., Levine, J. L., & Wetzel, R. D. (1986). Cognitive therapy and pharmacotherapy for depression: Sustained improvement over one year. *Archives of General Psychiatry, 43,* 43–48.

Smith, M. L., Glass, G. V., & Miller, T. I. (1980). *The benefits of psychotherapy.* Baltimore: Johns Hopkins University Press.

Spitzer, R. L., Endicott, J., & Robins, E. (1978). Research diagnostic criteria: Rationale and reliability, *Archives of General Psychiatry, 35,* 773–782.

Stenn, P. G., Mothersill, K. J., & Brooke, R. I. (1979). Biofeedback and a cognitive behavioral approach to treatment of myofascial pain dysfunction syndrome. *Behavior Therapy, 10,* 29–36.

Steuer, J. L., Mintz, J., Hammen, C. L., Hill, M. A., Jarvik, L. F., McCarley, T., Motoeke, P., & Rosen, R. (1984). Cognitive-behavioral and psychodynamic group psychotherapy in treatment of geriatric depression. *Journal of Consulting and Clinical Psychology, 52,* 180–189.

Straatmeyer, A. J., & Watkins, J. T. (1974). Rational-emotive therapy and the reduction of speech anxiety. *Rational Living, 9,* 33–37.

Tan, S., & Bruini, J. (1986). Cognitive-behavior therapy with adult patients with epilepsy: A controlled outcome study. *Epilepsia, 27,* 225–233.

Taylor, F. G., & Marshall, W. L. (1977). Experimental analysis of a cognitive behavioral therapy for depression. *Cognitive Therapy and Research, 1,* 59–72.

Teasdale, J. D., & Fennel, M. J. V. (1982). Immediate effects on depression of cognitive therapy interventions. *Cognitive Therapy and Research, 3,* 343–352.

Teasdale, J. D., Fennell, M. J. V., Hibbert, G. A., & Amies, P. L. (1984). Cognitive therapy for major depressive disorder in primary care. *British Journal of Psychiatry, 144,* 400–406.

Truax, C. B., & Carkhuff, R. (1967). *Towards effective counseling and psychotherapy.* Chicago: Aldine.

Turner, R. W., & Wehl, C. K. (1984). Treatment of unipolar depression in problem drinkers. *Advances in Behavior Research and Therapy, 6,* 115–125.

Vallis, T. M., & Shaw, B. F. (1987). *An investigation of patient difficulty and its relationship to therapist competence in cognitive therapy for depression.* Manuscript submitted for publication.

Vallis, T. M., Shaw, B. F., & Dobson, K. S. (1986). The Cognitive Therapy Scale: Psychometric properties. *Journal of Consulting and Clinical Psychology, 54,* 381–385.

Watkins, J. T. (1977). The rational-emotive dynamics of impulsive disorders. In A. Ellis & R. Grieger (Eds.), *Handbook of rational-emotive therapy* (pp. 135–152). New York: Springer.

Watkins, J. T. (1983). Treatment of impulse control disorders. In C. E. Walker (Ed.), *Handbook of clinical psychology: Therapy, research and practice* (pp. 590–632). Homewood, IL: Dow Jones-Irwin Press.

Watkins, J. T., & Rush, A. J. (1983). The Cognitive Response Test. *Cognitive Therapy and Research, 7,* 425–436.

Watkins, J., Leber, W., Imber, S., & Collins, J. (1986, May). *NIMH Treatment of Depression Collaborative Research Program: Temporal course of symptomatic change.* Paper presented at the meeting of the American Psychiatric Association, Washington, DC.

Weissman, A. N., & Beck, A. T. (1978). *Development and validation of Dysfunctional Attitude Scale.* Paper presented at the twelfth annual meeting of the Association for the Advancement of Behavior Therapy, Chicago, Illinois.

Williams, J. M. G. (1984). Cognitive-behavior therapy for depression: Problems and perspectives. *British Journal of Psychiatry, 145,* 254–262.

Williams, S. L., & Rappoport, A. (1983). Cognitive treatment in the natural environment for agoraphobics. *Behavior Therapy, 14,* 299–313.

Wilson, P. H., Goldin, J. V., & Charbonneau-Powis, M. (1983). Comparative efficacy of behavioral and cognitive treatments of depression. *Cognitive Therapy and Research, 7,* 111–124.

Young, J., & Beck, A. T. (1980). *Cognitive Therapy Scale: Rating manual.* Unpublished manuscript, University of Pennsylvania, Philadelphia, PA.

Young, J., Shaw, B. F., Beck, A. T., & Budenz, D. (1981). *Assessment of competence in cognitive therapy.* Unpublished manuscript, University of Pennsylvania.

Zeiss, A. M., Lewinsohn, P. M., & Munoz, R. F. (1979). Nonspecific improvement effects in depression using interpersonal skills training, pleasant activity schedules, or cognitive training. *Journal of Consulting and Clinical Psychology, 47,* 427–439.

Zettle, R. D. (1987). Component and process analysis of cognitive therapy. *Psychological Reports, 61*(3), 939–953.

# 5

# Cognitive Therapy and Cognitive Science

D. J. TATARYN, L. NADEL, AND W. J. JACOBS

> the empty rooms
> where the memory is protected
> where the angels' voices whisper
> to the souls of previous times
> —Bob Dylan ("Street Legal")

## WHY DO WE DO AS WE DO?

The doctrine of free will supposes that human behavior is the result of rational deliberation and conscious choice. Two recently formulated doctrines—psychoanalysis and behaviorism—that disavow free will for rather different reasons, disagree about what should be put in its place. Cognitive science, the modern study of the mind, offers yet another view on where our behavior comes from and what has to be done to effectively modify it. At stake in all this are matters absolutely central to our understanding of what it is to be human: to think, to feel and to act. The basic question seems to be: *What are the causes of our behavior?* Other questions arise immediately: *Are we, or can we be, consciously aware of these causes? If not, why not? If so, how, and to what avail?* The debates among proponents of the various views just noted are more than dry academic affairs; each view suggests a rather different approach to the treatment of people with clinical disorders. This chapter will consider first, and rather briefly, the nature of cognitive therapy and then the emergence and evolution of cognitive science. We will see that the two domains have converged on similar views of cognition and that fruitful collaboration is beginning.

Cognitive therapy emerged at a time of dissatisfaction with traditional psychoanalytic and behaviorist thinking. Psychoanalysts assumed that a person's thoughts and actions could

D. J. TATARYN AND L. NADEL • Department of Psychology, University of Arizona, Tucson, Arizona 85721    W. J. JACOBS • Department of Psychology, University of Lethbridge, Lethbridge, Alberta T1K 3M4, Canada.

reflect drives and motivations forcibly held out of his or her consciousness by an active process—*repression*. Thus they asserted, we can be unaware of the true sources of much of our behavior, with no easy remedy, because these sources are only rarely directly revealed. Behaviorists, for their part, supposed that the critical determinants of action lay in the complex web of environmental contingencies to which a person had been exposed throughout life. We are not typically aware of these deep external regularities "shaping" our behavior, much as we are not aware of the rules of grammar that shape speech production and comprehension.

Though in strong disagreement on many issues, psychoanalysts and behaviorists agreed that the true causes of behavior remain hidden from conscious view, and *it was this assertion that cognitive therapy disputed*. In contrast to established tradition, it proposed that one *could* fairly readily gain conscious access to thoughts and processes influencing how we feel and what we do.

## HISTORICAL ROOTS OF COGNITIVE THERAPY

The idea that cognitions play a critical, even central, role in psychological well-being is not a new one, as many authors have pointed out (e.g., Beck, Rush, Shaw, & Emery, 1979; Ellis, 1962; Goldstein, 1982). Ellis claimed that religious leaders such as Guatama Buddha, Lao-tse, and Jesus Christ were advocates of "self-help" systems essentially cognitive behavioral in nature. Classical philosophers such as Socrates and Epictetus felt that "people are disturbed not by things, but by the views they take of them". In their view, the development of a harmonious and balanced psychological state demanded self-knowledge, and the adoption of more objective, less egocentric points of view. In these ideas one can clearly see the outlines of cognitive theory. Though there are several readily identified precursors (e.g., Adler's *individual psychology,* 1927; Dubois's *rational psychotherapy,* 1906, 1908; Frankl's *logotherapy,* 1965, 1969), the works of Beck (1963, 1972) and Ellis (1958, 1962) are the generally accepted starting point for any analysis of "cognitive therapy" as it is understood today.

### BECK'S COGNITIVE PSYCHOTHERAPY

Beck was dissatisfied with psychoanalytic theory because he felt that it could not account for the content of his depressed clients' dreams (Beck & Rush, 1978). Beck's attention was drawn to the simultaneous, reactive speech—the "stream of consciousness"—going on "behind" a client's free associations. He trained his clients to increase their awareness of this ongoing stream and to freely verbalize it in their sessions. These cognitions were *automatic*— "without any apparent antecedent reflection or reasoning" (Beck, 1963, p. 329); *involuntary* —"would occur even when they had resolved 'not to have them' or were actively trying to avoid them" (p. 329); and, *plausible* to the client, who accepted "the validity of the cognitions uncritically" (p. 330). Beck felt that this rigid, automatized, form of thinking preceded many of his clients' characteristic emotional problems, and he devised a theoretical framework in which these types of thoughts were significant in the etiology of affective and psychotic disorders. The possibilities this perspective held for the client were dramatic:

> Rather than viewing himself as a helpless creature of his own biochemical reactions [*neuro-psychiatry*], or of blind impulses [*psychoanalysis*], or of automatic reflexes [*behaviorism*], he can regard himself as prone to learning erroneous, self-defeating notions and capable of unlearning or correcting them as well (Beck *et al.,* 1979, p. 4; parenthetic material ours).

Beck (1963) used *cognition* to "refer to a specific thought, such as an interpretation, a self-command, or a self-criticism. The term is also applied to wishes (such as suicidal desires) which have a verbal content'' (p. 326). Later, this definition was expanded to include non-verbal ''events'' in the stream of consciousness (Beck *et al.,* 1979).

What distinguished Beck's approach from the psychoanalytic framework was its rejection of the role of *active* repression in creating the autonomous habits at the root of a client's clinical problem. Beck did not dispute the central psychoanalytic claim of unconscious determinants of behavior. Core assumptions about the self and the world according to which a person functions are formed early in life, it is assumed, and these ''schemata'' remain largely unquestioned and out of awareness. These ''cognitions'' are unconscious because of the normal mechanisms by which patterns of thought and oft-repeated habits become automatized, not because they are subject to active repression. This difference in how unconscious factors were assumed to be created led Beck to very different therapeutic procedures than those used by psychoanalysts.

## RATIONAL-EMOTIVE PSYCHOTHERAPY

Ellis (1962) argued that mere insight into the origin of a client's problem would not by itself bring about change. Even assuming (as Beck was clearly unwilling to do) that the psychoanalytic framework could provide a basis for understanding the genesis of the problem, would this knowledge by itself effectively change a client's behavior or neurotic life patterns? The problem was that

> neurotic behavior is not merely externally conditioned or indoctrinated at an early age, but that it is also internally indoctrinated or autosuggested by the individual to himself, over and over again, until it becomes an integral part of his presently held (and still continually self-reiterated) philosophy of life. (p. 22)

Perhaps people could find alleviation from their neuroses by consciously ''catching'' their self-debasing sentences and questioning their validity; it was in this sense that Ellis was advocating a ''cognitive'' therapy.

## COGNITIVE-BEHAVIORAL PSYCHOTHERAPY

The cognitive orientation of Beck and Ellis has been conjoined with the clinical techniques of behaviorist tradition in the past decade, giving rise to a hardy and productive hybrid—*cognitive-behavioral therapy.* Two broad ''causes'' of this evolution can be discerned. There was, first of all, marked dissatisfaction with theoretical positions that disregarded cognitive influences upon learning and behavior (Beck *et al.,* 1979; Goldstein, 1982). Research with both human and nonhuman subjects indicated that learning could not be explained simply with reference to the formation of associations via temporal contiguity. In many cases, explanations that included such concepts as *awareness, expectations,* and *predictions* were needed (Bandura, 1969; Mahoney, 1974; Rescorla, 1969). Second, there was growing awareness that behaviorist learning principles did not apply to clinical populations as well as might have been hoped. Controlled research with these populations revealed interesting anomalies in many behavioral paradigms (e.g., anxiety relief conditioning, systematic desensitization, thought blocking); the interventions seemed effective, but the control conditions appeared to be just as effective (see Meichenbaum, 1977, for a review). Many researchers were forced to conclude that although environmental events were important in the etiology of psychological disorders, it seemed that it was the person's thoughts in reaction to these events that were critical in determining behavior.

The strength of the behaviorists—their methodologically oriented, technique driven approach to therapy—was now conceptualized in a new light. Bandura (1977) summarized thinking at the time:

On the one hand, the mechanisms by which human behavior is acquired and regulated are increasingly formulated in terms of cognitive processes. On the other hand, it is performance-based procedures that are proving to be the most powerful for effecting psychological changes. (p. 191)

This type of thinking gave rise to a new lineage of therapy—cognitive-behavior therapy. Meichenbaum (1977) defined what would become the major foci for such therapies: behavior, cognitive structures, and the "inner dialogue." Where behaviorists aimed solely at the acquisition of coping behaviors, cognitive-behavioral therapy would aim to alter the inner dialogue and perhaps tacit "cognitive" structures as well.

SUMMARY OF CRITICAL ASPECTS OF COGNITIVE THERAPIES

It has been argued that cognitions have always played at least an implicit role in most traditional psychological treatments (Goldstein, 1982). What seems to mark cognitive therapy off as different is the extent to which the uncovering and transformation of cognitive structures/functions takes on an explicit role in treatment. In specific contrast to a psychoanalytic orientation, which assumes that we are driven by unconscious motivations and impulses and the behavioral tradition that assumes that we are governed by external contingencies, cognitive therapies assume that factors of which we could become conscious guide most of our behavior. Though they *are* typically out of the normal stream of awareness, these causal antecedents are not, as Freud asserted, actively repressed; rather they could, with appropriate techniques, be accessible to observation and reflection.

This interest in the role of cognitive factors creates a dependence upon the scientific understanding of cognition itself. It is here, of course, that one would like some input from the cognitive scientist. What is the structure in human cognition? How are schemata formed, manintained, and transformed? Why do some forms of information processing become automatic, whereas others always remain in consciousness? Recent writing in the therapeutic community reflects these interests: Mahoney (1984), Guidano and Liotti (1982, 1985), and others (e.g., Meichenbaum & Gilmore, 1984; Safran, Vallis, Segal, & Shaw, 1986) have begun to explore the structure of human cognition, in the hope of determining where their efforts should be aimed. In what follows we briefly trace the historical foundations of cognitive science, some of the directions in which it has been evolving, and several implications of these new developments on our thoughts about the structure and function of the human mind.

# THE ROOTS OF MODERN COGNITIVE SCIENCE

Diverse forces have contributed to the rebirth of interest in cognition in the 1950s and the emergence, in this decade, of the interdisciplinary field of cognitive science. *Information processing* is the cognitive scientist's central dogma: Stimulation received at the periphery is *coded* by receptors, *represented* in some spatiotemporal set of brain activities, and then *processed, transformed,* and perhaps *stored* in the service of specific ends. Electronic computers show that the coding, representation, transformation, and storage of information can be carried out in purely mechanical devices. This, in turn, suggests that the cognitive processes of a living organism could be studied in a rigorous and objective fashion, revealing the underlying structures and transformational rules of biological thought itself.

In essence, the computer model suggests a view of cognition involving *manipulations* performed on symbolic *representations*, where the form of the representations is something like the form of sentences in an internal language, and manipulations are viewed as rule-governed transformations of these mental "phrases." Central to this view of cognition is the idea that thought processes are "rational," following logical rules. (It has been suggested that this reflects the fact that digital computers were conceived of by mathematicians—Turing and von Neumann.) The paradigm example of such rule-governed behavior is human language, which has received quite extensive analysis. This approach to cognition has proven quite successful, providing a framework within which to study one of the key features of the human mind: its capacity to handle thoughts, images, and language in what appears to be a highly structured, rule-based fashion.

Thoughts, however, have more than formal structure. They are always *about* things, referring to specific objects, their features, their changes of state and/or location, their interaction with other objects. Additionally, our thoughts often reflect subjective feelings, of pain, of hunger, of ecstasy, of despair, of hope. The inability, or unwillingness, of behaviorism to account for the influence or conscious experience of these, or indeed any, thoughts was one of the driving forces behind the cognitive renaissance. Cognitive science has, however, had relatively little to say about the "subjective" activities of the mind/brain, as they reflect beliefs and desires about the world we live in. The relative lack of attention given to these subjective aspects of cognitive function reflects the fact that modern cognitive science is ruthlessly mechanistic; the computing machine is after all its guiding metaphor.

What, then, does modern cognitive science tell us about the sources of behavior and a person's access to those sources? It has recently begun to say quite strongly that much that qualifies to be called cognitive is now thought to lie beneath awareness. This statement reflects the growing number of demonstrations of nonconscious mental processing, both within the cognitive (Marcel, 1983; see Kihlstrom, 1987, for a review) and neuropsychological (Schacter, 1987; Weiskrantz, 1986) literatures. These data indicate that at least some of the antecedent causes of our behavior could be cognitive—the result of complex mental processes—yet not be automatically open to conscious introspection. It is worth describing some of this work in more detail.

## Nonconscious Mental Processing

One of the first demonstrations of complex nonconscious processing emerged from the study of visual function after brain lesions in monkeys. In the initial demonstration of what has since come to be called "blindsight," Humphrey (1974; Humphrey & Weiskrantz, 1967) showed that extensive experimental lesions placed in the primary visual cortex of a monkey had a paradoxical effect. His monkey was able to locate and pick up even small objects with relative accuracy but was apparently unable to *identify* these objects. Thus, it appeared as though the animal "knew" that *something* was there but had no idea what it was. This form of "knowing" was clearly unusual, however; studying animals with the same brain damage, Cowey (1961; Cowey & Weiskrantz, 1963) had already shown that suspending a strange doll in the "blind" part of the monkey's visual world did not provoke the distress response easily observed when the doll was suspended where the monkey had complete sight. Taken together, these results indicate that the monkey without a visual cortex "knew" that there was an object present and where the object was located but "knew" nothing about its "meaning," not even whether it was new or old.

This unusual syndrome has now been observed and carefully studied in humans (Weiskrantz, 1986). Once again, evidence of both preserved and interrupted function has been obtained. The patient (D.B.) could both detect and locate visual stimuli but had difficulty identifying them. What is more, and most intriguing, is the fact that D.B. is *not consciously aware* of the presence of these stimuli. It is only through careful testing that his residual capacities of detection and location can be uncovered. In these tests, clearly, D.B.'s behavior is influenced by forces of which he is apparently unaware. In addition to these reports from the study of disordered vision, similar findings have been reported for other domains, such as face recognition ("prosopagnosia," Tranel & Damasio, 1985) and touch (Paillard, Michel, & Stelmach, 1983).

Perhaps the best-known demonstration of a separation between two forms of "knowing" comes from the study of amnesia. Many studies have now shown that amnesic patients are capable of considerable new learning, (see Squire, 1987, for a review) but that in all such cases they seem unaware of the fact that they have learned anything at all. Once again, careful tests must be used to demonstrate what the patient "knows." One interesting, and clinically important, example concerns what has been called "priming." There are many ways to demonstrate this phenomenon, but they all share the feature that *some experience A exerts a measurable effect upon the subject's response to a subsequent experience B*. Thus a stimulus flashed quite briefly in the visual field can impact upon what one perceives shortly thereafter, whether or not one was aware of the first stimulus, or even aware that there *was* a first stimulus. Intact "priming" effects have now been observed in amnesic patients in a wide variety of situations (Graf, Squire, & Mandler, 1984; Schacter, 1985; Schacter & Graf, 1986; Warrington & Weiskrantz, 1968), conjoined with total lack of awareness.

It is important to note that these disjunctions between having information, yet being unaware that one has it, are not restricted to cases of organic brain damage. Marcel (1983), for example, has shown much the same thing with normal people in a series of studies using tachistoscopically presented visual stimuli amid various kinds of "masking" stimuli. These masks obliterate the subject's ability to become aware of very briefly presented stimuli (4 msec), but they do not interrupt the impact of the brief stimuli on subsequent perception. Schacter (1988) has discussed many of these data, providing details of other studies in normal subjects that demonstrate the reality of information acquisition without any sign of awareness.

It is becoming clear that we are not conscious of much of the cognitive processing underlying our perceptions, thoughts, feeling, and actions. Interest in these nonconscious mental processes has benefitted from the recent emergence of two major themes in cognitive science: the *modularity* doctrine and what has been called the *connectionist* paradigm. Discussion of these two will provide some examples of what cognitive science might be able to offer clinical theory and, consequently, practice.

## MODULARITY

Cognitive science is, at base, the study of minds, their structure and modes of interaction with the external world. That the adult human mind is a rich and varied tapestry no one would deny. But debates continue over the source and nature of this variety. Some suggest that this heterogeneity is "hard-wired" into the structure of the nervous system itself, such that distinct cognitive "modules" simply unfold during brain maturation. Others see it as emerging from a rather uniform neurobiological base, in contact with a heterogeneous environment. There are two quite different kinds of "modularity" theories. One asserts that there are varied cognitive modules concerned with specific "processes" such as *short-term memory*, or *rehearsal*, or the like. Here, cognitive modules are defined by the kind of information processing they engage in. The other type of modularity theory asserts that modules differ from one another not in terms of the processes they engage in but rather in terms of the *contents* of the information being processed.

Janet's analysis of "dissociation," and Freud's separation between preconscious, conscious, and unconscious, indicated the allegiance of these two pioneers to a *modularity* view, though it is hard to be certain if they were suggesting "process" or "content" modules. In refusing to concern itself with anything under the organism's skin, and hence locating the mechanisms responsible for the rich variety of behavior in the environment, behaviorism implicitly accepted an undifferentiated view of the mind. Much of early cognitive science was surprisingly consistent with this view of the mind, giving rise to models within which apparently diverse cognitive capacities emerge from a single underlying functional system (e.g., Anderson, 1976; but see Nadel & Wexler, 1984).

More recently, converging evidence from several domains seems to have shifted the debate against this homogeneity view. It now appears certain that the cognitive system is "modularized"—composed of separate systems that represent and transform specific kinds of information, and perhaps operate under different rules (Fodor, 1983; Mishkin, 1982; O'Keefe & Nadel, 1978). Aspects of language function, those that are taken to be unique to humans, constitute one such system. Modularity accounts for the existence of nonconscious mental processing quite simply: The workings of some modules are accessible to consciousness, the workings of others are not. Some of the best evidence for the notion of modularity has already been discussed: the disjunctions in several clinical syndromes between preserved capacities and absent awareness.

The modular structure of mind is suggested also by the discontinuous way in which cognitive function unfolds during development. Freud and many others have observed that we have few if any personal memories from the earliest years of life, a phenomenon known as "infantile amnesia." Freud hedged his bets on whether this "absence" reflected present, but repressed, memories, or a biologically immature system. We, and others, have suggested that different learning/memory systems mature at different ages of life and that the system responsible for autobiographical memories matures late (Bachevalier & Mishkin, 1984; Nadel & Zola-Morgan, 1984; Schacter & Moscovitch, 1984). The relevance of this to infantile amnesia seems clear, and it provides an example of how modern neurobiology can address issues that were formerly in the province of psychotherapy. Jacobs and Nadel (1985) have applied these ideas to an analysis of *phobias,* in ways that address more directly the sources of what Freud labeled *repression.* We look more closely at this work later.

## THE CONNECTIONIST PARADIGM

When we recognize a face or a situation within a split-second, we are accomplishing something which the fastest, most powerful electronic computers remain incapable of doing with any degree of "flexibility." Because modern supercomputers can execute sequences of millions of operations per second, this suggests that the brain must be performing a staggering number of operations in the merest blink of an eye. Information is represented in the nervous system in the activity of *neurons,* which influence one another at *synaptic junctions.* Operations within this biological hardware are carried out orders of magnitude more slowly than in electronic "microchips." In the time available to recognize a face only a small number (<50) of sequential information-processing steps could be carried out in the nervous system. Such considerations indicate that much information processing in the brain must be proceeding *in parallel,* rather than in sequence.

The *connectionist* perspective (McClelland & Rumelhart, 1986; cf. Rumelhart & Mc-Clelland, 1986) provides a paradigm that can apparently accommodate the need for parallel processing. It starts with the assumption of a densely interconnected network of processing elements, which can effect one another through their connections. The "activation" strength of a particular connection, or pattern of connections, can be viewed as the strength with which a certain "hypothesis" about the world is being entertained. Cognitive processing involves changes in the strength of the connections among elements, until the network "relaxes" or settles into a dynamic equilibrium that satisfies the multiple "constraints" embodied in the connection patterns.

What is most relevant about connectionism is the way it talks about the representation of information, basing its principles upon what is known about such representation in the brain. First, information is assumed to be represented in the brain in a highly *distributed* fashion. This means that individual memories (thoughts, images, etc.) are not likely to be easily localized to discrete brain circuits. Second, connectionist networks represent knowledge in a fundamentally continuous fashion. The "connection weights" relating processing elements can take many "values" (or strengths), which permits a whole range of partial states of activation, or "knowledge." When conjoined with the notion of parallel processing, this property of partial activation provides a means by which information of which the person is unaware can exert effects upon later processing stages and even overt behavior. This property of the connectionist cognitive architecture provides a principled basis for understanding such phenomena as perceptual defense, priming without awareness, and a broad class of nonconscious mental phenomena. Consider, for example, its implications for understanding the relation between cognition and emotion.

Most authors approach this topic gingerly, as well they might. Most agree that whatever else is true, cognition and emotion are *different* things. The relation between the two has been debated for the better part of a century, often concerning the issue of which had causal primacy (Lazarus, 1982; Zajonc, 1980). In this debate, emotion was typically viewed as the "raw feel" of something, its unanalyzed direct impact. On the other side, cognition was viewed as that which one could be conscious of, typically could verbalize. Under this definition, it probably made sense to discuss the relation between the two. Unfortunately, the debate appears futile. It is based on views of emotion and cognition that are far too narrow. Here, Ellis seems to have been on the right track, refusing to see a clear distinction between emotions and cognitions:

> Thoughts and emotions are not two entirely different processes . . . they significantly overlap in many respects and . . . therefore disordered emotions can often (though not always) be ameliorated by changing one's thinking (Ellis, 1958, p. 3).

If our view of cognition is based on "symbol-manipulating" digital computers, we will, in all likelihood, conceive of thought and emotions as quite different things. The dominance of this perspective in the cognitive science community for much of the past 30 years accounts for the persistence of the cognition versus emotion debate, as well as the relative lack of attention given to the study of the "hot" side of cognitive function. In contrast, connectionism does not distinguish between the processing of so-called emotional and cognitive information. Nor, we might add, does there seem to be any basis for claiming such a distinction in the nervous system.

Not all is perfect with connectionism, however. Problems have arisen in its ability to account for the sequential aspects of behavior and for some of the detail of complex cognitive (language) behavior (Pinker & Prince, 1988). Though doubt remains as to the ability of this new conceptual framework to explain *all* of cognition, its successes at accounting for a variety of phenomena of particular interest to clinicians indicates that it will prove important in the future.

## PSYCHOPATHOLOGY, COGNITIVE STRUCTURE, AND NEUROBIOLOGY

Cognitive science has ignored the hot topics—feelings, desires, pains, and joys—much as it has until recently ignored the neurobiological bases of cognition. This lack of interest in neurobiology reflects the fact that the dominant metatheory in cognitive science—functionalism—supposes that mental function could be realized in any suitably complex physical system, as long as all the parts are hooked up properly. Cognitive processes, it is asserted, result from the relations among the physical entities of which the system is composed—neurons, or perhaps silicon chips, rather than from the nature of the materials of which they are composed. Though this argument satisfies many philosophers (but see Churchland, 1986), it is of scant help to the psychologist or psychiatrist who must deal with the doing and undoing of biologically based cognition. A renewed interest in the biology of cogntiion is, in fact, partly responsible for the emergence of notions like modularity and connectionism.

Much of what we know about the neurobiological structure of cognition comes from the careful study of individuals with some form of brain damage. The study of patients with focal brain damage has progressed in part because of the assumption that such damage might "carve nature as its joints," revealing aspects of the modular structure and function of the human brain. As Marshall (1987) has put it: "Pathology, by rudely tearing apart and isolating the elements of an integrated mechanism, will throw light upon the structure of the normal system" (p. 583). In combination with controlled studies of similar brain damage in nonhuman experimental subjects, such research has contributed to the resurgence of the notion of modularity. Support has also come from studies of patients with "functional" rather than "organic" disorders. For example, analysis of posthypnotic amnesia (Kihlstrom & Evans, 1979) has provided evidence on distinctions between *episodic* and *semantic* memory systems. The careful study of what Janet first referred to as "dissociations" should shed light on the modular structure of the mind, and the beginnings of such work with "multiple personality" cases can already be discerned. It is important to note that psychiatric disorders might be more likely than somewhat "random" organic brain damage to actually find "nature's joints." Thus a conceptually based, carefully conceived research program focusing on these dissociations could make a major contribution to our understanding of the mind (but see Miller, 1986). In this sense, psychotherapists could once again play a leading role in our study of the mind.

## BRINGING IT ALL BACK HOME

Modern cognitive therapy and cognitive science seem to be saying many of the same things: Behavior reflects both conscious and nonconscious factors; the distinction between emotion and cognition is not all that clear. In these broad areas of agreement, there should reside possibilities for useful interaction. The cognitive therapist's interest in *automatic* cognitions is matched by the cognitive scientist's study of the distinction between automatic and controlled processing (e.g., Schneider & Shiffrin, 1977). Philosophers (Dennett, 1987) have joined with James Joyce and cognitive therapists in looking to the stream of consciousness for clues about the causes of behavior. Many other examples could be cited of areas in which fruitful collaborations between clinicians and basic scientists could, and should, emerge. In the remainder of this chapter, we focus on a promising area for collaboration—the notion of *repression,* or more precisely, the means by which certain controlling features of a person's cognitive makeup become unconscious. We have already seen that there are many different views on this central issue. In what follows we briefly summarize the traditional position, and then offer two new ways of thinking about "repression," ways that emerge out of modern biological science.

## WHY DON'T WE KNOW WHY WE DO AS WE DO?

We began this chapter by raising several questions about the sources of our behavior and our knowledge of those sources. Our survey makes clear that, in many instances, we are governed in our perceptions, thoughts, and actions by factors of which we are not aware. This once-radical notion is now quite respectable, buttressed by data from several converging sources. However, little light has been shed on the matter of why we are unaware, how general this unawareness is, and so on. There are many things one would like to know about nonconscious mental processing. Why are some things "buried" and other things not? What are the best methods for revealing this buried stuff? How can these buried processes by changed?

In a sense, traditional psychotherapeutic approaches provide some answers to these questions, answers that have had only scattered success to date. Materials were buried by *repression* and could only be uncovered when the sources of that repression were uprooted.

Behaviorism provided a quite different kind of answer, one that suggested very different kinds of therapies. Little attention was given to what we were, or were not, aware of. Behavior was presumed to be shaped by environmental contingencies of which we were often quite unaware, and there was no need for the notion of repression. The way to change behavior was to alter the contingencies. Cognitive therapy, and its modern cousins, presents yet another set of answers. Behavior is governed by tacit schemata and automatic ways of thinking that go off the track, leading the client into maladaptive patterns of behavior. The underlying, faulty cognitions must be unearthed if therapy is to succeed. Providing a principled basis for this unearthing process remains a central task for any cognitive therapy. Cognitive scientists could provide information the clinician needs in order to generate such a base. Brief discussions of our own work will provide an idea of some of the possibilities.

### EARLY LEARNING, STRESS, FEARS, AND PHOBIAS

The lack of conceptual principles encompassing the peculiar features of phobic states provided the starting point for a neurobiological approach. Jacobs and Nadel (1985) noted: (1) the inability of the patient to recall a critical event leading to the phobia; (2) the persistence of the phobia in the face of reality; (3) the expression of the phobia in a wide range of environments; and (4) the broad generalization of the phobic reaction to similar stimuli. Their explanation rests on the assertion, already noted, that there are two broad classes of learning with rather different properties. These forms of learning are dependent upon different underlying brain systems, which in turn have separate maturational time courses. Thus, as we pointed out earlier in our brief discussion of "infantile amnesia," learning early in life bears the features of those brain systems that mature early, whereas that later in life bear the features of both early and late maturing systems. This is of importance in the present context because learning in the early-maturing systems has features quite reminiscent of the peculiar attributes of many phobias. For example, we do not have conscious access to specific early episodes because such episodic (autobiographical) aspects of our memories clearly depend upon a late-maturing brain system. If there were a critical pairing of the phobic stimulus/situation with some negative consequences early in life, the client would not be able to recall the specifics of the event, even if it were to have an impact on the person's subsequent behavior.

Recent neuroendocrinological research (e.g., McEwen, De Kloet, & Rostene, 1986) has shown that the late-maturing system, responsible for autobiographical memory—the hippocampal formation—is densely populated with "stress hormone" receptors, a subtype of which is quite selective to this particular system. Jacobs and Nadel used these facts to suggest that, under conditions of extreme stress, the late-maturing system will be atypically suppressed. The result will be a return, in many ways, to styles of behaviors appropriate to early life. For present purposes, the important implication of this "regression" is that it seems to create conditions of unusual accessibility to information stored in early-maturing systems, prior to the onset of hippocampal function. Such information, of which the person is not consciously aware and which to that point has had no behavioral impact, can then be brought to the surface. This "reinstatement" can only occur, of course, when part of the original situation—*that part that will determine the phobic stimulus*—occurs. Thus, it takes an unusual conjunction of life events to trigger a phobia by this mechanism: First, a traumatic event must occur in early life, say a painful insect bite; second, at some later time, severe stress disables the hippocampal system; and, third, during this stress period a portion of the original traumatic event, say a (harmless) encounter with a similar insect, is experienced. Under these conditions, it is claimed, phobias with "no" source, bearing the features of infantile learning, can emerge. Jacobs and Nadel provide explanations for many of the features of phobic states within this neurobiological framework and go from there to an analysis of the kinds of treatments that might make sense (see Jacobs & Nadel, 1985, for a fuller discussion of this notion, and references to the many others whose work contributed to this story; see O'Keefe & Nadel, 1978, for background).

93

COGNITIVE THERAPY
AND COGNITIVE
SCIENCE

## A MUSCULAR INTERFERENCE PARADIGM OF REPRESSION

Work with amnesic patients supports another distinction between forms of learning that is of interest here. It has been known for some time that even densely amnesic patients retain the ability to acquire "motor skills" (e.g., Corkin, 1968). Cohen and Squire (1980), in agreement with O'Keefe and Nadel (1978), argue from the study of amnesia that the brain honors a distinction between "knowing that" and "knowing how," a distinction given extensive treatment by the philosopher Ryle (1949). This distinction refers to two kinds of knowledge: *knowing that* is factual, propositional knowledge, whereas *knowing how* is implicit, dispositional knowledge. One knows "that' Tucson is in Arizona but "how" to play poker. Fascinating anecdotes abound of patients capable of impressive feats of learning, such as a new piece of piano music, but with no conscious awareness of the situation in which the learning transpired. This *procedural* learning, as Squire (1987) calls it, seems to rely on brain systems separate from those involved in the autobiographical memories of which we are typically aware. What implications might this independence between the two learning systems have for the etiology of psychopathologies?

As we have just seen, stress can serve to release hormones that temporarily disable the "knowing-that" system, leaving only the "knowing-how" (procedural) systems operational. We suggested that the cognitive system is highly sensitive to stress and is rather easily disabled by it. There are reasons to think that influences other than stress can alter the functional balance between these two kinds of systems. One of us (D.J.T.) has been exploring the well-known inverted U-shaped relation between muscle tension and cognitive function; too little or too much muscle tension will result in less-than-optimal performance (Courts, 1942).

The tensing of peripheral musculature results in a diminished capacity to process information. If a group of muscles were to become tense during a time of extreme anxiety, it could result in an abatement of experienced anxiety. By any of the myriad of models offered by Freud, Hull, and others, whatever action results in a decrease in anxiety must increase in probability. Thus a person afflicted with an environmentally based anxiety attack could react to this attack by tensing the muscles, which would then be reinforced in much the same way that escape behaviors are reinforced in a standard operant escape paradigm (Jacobs & Harris, 1985). It is known that under circumstances such as these, conditioning can occur without the person's complete awareness of the controlling contingencies or even of the behaviors that are involved (see Corteen & Wood, 1972; Martin, Stambrook, Tataryn, & Beihl, 1984; Wilson, 1979).

We can see how learned muscular reactions, governed by systems outside of normal adult awareness, could serve as a mechanism for "repression." The conditioned muscular response could chain to "more distant" stimuli, either through stimuli that "occasion set" (Rescorla, 1985; Ross & LoLordo, 1987), or through "second-order" stimuli (Rescorla, 1980). These higher-order stimuli could be either external environmental cues, or internal cognitive ones. In either case, the presence of tension in muscles could serve to decrease the efficiency of information processing, prevent critical information from entering the cognitive system, and thereby interfere with the occurrence of the upcoming emotional/cognitive reaction. Over repeated experiences (trials), as the organism acquires the conditioned reaction of muscular tension, this reaction, like any conditioned response, begins to move forward in time, closer to the onset of the higher-order conditioned stimuli. As it does so, the actual amount of activation of the cognitive/emotional system becomes relatively smaller and hence requires less muscular "interference." By the time the process is happening at the unconscious level, only minimal muscular tension is needed to interfere with the cognitive/emotional system. Because this muscular tension is specific to the information processing concerned with the conditioned stimulus precursors, there is only minimal interference with information processing in general.

Thus an emotional state might, in time, be subject to interference "in advance," before the state is consciously experienced. This, of course, would constitute a mechanism for *repression*. (Note that Freud also postulated that muscles played a role in repression and that Reich gave muscles a central role in the process he termed *armoring*). As conscious aspects of the particular emotions or cognitions surrounding a stimulus could now only be experienced in the absence of the conditioned muscular response and these emotions and thoughts are aversive, the contingencies of the situation set up the muscles to become chronically tense. The absence of awareness produced by this chain of events does not imply the cessation of all forms of neural processing. Autonomic correlates of emotion, such as altered heart and respiratory rate, sweating palms and cold feet, can be observed in the absence of conscious cognitions/emotions about the triggering event and may also become chronic, though unseen, reactions.

This idea leads to a series of questions that are important to both theoretician and cognitive therapist. Does tensing of the muscles diminish awareness of critical environmental or subjective events: events that control or trigger emotional responses? If so, are these tensions under the control of reinforcement (i.e., learned), or are they a by-product of a more central process? If muscular tension serves partially to control awareness, is it efferent feedback from these muscles, or the control mechanism that is involved? If feedback is involved, are the muscles that produce greater central feedback (e.g., face and hands) more often subjected to tensing in situations where we would expect repression to occur? The large, constantly activated muscles involved in maintaining an upright posture, (e.g., the muscles of the upper and lower back) may be activated during postural compensations associated with the various emotions and may thereby be subjected to the contingencies that interfere with these emotions. If the muscles prove to be intimately involved in the disruption of emotional processing, could specific patterns of muscular tension (or the activation of the autonomic nervous system) serve as diagnostic markers for particular kinds of emotional repressions? If it were possible to diagnose various disorders through examining patterns of muscular tension, could the therapist track the progress of a client by monitoring muscle tension during treatment?

These and other questions suggest themselves within the framework of this modular approach to repression. Although the idea offers new possibilities to the psychoanalyst, it carries a caution both for the behaviorist and the cognitive therapist. Techniques such as systematic desensitization may become more successful and efficient if they deal with the unconscious precursors now believed to influence behavior. Unless this is done, remnants of the problem can remain, coming to the fore at unexpected and unplanned-for moments. Techniques such as the manipulation of thoughts available to introspection cannot be fully successful unless and until they deal with precursors of behavior and emotional states that are not handy to direct introspection. What the muscles know is not necessarily open to the rest of the brain; what the "early brain" knows is not open to the "mature brain." Partial states of knowledge can remain, unbeknown to the bearer or the therapist. Problems will remain, often caught in modules not easily manipulated by direct, behaviorally based techniques.

## CONCLUSIONS

We have argued that the notion of cognition has undergone extensive alteration in the 30 years or so since its reemergence. What began in response to the need to account for phenomena such as conscious awareness has evolved into something considerably broader. Shifts in the way cognitive scientists conceive of the representation of knowledge, and the internal organization of knowledge systems, has focused attention on the important role played by nonconscious, yet cognitive, processes.

The supposed separation between emotion and cognition reflects this history, as noted earlier. The separation was predicated on narrow views of both: cognition seemingly limited to those aspects of mental life we can be conscious of and emotion limited to the *unanalyzed* impact of thoughts or experiences. Cognitive science, armed with the apparently nonconscious computer as its metaphor, has exchanged "information processing" for "consciousness" as the defining feature of cognition. There is no *a priori* reason to view the information processing that underlies feelings and desires as any different from that underlying thoughts, ideas, and beliefs; certainly there is nothing in the brain to suggest such a distinction.

Though cognitive psychology has made progress in the study of what we can call "cold" cognition, typified by rationality, logic, and language, it has with some notable exceptions ignored the evaluative, nonrational, illogical processes and experiences that populate our emotional life. Shifts in defining the nature of cognition within cognitive science open up the possibility of bringing cold and hot topics together. Emotions, as we have seen, are not separate from cognitions, nor does it seem appropriate to think of either one causing the other (Kuiper & MacDonald, 1983). Rather, emotional information processing is one species of cognition, perhaps based on a distinct processing module but no less cognitive for that.

This change in cognitive science has interesting ramifications for the pursuit of "cognitive" therapies. Recent data supporting the "modular" view of mind provide a new basis for understanding a whole class of phenomena characterized by *unaware knowing*: cases where a person's behavior reflects the presence of some knowledge of which he or she is not consciously aware. In attempting to come to grips with such phenomena, Freud and Janet were both led to postulate the reality of "psychological" modules; cognitive science and neurobiology are beginning to suggest ways in which this modular structure could be realized. We discussed two new approaches, based on modern psychobiological research, which provide ways of understanding how a client's behavior could be powerfully influenced by such "unaware knowledge." Each approach offers possible directions for future therapies whose central aim would be the uncovering of this "buried" knowledge. We could have chosen to discuss a range of other approaches, which clearly makes the point that fruitful interaction between cognitive science and cognitive therapy has already begun and can be counted on to provide new ways of thinking about why we are as we are.

ACKNOWLEDGMENTS. We would like to thank our colleagues through the years for their contributions—witting or unwitting—to these ideas. In particular, we thank Dick Bootzin, John Kihlstrom, and Jeff Willner for their thoughts on earlier versions of this chapter. We thank Hal Arkowitz for encouraging us to take on what turned out to be a fascinating task, for giving us time enough to carry it out, and for his continuous input. D.J.T. would like to thank his wife, Darlene, for her continuous patience, support, and many conversations. L. N. would like to apologize to his children, Melissa, Kenny, Misha, Leila, and Yael, for the theft of time this work represents. He hopes they decide it was worth it.

# REFERENCES

Adler, A. (1927). *The practice and theory of individual psychology.* New York: Harcourt.

Anderson, J. R. (1976). *Language, memory and thought.* Hillsdale, NJ: L. Erlbaum Associates.

Bachevalier, J., & Mishkin, M. (1984). An early and a late developing system for learning and retention in infant monkeys. *Behavioral Neuroscience, 98,* 770–778.

Bandura, A. (1969). *Principles of behavior modification.* New York: Holt, Rinehart & Winston.

Bandura, A. (1977). Self-efficacy: Toward a unifying theory of behavioral change. *Psychological Review, 84,* 191–215.

Beck, A. T. (1963). Thinking and depression. *Archives of General Psychiatry, 9,* 324–333.

Beck, A. T. (1972). *Depression: Causes and treatment.* Philadelphia: University of Pennsylvania Press.

Beck, A. T., & Rush, A. J. (1978). Cognitive approaches to depression and suicide. In G. Serban (Ed.). *Cognitive defects in development of mental illness* (pp. 235–257). New York: Brunner/Mazel.

Beck, A. T., Rush, A. J., Shaw, B. F., & Emery, G. (1979). *Cognitive therapy of depression.* New York: Guilford Press.

Churchland, P. S. (1986). *Neurophilosophy: Toward a unified science of the mind/brain.* Cambridge, MA: Bradford Books/MIT Press.

Cohen, N. J., & Squire, L. R. (1980). Preserved learning and retention of pattern analyzing skill in amnesia. Dissociation of knowing how and knowing that. *Science, 210,* 207–209.

Corkin, S. (1968). Acquisition of motor skill after bilateral medial temporal excision. *Neuropsychologia, 6,* 255–265.

Corteen, R. S., & Wood, B. (1972). Autonomic responses to shock associated words in an unattended channel. *Journal of Experimental Psychology, 94,* 308–318.

Courts, F. A. (1942). Relation between muscular tension and performance. *Psychological Bulletin, 39,* 347–367.

Cowey, A. (1961). Perimetry in monkeys. Unpublished doctoral dissertation, University of Cambridge.

Cowey, A., & Weiskrantz, L. (1963). A perimetric study of visual field defects in monkeys. *Quarterly Journal of Experimental Psychology, 15,* 91–115.

Dennett, D. (1987). Invited address, Philosophy and Psychology Society Meetings, San Diego.

Dubois, P. (1906). *The influence of the mind on the body.* New York: Funk and Wagnalls.

Dubois, P. (1908). *The psychic treatment of nervous disorders.* New York: Funk and Wagnalls.

Ellis, A. (1958). Rational psychotherapy. *Journal of General Psychology, 59,* 35–49.

Ellis, A. (1962). *Reason and emotion in psychotherapy.* New York: Lyle Stuart.

Fodor, J. A. (1983). *The modularity of mind.* Cambridge, MA: The MIT Press.

Frankl, V. E. (1965). *The doctor and the soul.* New York: Alfred A. Knopf, Inc.

Frankl, V. E. (1969). *The will to meaning.* New York: New American Library.

Goldstein, H. (1982). Cognitive therapies: A comparison of phenomenological and mediational models and their origins. *The Journal of Mind and Behavior 3,* 1–16.

Guidano, V. F., & Liotti, G. (1982). *Cognitive processes and emotional disorders.* New York: Guilford.

Graf, P., Squire, L. R., & Mandler, G. (1984). The information that amnesic patients do not forget. *Journal of Experimental Psychology: Learning Memory, and Cognition, 10,* 164–178.

Guidano, V. F., & Liotti, G. (1985). A constructivistic foundation for cognitive therapy. In M. J. Mahoney & A. Freeman (Eds.), *Cognition and psychotherapy* (pp. 101–142). New York: Plenum Press.

Humphrey, N. K. (1974). Vision in a monkey without striate cortex: A case study. *Perception, 3,* 241–255.

Humphrey, N. K., & Weiskrantz, L. (1967). Vision in monkeys after removal of the striate cortex. *Nature, 215,* 595–597.

Jacobs, W. J., & Harris, C. (1985). Escape responding in a shuttle-box. *Learning and Motivation, 16,* 334–340.

Jacobs, W. J., & Nadel, L. (1985). Stress-induced recovery of fears and phobias. *Psychological Review, 92,* 512–531.

Kihlstrom, J. F. (1987). The cognitive unconscious. *Science, 237,* 1445–1452.

Kihlstrom, J. F., & Evans, F. J. (1979). Memory retrieval processes in posthypnotic amnesia. In J. F. Kihlstrom & F. J. Evans (Eds.), *Functional disorders of memory* (pp. 179–218). Hillsdale, NJ: L. Erlbaum Associates.

Kuiper, N. A., & MacDonald, M. R. (1983). Reason, emotion and cognitive therapy. *Clinical Psychology Review, 3,* 297–316.

Lazarus, R. (1982). Thoughts on the relations between emotion and cognition. *American Psychologist, 37,* 1019–1024.

Mahoney, M. J. (1974). *Cognition and behavior modification.* Cambridge, MA: Ballinger.

Mahoney, M. J. (1984). Behaviorism, cognitivism, and human change processes. In M. A. Reda & M. J. Mahoney (Eds.), *Cognitive psychotherapies: Recent developments in theory, research and practice.* Cambridge, MA: Ballinger.

Marcel, A. J. (1983). Conscious and unconscious perception: Experiments on visual masking and word recognition. *Cognitive Psychology, 15,* 197–237.

Marshall, J. C. (1987). Is seeing believing? *Nature, 325,* 583–584.

Martin, D. G., Stambrook, M., Tataryn, D. J., & Beihl, H. (1984). Conditioning in the unattended left ear. *International Journal of Neuroscience, 23,* 95–102.

McClelland, J. L., Rumelhart, D. E. (and the PDP Research Group). (1986). *Parallel distributed processing: Explorations in the microstructure of cognition. Volume 2: Psychological and biological models.* Cambridge, MA: Bradford Books/MIT Press.

McEwen, B. S., De Kloet, E. R., & Rostene, W. (1986). Adrenal steroid receptors and actions in the nervous system. *Phsyiological Reviews, 66,* 1121–1188.

Meichenbaum, D. (1977). *Cognitive-behavior modification: An integrative approach.* New York: Plenum Press.

Meichenbaum, D., & Gilmore, B. (1984). The nature of unconscious processes: A cognitive-behavioral perspective. In K. S. Bowers & D. Meichenbaum (Eds.), *The unconscious reconsidered* (pp. 273–298). New York: Wiley.

Miller, L. (1986). 'Narrow localizationism' in psychiatric neuropsychology. *Psychological Medicine, 16,* 729–734.

Mishkin, M. (1982). A memory system in the monkey. *Philosophical Transactions of the Royal Society of London [Biology], 298,* 85–95.

Nadel, L., & Wexler, K. (1984). Neurobiology, representations and memory. In G. Lynch, J. L. McGaugh, & N. Weinberger (Eds.), *The neurobiology of learning and memory* (pp. 125–134). New York: The Guilford Press.

Nadel, L., & Zola-Morgan, S. (1984). Infantile amnesia: A neurobiological perspective. In M. Moscovitch (Ed.), *Infant memory* (pp. 145–172). New York: Plenum Press.

O'Keefe, J., & Nadel, L. (1978). *The hippocampus as a cognitive map.* Oxford: The Clarendon Press.

Paillard, J., Michel, F., & Stelmach, G. (1983). Localization without content: A tactile analogue of "blind sight". *Archives of Neurology, 40,* 548–551.

Pinker, S., & Prince, A. (1988). On language and connectionism: Analysis of a parallel distributed processing model of language acquisition. *Cognition, 28,* 73–193.

Rescorla, R. A. (1969). Conditioned inhibition of fear. In N. J. Mackintosh & W. K. Honig (Eds.), *Fundamental issues in associative learning* (pp. 65–89). Halifax: Dalhousie University Press.

Rescorla, R. A. (1980). *Pavlovian second-order conditioning: Studies in associative learning.* Hillsdale, NJ: L. Erlbaum Associates.

Rescorla, R. A. (1985). Inhibition and facilitation. In R. R. Miller & N. E. Spear (Eds.), *Information processing in animals: Conditioned inhibition* (pp. 299–326). Hillsdale, NJ: L. Erlbaum Associates.

Ross, R. T., & LoLordo, V. M. (1987). Devaluation of the relation between Pavlovian occasion-setting and instrumental discriminative stimuli: A blocking analysis. *Journal of Experimental Psychology, Animal Behavior Processes, 13,* 3–16.

Rumelhart, D. E., McClelland, J. L. (and the PDP Research Group). (1986). *Parallel distributed processing: Explorations in the microstructure of cognition. Volume 1: Foundations.* Cambridge, MA: Bradford Books/MIT Press.

Ryle, G. (1949). *The concept of mind.* New York: Barnes and Noble.

Safran, J. D., Vallis, T. M., Segal, Z. V., & Shaw, B. F. (1986). Assessment of core cognitive processes in cognitive therapy. *Cognitive Therapy and Research, 10,* 509–526.

Schacter, D. L. (1985). Multiple forms of memory in humans and animals. In N. M. Weinberger, J. L. McGaugh, & G. Lynch (Eds.), *Memory systems of the brain* (pp. 351–379). New York: Guilford Press.

Schacter, D. L. (1987). Implicit memory: history and current status. *Journal of Experimental Psychology: Learning, Memory and Cognition, 13,* 501–508.

Schacter, D. L. (1989). On the relation between memory and consciousness: Dissociable interactions and conscious experience. In H. L. Roediger & F. I. M. Craik (Eds.), *Varieties of memory and consciousness: Essays in honor of Endel Tulving* (pp. 355–389). Hillsdale, NJ: Erlbaum Associates.

Schacter, D. L., & Graf, P. (1986). Preserved learning in amnesic patients: Perspectives from research on direct priming. *Journal of Clinical and Experimental Neuropsychology, 8,* 727–743.

Schacter, D. L., & Moscovitch, M. (1984). Infants, amnesics, and dissociable memory systems. In M. Moscovitch (Ed.), *Infant memory* (pp. 173–216). New York: Plenum Press.

Schneider, W., & Shiffrin, R. M. (1977). Controlled and automatic human information processing: I. Detection, search and attention. *Psychological Review, 84,* 1–66.

Squire, L. R. (1987). *Memory and the brain.* New York: Oxford University Press.

Tranel, D., & Damasio, A. R. (1985). Knowledge without awareness: An autonomic index of facial recognition by prosopagnosics. *Science, 228,* 1453–1455.

Warrington, E. K., & Weiskrantz, L. (1968). New method of testing long-term retention with special reference to amnesic patients. *Nature, 217,* 972–974.

Weiskrantz, L. (1986). *Blindsight: A case study and implications*. Oxford: The Clarendon Press.

Wilson, W. R. (1979). Feeling more than we can know: Exposure effects without learning. *Journal of Personality and Social Psychology, 37*, 811–821.

Zajonc, R. B. (1980). Feeling and thinking: Preferences need no inferences. *American Psychologist, 35*, 151–175.

# 6

# Constructs of the Mind in Mental Health and Psychotherapy

## Richard S. Lazarus

Some years ago, when I was thinking about cognitive appraisal as the central process in emotion, I realized that the cognitive revolution in psychology did not create new constructs with which to understand the human mind but only changed the definition and arrangement of old constructs. The basic theoretical constructs have always consisted of *motivation, emotion,* and *cognition*. In an interesting discussion of the origins of faculty psychology, Hilgard (1980) questions whether this "trilogy of mind" describes fundamental faculties or is merely a convenient classification of mental activities. To the trilogy we must add two other fundamental concepts, namely *actions* and the *environmental stimulus* array, making a total of five concepts to juggle in our theories.

This chapter was originally intended to present my latest thoughts about cognition–emotion relationships. The first part of the chapter does this and more, adding the construct of motivation as well as those of action and environment. In the second part, I discuss the relevance of these relationships to psychotherapy. I have taken on the additional task because the cognitive and relational theories of emotion and coping developed by my colleagues and me, and our programmatic research, provide a comprehensive language and way of thinking about the constructs of the mind and how they relate to each other in adaptation. I would, therefore, like to try out these ideas in the clinical context.

Because the argument is complex and comes to its conclusions very late in the chapter, there is wisdom in adopting an anticlimactic style with conclusions stated at the outset. The reader will know where I am heading if I now ask and answer three searching questions:

First, can integrated or harmonious functioning, which I regard as the hallmark of mental health, ever be generated through psychotherapy without changing cognitive activity? My answer is no. Cognition is the key to functioning and change; it provides motivational direction, emotional significance, and the justification of action, and it connects action to the environmental context by the principle of feedback.

Richard S. Lazarus • Department of Psychology, University of California, Berkeley, California 94720.

Second, is cognitive change capable of producing integrated functioning? My answer to this, too, is no. Cognition is a necessary condition of motivation and emotion, and of change, but not a sufficient condition. Without motivational and emotional conformance, the constructs of mind remain disconnected. In short, for integrated functioning to occur, people must want to do what their appraisals imply and experience the emotions consonant with them. When motives, emotions, and cognitions dance to different drummers, there is disconnection and the risk of dysfunction.

Third, can we understand optimal functioning when attention is directed only to the structure or components of the mind, that is, cognition, emotion, and motivation, without reference to the way the person acts in a particular environment? The answer to this question must also be no. The mind cannot be divorced from the environmental conditions under which it operates or develops, or from situated actions.

## RECENT HISTORY

In the 1940s and 1950s, Freudians and reinforcement learning theorists placed drives early in the S-O-R sequence. Drives that were in conflict or blocked from discharge produced tension or anxiety, which was reduced by adaptive or ego-defensive behavior learned through the principle of reinforcement.

Figure 1 contains the concepts of motivation (as drive), emotion, and action. Thought is not mentioned. Freud regarded thought as an outcome of delayed or blocked primary drives. The safe discharge of drive tensions required that a secondary ego process be developed by the child to facilitate the inhibition or discharge of impulses based on the test of reality. Although Freud made thought secondary to drive and emotion, so-called ego psychologists came along later to once again enthrone cognition as independent and perhaps even primary.

This shift returned us to a position that had been well articulated as long ago as Aristotle, who suggested that people are made angry by the thought that they have been insulted or demeaned. Mainstream psychology has once again resurrected cognition—like the biblical Lazarus—in the form of judgments, expectations, attributions, or appraisals of the significance of what is happening for well-being. German action theory, which Frese and Sabini (1985a) define as a conception of human behavior directed toward the accomplishment of goals, governed by plans that are hierarchically arranged, and responsive to feedback from the environment, is a good example.

Psychology has also turned from structural S-R and S-O-R formulations toward a *systems approach* that focuses on temporal relations and the flow of behavior involving many interdependent variables and processes (see also McGuire, 1983). A systems arrangement of variables and processes in emotion is portrayed in Figure 2. Here the stimulus is buried in a person–environment transaction, still important but only in relationship with person characteristics; cognitive appraisal and coping are mediators of emotion; motivation, which comprises means,

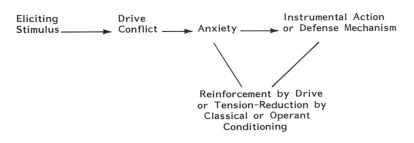

FIGURE 1. The drive-reinforcement view of adaptation.

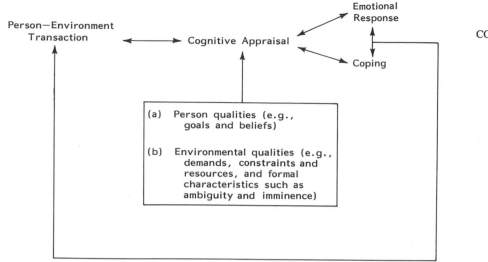

FIGURE 2. A cognitive-rational systems view of adaptation.

ends, and cognitive concerns as well as drives, is identified as goals, which in this system are antecedent variables that interact with personal beliefs and environmental events in shaping appraisal and coping. The system is in constant flux, and because it is recursive, the arrows go in many directions, with any variable capable of being antecedent, mediating process, or outcome depending on the point in time at which one enters the flow. Bandura (1978) uses the term *reciprocal determinism* (cf. also Phillips & Orton, 1983) for this metatheoretical concept, whereas I use the term *transaction*.

Although Figure 2 (cf. Lazarus, DeLongis, Folkman, & Gruen, 1985; Lazarus & Folkman, 1984) centers on cognitive appraisal and coping and contains antecedents I emphasize, comparable analyses with different language and detail are possible. For example, Bandura uses the term *self-efficacy* (Bandura, 1977, 1982) where I speak of *secondary appraisal* to denote the person's situational appraisal of control over the encounter and its outcome. Secondary appraisal is a broader concept than self-efficacy, however, because it includes coping options, resources, and constraints that the person must consider before acting or reacting. Although there are numerous controversies, one finds a remarkable degree of convergence of basic concepts across diverse cognitive-relational theories of emotion and adaptation.

## BASIC PRINCIPLES

Very briefly stated, cognitive and relational theories of emotion contain two basic themes: First, emotion is a response to evaluative judgments or *meaning;* second, these judgments are about ongoing *relationships* with the environment, namely how one is doing in the agendas of living and whether an encounter with the environment is one of harm or benefit. This judgment reflects the "motivational principle," which is that one's goal hierarchy or what is most and least important to the person, as well as the specific external conditions of an encounter, determine the potential for harm or benefit.

Emotion theorists are divided on a number of major issues, many of which are beyond what can be covered here. However, a few dealing with terminology should be addressed for purposes of clarification. *Acute emotions* such as anger, fear, joy, and pride are reactions to specific encounters of the moment; acute means they are short-lived and distinguished from longer-term emotions called *moods*. Acute emotions tend to be centered on the immediate encounter, whereas moods involve broader, longer-term, and more existential concerns. Each emotion, whether acute or a mood, expresses the particular harm or benefit that is cognized to be at stake in an ongoing relationship with the environment.

Psychologists commonly speak of *affect* as a synonym of emotion; however, the term *affect* emphasizes the cognitive, subjective state and deemphasizes the motor-behavioral and physiological aspects of an emotion. I prefer the term *emotion* because it includes these latter processes without which the emotion concept is shorn of essential components, despite the fact that the function of physiological changes in emotion, and whether such changes are necessary to the definition of emotion, remain unsettled.

Psychologists also distinguish between trait and state emotions, referring to the extent to which the origins of the reaction reside in the person (trait) or in the situational context (state). One speaks of *emotion as a trait* when the emotional pattern is recurrent; for example, in Ellis's (Ellis & Bernard, 1985) and Beck's (1976) therapeutic approach, attention is directed at the irrational assumptions about social relationships that (as a trait) characterize the person in trouble and generate the same type of emotional distress repeatedly. The therapy is designed to overcome the cognitive tendency that causes manifestations of distress such as anxiety or depression. *State emotions,* on the other hand, are largely contextual and evanescent and therefore are not of great interest to the clinician, though they are nevertheless important to understand.

The transactional themes of meaning and relationship are expressed theoretically in the concept of cognitive appraisal (cf. Lazarus, 1966, 1981; Lazarus & Launier, 1978; Lazarus & Folkman, 1984) and coping (Folkman & Lazarus, 1980, 1985; Lazarus & Folkman, 1984; Folkman, Lazarus, Dunkel-Schetter, DeLongis, & Gruen, 1986a; Folkman, Lazarus, Gruen, & DeLongis, 1986b). *Primary appraisal* concerns whether what is happening in a relationship is relevant for one's well-being. This is assessed as the stakes one has in an encounter. *Secondary appraisal* concerns the options and resources for coping with troublesome relationships.

The task of cognitive appraisal is to assimilate two sometimes contradictory sets of forces operating in a person's transactions with the environment: The goals and beliefs brought to the scene by the person *and* the environmental realities that affect the outcome of the transaction must be synthesized in the appraisal. To overemphasize personal agendas, however, is autism and to overemphasize the environment is to abandon one's personal identity. Survival would be impossible if appraisals were constantly in a bad fit with the environmental realities. It would be equally in jeopardy if we failed to take personal stakes into account in our appraisals.

*Coping* is important in the emotion process because it can change the significance for well-being of what is happening in the encounter in one of two ways: (1) by actions that alter the actual terms of the person–environment relationship, or (2) by cognitive activity that influences either the deployment of attention (e.g., by avoidance) or the meaning of the encounter (e.g., denial or distancing). The latter process has also been referred to as emotion-focused coping, whereas the former is problem-focused coping (e.g., Folkman & Lazarus, 1980; Lazarus & Folkman, 1984). Throughout the remainder of this chapter, I will use the term *cognitive coping* for the latter because emotion-focused coping is essentially a cognitive process.

## CONTROVERSIES ABOUT THE COGNITION-EMOTION RELATIONSHIP

Many theorists and researchers accept the premise that adult human emotion can best be understood in cognitive terms. Indeed, the term *appraisal* has been adopted by a large number of writers, though it is often used imprecisely. My colleagues and I distinguish between *information* or knowledge and *appraisal,* which refers to an evaluation of the significance of information for personal well-being and action (cf. Kreitler & Kreitler, 1976).

Although few seem to challenge that appraisal can affect emotion quality and intensity, current controversies tend to focus on three closely intertwined questions: (1) Is appraisal necessary for emotion? (2) Are there conditions, for example, in animals or infants, under which emotions can occur without appraisal? (3) Are cognition and emotion best regarded as separate processes or as indissolubly bound together and only separated with difficulty, as in psychopathology?

The separatist position has been debated by Zajonc (1980, 1984) and me (Lazarus, 1982, 1984). Zajonc's position appealed to many because of the false belief that cognitive theories leave emotion bloodless and cold by subsuming it under thought. As Tomkins (1981, p. 306) put it using the images of Shakespeare, "a remedy [is needed] for affect 'sicklied o'er with the pale cast of thought.'" The belief that cognitive theories take the heat out of emotion is encouraged by the imprecise equation of emotion and cognition as illustrated by Solomon's (1980, p. 271) comment that "emotions are akin to judgments," or Sartre's (1948, p. 52) statement, taken out of context, that "emotion is a certain way of apprehending the world."

Zajonc argued that there are separate anatomical brain structures for emotion and cognition and, therefore, that emotion could precede cognition as well as the other way around. This position is especially appealing to those who think of emotion as a hard-wired, innate process. Separatists also tend to reduce mental activity to neurophysiological processes. Reduction leaves an unresolved mind–body problem in which key mental concepts such as appraisal and coping are not parallel to concepts at the body level. This lack of adequate mapping makes the two levels of analysis, neurophysiological and psychological, difficult to connect in a meaningful way. It is also risky to make a decision about psychological concepts on the basis of what we currently know about the anatomy and physiology of the brain (see also Burghardt, 1985).

I favor a *yes* answer to the question of whether appraisal is necessary to emotion, which is not the same as saying that the appraisal is always conscious, deliberate, or rational (Lazarus, 1982, 1984). For the garden variety of human emotions, no other principle of emotion generation is necessary. Given what evidence is available, the burden of proof of another mechanism rests on anyone who would so claim. A statement by Sartre (1948, pp. 51–52) points up the essential connection of emotion and cognition as convincingly as any I have seen:

> It is evident, in effect, that the man who is afraid is afraid *of* something. Even if it is a matter of one of those indefinite anxieties which one experiences in the dark, in a sinister and deserted passageway, etc., one is afraid *of* certain aspects of the night, of the world. And doubtless, all psychologists have noted that emotion is set in motion by a perception, a representation-signal, etc. But it seems that for them the emotion then withdraws from the object in order to be absorbed into itself. Not much reflection is needed to understand that, on the contrary, the emotion returns to the object at every moment and it's fed there. For example, flight in a state of fear is described as if the object were not, before anything else, a flight *from* a certain object, as if the object fled did not remain present in the flight itself, as its theme, its reason for being, *that from which one flees.* And how can one talk about anger, in which one strikes, injures, and threatens, without mentioning the person who represents the objective unity of these insults, threats, and blows? In short, the affected subject and the affective object are bound in an indissoluble synthesis. Emotion is a certain way of apprehending the world.

Expanding on Sartre, I offer the following manifesto for cognitive theorists that sums up the issue: Emotion and cognition are inseparable. If the personal meaning, however primitive or inchoate it might be, vanishes, so does the emotion. Emotion without cognition would be mere activation without the differential direction manifested in the impulse to attack in anger or to flee in fear. What would motivation be without cognition? It, too, would be merely a diffuse, undifferentiated state of activation, as in a tissue tension that does not specify the consummatory goal or the means required to attain it (cf. Gallistel, 1980, 1985; Klein, 1958; Stadler & Wehner, 1985; White, 1960). Integration of behavior would be impossible without cognitive direction (Miller, Galanter, & Pribram, 1960). There could be no possibility of the feedback control of behavior without the ability to take cognizance of what is happening. Cognition is thus the key to emotion and integrated human functioning.

Yet, because there is so much misunderstanding here, I emphasize that cognition and emotion are not the same thing. The information that one has been threatened or insulted does not *per se* produce or constitute the emotion of fear or anger. In order to feel fear or anger, one must also appraise the information as signifying harm, in the past, present, or future. If the person who insults us has no personal or social power to harm, the insult will probably not result in anger. Similarly, if the potential danger is totally within our power to neutralize or avoid, we are not apt to react with fear. In other words, the environmental information must be seen as relevant to our well-being to generate involvement in the transaction (Singer, 1974); detached knowledge is not enough to generate emotion. This view has a parallel in Arnheim's (1958) analysis of aesthetic emotions; to feel emotion, one must be actively engaged in appreciating a painting or a piece of music, not merely looking at it in a detached fashion.

There are many who agree with the preceding theorem yet still question the principle that emotion is *always* a response to meaning. As Hoffman (1985) puts it, "we gain very little by postulating in advance, as Lazarus does, that cognitive evaluation is always necessary." There is doubt that a single cognitive principle works for simple animals and infants. Leventhal (1984; Leventhal & Tomarken, 1986) speaks of a sensorimotor level of emotional processing and regards as innate the newborn's receptivity to emotional cues such as voice tone and facial expression. Leventhal and Tomarken (1986, p. 275) write, for example, that "the variety of expressive reactions produced just hours after birth provide strong evidence to the preprogrammed nature of expression and its associated set of emotional experiences, though evidence for the latter half of the assumption is lacking." Therefore, even though infants grow into adults for whom cognitive activity mediates emotional responses, the nay-sayers argue that infants are unable to engage in the complex meaning-building activity on which emotions later depend.

The evidence on which to resolve this issue is difficult if not impossible to obtain, mostly for methodological reasons (cf. Lazarus, 1984). Any decision must therefore be made tentatively and by surmise from whatever is known about cognitive appraisal in infants and young children. Emde's (1984, p. 82) observation that smiling in the newborn is uncommonly related to external events should make us wary of statements that infants display emotions before they are capable of making even the most primitive kinds of appraisals.

On this issue, research by Campos and his colleagues (Bertenthal, Campos, & Barrett, 1984) suggests that an infant's appraisal of the dangers of height depends on experience with locomotion (crawling) and that such appraisals could develop very early. Other research (e.g., Harris, 1988; Harter, 1982; Ridgeway, Bretherton, & Barrows, 1985; Schwartz & Trabasso, 1984; Stein & Levine, 1988) suggests that young children understand much more about the significance of social relations underlying emotion than has hitherto been assumed. The development of the concept of self (cf. Lewis, 1988) appears relevant here too. We may well be understating an infant's appraisal capacities and also mistaking very early expressive activity as evidence of emotion. Therefore, it may not be so intemperate to propose that emotion is "always" (a high-risk word) a response to meaning and that no other mechanism of emotion generation is required.

The case for emotion in infrahuman animals may be similar. Animals may have much more cognitive capacity to make rough categorical appraisals than is ordinarily acknowledged. Small changes in another animal's bodily comportment can rapidly change defensive rage or a feeling of security into fear, or vice versa. It is not enough to label these patterns as *hard-wired* in the nervous system without identifying the neurophysiological process. Some of these reactions, especially in very simple animals such as the fowl and fish studied by Tinbergen (1951), could well be hard-wired and therefore not subject to learning or cognitive mediation, but I remain impressed by Beach's (1955) famous admonitions about "either/or" treatments of genetics and learning in trying to understand adaptive behavior.

I now realize that I made a tactical error in my argument with Zajonc (1980, 1984) by seeming to overextend the meaning of cognition to include inborn discriminations between dangerous and benign stimulus configurations. I had intended this to be an analogy, not an example, of cognitive activity. However, in including hard-wired processes in the definition of cognitive appraisal, I confused the issue by overextending the boundaries of cognition (cf. Ellis, 1985; Kleinginna & Kleinginna, 1985). It is difficult to evaluate the limits of cognitive activity in simple animals, as well as in human infants. To argue that meaning is necessary to emotion is to presume, by definition, that when an animal or infant is not capable of generating meaning of the most elementary sort—if this could ever be demonstrated—it is also unable to experience an emotion even when it acts expressively (e.g., with a smile) as though an emotion is taking place.

Even if one accepts the preceding as tenable, the issue about how meaning arises—via appraisal—in the generation of an emotion remains nevertheless unsettled. The initial appraisal is often hasty, incomplete, and even inaccurate, in which case a judgment that one is in danger or safe can be changed by further input or deliberation (Folkins, 1970), a process I have called *reappraisal*. Zajonc was correct in arguing that an emotion can be instantaneous and contain very little in the way of complex information processing. But this is not to say that emotion is entirely free of cognitive activity.

The approach to appraisal I have advocated before seems to have a parallel in Buck's (1985) concept of *syncretic cognition,* which is analogous to Gibson's (1966, 1979) view of perception as the analog-detection of ecologically significant information. In *analytic cognition,* on the other hand, the mind is viewed as a digital computer that engages in the linear scanning and buildup of meaning from originally meaningless bits in a stimulus display. This is the approach to knowledge that characterizes much of the field of cognitive psychology and is called information processing.

LeDoux (1986) has suggested that there is a neural pathway for affective processing from the thalamus to the amygdala, which can function independently of the neocortex; this pathway permits rapid, crude, and even hasty judgments of danger in the environment, a defensive reaction that later can be aborted on the basis of more detailed cognitive analysis. It is tempting to think of this thalamo-amygdala neural circuit as the analog of a primitive, instantaneous, unreflective, and perhaps unconscious stimulus evaluation process in contrast with appraisals and reappraisals that are complex, deliberate, conscious, and reasoned and which must, therefore, involve the neocortex (see also Lazarus, 1986).

Although my position is that the personal significance of an encounter is a necessary condition for emotion and although I have emphasized a holistic process of appraisal akin to Buck's syncretic cognition, I need not take a stand on which meaning-generating process is involved in any particular encounter. Both could be involved, and the process could vary with the type of creature (human vs. nonhuman), the stage of human development, and the temporal stage of the encounter when the observations are made.

I believe we should also be wary about a doctrine of separatism as a model of the mind. In addition to the dangers of reducing psychological processes to neurophysiological, the proper psychological and neurophysiological units or subsystems to identify remain elusive. To divide the mind into cognition and emotion segments seems to me strangely out of touch with the way we function. Emotion involves portions of the brain that extend from the relatively primitive, such as the brain stem (e.g., the reticular activating system), the hypothalamus, and thalamus, to phylogenetically much more advanced units such as the limbic system and cortex. I wonder whether it makes sense to combine such diverse portions of the brain's anatomy into a single process with the diversity and complexity of emotion and to regard it as operating separately from cognitive activity, which includes sensory, perception, memorial, and analytic processes that take place all over the brain.

Although thought and emotion are normally conjoined, as my earlier quote from Sartre about fear implies, they can, of course, be kept apart, as in what is clinically referred to as *distancing, isolation, depersonalization, repression, denial,* or *dissociation.* We think of these "defensive" processes as pathological or pathogenic, the result of intentional effort at regulating distressing emotions. When people use them, they are said to be out of touch with their actions and feelings and with the environmental conditions they face. However, it is one thing to say that separation is *possible* under certain conditions and another thing to say that it is *normative.*

Dissociative theories of hypnosis, for example, imply the splitting of sensory and other mental processes, suggesting that a single, central cognitive control process is not always firmly in the saddle (cf. Ahsen, 1985). However, when splitting occurs, there is still some degree of mutual awareness of interaction among split thoughts and images in the normal waking state. Thus all such dissociations are relative rather than absolute, if care is taken to detect interactions (Hilgard, 1975, 1977).

To give the separation between motivation, cognition, and emotion the status of a biological principle is to turn the mind, which is usually coordinated and directed, into an uncoordinated arrangement in which each function operates on its own. This can also be a dysfunctional arrangement. Instead, we should be seeking the *organizing principle* or principles that make the components of the mind a unit operating in harmony with the adaptational requirements of the environment and the personal agendas that create the story lines of our lives.

Although it is convenient for analysis to separate diverse mental functions, we must also be able to visualize how the parts work in synthesis. When we take literally what our penchant for analysis creates, namely breaking down the whole into separate components, we are in danger of failing to put the parts back together as an organized whole (Lazarus, Coyne, & Folkman, 1982). This was one of the messages of gestalt psychology and is a premise held dear by systems theorists, as stated recently by Evered (1980, p. 7):

> Traditional causal thinking which underlies much of modern science has not proved adequate for the task of understanding change, and increasingly one senses that it never can. The assumption of an *independent, external,* and *antecedent* factor, a set of factors that "causes" changes seems far too simplistic. . . . As von Bertalanffy puts it: "We may state as characteristic of modern science that this scheme of isolable units acting in one-way causality has proved to be insufficient. Hence the appearance, in all fields of science, of notions like wholeness, holistic, organismic, gestalt, etc., which all signify that, in the last resort, we must think in terms of systems of elements in mutual interaction. . . .
>
> Until quite recently the prevailing view of science . . . incorporated a bias to generic, past-oriented, antecedent explanation. In the past two or three decades, however, the culturally infectious influences of existentialism, phenomenology, gestalt psychology and systems thinking have influenced science toward a more present-oriented, interactive and perceptual view of science—at least in some areas of the social sciences.

## DISCONNECTION AS AN EXPLANATION OF MALADAPTATION

The components of the mind control adaptational commerce with the environment. For optimal functioning and mental health, there must be integration and harmony among these components. Disconnection among them places the person at risk for psychopathology. Bear in mind that integration is not good or bad *per se;* zealotry, xenophobia, and the acceptance of societal evil can be one of its follies. We must recognize, too, that a person comes to treatment not because of a single occurrence of difficulty but for sustained trouble. Although disconnection among the five constructs in a single life encounter could be of value for the person, its presence as a recurrent pattern is likely to pose adaptational problems.

The case for the normal integration of the constructs of the mind requires qualification. For example, mental development involves gaining gradual freedom from the concrete environmental stimulus and from the tyranny of drives or impulses in action. With respect to the *environmental stimulus,* as children mature, they become increasingly capable of manipulating concrete objects and events symbolically, thus becoming free of concrete dependency on them. Piaget (1952) regarded the development of intelligence as always moving in the direction of increasing spatial and temporal distance between the person and the objects of the environment. With respect to *action,* Werner (1948) pointed out that, although very young children cannot inhibit the expression of impulses, in the course of their development they become capable of doing so by interposing thought between impulse and action; this allows them to control action by delaying it and attuning it to the requirements of the situation.

At the same time, however, development brings with it increasing integration of the constructs of the mind. Cognition, emotion, and motivation become welded into a system that, though under tension, must remain in touch with the environment and in control of actions in the interests of helping the person survive and flourish. The links between action and the demands, constraints, and resources of the environment, as well as among the components of the mind, are forged and changed developmentally and dialectically by continuous adaptational transactions. For example, Block (1982; see also Piaget, 1952) has emphasized not a smooth movement toward integration but the occurrence of periodic crises in which the established psychological structure, when it is no longer viable, requires a reorganization that works better. Fischer and Pipp (1984, p. 89) put the matter a bit differently, emphasizing more than I the need for constant effort to maintain integrity:

> With development, the capacity for integrating components of thought and behavior grows, and at the same time the capacity for active fractionation increases (e.g., dissociation and repression). The mind is therefore both fractionated and integrated; there is neither a unitary conscious system nor a unitary unconscious one, but there are conscious and unconscious components that can be coordinated or kept separate.

Later they state that "the mind is naturally fractionated, and people must work to integrate its pieces" (p. 138). But listen to some other voices. von Hofsten (1985, p. 95) writes:

> It has been argued in the present chapter that perception and action are functionally inseparable. The function of perception is to guide action in setting goals as well as in supporting movements. This is done by making knowledge about critical task-related properties of the world (i.e., affordances) immediately available to the action system.

And Neisser (1985, p. 97) says that

> under normal circumstances perception and action are simultaneous and well coordinated. The links between them are very close. Indeed, von Hofsten finds them all but inseparable. "It is . . . difficult to speak of one of these two aspects of biological functioning without referring to the other" (von Hofsten, 1985, p. 8). But unfortunately it is *not* difficult; we have been doing it for a century.

What do I mean by *disconnection*? Disconnection refers to a condition in which the components of the mind are responsive to divergent influences and generate contradictory actions. For example, what the person thinks may be out of touch with the emotions that are experienced or the motives that shape action. Epstein (1985, p. 288) makes a similar point in citing cases in which "the person does not 'feel' like doing what intellectually he or she 'thinks' should be done"; "the person may state . . . 'I made myself do it.'" Epstein emphasizes that an overall self attempts to integrate various subselves, but when there is complete insulation among the subsystems, there is psychopathology. Schwartz (1979) seems to mean something similar by his use of the term *disregulation* to refer to the loss of communication among the parts of the brain, which allows the normally integrated system of feedback loops to go out of control.

Disconnection overlaps cognitive dissonance (Festinger, 1957), a concept that was once all the rage in psychology, especially social psychology. However, *dissonance* refers to cognitive contradictions—for example, between thoughts—whereas disconnection involves contradictions among cognition, emotion, and motivation and between mind on the one hand and environment and action on the other. Disconnection is, therefore, a broader concept. Dissonance is also a motivational principle—its presence motivates efforts to resolve the contradiction—and so it is said to play a causal role in thought and action. The concept lost favor, I believe, because there were no principles capable of predicting whether or how the person would seek resolution of a contradiction. On the other hand, I view disconnection as an effect of efforts to cope with a troubled person–environment relationship, not a cause of such efforts, as will be seen shortly in the section on ''seeking disconnection.''

For the opposite of disconnection to occur, short-term goals must be in harmony with long-term goals and contribute to them as means to ends. Conflict among goals is obviously disruptive of harmony and results in the system components pulling apart rather than working together. Motivation must accord with (cognitive) understandings of what is possible, likely, reasonably safe, properly timed, properly sequenced. Emotions must be accurate reflections of the significance of encounters for well-being. All conflict theories of psychopathology and mental health treat this as a basic assumption. Integration is a common term for harmony and mental health and fragmentation or ego failure for disharmony and mental illness (cf. Haan, 1969, 1977; Menninger, 1954).

## TYPES OF DISCONNECTION

Figure 3 presents a simple schematization of the five basic concepts I have been discussing, perusal of which will help the reader follow the various forms of disconnection I will identify and discuss next.

### BETWEEN MIND AND ENVIRONMENT

Two fundamental subtypes of disconnection between mind and environment are common. The first involves an inappropriate appraisal of harm or threat; examples include depression, anxiety states, panic, and phobia in the apparent absence of realistic provocation. One might also include shame and guilt-centered neuroses (cf. Lewis, 1971), though Mowrer (1975) argued that guilt reactions were not, as Freud suggested, based on imaginary, nonexistent sins but were the product of genuine moral wrongs. The second subtype is the absence of appraisal

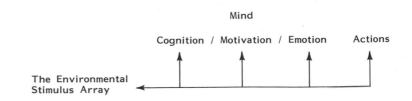

FIGURE 3. The five basic variables of adaptation.

of harm or threat when there is good reason for it. The theory of "delayed stress syndrome" or "posttraumatic stress disorder" may be an example because it is assumed that the trauma or grief connected with the high stress period (in Vietnam or in a personal or natural disaster) was blocked during the trauma, which is why the person displayed little or no disorder during the traumatic encounter but does so much later when suitably triggered. In both subtypes, when the process of cognitive appraisal has gone wrong, there are counterproductive and inappropriate patterns of emotional distress in which people who are neurotically vulnerable judge, incorrectly, that they are exposed to threatening or nonthreatening environmental conditions. There is, therefore, disconnection between mind and environment.

The fault could center either on primary or secondary appraisal processes. As an example of the former, persons with an exaggerated commitment to seeking approval may see themselves recurrently or chronically as being unloved or unappreciated; they are apt to be threatened and anxious when meeting people socially and react excessively to the slightest sign of disapproval with anxiety, guilt, humiliation, or shame. Persons with an exaggerated commitment to competition or achievement may feel recurrently or chronically that they are failures, evaluated as inadequate by others as well as themselves, and threatened and anxious when giving a performance, taking a test, or being interviewed for a job. Ellis's (1958; see also Ellis & Bernard, 1985) well-known list of "irrational" beliefs that result in chronic or recurrent emotional distress is illustrative (see also Lazarus, in press), as is Beck's (1976) cognitive triad in depression. In these examples, the persons involved accept an unreasonable stake in relationships with others, which makes them vulnerable to emotional distress in many social contexts. The treatment is designed to help such people give up these counterproductive goals and ways of thinking about what is important or essential (*mustabatory* in Ellis's terms) in daily living.

Alternatively, some persons have acquired the (secondary appraisal) tendency to exaggerate malevolence in the environment and evaluate themselves as inadequate to deal with it. This is an example of faulty secondary appraisal. Overprotective and solicitous parents encourage fear in their children about what will happen in the absence of parental protection; other parents push their children to "sink or swim" even before they have acquired competence (cf. Baumrind, 1975; Harlow, 1953; Levy, 1943). A common consequence of these pathogenic child-rearing patterns is early stunting of social skills and chronic or recurrent fearfulness and dependency.

These faulty appraisal patterns can also be a consequence of *hidden agendas,* for example, motives and beliefs (or thoughts) that are not acknowledged because of defense mechanisms. For example, Lewis (1971) interprets recurrent shame emotions (e.g., the tendency to react with humiliation, chagrin, embarrassment, or shyness) as an expression of an unconscious fear of abandonment. In this syndrome, the feeling of shame is experienced by a person who does not recognize the concern that underlies it, namely failing to live up to a demanding parent's standards and, therefore, being disapproved or abandoned.

When faulty appraisals and the emotions they produce involve hidden agendas, they are difficult to evaluate and treat because the coping process on which they are based conceals or distorts the underlying goals and beliefs generating the distress. The person overreacts with humiliation, for example, to many situations whose threat content is not readily apparent. The reaction, and the obscure appraisal process on which it is based, seems inappropriate to or disconnected from the environment that elicits it. The pattern can only be understood from the vantage point of the hidden agenda.

## BETWEEN MIND AND ACTION

The two major logical possibilities in this form of disconnection are actions that do not conform to intentions and intentions that are not expressed in action. These patterns are usually explained by reference to one or another of the three constructs of mind. For example, we say that people are acting in ways that are inappropriate to their *wishes;* that they are acting inconsistently with their *feelings;* or that they *cognize* things in one way but act in another. The meaning of disconnection is roughly the same whether we refer to motivations, emotions, or cognitions because each component seems to stand for a unitary mind. In other words, depending on whether we incline toward cognition, emotion, or motivation, we use one construct of mind to stand for the whole mental process.

Without reference to a specific component of mind such as a wish, feeling, or thought, we have no satisfactory account of actions disconnected from mind except perhaps to refer to developmental immaturities, as when we speak of *disorders of impulse* in which the person acts before thinking or, like a child, fails to control impulse; or, like the sociopathic adult who has failed to internalize social proscriptions, the person does not experience guilt and is therefore not restrained by it. Another version of this is to speak of regression to a more primitive form of functioning.

Lack of *skills or knowledge* is another explanation. Within the framework of action theory, Semmer and Frese (1985) describe one organizational mode of action that is sequential, requiring a mental representation of the course of the action as well as continuous feedback. Sometimes, however, cognition runs ahead of action. Another mode is hierarchical in which smaller units of action can be summarized and contained or chunked within higher abstractions. When the higher units are too global, they may not be connected well with the specific actions that are called for, and there is a gap between plans and actions.

Semmer and Frese (1985, pp. 297–298) illustrate this with assertiveness:

> If one has command over the hierarchical system of behaviors that constitute "assertiveness," he or she is able to generate requisite actions merely by "triggering" the highest unit—for example, the strategic decision that in a given situation he or she should not yield but rather should assert him or herself. If, however, this system is not adequately developed, the code "assertiveness" is a mere verbal code. At best it contains lower levels in the form of verbal descriptions, but lacks serviceable action plans that entail behavioral skills and the adequate use of feedback. Because its connection to lower units is only vague and global, Volpert . . . calls this type of higher unit a *global code*. One goal of therapy is to replace global codes with supercodes. Neither the mere cognitive insight (e.g., "I should be more assertive") nor the mere teaching of specific behavioral skills (e.g., "assertive behaviors") will be sufficient. . . . Rather, it is necessary to connect general cognitions with appropriate actions, in such a way that a single command can regulate the entire action sequence.

The preceding is interesting and important. However, the typical clinical explanation of disconnection between mind and action is based on *conflict*. Reference to emotions that conflict with goals (as when fears get in the way of actions) or to cognitions that conflict with goals (as when we fail to act because of consequent dangers to our well-being) makes use of one or another type of disconnection among the three constructs of mind and their respective links to environment and action.

BETWEEN ENVIRONMENT AND ACTION

There is also no satisfactory explanation for disconnection between environment and action without recourse to what is going on in the mind. Adopting a totally behavioristic stance forces us to refer to a history of prior conditioning that is seldom actually identified and tracked. This was the explanatory strategy of the elegant theory of learned helplessness (Seligman, 1975; Seligman, Maier, & Solomon, 1971). Its main protagonists have now given up on the original radical behavioral formulation and have turned to neobehavioristic analyses that draw upon mediating cognitive, emotional, and motivational processes, especially cognitive ones (cf. Garber & Seligman, 1980).

The components of mind can be disconnected through neurological disease and disconnection sought as a solution to some of the harsh psychological dilemmas of living. Let us examine some of the conditions under which the latter might happen and consider the adaptational value and cost.

There are, of course, many strategies of cognitive coping. I will illustrate with two powerful and commonly used cognitive coping strategies that result in disconnection, deniallike processes, and distancing.

*Deniallike processes* are a common way of regulating emotional distress, especially when people are facing devastating harms and threats. Denial means *disavowal* of some distressing truth. The incidence of denial cannot be known with any accuracy because of confusion about how it manifests itself and should be measured. There is a long history of thought about denial from a psychoanalytic perspective (cf. Lazarus, 1983, for a brief review; and Sjöbäck, 1973). There are also divergent forms of denial itself; Weisman (1972) distinguishes denial of fact, denial of distress, and denial of implication; Breznitz (1983) discusses seven forms of denial.

Denial results in *disconnection* because knowledge that is available is warded off and not utilized in awareness. Such knowledge is, in some sense, still active in the mind, as in Weisman's (1972) concept of "middle knowledge," or Freud's concept of the "return of the repressed." Although denial is an attempt to wipe out the threat cognitively, the person is said to remain vulnerable to it emotionally and in action and must engage in continual vigilance to ward off the denied truth when triggered by appropriate conditions. The disconnection usually takes the form of not appraising threat at the surface level, but such an appraisal is nevertheless occurring below the surface, which results in contradictory emotions. The diagnosis is made by the clinician, who notices the contradiction.

Denial was originally regarded by Anna Freud (A. Freud, 1946) as a primitive process used by young children but abandoned later in life in favor of avoidance. When retained into adulthood, it was regarded as a psychotic process. Without careful clinical observation, it is easy to confuse denial with a host of other common forms of cognitive coping such as avoidance and illusion. In avoidance, a threatening thought is simply not attended to; the person refuses to talk or think about it but does not disavow. Measures of denial that are based heavily on avoidance (e.g., Hackett & Cassem's denial rating scale, 1974) confuse the two cognitive coping strategies. Another look-alike is *illusion,* which is probably a universal form of cognitive coping (Lazarus, 1973). To have illusions is to believe private or collective euphemisms and untruths designed to make us feel better. If we think of denial as a family of different cognitive coping processes including disavowal of reality, avoidance, positive thinking, and illusion, each form can be assessed as to whether it is useful or dysfunctional, which probably depends on the circumstances. The reason for using the overarching term *deniallike processes* is the real possibility that each is subject to its own rules of operation.

*Distancing* or detachment involves disconnection of a different type. It refers to a process in which a person appears to keep cool in the face of threat and not give reign to the emotions that would ordinarily be generated. Parallel concepts include intellectualization, isolation, and undoing, which are terms found in the psychoanalytic conceptualization of the obsessive-compulsive clinical syndrome (cf. Shapiro, 1965).

Distancing is also used by large numbers of people, perhaps universally in certain contexts. Social institutions are often designed to increase the likelihood of "achieving a healthy distance" from disturbing events. This is illustrated by the way autopsies are staged in medical school; the face, body, and hands are covered, a cool, detached, scientific demeanor is maintained, and any suggestions of a living person for whom there could be empathy are minimized.

Like denial, distancing creates disconnection because emotions are divorced from the threatening thoughts and environmental conditions to which they would ordinarily be tied. Unlike denial, the thoughts themselves are not blotted out but are allowed to occur in a cool and detached fashion. The environment is accurately, often vigilantly searched and comprehended intellectually, but its emotional significance is deleted. It is as if we say to ourselves, "I know it's terrible, but it does not have anything to do with me."

Disconnection created by both deniallike and distancing cognitive coping processes has great adaptational value. We try hard to make it happen in certain contexts, for example, when we would be traumatized psychologically by fully assimilating the reality and failing thereby to control the associated emotional distress. Not to do so could lead to impairment of functioning. When, indeed, there is nothing else constructive to do, distancing and denial are especially useful and are apt to have minimal costs.

The parents who manage to keep their distress under control and succeed in getting their bleeding child to the hospital will be thankful for their capacity to distance; likewise with the farm child who must cut the turkey's throat to make it available for Thanksgiving dinner. The parents and/or nurse who must speak encouraging words to a dying child (cf. Hay & Oken, 1972), or deal with handicapped or distressed friends, control their distress through distancing and perhaps function better in these normally distressing roles than they would have without distancing. However, detachment is sometimes achieved by dehumanizing people who are already victims (Bernard, Ottenberg, & Redl, 1971; Lazarus, 1985). Similarly, with regard to denial, the combat navigator is benefitted if he denies the danger because there is nothing he can do about it, and he will perform better if he believes he is not in danger. The spinal-cord-injured patient who has just become a quadraplegic can also gain at the outset by denying the extent of the neurological damage, thereby maintaining hope and avoiding total despair at a time when probably nothing else can be done.

There are, however, three conditions under which disconnection can be maladaptive. The first is when it prevents an essential adaptational act. For example, students who distance from or deny the threat of failure during the period of preparation for an important examination but who should instead be mobilized for study increase the actual danger of failure. Although distancing is quite effective when nothing can be done but wait, it is counterproductive when preventive action is needed.

The second is when disconnection becomes a habitual cognitive style. Although there may be no psychological cost in a particular encounter, deniallike processes and distancing can be damaging when not abandoned in the long run. Quadraplegics who do not ultimately acknowledge the realities of their situation cannot successfully learn to be independent. The person who constantly distances is prevented from experiencing the ups and downs of emotional attachments that are a normal feature of living.

The third condition under which disconnection can be maladaptive is when it prevents the person from learning how to cope more effectively with problematic situations or from unlearning a pathogenic coping pattern. Disconnection, as will be seen later, can defeat efforts at therapeutic change.

## OVERCOMING DISCONNECTION IN PSYCHOTHERAPY

It is beginning to be clear that clients must do more than merely learn intellectually what has been happening to them, though such insight can be useful and for some therapists is even regarded as necessary. In addition to thinking differently from before, clients must act differently in the presence of the troublesome environmental condition in order to change the dysfunctional emotions experienced and their underlying goals. This point is now being expressed in different ways by many present-day clinical theorists.

Meichenbaum (Meichenbaum & Cameron, 1983, p. 141) gives recognition to the futility of attempting to change thoughts without parallel emotional accompaniment:

> It is important to understand that [cognitive self-statements] are not offered as catch-phrases or as verbal palliatives to be repeated mindlessly. There is a difference between encouraging the use of a formula or psychological litany that tends to lead to rote repetition and *emotionless* patter versus problem-solving thinking that is the object of stress inoculation training. Formula-oriented thoughts that are excessively general tend to prove ineffective. [italics added]

Ellis (1984, p. 216) makes a comparable point about the unity of cognition, emotion, and motivation:

> RET assumes that human thinking and emotion are *not* two disparate or different processes, but that they significantly overlap and are in some respects, for all practical purposes, essentially the same thing. Like the two other basic life processes, sensing and moving, they are integrally integrated and never can be seen wholly apart from each other. . . . Instead, then of saying that "Smith thinks about this problem," we should more accurately say that "Smith senses-moves-feels-THINKS about this problem."

Beck (1987, p. 32) makes a similar point; he wants to tell us that affect is not enough and that cognitive processing and working through are crucial. For example, he states that (pp. 161–162)

> some type of intellectual framework is important if the cathartic, flooding, or emotional experience is to have a therapeutic effect. It is apparent that people go through catharses and abreactions, . . . continuously throughout their lives—without any benefit. What seems to be offered within a therapeutic milieu is the patient's ability to experience simultaneously the "hot cognitions" and to step back, as it were, and to observe this experience objectively. . . . When therapy is effective the essential components are the production of "hot cognitions" and affect within a therapeutic structure and the opportunity to reality-test these cognitions—whether the therapist is employing psychoanalysis, behavior therapy, cognitive therapy, or one of the experiential therapies.

And finally (p. 163):

> All systems work together in much the same way as do the heart and lungs. Thus, you can affect the cognitive systems through cognitive therapy, but you will also get a spread to the affective, motor, and physiological systems. Similarly, physiological systems may be directly affected through procedures such as relaxation, but this may lead to reverberation throughout all the other systems.

Another version is the old distinction between intellectual insight and emotional insight, the former referring to understanding without feeling. Real change requires that the client experience the feelings that are part of a given understanding, including those that stand in the way of emotional insight (cf. Wachtel, 1977). Implicit recognition of this is the reason most psychotherapists refuse to restrict their efforts to cognition alone, and why Freudians in the 1930s came to speak of "working through" or reeducation rather than focusing treatment on abreaction or insight alone. After the initial enthusiasm for insight as the key to successful treatment began to wane, psychodynamically oriented psychotherapists increasingly came to emphasize the emotional struggle of the client to draw on the new self-knowledge (cf. Freud, 1950). It was essential that knowing about oneself be reinforced by actions that would force persons to confront the realities of their environments and their conditional emotions, in effect, to turn intellectual insight into emotional insight. Actions are necessary to provide the basis of such knowledge. Most cognitive therapists, despite their focus on cognition, join with Arnold Lazarus (1981) in pressing simultaneously on all fronts, the cognitive, emotional, motivational, and in pushing the client to act in new ways under problematic environmental conditions.

Foa and Kozak (1986) make the same point as the "principle of exposure." Citing Lang (1977, 1979), they write (Foa & Kozak, 1986, p. 20):

> Anxiety disorders are continuous attempts to avoid confrontation with fear-evoking cues. . . . Indeed, if neurotics are avoiders who fail to recognize and/or retrieve discomfort-evoking information about themselves or their environment, psychotherapy might be construed as providing a setting in which *confrontation* with such information is promoted so that changes in affect can occur. [italics added]

They suggest, in short, that fearful people must learn that their fear-inducing expectations are wrong. To learn this, they must stop avoiding and *act* in a way that makes this discovery possible. In other words, cognitive change is not enough when it is disconnected from the other components of the mind.

In our book, *Stress, Appraisal, and Coping* (Lazarus & Folkman, 1984), Folkman and I argued that an implicit tenet of a cognitive and relational theory of emotion was that, to change, clients had to think differently about themselves and their environments. We also argued that because cognition, emotion, and motivation are interdependent and normally operate as a single unit, changing the way the client construes what is going on can be approached from the vantage point of any component of mind, cognition, emotion, or motivation. If the components of the mind are normally interdependent, and if the environmental stimulus and action are powerful influences, then changing one should also produce change in the others.

Now, however, I am arguing something more, namely that the task of treatment is often difficult because of chronic disconnection in troubled people. Changes in one component alone—for example, cognition—are insufficient if the others remain disconnected. And, because for most clients, there is chronic disconnection as a result of well-established forms of cognitive coping with powerful sources of threat, the client will continue to resist change that could bring with it mental harmony or integration.

What then are the implications for clinical practice of what I have been saying about the five concepts that must be juggled in psychological theory? I can see at least five that flow from the key themes of this chapter. These themes were that emotion is a complex system of variables and processes; that it must be understood as cognitive and relational; that coping is a key mediating factor; and that harmony or integration is tantamount to mental health, whereas disconnection, especially when it is continuing and pervasive, is tantamount to psychopathology and dysfunction. Although the implications, which are stated next, will not be new to psychotherapists and are to some extent honored in practice, they emerge from and are consistent with the metatheoretical and theoretical arguments I have been emphasizing.

1. *The therapeutic strategy should match the client's problem of living.* I reject the opposite premise that psychotherapy is a highly general procedure that is applicable to all problems of living, because I believe that future advances in treatment will attempt systematically to fit the treatment strategy to the client's problem. This position is consistent with a systems analysis of emotion and adaptation in which things can go wrong for the individual at different places in the system, for example, in antecedent beliefs and commitments, the person–environment fit, primary appraisal, secondary appraisal, and coping.

Imagine, if you will, that a therapist or stress management practitioner wants to teach assertiveness as a coping skill. If the reason for the lack of skill includes hidden agendas or neurotic conflicts that will continue to operate in the present to defeat skill acquisition, one must take a different approach than if the client has simply not had the appropriate opportunity or incentive to learn. Similarly, if the client suffers from an existential malady, for example, elderly depressed clients who believe their lives are finished, the task of helping them see that their cup is half full rather than half empty will require a very different approach than might be used in dealing with a phobia or for reducing job stress.

In the face of wide divergence in client problems and therapeutic requirements, psychotherapists have two main options: One is to be flexible in adapting the therapeutic approach to the specific problem; another is to treat only one, or several related problems, for example, depression, phobia, or traumatic life events such as bereavement or disabling illness. Some therapist specialization existed in the past, manifested in the more or less informal tendencies to prefer practice with certain kinds of clients, for example, children, family groups, schizophrenics, neurotics. What I am proposing, however, is that such specialization be based on conceptual principles of emotion and adaptation that would make possible the matching of problems to the therapeutic strategy. The system of thought I have presented here is not yet far enough advanced to permit this, but I believe that it—or some other version of it—might be a step in that direction.

2. *Matching the therapeutic strategy to the client's problem requires psychodiagnosis.* A corollary of the concept of strategy/problem fit is that psychotherapists once again become concerned with *diagnosis* at the outset or in the early stages of treatment. By diagnosis I do not mean the labeling of clients with the psychiatric categories of the *Diagnostic Statistical Manual* (DSM-III). A long-standing criticism of psychiatric labeling is that it does not provide an analysis of the psychological process that has gone wrong.

One reason the study of emotion is so important clinically is that a person's *emotional pattern* can serve as a basis of inference about what is going on in the person's life. The emotions a person displays in diverse life settings provide clues about appraisal and coping processes and how they have gone wrong. Recurrent anger, for example, suggests one kind of troubled person–environment relationship, whereas anxiety or depression suggests a different kind. Just as appraisal and coping processes shape the emotional reaction, the emotional reaction in turn can be used to help infer the causal psychological process that should be dealt with in treatment. We need to think more about how psychological theory about emotion and adaptation can be better employed in clinical practice and how practice can better inform the construction of such theory.

3. *Psychotherapists must bring new understanding to clients if therapeutic change is to occur.* Noncognitive therapists will say this is retrogression to what was once called by the Freudians *insight therapy*. Yet the premise of a cognitive and relational theory of emotion, and hence of psychological dysfunction, is that cognitive appraisal underlies all emotion, whether dysfunctional or not, and regardless of strategy and terminology the bottom line of therapeutic change is, therefore, still revised understanding. Whether this understanding must be conscious or not is an open question, though awareness and verbalization may indeed be critical and are certainly assets in producing therapeutic change. If psychotherapy fails to produce new understandings and expectations, or the person fails to act on them, it will have failed to produce viable and sustained changes in psychological functioning.

Cognitive change is produced in diverse ways. The methods include desensitization and implosion; or the therapist listens acceptingly and nondirectively; in some therapies, the client's understandings are vigorously disputed; in others, the therapist subtly interprets what is happening, has the client role-play, or attempts to inspire positive thinking. The so-called cognitive therapists such as Ellis, Beck, and Meichenbaum are the most explicit in their emphasis on changing cognitive assumptions and situational appraisals.

4. *Cognitive change alone is not sufficient to produce therapeutic change.* If cognitive therapy were no more than exhortation or efforts to influence or teach, it would offer clients little of lasting value. This thesis, which is based on my arguments about psychological integration and disconnection, has a number of practical consequences:

As in learning to drive a car, clients achieve much of their new understandings and expectations by acting in their natural environments, and they must try these discoveries out and experience the distress of failure and the positive emotions that go with success. One learns most firmly by doing and feeling. Those therapists who emphasize coping are, in effect, attempting to change how the client acts toward and thinks about the environment. This is evident in the writings of Goldfried (1980), who speaks of psychotherapy as coping skills training, in Rosenbaum (1988), who emphasizes resourcefulness, and D'Zurilla (D'Zurilla & Nezu, 1982), whose interest centers on social problem-solving skills. To phrase the preceding as a general implication for practice, the therapist must encourage the client to act in ways consistent with new understandings and expectations.

Overcoming disconnection by trying out thoughts and emotions in action to produce a new integration takes patience, fortitude, and time. Pressures for brief psychotherapy, and for dramatic solutions to long-standing problems, typically run counter to the realities. The therapist should cultivate in the client modest and realistic expectations about the process. Fortunately, much of the psychological work done by the client occurs in day-to-day living situations outside the psychotherapy sessions. The conditions of change are set in motion by treatment in clients positively disposed to do something about their problems, but most therapeutic change goes on elsewhere.

The emotional and coping patterns of some clients are simply not amenable to change, and these persons might be better helped to control distress and to accept the situation rather than be urged to seek change. Questions of what can be changed, to what extent, and under what conditions, continue to plague life-span developmental psychology, social psychology, personality psychology, and clinical psychology.

In this connection, effective coping is not just problem solving but also includes emotion-focused strategies, which I used to call *palliation*. Despite our cultural commitment to active mastery, the regulation of emotion is necessary for successful living, especially when the environment is hostile and refractory. Helping clients to see the realities of their life situation and to accept them is just as valid a goal of psychotherapy as problem solving and change.

5. *Psychotherapists should be wary of the pathology mystique.* A central theme of a relational conception of emotion is that the characteristics of the physical and social environment are just as important as person characteristics in the emotional life. The clinical bias that dysfunction and distress must be understood as personal failure understates the powerful role of the environment. Psychology has yet to evolve a successful conceptualization of mental health that takes adequate account of the environmental conditions under which the person develops and functions.

Some years ago, leadership and management programs in industrial psychology foundered because, after training in human relations, middle-level executives would return to organizational settings where they were unable to apply what they had learned. Similarly, psychotherapy clients return to or continue to live in social and work settings that are often hostile and unbending. The provocations to anxiety and depression that brought the client to treatment are apt to continue unless the environments themselves are changed or the person finds a new setting in which to live and function.

It is reasonable to try to teach the client how better to cope with hostile environments, but it is also destructive to imply thereby that only troubled, inadequate people cannot overcome the distress and dysfunction that arises in such settings. As in the case of divorce, the failure is that of relationship rather than of an individual. The bias that the client must manifest health and well-being regardless of the circumstances of living has to give way to one in which the psychotherapist and client recognize that it is the person–environment relationship that is dysfunctional.

It might also be useful to recognize that many clients are distressed because they are lonely in a societal context that isolates people and defeats group involvement and commitment. When such clients come into therapy, they are often seeking the social support missing in their lives, whether or not they are aware of it. Indeed, modern-day self-help groups probably depend to a high degree on the positive emotional value of social connection. Cognitive therapies and therapeutic programs geared to a mechanical, technical outlook similar to that found in modern medicine are in danger of compounding for some of their clients the impersonal, destructive features of our fragmented society by forgetting the unmet interpersonal needs that often lie beneath the surface problems for which they sought professional help.

Furthermore, a centerpiece of earlier psychodynamic approaches to treatment was an emphasis on the therapist–patient relationship rather than on a technology of treatment. The Freudians argued that the transference relationship was a central motivating factor in the client's willingness to sustain the painful struggle of self-discovery and change, as well as a basis for understanding the client.

Although what I have said before will sound to some like the party line of traditional psychodynamic theory, I believe it is neutral with respect to which therapeutic strategy is appropriate or creates the best strategy/problem fit. The diverse therapeutic strategies observed among cognitive and noncognitive therapists alike are all intended to set in motion an active examination of and confrontation with what is troubling the client. I do not view these strategies in either/or terms, that is, as methods to be compared but as diverse ways of making the same thing happen; psychotherapy must generate new understandings and expectations in the client, new patterns of action, and new motivational and emotional patterns in the interests of a more harmonious integration.

Clients do not fit a single model but consist of very diverse people with different problems, living under different circumstances, and best approached therapeutically with a strategy that should accord with what makes them distinctive individuals. Each client lies at the intersection of three complex variables—cognition, emotion, and motivation—which are the constructs of mind; these constructs govern actions in particular environments, making the five variables psychological theory must draw upon. The difficult tasks of finding out how these variables intersect and got disconnected, and moving the client toward a better working arrangement, make psychotherapy the truly remarkable professional challenge that it is. No other occupation demands more in the way of humanity, knowledge, and capacity for intellectual creativity.

## REFERENCES

Ahsen, A. (1985). Image psychology and the empirical method. *Journal of Mental Imagery, 9*(2), 1–40.

Arnheim, R. (1958). Emotion and feeling in psychology and art. *Confinia Psychiatrica, 1,* 69–88.

Bandura, A. (1977). *Social learning theory.* Englewood Cliffs, NJ: Prentice-Hall.

Bandura, A. (1978). The self-system in reciprocal determinism. *American Psychologist, 33,* 344–358.

Bandura, A. (1982). Self-efficacy mechanism in human agency. *American Psychologist, 37,* 122–147.

Baumrind, D. (1975). Early socialization and the discipline controversy. In *University programs modular studies.* Morristown, NJ: General Learning Press.

Beach, F. A. (1955). The descent of instinct. *Psychological Review, 62,* 401–410.

Beck, A. T. (1976). *Cognitive therapy and the emotional disorders.* New York: International Universities Press.

Beck, A. T. (1987). Cognitive therapy. In J. Zeig (Ed.), *Evolution of psychotherapy.* New York: Brunner/Mazel.

Bernard, V. W., Ottenberg, P., & Redl, F. (1971). Dehumanization. In R. N. Sanford & C. Comstock (Eds.), *Sanctions for evil* (pp. 102–124). San Francisco: Jossey-Bass.

Bertenthal, B. I., Campos, J. J., & Barrett, K. C. (1984). Self-produced locomotion: An organizer of emotional, cognitive, and social development in infancy. In R. N. Emde & R. J. Harmon (Eds.), *Continuities and discontinuities in development* (pp. 175–210). New York: Plenum Press.

Block, J. (1982). Assimilation, accommodation, and the dynamics of personality development. *Child Development, 53,* 281–295.

Breznitz, S. (1983). The seven kinds of denial. In S. Breznitz (Ed.), *The denial of stress* (pp. 257–280). New York: International Universities Press.

Buck, R. (1985). Prime theory: An integrated view of motivation and emotion. *Psychological Review, 92,* 389–413.

Burghardt, G. M. (1985). Animal awareness: Current perceptions and historical perspective. *American Psychologist, 40,* 905–919.

D'Zurilla, T. J., & Nezu, A. (1982). Social problem solving in adults. In P. C. Kendall (Ed.), *Advances in cognitive-behavioral research and therapy* (Vol. 1). New York: Academic Press.

Ellis, A. (1958). Rational psychotherapy. *Journal of General Psychology, 59,* 35–49.

Ellis, A. (1984). Is the unified-interaction approach to cognitive-behavior modification a reinvention of the wheel? *Clinical Psychology Review, 4,* 215–218.

Ellis, A. (1985). Cognition and affect in emotional disturbance. *American Psychologist, 40,* 471–472.

Ellis, A., & Bernard, M. E. (1985). What is rational-emotive therapy (RET)? In A. Ellis & M. E. Bernard (Eds.), *Clinical applications of rational-emotive therapy* (pp. 1–30). New York: Plenum Press.

Emde, R. N. (1984). Levels of meaning for infant emotions: A biosocial view. In K. R. Scherer & P. Ekman (Eds.), *Approaches to emotion* (pp. 77–107). Hillsdale, NJ: Erlbaum.

Epstein, S. (1985). The implications of cognitive-experiential self-theory for research in social psychology and personality. *Journal of the Theory of Social Behavior, 15,* 283–310.

Evered, R. (1980). Consequences of and prospects for systems thinking in organizational change. In T. G. Cummings (Ed.), *Systems theory for organizational development* (pp. 5–13). New York: Wiley.

Festinger, L. (1957). *A theory of cognitive dissonance.* Stanford, CA: Stanford University Press.

Fischer, K. W., & Pipp, S. L. (1984). Development of the structures of unconscious thought. In K. Bowers & D. Meichenbaum (Eds.), *The unconscious reconsidered* (pp. 88–148). New York: Wiley.

Foa, E., & Kozak, ]. J. (1986). Emotional processing of fear: Exposure to corrective information. *Psychological Bulletin, 99,* 20–35.

Folkins, C. H. (1970). Temporal factors and the cognitive mediators of stress reaction. *Journal of Personality and Social Psychology, 14,* 173–184.

Folkman, S., & Lazarus, R. S. (1980). An analysis of coping in a middle-aged community sample. *Journal of Health and Social Behavior, 21,* 219–239.

Folkman, S., & Lazarus, R. S. (1985). If it changes it must be a process: Study of emotion and coping during three stages of a college examination. *Journal of Personality and Social Psychology, 48,* 150–170.

Folkman, S., Lazarus, R. S., Dunkel-Schetter, C., DeLongis, A., & Gruen, R. (1986a). The dynamics of a stressful encounter: Cognitive appraisal, coping, and encounter outcomes. *Journal of Personality and Social Psychology, 50,* 992–1003.

Folkman, S., Lazarus, R. S., Gruen, R., & DeLongis, A. (1986b). Appraisal, coping, health status, and psychological symptoms. *Journal of Personality and Social Psychology, 50,* 571–579.

Frese, M., & Sabini, J. (1985a). Action theory: An introduction. In M. Frese & J. Sabini (Eds.), *Goal-directed behavior: The concept of action in psychology* (pp. xvii–xxv). Hillsdale, NJ: Erlbaum.

Frese, M., & Sabini, J. (Eds.). (1985b). *Goal-directed behavior: The concept of action in psychology.* Hillsdale, NJ: Erlbaum.

Freud, A. (1946). *The ego and the mechanisms of defence.* New York: International Universities Press.

Freud, S. (1950). Analysis terminable and interminable. In *Collected papers* (Vol. 5, pp. 316–357). (Originally published in German, 1937)

Gallistel, C. R. (1980). The organization of action: A new synthesis. In M. Frese & J. Sabini (Eds.), *Goal-directed behavior: The concept of action in psychology* (pp. 48–65). Hillsdale, NJ: Erlbaum.

Gallistel, C. R. (1985). Motivation, intention, and emotion: Goal directed behavior from a cognitive-neuroethological perspective. In M. Frese & J. Sabini (Eds.), *Goal-directed behavior: The concept of action in psychology* (pp. 48–65). Hillsdale, NJ: Erlbaum.

Garber, J., & Seligman, M. E. P. (1980). *Human helplessness: Theory and applications.* New York: Academic Press.

Gibson, J. J. (1966). *The senses considered as perceptual systems.* Boston: Houghton-Mifflin.

Gibson, J. J. (1979). *The ecological approach to visual perception.* Boston: Houghton-Mifflin.

Goldfried, M. R. (1980). Psychotherapy as coping skills training. In M. J. Mahoney (Ed.), *Psychotherapy process: Current issues and future directions* (pp. 89–119). New York: Plenum Press.

Haan, N. (1969). A tripartite model of ego functioning: Values and clinical research applications. *Journal of Nervous and Mental Disease, 148,* 14–30.

Haan, N. (1977). *Coping and defending: Processes of self-environment organization.* New York: Academic Press.

Hackett, T. P., & Cassem, N. H. (1974). Development of a quantitative rating scale to assess denial. *Journal of Psychosomatic Research, 18,* 93–100.

Harlow, H. F. (1953). Mice, monkeys, men and motives. *Psychological Review, 60,* 23–32.

Harris, P. L. (1985). What children know about the situations that provoke emotion. In M. Lewis & C. Saarni (Eds.), *The socialization of affect.* New York: Plenum Press.

Harter, S. (1982). Children's understanding of multiple emotions: A cognitive-developmental approach. In W. Overton (Ed.), *The relation between social and cognitive development.* Hillsdale, NJ: Erlbaum.

Hay, D., & Oken, S. (1972). The psychological stresses of intensive care unit nursing. *Psychosomatic Medicine, 34,* 109–118.

Hilgard, E. R. (1975). Neo-dissociation theory: Multiple cognitive controls in hypnosis. In L. Unsestahl (Ed.), *Hypnosis in the seventies.* Orebro, Sweden: Veje Forlag.

Hilgard, E. R. (1977). *Divided consciousness: Multiple controls in human thought and action.* New York: Wiley Interscience.

Hilgard, E. R. (1980). The trilogy of mind: Cognition, affection, and conation. *Journal of the History of the Behavioral Sciences, 16,* 107–117.

Hoffman, M. L. (1985). Affect, motivation, and cognition. In R. Sorrentino & E. T. Higgins (Eds.), *Handbook of motivation and cognition.* New York: Guilford.

Klein, G. S. (1958). Cognitive control and motivation. In G. Lindzey (Ed.), *Assessment of human motives.* New York: Holt, Rinehart & Winston.

Kleinginna, P. R., Jr., & Kleinginna, A. M. (1985). Cognition and affect: A reply to Lazarus and Zajonc. *American Psychologist, 40,* 470–471.

Kreitler, H., & Kreitler, S. (1976). *Cognitive orientation and behavior.* New York: Springer.

Lang, P. J. (1977). Imagery in therapy: An information processing analysis of fear. *Behavior Therapy, 8,* 862–886.

Lang, P. J. (1979). A bio-informational theory of emotional imagery. *Psychophysiology, 16,* 495–512.

Lazarus, A. A. (1981). *The practice of multimodal therapy.* New York: McGraw-Hill.

Lazarus, R. S. (1966). *Psychological stress and the coping process.* New York: McGraw-Hill.

Lazarus, R. S. (1981). The stress and coping paradigm. In C. Eisdorfer, D. Cohen, A. Kleinman, & P. Maxim (Eds.), *Models for clinical psychopathology* (pp. 177–214). New York: Spectrum (Medical & Scientific Books).

Lazarus, R. S. (1982). Thoughts on the relations between emotion and cognition. *American Psychologist, 37,* 1019–1024.

Lazarus, R. S. (1983). The costs and benefits of denial. In S. Breznitz (Ed.), *The denial of stress* (pp. 1–30). New York: International Universities Press.

Lazarus, R. S. (1984). On the primacy of cognition. *American Psychologist, 39,* 124–129.

Lazarus, R. S. (1985). The trivialization of distress. In J. C. Rosen & L. J. Solomon (Eds.), *Preventing health risk behaviors and promoting coping with illness* (Vol. 8, Vermont Conference on the Primary Prevention of Psychopathology, pp. 279–298). Hanover, NH: University Press of New England.

Lazarus, R. S. (1986). Commentary. *Integrative Psychiatry, 4,* 245–247.

Lazarus, R. S. (1989). Cognition and emotion from the RET viewpoint. In M. E. Bernard & R. DiGiuseppe (Eds.), *Inside rational emotive therapy* (pp. 47–68). Orlando, FL: Academic Press.

Lazarus, R. S., & Folkman, S. (1984). *Stress, appraisal, and coping.* New York: Springer.

Lazarus, R. S., & Folkman, S. (1986). Cognitive theories of stress and the issue of circularity. In M. H. Appley & R. Trumbull (Eds.), *Dynamics of stress* (pp. 63–80). New York: Plenum Press.

Lazarus, R. S., & Launier, R. (1978). Stress-related transactions between person and environment. In L. A. Pervin & M. Lewis (Eds.), *Perspectives in interactional psychology* (pp. 287–327). New York: Plenum Press.

Lazarus, R. S., Coyne, J. C., & Folkman, S. (1982). Cognition, emotion, and motivation: The doctoring of Humpty-Dumpty. In R. W. J. Neufeld (Ed.), *Psychological stress and psychopathology* (pp. 218–239). New York: McGraw-Hill.

Lazarus, R. S., DeLongis, A., Folkman, S., & Gruen, R. (1985). Stress and adaptational outcomes: The problem of confounded measures. *American Psychologist, 40,* 770–779.

LeDoux, J. E. (1986). Sensory systems and emotion: A model of affective processing. *Integrative Psychiatry, 4,* 237–248.

Leventhal, H. (1984). A perceptual motor theory of emotion. In K. R. Scherer & P. Ekman (Eds.), *Approaches to emotion* (pp. 271–291). Hillsdale, NJ: Erlbaum.

Leventhal, H., & Tomarken, A. J. (1986). Emotion: Today's problems. In M. R. Rosenzweig & L. W. Porter (Eds.), *Annual review of psychology* (pp. 565–610). Palo Alto, CA: Annual Reviews.

Levy, D. M. (1943). *Maternal overprotection*. New York: Columbia University Press.

Lewis, H. B. (1971). *Shame and guilt in neurosis*. New York: International Universities Press.

Lewis, M. (1986). Origins of self-knowledge and individual differences in early self-recognition. In J. Suls & A. Greenwald (Eds.), *Psychological perspectives on the self* (Vol. 3). Hillsdale, NJ: Erlbaum.

McGuire, W. J. (1983). A contextualist theory of knowledge: Its implications for innovation and reform in psychological research. In L. Berkowitz (Ed.), *Advances in experimental social psychology* (Vol. 16, pp. 1–47). New York: Academic Press.

Meichenbaum, D., & Cameron, R. (1983). Stress inoculation training: Toward a general paradigm for training coping skills. In D. Meichenbaum & M. E. Jaremko (Eds.), *Stress reduction and prevention*. New York: Plenum Press.

Menninger, K. (1954). Regulatory devices of the ego under major stress. *International Journal of Psychoanalysis, 35,* 412–420.

Miller, G. A., Galanter, E. H., & Pribram, K. (1960). *Plans and the structure of behavior*. New York: Holt.

Mowrer, O. H. (1960). *Learning theory and behavior*. New York: Wiley.

Mowrer, O. H. (1975). From the dynamics of conscience to contract psychology: Clinical theory and practice in transition. In G. Serban (Ed.), *Psychopathology of human adaptation* (pp. 211–230). New York: Plenum Press.

Neisser, U. (1985). The role of invariant structures in the control of movement. In M. Frese & J. Sabini (Eds.), *Goal-directed behavior: The concept of action in psychology* (pp. 80–96). Hillsdale, NJ: Erlbaum.

Phillips, D. C., & Orton, R. (1983). The new causal principle of cognitive learning theory: Perspectives on Bandura's "reciprocal determinism." *Psychological Review, 90,* 158–165.

Piaget, J. (1952). *The origins of intelligence in children*. New York: International Universities Press.

Ridgeway, D., Bretherton, L., & Barrows, L. (1985). *Children's knowledge and use of emotion language.* Paper presented at the Biennial Meeting of the Society for Research in Child Development, Toronto, April, 1985.

Rosenbaum, M. (1983). Learned resourcefulness as a behavioral repertoire for the self-regulation of internal events: Issues and speculations. In M. Rosenbaum, C. M. Franks, & Y. Jaffe (Eds.), *Perspectives on behavior therapy in the eighties*. New York: Springer.

Sartre, J. P. (1948). A sketch of a phenomenological theory. *The emotions: Outline of a theory*. New York: Philosophical Library.

Schwartz, G. (1979). The brain as a health care system. In G. C. Stone, F. Cohen, & N. Adler (Eds.), *Health psychology* (pp. 549–571). San Francisco: Jossey-Bass.

Schwartz, R. M., & Trabasso, T. (1984). Children's understanding of emotions. In C. E. Izard, J. Kagan, & R. B. Zajonc (Eds.), *Emotions, cognition, and behavior* (pp. 409–437). Cambridge, England: Cambridge University Press.

Seligman, M. E. P. (1975). *Helplessness*. San Francisco: W. H. Freeman.

Seligman, M. E. P., Maier, S. F., & Solomon, R. L. (1971). Unpredictable and uncontrollable aversive events. In F. R. Brush (Ed.), *Aversive conditioning and learning*. New York: Academic Press.

Semmer, N., & Frese, M. (1985). Action theory in clinical psychology. In M. Frese & J. Sabini (Eds.), *Goal-directed behavior: The concept of action in psychology* (pp. 296–310). Hillsdale, NJ: Erlbaum.

Shapiro, D. (1965). *Neurotic styles*. New York: Basic Books.

Singer, M. T. (1974). Engagement-involvement: A central phenomenon in psychophysiological research. *Psychosomatic Medicine, 36,* 1–17.

Sjöbäck, H. (1973). *The psychoanalytic theory of defensive processes*. New York: Wiley.

Solomon, R. C. (1980). Emotions and choice. In A. O. Rorty (Ed.), *Explaining emotions* (pp. 251–281). Berkeley: University of California Press.

Stadler, M., & Wehner, T. (1985). Anticipation as a basic principle in goal-directed action. In M. Frese & J. Sabini (Eds.), *Goal-directed behavior: The concept of action in psychology* (pp. 67–77). Hillsdale, NJ: Erlbaum.

Stein, N. L., & Levine, L. J. (1988). Thinking about feelings: The development and organization of emotional knowledge. In R. E. Snow & M. Farr (Eds.), *Aptitude, learning and instruction, Vol. 3: Conative and affective process analysis*. Hillsdale, NJ: Erlbaum.

Tinbergen, N. (1951). *The study of instincts*. London: Oxford University Press.

Tomkins, S. (1981). The quest for primary motives: Biography and autobiography of an idea. *Journal of Personality and Social Psychology, 41,* 306–329.

von Hofsten, C. (1985). Perception and action. In M. Frese & J. Sabini (Eds.), *Goal-directed behavior: The concept of action in psychology* (pp. 80–96). Hillsdale, NJ: Erlbaum.

Wachtel, P. (1977). *Psychoanalysis and behavior therapy: Toward an integration*. New York: Basic Books.

Weisman, A. D. (1972). *On dying and denying: A psychiatric study of terminality.* New York: Behavioral
  Publications.
Werner, H. (1948). *Comparative psychology of mental development* (rev. ed.). Chicago: Follett.
White, R. W. (1960). Competence and the psychosexual stages of development. In M. R. Jones (Ed.), *Nebraska
  Symposium on Motivation* (pp. 97–141). Lincoln: University of Nebraska Press.
Zajonc, R. B. (1980). Feeling and thinking: Preferences need no inferences. *American Psychologist, 35,* 151–
  175.
Zajonc, R. B. (1984). On the primacy of affect. *American Psychologist, 35,* 151–175.

# 7

# The Role of Cognitive Change in Psychotherapy

LARRY E. BEUTLER AND PAUL D. GUEST

Identifying the roles that cognitive change is thought to play among contemporary psycho-therapies represents a considerable challenge. This task assumes that one can recognize the commonalities among approaches that masquerade as differences and the differences that masquerade as similarities. Extracting meaningful similarities and differences confronts us with the thorny and multifaceted issue of assigning causal relationships among cognitions, emotional distress, and behaviors, as viewed both from the vantage point of diverse theories and from empirical literature.

In approaching this broad-ranging task, we urge the reader to keep two things in mind. First, any specific behavioral problem and the mechanisms for its remediation can be defined and interpreted from many different levels within the human system. These explanations range from the biological to the metaphysical. Second, any conceptual ordering of these levels of interpretation is somewhat arbitrary. For example, we often label functional systems such as *thinking, feeling, sensing,* and *behaving* as if they were physically distinct. In fact, the definitive distinctions among even such broad categories as the foregoing are fuzzy, and the defining boundaries for these domains of human experience vary from theory to theory. Therefore, any of the constructs by which we define our experience offer only an approximate description of the matrix of phenomenon to which we are exposed or which we create by the very processes that we are attempting to understand. Nonetheless, applying labels to experi-ence is crucial both for the communication and differentiation of those experiences and in order to enable experience to tolerate those types of observation that may pass as empirical research.

The integrative, multifaceted task of this chapter requires that we communicate with a broad constituency that includes the cognitive therapist, the dynamic therapist, the rela-tionship-oriented therapist, the behaviorist, and the cognitive scientist. To accomplish this, we

LARRY E. BEUTLER • Department of Psychiatry, College of Medicine, University of Arizona, Tucson, Arizona 85724. PAUL D. GUEST • Program 3, Patton State Hospital, Patton, California 92369.

LARRY E. BEUTLER
and PAUL D. GUEST

will attempt to find common meanings in the various linguistic and conceptual systems that characterize these diverse fields of inquiry.

It has become commonplace to point to the exponential increase in the number of psychotherapy theories as an indication both of confusion in the field and of the primitive level at which contemporary psychotherapy theory exists (e.g., London, 1986). It is often thought, for example, that theoretical differences reflect profound differences in views of reality that have powerful implications for treatment and even emotional survival. As easily, however, it could be argued that the diversity of theoretical viewpoints and concepts reflects primary differences in the labels that are applied to the basic phenomena rather than to actual disagreements about foci and targets. Whether or not the variety of theories available represents irrelevant and esoteric disagreements among theorists, merely differences in the labels attached to similar processes or practical differences of focus and procedure cannot be determined until theorists will permit themselves to sit in the same room with one another. observe the same phenomenon, and discuss its implications. In recent years, we note an increasing willingness for such interchanges to occur. A series of workshops on the development of a common language for psychotherapy has taken place at a number of the annual conventions of the Society for Psychotherapy Research since 1983 (Beutler, 1983a; Goldfried, 1983; Norcross, 1986c), a new society designated specifically for the consideration of integrating approaches and conceptual systems in psychotherapy has evolved (The Society for the Exploration of Psychotherapy Integration), a journal (*Journal of Eclectic and Integrative Psychotherapy*) devoted to such exchange has appeared and recently, the National Institute of Mental Health has convened a special study group to consider issues of theoretical and technical integration. Complementing these movements has been a consistent increase in the amount of empirical and theoretical attention given to eclectic movements in psychotherapy research and practice (e.g., Beutler, 1983b; Garfield, 1980; Lazarus, 1981; Norcross, 1986b; Prochaska, 1984). Nonetheless, fierce debate still exists as to whether integration is a meaningful goal and even if it is, whether such integration either does or should represent a simple translation of theoretical concepts to a common perspective, a true marriage of theoretical priorities and values, or a merging of practical interventions, irrespective of theoretical underpinnings.

Recently, the Society for Psychotherapy Research (SPR) sponsored the third of a series of workshops on the development of a common language, considering a variety of alternative language systems from which diverse psychotherapy theories could be evaluated (Norcross, 1986c). Theories of natural language, cognitive therapy, social persuasion, and systems theory all offered important perspectives on this problem. If nothing else has emerged from such activities, psychotherapists are becoming aware that language determines a great deal of what one sees in psychotherapy as well as how one thinks about, interprets, and infers the presence of change. The diversity of viewpoints that has contributed to these several movements as well as the conflicts that derive from efforts to develop a common language underline the many ways in which psychotherapy processes are conceptualized by different theoretical approaches. An inspection of these viewpoints also emphasizes that cognitive constructs are applied to psychotherapy processes by virtually all therapies, even though theorists cannot agree upon the nature of cognition itself, its role in the development of psychopathology, or its contribution to therapeutic change. One may conclude that cognitive constructs paradoxically are at once arbitrary, unvalidated, and necessary in psychotherapy.

The advent of a host of viewpoints under the title of ''cognitive therapies'' has brought into high relief the various curative roles assigned to cognition by various psychotherapies. These roles range from ''insight'' to that of providing a ''substitute image'' of external, frightening events. However, in spite of their impact upon theories of psychotherapy generally, their wide appeal to psychotherapists, and their increasing ascendance in clinical practice, cognitive therapy theories themselves have remained surprisingly insulated from the broader concepts and methods of cognitive science. Even a cursory review of the literature will impress one that the spectrum of cognitive therapies employs a much more constricted and exclusive notion about "cognition" than does cognitive psychology more generally. This limiting view of cognition applies not only to the assumed relationship of inner language and/or images to the development and maintenance of psychopathology but to the more general relationship proposed to exist between "cognition" and cognitive change.

More specifically, from the perspective of cognitive therapy, the term *cognition* largely is restricted to the concept of an inner, verbal language. Only occasionally has cognitive therapy extended its definition of cognition to include images, and even more rarely has it included experience that is not within easy access to conscious awareness (Beidel & Turner, 1986; Kuiper & MacDonald, 1983). In view of their behavioral heritage, it is even more interesting that cognitive therapies have given relatively little attention to the roles of conditioning environments and learning principles in the development of cognitive patterns.

Cognitive science, in comparison to the more narrow perspective of cognitive therapy, places few limitations upon the structures and functions that are included in the term *cognitive*, gives great credence to the roles of conditioning and evoking environments in the development of cognitive structures, and is very flexible in the assignment of the causal roles played by cognition in psychopathology, normal behavior, and therapeutic change (Lazarus, 1984, Chapter 6 in this volume).

In organizing the complex task of assessing the role of cognitive change in psychotherapy, we have divided this chapter, somewhat arbitrarily, into three general sections. The first section represents a descriptive comparison of the roles assigned to cognition by cognitive scientists and diverse schools of psychotherapy. The second section provides a review of empirical findings about the relationship between cognitive change and psychotherapy outcome, and the third section offers an integrative perspective of how cognition might be viewed within the field of psychotherapy research.

## THEORETICAL DIVERSITIES

In this section, we will explore and delineate the different ways that the cognition–emotion–behavior link has been viewed. This presentation will include perspectives from cognitive psychology, cognitive therapies, and from therapies that normally are not considered to be primarily cognitive.

### Cognitive Psychology

A delineation of the relationship between cognition, emotion, and behavior requires that we define the limits and restricting conditions of each of these concepts. In general psychology, "cognition" encompasses the spectrum of processes extending from the organization of sensory input to the initiation of behavior (Kuiper & MacDonald, 1983; Lazarus, 1984; Mandler, 1975). Within this broad perspective, the construct of cognitive schemata occupies a central position. Schemata are defined as mental structures that serve to help us organize past experiences (Mandler, 1982). These structures vary in their level of specificity, ranging from the relatively concrete to the very abstract, and are taken to operate interactively with one another. The interpretive processes of perceiving experience procedes by activating relevant schemata. Concurrently, the schemata themselves are reciprocally modified by exposure to specific experiential events that constitute instances of that class of events that initially contributed to the development of the schema. The development and utilization of schemata are generally held to be data-driven processes. That is, they are activated and maintained by the infusion of information. This activity is presumed to occur automatically and generally outside of awareness. In fact, one view holds that the awareness of one's own cognitive structures arises from the process of integrating the contributions of two or more active schemata (Marcel, 1983).

The foregoing definitions of cognition and associated functions have a number of implications that distinguish them from those of cognitive therapy:

1. Cognition and conscious awareness are not assumed to be equivalent. Much of the process of apprehending, selecting, encoding, storing, retrieving, and transmitting experiential data is outside of and inaccessible to conscious awareness but is, nonetheless, "cognitive."

2. Schematic structures are assumed to transcend the auditory/verbal and visual or imagery-based constituents that contributed to their formation. Although individual structures may differentially mediate the data of experience encountered through specific sensory modalities, the creation and modification of these structures represent processes that are common to all sensory modalities.

3. A distinction is made between cognitive *process* and cognitive *content,* each of which is a legitimate focus in the investigation of cognitive functioning. This distinction parallels that made between "episodic" and "semantic" memory (Craik, 1979; Rumelhart & Ortony, 1978; Tulving, 1972). The concept of *semantic memory* closely corresponds to the concept of *schematic structures,* whereas *episodic memory* refers to the recordings made of specific experiential events. Cognitive content may directly reflect memory for specific experiences and is likely to reflect schematic structures in a derivative fashion. Cognitive dysfunction, seen within this framework, generally refers to impairment of the processes underlying the encoding, storage, and retrieval of experiential data rather than to the specific content of those data.

4. Most important to our discussion of differences between general cognitive theory and psychotherapy theory, "emotion" is considered by cognitive psychology to be a cognitively mediated experience, though its physiological correlates are not. Cognitive theory assumes that schemas contribute to the interpretation of experience after the same fashion that other forms of experiences are mediated. *Emotion,* therefore, is a term that jointly reflects both the activity of cognitive schemas and concomitant physiological experience without assigning causal priority to either component (e.g., Bower & Cohen, 1982; Candland *et al.,* 1977; Lazarus, 1982; Leventhal, 1982; Linville, 1982). The separable processes of *cognitive appraisal* and *physiological arousal* are jointly expressed as *emotion,* which itself is viewed as a form of cognitive experience. However, the chain of interactive events among these phenomena may be initiated from any of the separate domains. Thus, emotions may parallel cognitions, produce cognitions, or be produced by cognitions. As suggested by the pioneering work of Schachter and Singer (1962), the meaning given to any defined physiological event depends upon a process of appraisal, attribution, and response selection. The emotion, in other words, is dependent upon the appraised characteristics of the environment in which one exists, the causal attribution assigned to this environment as well as the available response alternatives that are judged to be present. In terms of our current framework, the variability of emotions that occur in response to a given set of environmental stimuli would be accounted for by the activation of contrasting sets of schemata. Although schema activation tends to be data driven, in those cases where the major stimulus is ambiguous, conceptual cues may become more salient than the primary stimulus in determining the nature of the interpretive cognitive processes.

Lazarus (Chapter 6), in this volume, makes a case for the inseparability of cognition and emotion, suggesting that to view them as separate entities is "strangely out of touch with the way we function." In fact, he maintains that separation or fragmentation (his word is *disconnection*) of experienced emotion from cognitive appraisal is the basis for psychopathology. This is an approach that is in concert with the general views of cognitive psychology. Moreover, Lazarus emphasizes a systems orientation for considering the interactive effects of various conceptually defined dimensions such as *interpersonal relationship, emotion, sensation, physiological response,* and the like.

Although natural language discriminates among a large number of emotional experiences, most cognitive and developmental theorists suggest that there is a small and finite number of emotions that can be reliably identified. The number and type of these emotions range from as few as two to as many as eight (Kuiper & MacDonald, 1983). To qualify as a primary emotion, a constant behavioral form must be traced through all levels of phylogenetic development and must be associated with a discriminating biological or physiological experience—for example, lust, rage, fear.

These so-called "primary emotions" form the basis for subsequent experiences that vary in intensity and purity and that are defined as "secondary emotions." These latter experiences cannot be dissected by reductionist efforts and are often differentiated only by variations in one's interpretations of external events. The available natural language labels that are commonly applied to the experience of "feelings" probably reflect these latter variations among the interpretations given to general arousal states more than they define discretely different arousal patterns (Clark, 1982).

Cognitive theorists do not uniformly agree either on the nature of these primary emotions or the specificity of the cognitive schemas that are associated with each of them. Within some limits, however, it is logical to assume that there is correspondence between the structure of the cognitive schema and the nature of a given emotion. For example, it would be difficult to imagine anger without a concomitant cognitive process that includes an external attribution and a statement of demand (e.g., "He shouldn't do that"), or anxiety without the expectation of danger or a remembrance of hurt (e.g., "Something bad is about to happen"). Secondary emotional reactions such as depression, hurt, and anxiety are derived through the activation of multiple schemata. A cardinal task of cognitive research is to define the specific cognitive structures and processes that are associated both with primary and secondary emotions and, reciprocally, to define the effect of these primary and secondary emotions on subsequent cognitive content and processes. One sees in this literature, for example, both research on the effect of induced emotions upon memory and information recall and research on the effect of memory enhancement or impairment upon subjective distress (e.g., Bower, 1981; Bower & Cohen, 1982; Mathews & Bradley, 1983). From this literature, we know that the environmental context in which a given physiological arousal process occurs is likely to activate either positive or negative schematic networks that, in turn, determine the valence of and select which collateral schemata will be activated. In other words, a given mood or feeling state will determine the accessibility of pleasant and unpleasant material to memory and attention (Clark, 1982). Concomitantly, the nonspecificity of most autonomic arousal states allows the valences of preexisting schemata (expectations, attributional sets, memories) to assume great power in determining the nature of current subjective states.

The study of cognitive development also has extended our understanding of socialization processes. Although children's external speech develops in a consistent and progressive manner, children who are the most socially active, advanced, and popular place high reliance upon private speech that they use to direct their behavior and to solve complex problems (e.g., Luria, 1961; Vygotsky, 1962). As young as age 5, a close correspondence has been noted between the use of language as a social medium and the use of private language or self-talk (Berk, 1986). Moreover, the use of self-talk among socially advanced children increases with stress and problem difficulty. Apparently, children use such self-talk to help control their anxiety and to direct their behavior. This finding suggests that inner language is a reflection of prior socialization experiences and precipitates both the development and maintenance of social skills, impulse controls, and abstract problem-solving efficiency. As such, findings such as these have a direct bearing on clinical interventions and pathology.

## COGNITIVE THERAPIES

The proliferation of psychotherapy theories and approaches has been well documented (Beutler, 1983b; Corsini, 1981; Smith, Glass, & Miller, 1980). With the relatively recent

LARRY E. BEUTLER
and PAUL D. GUEST

advent of cognitive therapies have come a plethora of treatment packages and specific techniques, each of which espouses to produce cognitive or emotional change. These approaches range from early rational-emotive therapy (Ellis, 1962), to more recent RET technical developments such as rational restructuring (Goldfried, DeCanteceo, & Weinberg, 1974), and to purer cognitive interventions like self-instruction training (Meichenbaum, 1974, 1977) and Beck's cognitive therapy (Beck, Rush, Shaw, & Emery, 1979). A cursory review of the literature will reveal at least two dozen different approaches or technologies that, at one time or another, have been identified with cognitive therapy. Some of these approaches represent comprehensive interventions, whereas others are relatively isolated techniques.

Although both behavior therapies and insight-oriented therapies can be seen as cognitive insofar as they affect and focus upon cognitive processes and structures, for most purposes it is convenient to adopt the more restrictive definition of cognitive therapy provided by Hollon and Beck (1986):

> [Cognitive therapies are] those approaches that attempt to modify existing or anticipated disorders by virtue of altering cognitions or cognitive processes. The emphasis in this definition is on the nature of the presumed causal mediators targeted by the therapist for modification. This definition excludes various approaches relying more exclusively upon techniques such as systematic desensitization. . . . since the intended intermediate goal of systematic desensitization is typically not to alter cognitions per se. (pp. 443–444).

One can see in this definition that ''cognition,'' in cognitive therapy theory is principally viewed as both the instigator of emotional distress and the object of change. In other words, cognitive therapy gives little attention to the dynamic process of memory and information recall and is defined as a methodology for *intervening* rather than understanding. In an effort to bring some order to the interventions that comprise this methodology, Hollon and Beck (1986) suggest that there are three basic mechanisms of therapeutic change. These include rational analyses, logical/empirical assessment, and repetition or practice. An exploration of these methodologies will help us understand the various ways in which cognition is defined and employed within the realm of cognitive therapies.

*Rational* approaches emphasize procedures for disconfirmation and reconceptualization (Ross, 1977); *empirical* approaches emphasize the role of systematic analysis of evidence toward the goal of constructing disconfirming experiences; and *repetition* emphasizes the role of directed practice. Although acknowledging that these distinctions cannot be maintained completely by virtue of the sheer diversity of available and overlapping procedures, Hollon and Beck maintain that the more integrated and comprehensive cognitive theories can be differentiated by their relative emphasis on these three mechanisms. For example, rational-emotive therapy (RET) (Ellis, 1962) relies on disconfirmation and rational appeal, whereas Beck *et al.* (1979) emphasize empirical procedures, and self-instruction training (Meichenbaum, 1977) capitalizes on repetition.

Although early philosophers in Western civilization seem to have been aware of the relationship between one's assumptions and attitudes, on one hand, and one's disordered and disturbed behavior on the other, Ellis can properly be credited, in contemporary times, with having first described psychopathology as a disturbance of beliefs and values. By his systematic description of the relationship between assumptive sets and both disturbed feelings and behavior, Ellis initially articulated the premises from which other cognitive therapy theories and approaches subsequently developed. As observed by Hollon and Beck (1906), criticisms of rational-emotive therapy have consisted less of attacks on the theoretical rationale than on the technical procedures to which RET subscribes, the theoretical rationale having achieved the state of implicit acceptance in today's zeitgeist. Most cognitive interventions and theories accept the basic premises of psychopathology established by Ellis, although varying in the labels used and the relative importance assigned to the roles of rational assessment and directed experience. An explanation of these differences may illucidate both the common assumptions of various cognitive-therapy models and their distinctiveness from other cognitive and psychotherapy theories.

Hollon and Beck (1986) observe that cognitive therapy (Beck *et al.*, 1979) incorporates both behavioral and cognitive interventions and, in contrast to rational-emotive therapy, emphasizes empiricism and reconceptualization rather than rational disconfirmation. Beck's cognitive therapy differs from that of Ellis, in its emphasis upon initiating change through facilitating and testing new understandings or appraisals of emotional experience. Clients are encouraged to assume the role of personal scientist in exploring and attempting to validate their personal belief systems in much the same way as that advocated by George Kelly (1955). The therapist assumes the role of collaborator, in contrast to that of counterpropagandist as advocated by Ellis. As such, the therapists' task is to assist the patient in identifying disorganized or dysfunctional ideas, evaluating the usefulness and truthfulness of these ideas, and developing more practical ideas and procedures for resolving life dilemmas. Aside from identifying the contents of thought, little attention is given to the nature of perception, retrieval, and memory.

Finally, in Hollon and Beck's formulation, self-instruction training (Meichenbaum, 1977) and stress inoculation training are both designed to exert their influence through systematic repetition and practice, less in the interest of correcting underlying psychopathology or dysfunction than in the interest of developing and building skills that were not heretofore present. They propose that these repetition interventions are more useful interventions than either empirical analysis or rational argument when the psychopathology derives, not from dysfunctional or inaccurate thoughts, but from the absence of systematic problem-solving and coping skills. Hence, in a move toward prescribing specific interventions for specific types of disorders, Hollon and Beck propose a dimension similar to that proposed both by Beutler (1983b) and Kendall and Braswell (1985). Although Kendall and Braswell's formulation is specific to cognitive therapy, Beutler (1983b) has extended the concept to other therapies. In both instances, the authors differentiate between neurotic distortions or neurotiform patterns, on one hand, and absence of skills or the presence of dysfunctional habits, on the other, and propose that this dimension is an indicator for the type of intervention to be used.

We also can observe parallels between the three intervention mechanisms described by Hollon and Beck and the general cognitive model explicated earlier. For example, assume that: (1) the cognitive schemas that serve to organize present experience are hierarchically arranged and associatively linked in networks along dimensions of concreteness/abstractness or specificity/generality; and (2) network activation spreads along these associative lines in both top-down (i.e., knowledge and expectations activate retrieval of responses) and bottom-up (i.e., sensory and informational data activate the acquisition of expectancies and knowledge) directions. Within this framework, *rational* approaches to intervention are aimed at superordinate, cultural attitudes that represent a relatively high or abstract level of cognitive activity. These approaches assume that modification of these high-level schemata will necessarily ripple down and produce concomitant change in the more specific, idiosyncratic, and concrete cognitive structures within each individual's associative chain. The conceptual difficulty with this assumption is that the *irrational ideas* targeted for alteration necessarily represent a simplified condensation of the very complex and specific cognitive structures that have been developed over the course of any individual's unique experiential history. Although abstract *irrational ideas* may be identified as general or common elements in one's cognitive hierarchy, they are unlikely adequately to encompass the range of functional meanings and specific experiences that comprise dysfunctional thoughts for different individuals.

On the other hand, an *empirical* approach to intervention targets cognitive structures within the lower (specific) and midlevel range of the schematic hierarchy. This approach takes advantage of the salience associated with experiences that are unique to individuals. Such unique and novel experiences are those that cannot be automatically and unconsciously processed by existent and general schemas. Because they cannot be processed automatically, these new experiences produce arousal and in turn motivate attempts to realign schematic structures in a manner that will allow incorporation of the novel data.

Finally, *repetition*-based interventions target the bottom-up (from specific data to general knowledge) systematic creation of new structures that are designed ultimately to compete with prior dysfunctional schematic networks. Of the interventions, therefore, these are the most responsive to individual differences, exert the least direct effect on higher order structures, and are the most likely to be identified with specific behaviors.

*Critique*

As we have seen, the several theories of cognitive therapy emphasize interventions rather than descriptive relationships. To the degree that descriptive data about cognitive function is provided, there is greater reliance upon the contacts or structure of cognition than upon the processes of cognitive function. Few distinctions are made by any one cognitive therapy theory between the contents or attitudes that influence psychopathology and those processes of solving problems or retrieving information that may underlie psychopathology. In this respect, cognitive therapy theory is at variance with most of the information-processing models that have been applied to clinical phenomena. These latter models propose a more complex role for cognition in psychotherapy than do more existant cognitive therapy theories. For example, Kuhl (1984) has attempted to address the apparent perseverance of depressive affect beyond that of an existent depressogenic environment. He suggests that depression represents a dynamic and active interplay between intentional states and memory storage. Depression may be maintained, for example, if unfulfillable intentions occupy long-term memory to the point of excluding access to the short-term memory processes that are needed to develop and enact new, and more fulfillable expectancies (Kuhl & Helle, 1986). Such sophisticated formulations about depression pose a dominant role for cognitive processes in the development and maintenance of psychopathology and stand in sharp contrast to the relatively static role posed for cognitive contents and ideas by most theories of cognitive therapy. Here again we are reminded that conscious representations of information-processing schemata are themselves the products of schema activation. The natural fallacy that occurs here is to mistake the semantic label (constructed representation) for the thing itself (cognitive schema).

In spite of their overall emphasis on static, cognitive states in the application of therapeutic procedures, one does see some distinctions in the relative emphasis placed on dynamically active constructs by the various cognitive therapies. For example, procedures like self-instruction and stress inoculation that rely upon repetition tend to concentrate upon the development of new problem-solving *processes* as means to instigate change. Attitudinal content change is an indirect, albeit important, effect of this alternative process. On the other hand, the cognitive therapies of Beck and Ellis concentrate directly upon disconfirming or altering the *content* of dysfunctional attitudes either through the presentation of rational arguments or through quasi-empirical observations. Although it must be emphasized that Beck's cognitive therapy places more emphasis upon the evaluation and development of new cognitive processes than does that of Ellis, a primary role still is given by Beck's approach to understanding and replacing relatively constant dysfunctional ideas.

It is to be noted in the foregoing that, although cognitive therapies share common views of psychopathology and of the emotion/cognition link, these theories give little attention to the particular ways in which pathological cognitions have developed. Although there is an implicit assumption that cognitions evolve from a history of learning and environmental experience, this point is not clear in most theories. Beidel and Turner (1986), for example, point out that cognitive therapists assume that initial and triggering cognitions may develop independently of the normal laws of learning and may be bound to biological and physiological events. The point here is that, although the specific structure of schemata themselves are developed in concert with learning principles, the more fundamental existence of schemata as a class of cognitive structures is often assumed to be more closely tied to laws governing the biological substrate than to psychological principles. This view is discrepant, if not qualitatively then in the relative weight given to environmental and biological variables, from the operating assumptions of most information-processing theories.

Aside from conceptual and theoretical differences between cognitive therapy theory and cognitive science theory, there are also empirical criticisms of the former that demand attention. For example, we would anticipate, following cognitive therapy theory, that (1) disturbed cognitive patterns or distortions will occur more frequently in pathological groups than in normals; (2) disturbed cognitive content will predict the nature of psychopathology that will appear in times of stress; (3) cognitive therapies that are designed to impact these cognitive contents and dysfunctional process will do so at a faster rate than therapies that are not so designed; and (4) changes in cognitive patterns will coincide with changes in symptoms and signs of emotional disturbance.

None of the foregoing hypotheses is strongly supported by current research. To the contrary, evidence suggests that normals may have more distorted cognitions than either depressed individuals or those with other types of psychopathologies (Alloy & Abramson, 1979, 1982). Surprisingly, depressed individuals seem to be more accurate than their normal counterparts in assessing their own social skills, whereas normals tend to imbue their observations with a ''positive glow'' (Alloy & Abramson, 1982; Kuiper & McDonald, 1982; Lewinsohn, Mischel, Chaplin, & Barton, 1980). Further, the presence of disturbed cognitive patterns do not observably precipitate the development of psychopathology during times of stress, suggesting that depressive cognitive patterns may be only correlates of depression rather than causative agents (Beidel & Turner, 1986; Coyne & Gotlib, 1983). Indeed, it is quite uncertain even that specific forms of cognitive distortions differentiate depression from other types of psychopathologies (Coyne & Gotlib, 1983).

To date, the failure of cognitive therapy researchers to specifically define the cognitive elements and structures that are specific to certain types of psychopathologies may result from the theory-specific nature of the measurement instruments currently available. Hollon, Kendall, and Lumry (1986) compared the most used assessment devices, the Automatic Thoughts Questionnaire and the Dysfunctional Attitudes Scale. Their analysis revealed that the two scales were differentially sensitive to depression. Contrary to other research (e.g., Derry & Kuiper, 1981), ruminations and thoughts (he Automatic Thought Questionnaire) and beliefs and attitudes (the Dysfunctional Attitudes Scale) were found to differentiate depressives from normals. Neither cognitive pattern selectively differentiated among various types of depressions, however, and neither had more than modest ability to differentiate depression from other psychopathological disorders (e.g., substance abuse, general psychiatric disorders, medical control groups).

Similar concerns with what is measured by available instruments may account for why changes in cognitive patterns are not observed to occur in cognitive therapy to any remarkable degree (Beutler et al., 1987) in spite of therapy induced changes in depressive symptoms. This observation is made more telling by the observation that when cognitive changes do coincide with changes in symptoms, they are no more likely to occur in response to cognitive therapy than they are to pharmacotherapy (Silverman, Silverman, & Eardley, 1984; Simmons, Garfield, & Murphy, 1984). To emphasize the probable role of theory-bound instrumentation (Goldberg & Shaw, Chapter 3), it is important to observe, at this point, that the lack of correspondence between cognitive change and improvement is reflected only in those cognitive contents that have been seen as important to cognitive therapy. As we will observe shortly, there is ample evidence that certain types of cognitive contents systematically change with psychotherapy, particularly those cognitions reflecting evaluative attitudes (Beutler,

1981). Instruments that are less specific to the theoretical concepts of cognitive therapy may ultimately prove to be more useful in psychotherapy research than are those now available.

## NONCOGNITIVE THERAPIES

Beidel and Turner (1986), in concert with Schwartz (1982), have observed that cognitions have been treated in various psychotherapy theories in one of three ways: as precipitators of events, as mediators between causative antecedants and subsequent behaviors, and as responses to other precipitators. These three roles of cognition correspond with three general approaches to psychotherapy. Like cognitive therapies, dynamic/insight therapies propose that cognitions *precipitate and cause* pathological behaviors and feelings. In contrast, behavioral interventions propose that cognitions serve only as *mediators* between controlling stimuli and evoked behavior, and experiential therapists view cognitive processes as *organizers of experience* that in turn derive from experiential learning (Greenberg, Safran, & Rice, Chapter 10 in this volume).

### Psychodynamic Therapies

Whether dynamic conflicts, schemata, or automatic thoughts are proposed as precipitators of psychopathology, all therapies that search for cognitive disturbances assume that cognitive structures are partially precipitated by experience with a hostile environment and that psychopathology derives from nonoptimal cognitive processes and contents. These processes are called "ego defenses" and serve to distort views and beliefs in order to protect against anxiety emanating either from basic impulses (classical psychoanalytic theory) or interpersonal relationships (object relations theories). The process of containing or avoiding anxiety evokes or fosters specific attitudes and belief systems that further this aim. Hence, psychic disturbances are assumed to reflect faulty or inaccurate conclusions that have been drawn about oneself and others as a consequence of nonrepresentative experience, and that are maintained because of their protective function. In turn, symptoms are consequences of perceiving current environments through the tainted or distorted lenses that develop from this accumulated experience and corollary defense against anxiety. Moreover, these patterns of disturbance in the process (ego defense) and content (distortions) of cognitions are thought to become exaggerated with stress, provoking an increase in the overt manifestations of psychopathological feelings and behaviors.

Like us, Beidel and Turner (1986) find some common ground between cognitive therapy and psychodynamic theories. Both systems view psychopathology as a disturbance of cognitive structures and contents (e.g., repressed memories or automatic thoughts), and both aim to change cognitive experience. In psychodynamic theories, this process is called "insight," and it is assumed to be facilitated by abreactive experience of emotions, a condition that is not emphasized by cognitive therapy theory. Nevertheless, this common reliance on cognitive content change binds both theories to the strengths as well as to the weaknesses of the assumption of cognitive determinism. Like their cognitive-therapy cousins, psychodynamic therapies emphasize the role of insight into the conflicts that exist among cognitive structures (in this latter case, dynamic conflicts) that have been heretofore hidden. The process of therapy may offer the opportunity for novel semantic constructions, which parallel the underlying structures to be rediscovered. Unlike their cognitive therapy counterparts, however, psychodynamic theorists consider the mechanisms of pathology to be active and protective processes of moving anxiety-laden material out of awareness through repression and denial, rather than simply being the result of inaccurate information storage. Additionally, psychodynamic theories place a reliance on the emotional processes (i.e., corrective emotional experiences) associated with changing cognitions, a view that is not shared by cognitive therapists. Nonetheless, the implicit assumption is that once the content of consciousness is changed, process changes (defensive patterns) will follow, and symptoms will be relieved (London, 1986). Beidel and Turner identify the cardinal theoretical issue in these theories as that of determining whether mere awareness of previously hidden cognitive contents and the replacement of these contents, even in the presence of abreaction, themselves, with adaptive alternatives, will control subsequent behavior or whether it is only through placing contingencies upon subsequent behavior that observed changes in psychopathology will occur. If contingencies are necessary and sufficient for change, they could be effectively applied independently of changes in cognitive contents (i.e., insights).

Citing the results of seat-belt campaigns, Beidel and Turner argue that the threat of punishment or reprisal for not altering one's behavior, rather than the ability accurately to appraise the presence of danger, are more likely to motivate change in behavior. Although persuasive, this latter argument fails to recognize that the "threat of punishment" is itself a cognitive construct rather than an actual consequence because most drivers do not experience the threatened punishment. Nonetheless, such evidence suggests that, aside from simple insight or change in cognitive content, specific aspects of that content (e.g., fear of reprisal) are apparently more important motivators for subsequent behavior change than passive substitutions or the addition of information.

## Behavior Therapies

Unlike cognitive and insight-oriented therapists, behavior therapists view cognitive processes as covert behaviors that are simple *mediators* of overt behavior rather than as causative elements. Actual behavioral contingencies, rather than cognitions *per se,* are assumed to produce and evoke behavioral changes. But cognitions may be used to symbolize external consequences. For example, in systematic desensitization, the task of intervention is not directly to change existing images or cognitions in the hope of changing behavioral pathology but to utilize the covert image as a representation of some external reinforcing event from which the subject/patient can generalize. The external event, not the image itself, is assumed concomitantly to exert the most powerful behavioral influences (Hollon & Beck, 1986). Again, this approach emphasizes the bottom-up approach to change, in contrast to the top-down approach of insight theorists.

The viewpoint that cognitions serve as mediators of overt behavior, rather than as direct, causal agents is consistent with the observation that dysfunctional attitudes (conscious representations of underlying structures) characterize general psychological disturbance but do not clearly differentiate among specific types of psychopathologies (Hollon & Beck, 1986). Another argument in favor of considering cognitions as mediators rather than as instigators of behavior is to be found in the observation that cognitive change tends to follow behavior change in many instances (e.g., Bandura, 1977; Beidel & Turner, 1986). Self-efficacy theory, for example, emphasizes the importance of mastery experiences in overcoming feared situations. The cognitive experience (content) of self-efficacy follows the experience of behavioral mastery. Although, in covert rehearsal procedures and in overt practice procedures, both the experience of self-efficacy and its precipitating cognitive rehearsal represent classes of cognitive experiences, rather than of external behaviors (Bandura, 1977).

Bootzin (1985) has observed that the advent of biofeedback forced a revolution in behavior therapy by underlining the need to recognize the role that cognitive mediation has upon even automatic and reflexive behaviors. He has further observed that behavioral research has led us to an appreciation of how such symbolic processes as expectancies, goals, plans, motives, and values may affect the nature and expression of emotions. On the other hand, the behavioral view of cognitions as passive reflections of external experience fails to account for the apparent motivational properties of certain cognitions (Clark, 1982; Ross & Olson, 1981). Schacter and Singer (1962) first drew attention to the motivational role of attributional beliefs when they observed that a single, artificially induced physiological arousal state could be associated with a wide range of reported emotions. Clark and her colleagues (Clark, 1982) have emphasized this point in observing that nonspecific and general arousal states activate pleasant or unpleasant schematic networks, depending upon the nature of the environment in which they occur. In turn, these activated schemata may serve as cues for the selective memory recall and selective attribution that give meaning to the arousal, define the nature of the emotion, and determine subsequent behaviors. If the situation evoking the initial arousal is one that is easily interpreted from a positive dispositional set, other memories associated with similar positive states are more accessible to recall, and responses attendant upon such emotional states tend to rise in the response hierarchy. The emotional response and subsequent behavior are less dependent upon the specific nature of the physiological arousal pattern than upon either the context or the meaning given to external events. The same physiological response pattern can evoke euphoria or anger, depending upon the interpretation given to it. Moreover, selective modification of attributional processes has been found to override the physical effects of psychoactive medication in facilitating (motivating) or maintaining change in disordered behavior. For example, when sleep-disordered subjects were administered 500 mg of chlorohydrate but were later told that they had been given a placebo and that changes in sleep pattern observed in the intervening period was the result of self-management training, withdrawal of the medication produced little loss of improved sleep patterns (Davison, Tsujimoto, & Glaros, 1973). Those for whom the medication had been interpreted as the cause of improved sleep, on the other hand, reverted to prior levels of sleep disturbance when medication was withdrawn. Such observations have led Valins and Nisbitt (1972) to suggest intervention procedures that challenge patients to attribute improvements to dispositional traits, whereas encouraging situational interpretations of disturbances.

A partial reconciliation of the disparate views of cognitions as mediators versus precipitators of behavior has been proposed by several cognitive scientists. Candland (1977) suggests that cognitive appraisal, emotional experience, and physiological responses are interrelated in a continuous loop. This interpretation is consistent with the proposal of Bower (1981) who suggests that cognitive and emotional aspects of experiences are subsets of an organizing system that includes both internal and external experiences. Each emotion may be stimulated and provoked by a variety of cognitive, physiological, and situational factors. Hence, at times, cognitions may passively reflect emotional experience, and, at other times, they may motivate and evoke emotional as well as behavioral experience.

*Experiential Therapies*

The view of cognition held by experiential therapists emphasizes their role as responses rather than as either mediators or motivators (Greenberg, Safran, & Nice, Chapter 9, this volume). In this view, cognitive sets or beliefs are reorganized with every new experience to retain balance, relative harmony, and congruity among them. In other words, emotional experiences produce schema development rather than vice versa as usually proposed by theories of cognitive therapy. From an experiential point of view, cognitive distortions are the result of fragmented experience. Phenomenologically, new experiences are excluded from incorporation and fail to impact existant views if they are either very discrepant from prior information or challenge fundamental concepts and beliefs about self and others. Once excluded, they interfere with the processing of new information, providing a restrictive filter through which new experience is selected with the consequence of impairing the adaptability of the organism. More important than the content of one's cognitive life, therefore, is the process by which one disowns or reincorporates these new experiences. Such experiences are disowned and isolated from incorporation into ongoing cognitive structures through a process of selective matching. Matching determines whether important elements of the new experience fit with prior beliefs. This is not a conscious process, but, to the degree that the new experience fails to conform with prior beliefs (cognitive contents), the new information is occluded (a cognitive process), and one's emotional life becomes fragmented due to a failure of schemata to undergo natural reorganization (Greenberg, Safran, & Rice, Chapter 9, this volume).

In their systematic efforts to provide rapproachement of cognitive and experiential views of psychotherapy, Greenberg and Safran (1980, 1981, Chapter 9 in this volume) have emphasized the role of attention and inference in both psychopathology and psychotherapy. In so doing, these authors emphasize the reliance placed upon cognitive constructs by cognitive therapy theory and advocate paying more systematic attention to patients' characteristic processes of attending to relevant stimuli, storing these stimuli for future reference and retrieving this information when called upon to assess causality. They propose that therapeutic procedures could well focus upon such information-processing deficits and variations by constructing therapeutic experiments that would facilitate the acquisition of new information and the reappraisal of old beliefs. When certain experiences are defensively protected from other experiences, such as may happen when the cognitions that arise in a given situation are incongruous with the emotional qualities ordinarily associated with that experience, psychopathology is thought to be the result. Experiential interventions are designed to break down the barriers between various experiences, thus evoking emotional realignment and the reestablishment of harmony. Hence, *discrepancy among cognitive contents* rather than any specific content itself may motivate an integration of cognitive structures, which in turn provokes the development of new cognitive contents (i.e., the semantic representation of these structures).

The most usual form of fragmentation that manifests in cognitive distortion, is the separation of emotional and sensory experience from thought and awareness. Treatment is designed to break down these barriers, reimplement the process of incorporation, and to evoke a changed cognitive set or perspective. A truly therapeutic experience is one that induces sufficient discord in cognitive processing to evoke an emotional response, with the result that one reappraises experience and incorporates more of that which has been disowned, abandoned, or discarded from awareness.

Support for the assertion that emotional experiences are sufficient to evoke a cognitive process is to be found in investigations of mood induction. Systematic induction of a depressed mood through role playing and/or hypnosis have been observed to change both the cognitive content of one's beliefs and to motivate the selection of a particular process of memory recall or information processing (Bower, 1982; Mathews & Bradley, 1983; Teasdale & Fogarty, 1979). Similar support for the role of cognition as an inseparable response class with "emotion" is to be observed in the proposal that cognitive changes often are facilitated by the presence of intense emotional arousal. Hoehn-Saric *et al.*, (1972), for example, found that cognitive beliefs were more easily changed if individuals were artificially induced to high levels of emotional arousal before presenting them with new information in psychotherapy. In a comprehensive review of the functions of state-dependent learning and mood-congruent storage, Blaney (1986) also highlights extensive work that has suggested that certain cognitive material that evokes high levels of arousal is more likely to be stored and recalled when one's mood is congruent with that present when the affectively laden material initially was learned. This observation supports the role of affect in facilitating the realignment of cognitive structures. These latter findings set the stage for our review of cognitive change as a therapeutic experience.

LARRY E. BEUTLER
and PAUL D. GUEST

This section will explore the role of cognitive change in psychotherapy from an empirical perspective. We will briefly address some issues related to the differences between the ways cognitive structures and contents relate to therapeutic effectiveness. We also will explore psychotherapy in the context of similarities, differences, and areas of convergence of patient and therapist belief systems. From a foundation in these findings, we will attempt partially to address the question of what actually changes in psychotherapy and the degree to which these changes are causally related to therapeutic outcomes.

The foregoing pages have elucidated the importance of distinguishing between cognitive processes and cognitive contents. As we explore some of the empirical findings relative to the roles of cognition in psychotherapy, a clear distinction between process and content must be kept in mind. Cognitive content refers to conscious representations of secondarily derived and quite specific attitudes and belief systems; cognitive process refers to the structures from which those concepts are derived and that are employed as one appraises the environment. The process of attribution, judgments of efficacy, and styles of coping all reflect cognitive processes and their associated structures more than they index the presence of discrete cognitive contents. The question facing us at this point in our discussion is, "What changes in psychotherapy?"

The content–process distinction is rarely made either in psychotherapy research or in psychotherapy itself. At a practical level, cognitive therapists have typically concentrated more upon changing cognitive contents than processing styles (e.g., Beck et al., 1979; Ellis, 1970). On the other hand, cognitive theorists have paid much closer attention than cognitive therapists to the cognitive processes of information management that accompany human experience (e.g., Blaney, 1986; Bower, 1981). When psychotherapy change is inspected in terms of various cognitive dimensions, some interesting correlates emerge. For example, Beutler (1981) reviewed 21 studies in which attitude changes were evaluated in relation both to the attitudinal content espoused by therapists and to subsequent psychotherapy improvement. He also reviewed 18 studies in which variation in cognitive processes (e.g., personality-, attributional-, and cognitive-style variables) were evaluated both with respect to outcomes of psychotherapy and to the roles of initial similarity between patients and their therapists. Beutler concluded that psychotherapy, regardless of the particular theoretical orientation assumed by the therapist, constituted a social persuasion process in which convergence of specific attitudes and values was frequently found to occur over the course of therapy. Patient's attitudes changed in a direction to be more consistent with the attitudes and values presented by the therapist. Of 16 studies reviewed, 12 observed that an increasing convergence among the attitudinal contents of patient and therapist was related to improvement. That is, as patients adopted the attitudinal contents of their therapists, they became less symptomatic and felt better. Surprisingly, changes in processing structures did not follow the same pattern as changes in the beliefs and attitudes. Changes in cognitive processes and their underlying structures were observed to accrue with successful psychotherapy, but these changes were not dependent on, and did not come to be similar to, the type of cognitive process utilized or valued by the therapist. Indeed, the most consistent observation arising from a review of changes in processing mechanisms is that psychological improvement corresponds with increases in patient attributions of self-control and responsibility (Baker, 1979), seemingly irrespective of how little or much their therapists value such attributions.

Hence, one sees that the conscious contents of patient's ideation tends to become more similar to those of their therapists over the course of successful treatment. At the same time, patients who have a positive treatment response tend to adopt cognitive processes and develop cognitive structures that allow them to perceive more of their world as being under personal control and more of their behavior as being self-determined. We know of no persuasive evidence that these changes reflect a convergence with a particular therapist rather than an adaption of a more functional pattern. Initial attributional patterns and styles also seem to determine the relative efficacy with which different types of therapeutic procedures can be implemented. For example, individuals who initially adopt an external explanation for and attribution of their own behavior seem to be quite responsive to therapeutic directions and therapist control, producing subsequent symptom relief and greater subjective improvement than their internally oriented counterparts. On the other hand, individuals who initially manifest cognitive processes and structures that allow internal attributions tend to respond better to therapeutic procedures that are nondirective and nonconfrontive than they do to directive and confrontive ones (Beutler, Crago, & Arizmendi, 1986; Beutler, 1983b). This finding parallels the conclusion of Hollon and Beck (1986), who propose that certain deficits in methods of processing information may be indicative of the type of cognitive interventions to be utilized. However interesting, these conclusions leave us with the question of their importance to our consideration of integrative views in the role of cognition in psychotherapy from which this chapter began.

## AN INTEGRATIVE VIEWPOINT

In the last section of this chapter, we will attempt to bring together some of the theoretical and empirical perspectives that have been explored in the foregoing pages within an integrative language system and theory of change. The viewpoint presented is designed to be sufficiently flexible as to consider the role of cognitive change within a variety of theoretical models.

Our review leads us to suggest that cognitive therapists have been misguided in placing greater emphasis upon cognitive content than upon cognitive process and structures. The attempt to define a linear relationship between discrete types of cognitive contents and specific varieties of psychopathologies (e.g., depression vs. anxiety; Hollon, Kendall & Lumry, 1986; Ross, Mueller, & De La Torre, 1986) is ill conceived and, not surprising, has not been very successful. Because depressed patients appear to have ideas and beliefs that are similar to those of normals, a therapy that focuses upon the cognitive contents of beliefs as a *therapy-specific* goal begs more important questions. Again we are drawn to recall the fallacy of equating the label with the structure itself and maintain that the cognitive phenomena that are important to psychotherapy cannot be considered to be solely products of the patient. Psychotherapy, and particularly cognitive therapy, can be seen as a social persuasion process. We conclude, that the patient's attitudes and belief systems must be observed in juxtaposition with those of the therapist. Rather than attempting to define certain finite attitudinal systems that universally characterize certain psychopathologies and then setting out to modify these beliefs in a prescribed direction through psychological intervention, one's efforts might better be directed to the role of patient merging with therapist beliefs as a defining goal of treatment. The ethics of such an approach as well as defining the therapy relevant beliefs is increasingly drawing the attention of writers but deserves more empirical effort (Tjeltveit, 1986).

We maintain that all forms of psychotherapies are *processes* of conveying philosophies and viewpoints. Hence, cognitive change is a *nonspecific* outcome of effective therapy. That is to say, all therapies promote organizational frameworks for experience and new ideas or attitudes. Some of these philosophies embody world views, whereas others are more situation-specific. In either case, therapist viewpoints represent the overt manifestations of the organizing structures (philosophies) that will be communicated and the adoption of which will be correlated with improvement. Effective promotion of these philosophies is made possible by the quality of the therapeutic contact. By identifying with the therapist, valuing the therapist's opinion, and modeling one's own belief systems after those espoused by the therapist, the patient's cognitive schemata are changed to become more like those of the therapist. The

LARRY E. BEUTLER
and PAUL D. GUEST

attitudes of the patient come to parallel the beliefs and values held by the caring, sensitive, and responsive therapist.

Earlier in this chapter, we discussed the necessity of a common language to understand psychotherapy and psychotherapy process. Strong (1986) recently has reemphasized the potential of social influence language for such a purpose. Broadly defined, social influence theory defines the conditions under which one individual will exert an impact upon another individual. Social influence theory emphasizes that the power of the persuader (therapist) is a function of how that individual is perceived by the recipient (client/patient) and how the process of change is justified or attributed. Hypothetically, dispositional characteristics of the client, similarities in cognitive structure between patient and therapist, and environmental influences will all determine what is persuaded, the mechanism by which it can be persuaded, and the role that various aspects of cognitions (sensory experience, emotional experience, etc.) play.

If one views psychotherapy from this broad social persuasion perspective, then the empirical questions facing cognitive therapy broaden to include investigation of the conditions and problems for which cognitive change: (1) merely reflects or correlates with behavior change, (2) provokes or maintains behavior and emotional change, and/or (3) is a product or criterion of successful treatment. The relatively close relationship between convergence of patients' and therapists' conscious beliefs and subsequent improvement in affect and mood (Beutler, 1981) at least suggests that cognitive changes should be included among the array of dependent variables studied by all therapies. Assessing the degree to which the therapists' cognitive belief structures are assumed by the patients may complement an understanding of symptom change and can index therapists' influence power in ways not captured by other dependent variables. Such convergence may be an especially sensitive index of the power of the nonspecific factors in psychotherapy.

Changes in cognitive contents, toward some predetermined notion of what constitutes ''realistic'' ideas, when considered independently from the ideas held by therapists, do not relate strongly to important outcomes of psychotherapy and do not seem to provoke large changes in symptoms. To the degree that we find that the beneficial and symptomatic effects of therapy are causally related to convergence of specific attitudes, we may be able to enhance these effects directly by encouraging new and adaptive problem-solving methods and attributional processes that are valued by the therapist. This tactic is to be preferred over working toward theory-specific attitudinal sets that have no apparent, direct relationship either to patient distress or improvement.

Although changes in general cognitive attitudes reflect the power of the therapist's persuasiveness, changes in specific cognitive processes may be therapy-, rather than therapist-, specific. Different therapy procedures may facilitate the development of different processes. Valins and Nisbitt (1972) have proposed, for example, that attention be given to the propensity to make situational versus dispositional attributions among different patients when selecting interventions. Those who are prone to interpret failure situations dispositionally may be provided with procedures that force the development of more situational interpretations. In contrast, those who are prone to interpret their behavior as situationally determined, may be differentially susceptible to strategies that encourage dispositional attributions.

Kuiper and McDonald (1983) give examples of the prescriptive assignment of interventions in which some systematic procedures work to change one's attributional processes from situational to dispositional, whereas others auger to shift attributional process from dispositional to situational. Forsterling (1986) has expanded upon the notion that specific therapies can be designed to alter attributional processes. He rightly observes that most efforts to systematically retrain attributional processes in psychotherapeutic settings draw heavily upon studies of achievement motivation (e.g., Weiner, 1979), but that this approach emphasizes changing the attributions that one applies *following* either successful or unsuccessful experiences. For example, attributional models of success and failure (e.g., Abramson, Seligman, &

Teasdale, 1978) have been applied widely to an understanding of how depression may derive from differential ascriptions of temporality, causality, and generality following successful and unsuccessful experiences. Although persuasive, these models say little about the wide variety of problematic and pleasant emotions that exist, or how these emotions may arise or be changed in situations that do not involve experiences that are easily classified as "successful" or "unsuccessful." Indeed, these applications give little attention to the attributions that are ascribed to the *antecedents* of emotional experience. By extending concepts of attribution and attribution training to antecedents of behavior, Forsterling (1986) proposes the application of attributional retraining to a host of new situations and therapeutic experiences. We believe that these possibilities deserve greater attention and amplification.

In applying concepts of social and interpersonal persuasions to the language of psychotherapy, concepts of sensitivity to external control (i.e., reactance, Brehm & Brehm, 1981), attribution of influence, and coping styles should be considered. We have already elucidated data to suggest that certain types of cognitive interventions might be most appropriately applied when the problems of individuals are the result of deficits in social skills rather than inappropriate or dysfunctional cognitive beliefs (Beutler, 1983b; Hollon & Beck, 1986). Greater degrees of specificity need to be applied to these dimensions, both within cognitive therapy and psychotherapy more generally, in order to define the particular interventions required for specific purposes at given times (Beutler, 1983b; Norcross, 1986a,b).

Although still in its rudimentary forms, various models of technical integration are available for applying social persuasion concepts to psychotherapy process and outcome. The model of systematic eclecticism proposed by the senior author (Beutler, 1983b) specifically considers the role of matching patient and therapist to obtain optimal change of conscious ideas and attitudes, whereas at the same time applying strategic procedures that are selected on the basis of patients' reactance levels and coping styles to facilitate change in problem-solving structures and attributional dispositions. For example, this model proposes that the patient's defensive style is an important consideration in selecting whether direct efforts at change are initiated toward cognitive contents and structures, affective tone and quality, or behavioral repertoires. Like Beck and Hollon (1986), moreover, it is anticipated that habitual deficits or excesses are indicators for the application of different treatment modalities, from those that are appropriate when symptoms merely represent indirect symbols of their initiating events. By developing greater specificity in integrative models, it may be possible for research to gradually clarify the conditions under which cognitive content should be a principal focus of intervention as opposed to conditions under which the underlying processes that mediate one's interpretation of experience ought to become targets of therapeutic influence.

# REFERENCES

Abramson, L. Y., Seligman, M. E. P., & Teasdale, J. J. (1978). Learned helplessness in humans; critique and reformulation. *Journal of Abnormal Psychology, 17*, 56–67.

Alloy, L. B., & Abramson, L. Y. (1979). Judgement of contingency in depressed and non-depressed students: Sadder but wiser? *Journal of Experimental Psychology: General, 108*, 441–485.

Alloy, L. B., & Abramson, L. Y. (1982). Learned helplessness, depression and the illusion of control. *Journal of Personality and Social Psychology, 42*, 1114–1126.

Baker, E. K. (1979). The relationship between locus of control and psychotherapy: A review of the literature. *Psychotherapy: Theory, Research and Practice, 16*, 351–362.

Bandura, A. (1977). Self-efficacy: Towards a unifying theory of behavioral change. *Psychological Review, 84*, 191–215.

Beck, A. T., Rush, A. J., Shaw, B. F., & Emery, G. (1979). *Cognitive therapy of depression.* New York: Guilford Press.

Beidel, D. C., & Turner, S. M. (1986). A critique of the theoretical bases of cognitive-behavioral theories and therapy. *Clinical Psychology Review, 6*, 177–197.

Berk, L. E. (1986, May). Private speech: Learning out loud. *Psychology Today, 34–36*, 38–39, 42.

Beutler, L. E. (1981). Convergence in counseling and psychotherapy: A current look. *Clinical Psychology Review, 1,* 79–101.

Beutler, L. E. (1983a, July). (Moderator). *Eclecticism: A neutral theory of therapy.* A paper presented at the 14th Annual Meeting of the Society for Psychotherapy Research, Sheffield, England.

Beutler, L. E. (1983b). *Eclectic psychotherapy: A systematic approach.* New York: Pergamon Press.

Beutler, L. E., Crago, M., & Arizmendi, T. G. (1986). Research on therapist variables in psychotherapy. In S. L. Garfield & A. E. Bergin (Eds.), *Handbook of psychotherapy and behavior change* (3rd ed., pp. 257–310). New York: Wiley.

Beutler, L. E., Scogin, F., Kirkish, P., Schretlen, D., Corbishley, A., Hamblin, D., Meredity, K., Potter, R., Bamford, C. R., & Levenson, A. I. (1987). Group cognitive therapy and alprazalam in the treatment of depression in older adults. *Journal of Consulting and Clinical Psychology, 55,* 550–556.

Blaney, P. H. (1986). Affect and memory: A review. *Psychological Bulletin, 99,* 229–246.

Bootzin, R. R. (1985). Affect and cognition in behavior therapy. In S. Reiss & R. R. Bootzin (Eds.), *Theoretical issues in behavior therapy* (pp. 35–45). New York: Academic Press.

Bower, G. H. (1981). Mood and memory. *American Psychologist, 36,* 129–148.

Bower, G. H., & Cohen, P. R. (1982). Emotional influences in memory and thinking: Data and theory. In M. S. Clark & S. T. Fiske (Eds.), *Affect and cognition: The seventeenth Annual Carnegie Symposium On Cognition* (pp. 291–232). Hillsdale, N.J.: Lawrence Erlbaum.

Brehm, S. S., & Brehm, J. W. (1981). *Psychological reactance: A theory of freedom and control.* New York: Academic Press.

Candland, D. K. (1977). The persistence problems of emotion. In D. K. Candland, J. P. Fell, E. Keen, A. I. Leshner, R. Plutchik, & R. M. Tarpy (Eds.), *Emotion* (pp. 1–84). Belmont, CA: Brooks/Cole.

Candland, D. K., Fell, J. P., Keen, E., Leshner, A. I., Plutchik, R., & Tarpy, R. M. (Eds.). (1977). *Emotion.* Belmont, CA: Brooks/Cole.

Clark, M. S. (1982). A role for arousal in the link between feeling states, judgements and behavior. In M. S. Clark & S. T. Fiske (Eds.), *Affect and cognition: The 17th Annual Carnegie Symposium on Cognition* (pp. 263–289). Hillsdale, NJ: Lawrence Erlbaum.

Corsini, R. J. (Ed.). (1981). *Handbook of innovative psychotherapies.* New York: Wiley.

Coyne, J. C., & Gotlieb, I. H. (1983). The role of cognition and depression: A critical appraisal. *Psychological Bulletin, 94,* 472–505.

Craik, F. I. M. (1979). Human memory. *Annual Review of Psychology, 30,* 63–102.

Davison, G. C., Tsujimototo, R. N., & Glaros, A. G. (1973). Attribution and the maintenance of behavior change in falling asleep. *Journal of Abnormal Psychology, 82,* 124–133.

Derry, P. A., & Kuiper, N. A. (1981). Schematic processing and self reference in clinical depression. *Journal of Abnormal Psychology, 90,* 286–297.

Ellis, A. (1962). *Reason and emotion in psychotherapy.* New York: Lyle Stuart Press.

Ellis, A. (1970). *The essence of rational psychotherapy: A comprehensive approach to treatment.* New York: Institute for rational living.

Forsterling, F. (1986). Attributional conceptions in clinical psychology. *American Psychologists, 41,* 275–285.

Garfield, S. L. (1980). *Psychotherapy: An eclectic approach.* New York: Wiley.

Goldfried, M. (1983, July). *Eclecticism: A neutral theory of psychotherapy.* A symposium presented at the Annual Meeting of the Society for Psychotherapy Research, Sheffield, England.

Goldfried, M. R., DeCanteceo, E. T., & Weinberg, L. (1974). Systematic rational restructuring as a self control technique. *Behavior Therapy, 5,* 247–254.

Greenberg, L. S., & Safran, J. D. (1980). Encoding, information processing and the cognitive behavioural therapies. *Canadian Psychologist, 21,* 59–66.

Greenberg, L. S., & Safran, J. D. (1981). Encoding and cognitive therapy: Changing what clients attend to. *Psychotherapy: Theory, research and practice, 18,* 163–169.

Hoehn-Saric, R., Lieberman, B., Imber, S. D., Stone, A. R., Pande, S. K., & Frank, J. D. (1972). Arousal and attitude change in neurotic patients. *Archives of General Psychiatry, 26,* 51–56.

Hollon, S., & Beck, A. T. (1986). Research on cognitive therapy. In S. L. Garfield & A. E. Bergen (Eds.), *Handbook of psychotherapy and behavior Change* (3rd ed., pp. 443–482) New York: Wiley.

Hollon, S. D., Kendall, P. C., & Lumry, A. (1986). Specificity of depressogenic cognitions in clinical depression. *Journal of Abnormal Psychology, 95,* 52–59.

Kelly, G. A. (1955). *The psychology of personal constructs* (Vol. 1). New York: Norton.

Kendall, P. C., & Braswell, L. (1985). *Cognitive-behavioral modification with impulsive children.* New York: Guilford Press.

Kuhl, J. (1984). Volitional aspects of achievement motivation and learned helplessness: Toward a comprehen-sive theory of action control. In B. A. Maher (Ed.), *Progress in experimental personality research* (Vol. 13, pp. 99–170). New York: Academic Press.

Kuhl, J., & Helle, P. (1986). Motivational and volitional determinants of depression: The degenerated-intension hypothesis. *Journal of Abnormal Psychology, 95,* 247–251.

Kuiper, N. A., & MacDonald, M. R. (1983). Reason, emotion, and cognitive therapy. *Clinical Psychology Review, 3,* 297–316.

Lazarus, R. S. (1982). Thoughts on the relations between emotion and cognitive. *American Psychologist, 37,* 1019–1024.

Lazarus, R. S. (1984). On the primacy of cognition. *American Psychologist, 39,* 124–129.

Leventhal, H. (1982). The integration of emotion and cognition: A view from the perceptual-motor theory of emotion. In M. S. Clark & S. T. Fiske (Eds.), *Affect and cognition: The seventeenth annual symposium on cognition* (pp. 121–156). Hillsdale, NJ: Lawrence Earlbaum.

Lewinsohn, P. M., Mischel, W., Chaplin, W., & Barton, R. (1980). Social competence and depression: The role of illusory self perception. *Journal of Abnormal Psychology, 90,* 213–219.

Linville, P. W. (1982). Affective consequences of complexity regarding the self and others. In M. S. Clark & S. T. Fiske (Eds.), *Affect and cognition: The seventeenth annual symposium on cognition* (pp. 79–110). Hillsdale, NJ: Lawrence Earlbaum.

London, P. (1986). *The modes and morals of psychotherapy* (2nd ed.). New York: Hemisphere Publishing Corporation.

Luria, A. R. (1961). *The role of speech in the regulation of normal and abnormal behavior.* New York: Liverwright.

Mandler, G. (1975). *Mind and emotion.* New York: Wiley.

Mandler, G. (1982). The structure of value: Accounting for taste. In M. S. Clark & S. T. Fiske (Eds.), *Affect and cognition: The seventeenth annual carnegie symposium on cognition* (pp. 3–36). Hillsdale, NJ: Lawrence Earlbaum.

Marcel, A. J. (1983). Conscious and unconscious perception: An approach to the relations between phenomenal experience and perceptual processes. *Cognitive Psychology, 15,* 238–300.

Mathews, A., & Bradley, B. (1983). Mood and the self-reference biases in recall. *Behaviour Research and Therapy, 21,* 233–239.

Meichenbaum, D. (1974). *Cognitive behavior modification.* Morristown, NJ: General Learning.

Meichenbaum, D. (1977). *Cognitive-behavior modification: An integrative approach.* New York: Plenum Press.

Norcross, J. C. (1986a). *A casebook of eclectic psychotherapy.* New York: Brunner/Mazel.

Norcross, J. C. (1986b). *Handbook of eclectic psychotherapy.* New York: Brunner/Mazel.

Norcross, J. C. (1986c, June). *Toward a common language.* A paper presented at the Annual Meeting of the Society for Psychotherapy Research, Wellesley, MA.

Prochaska, J. O. (1984). *Systems of psychotherapy: A transtheoretical analysis* (2nd ed.). Homewood, IL: Dorsey Press.

Ross, L. (1977). The intuitive psychologist and his shortcomings. In L. Berkowitz (Ed.), *Advances in experi-mental and social psychology* (Vol. 10, pp. 173–220). New York: Academic Press.

Ross, M., & Olson, J. M. (1981). An expectancy-attribution model of the effects of placebos. *Psychological Review, 88,* 408–437.

Ross, M., Mueller, J. H., & De La Torre, M. (1986). Depression and trait distinctiveness in the self-schema. *Journal of Social and Clinical Psychology, 4,* 46–59.

Rumelhart, D. E., & Ortony, A. (1978). The representation of knowledge in memory. In R. C. Anderson, R. C. Spiro, & W. E. Montague (Eds.), *Schooling and the acquisition of knowledge.* Hillsdale, NJ: Lawrence Earlbaum.

Schacter, S., & Singer, J. E. (1962). Cognitive, social and physiological determinants of emotional states. *Psychological Review, 69,* 379–399.

Schwartz, R. M. (1982). Cognitive-behavior modification: A conceptual review. *Clinical Psychology Review, 2,* 267–293.

Silverman, J. S., Silverman, J. A., & Eardley, D. A. (1984). Do maladaptive attitudes cause depression? *Archives of General Psychiatry, 41,* 28–30.

Simons, A. D., Garfield, S. L., & Murphy, G. E. (1984). The process of change in cognitive therapy and pharmacotherapy for depression. *Archives of General Psychiatry, 41,* 45–51.

Smith, M. L., Glass, G. V., & Miller, T. I. (1980). *The benefits of psychotherapy.* Baltimore: Johns Hop-kins.

142

LARRY E. BEUTLER
and PAUL D. GUEST

Strong, S. R. (1986, June). *Interpersonal influence theory as a common language.* A paper presented at the Annual Meeting of the Society for Psychotherapy Research, Wellesely, MA.

Teasdale, J. D., & Fogarty, S. J. (1979). Differential effects of induced mood on retrieval of pleasant and unpleasant events from episodic memory. *Journal of Abnormal Psychology, 88,* 248–257.

Tjelveit, A. C. (1986). The ethics of value conversion in psychotherapy: Appropriate and inappropriate therapist influence on client values. *Clinical Psychology Review, 6,* 515–537.

Tulving, E. (1972). Episodic and semantic memory. In E. Tulving & W. Donaldson (Eds.), *Organization of memory* (pp. 382–402). New York: Academic Press.

Valins, S., & Nisbett, R. E. (1972). Attribution processes in the development and treatment of emotional disorders. In E. E. Jones, D. E. Kanouse, H. H. Kelley, R. E. Nisbett, S. Valins, & B. Weiner (Eds.), *Attribution: Perceiving the causes of behavior* (pp. 137–150). Morristown, NJ: General Learning Press.

Vygotsky, L. (1962). *Thought and language.* New York: Wiley.

Weiner, B. (1979). A theory of motivation for some classroom experiences. *Journal of Educational Psychology, 71,* 3–25.

Wolpe, J. (1973). *The practice of behavior therapy.* New York: Pergamon.

# 8

# Cognitive, Behavioral, and Psychodynamic Therapies
## Converging or Diverging Pathways to Change?

HAL ARKOWITZ AND MO THERESE HANNAH

Although the origins of cognitive therapy can be traced back in the history of philosophy and psychology (see Ellis, Chapter 1, this volume), it is still a relatively new arrival on the psychotherapy scene. Nonetheless, there already exists some very promising data for its effectiveness, particularly in the treatment of depression (e.g., Beckham & Watkins, Chapter 4, this volume; Elkin, Shea, Watkins, & Collins, 1986; Hollon & Beck, 1986). The recent proliferation of books, articles, and conferences on cognitive therapy, along with its inclusion in the NIMH Collaborative Study on Depression (Elkin, Parloff, Hadley, & Autry, 1985) point to the wide and rapidly growing acceptance of this approach. Given this, it seems particularly timely to consider the relationship between cognitive therapy and other major forms of psychotherapy. In this chapter, we will compare cognitive therapy with behavioral and psychodynamic therapies in an attempt to determine commonalities and differences among them.* In addition, we will present a formulation of change in psychotherapy based on factors that we believe are present in all three of these therapies. The argument will be advanced that the favorable outcome data for cognitive therapy may not be due to any particularly unique or novel elements but may instead be due to a more efficient and explicit use of factors that are present in these other forms of psychotherapies as well.

---

*Because Greenberg, Safran, and Rice's chapter (Chapter 9, this volume) examines the relationship between cognitive and experiential therapies, we decided to omit experiential therapies from the present analysis. This exclusion is not meant to imply any value judgment about these therapies that we believe represent a viable and exciting direction in the field of psychotherapy.

---

HAL ARKOWITZ AND MO THERESE HANNAH • Department of Psychology, University of Arizona, Tucson, Arizona 85721.

HAL ARKOWITZ and
MO THERESE
HANNAH

Historically, the three therapy approaches have developed along rather distinct paths, but there have been some significant points of overlap and influence. To cite just two examples, there has been a close and growing relationship between cognitive and behavior therapies (e.g., Beck, Rush, Shaw, & Emery, 1979), and there have been various attempts to integrate psychoanalytic and behavioral approaches to therapy (e.g., Arkowitz & Messer, 1984; Wachtel, 1977).

It is quite clear that many behavior therapy techniques have been incorporated into cognitive therapy. This is clearly acknowledged by Beck (e.g., Beck *et al.*, 1979; Beck & Weishaar, Chapter 2 in this volume). The use of such techniques as social skills training, relaxation training, and homework assignments in cognitive therapy reflects the very apparent influence of behavior therapy on the practice of cognitive therapy. Conversely, behavior therapy has become increasingly cognitive, particularly since Beck (1976) published his first major book on cognitive therapy.

To illustrate the increasing cognitive trend in behavior therapy, the authors conducted a survey of articles published in *Behavior Therapy* (the main journal of the Association for the Advancement of Behavior Therapy) in the 3 years just prior to the appearance of Beck's book (1974–1976), and once again a decade later (1984–1986). Each therapy paper was coded by the present authors to determine whether or not it had significant cognitive content. These judgments were based on the presence or absence of clear cognitive constructs or techniques described in the abstract of the article.

During 1974–1976, only 9% of the behavior therapy articles used cognitive constructs. However, this percentage almost quadrupled (32%) for articles appearing a decade later (1984–1986). It seems clear from this trend that the gap between behavior therapy and cognitive therapy has narrowed considerably in recent years.

Several major behavior therapies have become increasingly influenced by cognitive therapy as well. To cite just two examples, the early 1970s witnessed the development of new behavior therapies for depression (Lewinsohn, 1974) and for marital distress (Weiss, Hops, & Patterson, 1973). In the early publications on these therapies, cognitive constructs and techniques were either totally ignored or relegated to a trivial position. By contrast, later presentations of these two behavior therapies have become increasingly cognitive, using cognitive conceptualizations of the problem and incorporating cognitive strategies into the treatments (e.g., Lewinsohn & Arconad, 1981; Weiss, 1980). As early as 1978, Kazdin wrote that

> the inclusion of cognition-based treatment represents a new direction in behavior modification that evolved out of dissatisfaction with stimulus-response explanations of behavior and in response to research that has demonstrated the role of thought processes in controlling behavior. (Kazdin, 1978, pp. 307–308).

Thus, cognitive and behavioral approaches have had and continue to have a close mutual relationship since the middle 1970s.

Although cognitive and behavioral approaches have only recently become more intimate, psychodynamic and behavioral approaches might be characterized as having had a long history of casual affairs. The history of attempts to integrate behavioral and psychodynamic therapies has been reviewed by Arkowitz (1984) and Goldfried (1982a). It spans the work of Thomas French (1933), Dollard and Miller (1950), and Franz Alexander (1963). The most recent and extensive attempt at such an integration can be seen in the work of Paul Wachtel (1977, 1987). It appears to be the case that as behavior therapy becomes more cognitive and as psychoanalytic therapists show interest in short-term therapies and object relations and interpersonal analytic models, the opportunity for rapprochement increases.

Arkowitz and Messer (1984) invited a group of distinguished representatives of behavioral, psychodynamic, and integrationist orientations to address the feasibility and desirability of integration. The contributions to their book illustrate the strong interest and intense controversy that still surrounds the idea of a behavioral–psychodynamic integration. Despite the interest, it was quite apparent that there are still many clinical and empirical issues that need to be resolved before this integration can become a viable approach in the field of psychotherapy.

A broader interest in psychotherapy integration has been apparent in the past few years as well. Many researchers, theorists, and therapists from diverse orientations have begun to explore commonalities among their respective approaches. The 1980s witnessed the birth of a journal (*Journal of Integrative and Eclectic Psychotherapies*) and an organization (Society for the Exploration of Psychotherapy Integration) devoted to this purpose. Given these developments, it is likely that the future will hold further attempts to explore relationships among cognitive, behavioral, and psychodynamic therapies.

## SOURCES OF DATA FOR A COMPARATIVE ANALYSIS

In our analysis, we will distinguish between two sets of issues. Different psychotherapies can be compared on practical issues that reflect what the therapists of different orientations actually *do* in their practice. Such issues include the choice of patients and problems for the therapy, assessment procedures, the nature and role of the therapeutic relationship, and the role of technique. A comparison of the three therapies on these issues will be presented first. A second set of issues will also be discussed relating to philosophical and theoretical concerns that include visions of human nature and theories of how change occurs in therapy.

A question arises as to the best data base to use for our comparison. Obviously, the best source would be studies in which therapy sessions were observed and directly relevant dimensions of the patient–therapist interactions assessed. However, there have been very few studies of this type. In one such study, Luborsky, Woody, Lellan, O'Brien, and Rosenzweig (1982) compared drug counseling, supportive-expressive therapy, and cognitive-behavior therapy. Each of these three therapies had specific treatment manuals associated with them. Independent judges were quite accurate in discriminating the three therapies. In addition, analyses also revealed that the therapists conducted their therapies largely as the treatment manuals dictated. The raters determined that the therapists in each approach met the criteria for their respective therapies when their actual behavior was compared to the instructions in the therapy manual.

The finding that therapists using different manual-based therapies engaged in appropriate and discriminably different behaviors suggests that therapy manuals may be a reasonable starting point for our comparative analysis. Fortunately, the past decade has witnessed the increasing ''manualization'' of short-term psychotherapies for the purpose of conducting meaningful therapy outcome studies. Because of this, there are therapy manuals or near equivalents available for cognitive, psychodynamic, and behavioral therapies that can be used as the main source for our comparisons.

One aspect of the ''uniformity myth'' discussed by Kiesler (1966) is relevant to consider here. When speaking of cognitive therapy, one could refer to the work of Beck *et al.* (1979), Ellis (1962), Mahoney (1974), or Meichenbaum (1977). Behavior therapy could refer to such diverse approaches as Skinner's (1953) radical behaviorism, Wolpe's (1973) systematic desensitization, or Bandura's (1977, 1986) more cognitively mediated view. Likewise, psychoanalytic or psychodynamic therapies have numerous variations, ranging from formal psychoanalysis, based upon Freudian or interpersonal theories, to the short-term psychodynamic approaches of Luborsky (1984), Malan (1979), Mann (1973), Sifneos (1979), and Strupp and Binder (1984). Each orientation represents an approach that differs considerably from the others. Thus, when using the broad labels of *cognitive, behavioral,* or *psychodynamic,* we may be assuming a degree of homogeneity that simply does not exist.

To avoid this erroneous assumption and to simplify our task, we decided to draw from the work of one or two major proponents of each of the three approaches. This "exemplar" strategy will enable us to choose a specific and well-described version of each orientation, rather than discuss some nonexistent stereotype.

Considering the heterogeneity within each orientation, any choices we make must be somewhat arbitrary. Cognitive therapy offers the most obvious alternative. Although Ellis, Meichenbaum, and Mahoney have made significant contributions, Beck's therapy is the most clearly described and empirically supported cognitive approach (Beck *et al.*, 1979; Hollon & Beck, 1986). The inclusion of Beck's cognitive therapy in the NIMH outcome study on depression and the preliminary report of its effectiveness in that study (Elkin *et al.*, 1986) ensure that it will likely continue to be the most widely used of the cognitive therapies, at least in the near future. Behavior therapy cannot be well-represented by any single exemplar, but the writings of Kazdin (e.g., 1978) represent a thoughtful and articulate position that has won wide acceptance. We will also draw from O'Leary and Wilson's (1987) behavior therapy textbook and the clinical descriptions in Goldfried and Davison (1976). Psychodynamic therapies include a similar array of choices, but we selected Strupp and Binder's (1984) time-limited dynamic psychotherapy (TLDP) because of its attempt to describe the therapy in practical detail and because of the active research program that has accompanied this approach. We should note that Luborsky's (1984) manual for short-term psychoanalytic therapy is also thoughtful and explicit, and either of these two could have served equally well as an "exemplar" of short-term psychodynamic therapy.

At the outset, our three exemplar approaches immediately share one important feature in common. They are all short-term therapies. Our analysis might arrive at different conclusions, if, for example, we considered formal long-term psychoanalysis instead of short-term psychodynamic therapy. Brief therapies, by their very nature, share some characteristics in common despite differing theoretical orientations. Koss and Butcher (1986) have reviewed the area of brief therapy and concluded that their commonalities include such features as the setting of more limited goals than long-term therapy, a strong emphasis on the "here and now" instead of early life history and a therapeutic style that tends to be more active and/or directive than might be the case for the longer term version. Given these commonalities among the various forms of brief psychotherapies, let us now turn to a more specific comparison of cognitive, behavioral, and psychodynamic approaches to therapy.

## PATIENT SELECTION

All three approaches are viewed as generally appropriate for the same general class of patients, that is, those suffering from anxiety and depression. Only psychodynamic therapy stipulates certain *a priori* exclusionary criteria. Because this method is intended only for individuals whose difficulties are embedded in *long-term and primarily interpersonal maladaptive patterns,* chronicity and dysfunctional style as well as anxiety and depression are inclusionary criteria. The relearning that occurs in psychodynamic therapy takes place in the context of the therapy relationship in which the dysfunctional patterns are enacted and eventually discarded. A specific and relatively isolated problem such as a simple phobia may be judged to be inappropriate for psychodynamic therapy, unless it was a part of a broader interpersonal pattern that would likely manifest itself in the therapy relationship.

Although cognitive therapy continues to be extended to other clinical problems, most of the empirical evidence for its effectiveness comes from treatment outcome studies of depression (Hollon & Beck, 1986). Beck, Emery, and Greenberg (1985) have presented the details of a cognitive therapy for anxiety. There are no specific exclusionary criteria for cognitive therapy.

Likewise, there are no *a priori* exclusionary criteria for behavior therapy. In practice, this approach has also been applied to a wide variety of problems (see O'Leary & Wilson, 1987). The strongest data supporting the effectiveness of behavioral interventions are based on its use with anxiety problems, child and family problems, and rehabilitation of the chronically mentally ill (O'Leary & Wilson, 1987).

Psychodynamic and cognitive therapies differ from behavioral theory in the degree to which patients must be able and willing to comprehend and to verbally express themselves. Behavior therapy requires less of these verbal skills than do the other two approaches.

In summary, then, only psychodynamic psychotherapy excludes patients based upon some *a priori* criteria, and all three emphasize applications with anxiety and depression. However, extensions of all three have been made to a variety of other clinical problems as well.

## ASSESSMENT AND TARGETS FOR CHANGE

The question of what to assess is closely linked to the question of what to change in therapy. Because the different therapies target different change mechanisms, assessment in the three approaches has proceeded along somewhat different lines. However, there is some degree of similarity that we will consider first.

With the appearance of DSM-III in 1980, the reliability of psychiatric diagnoses has increased considerably. Structured interviews based on DSM-III criteria such as the SADS (Endicott & Spitzer, 1978) or the NIH-DIS (Robins, Helzer, Croughan, & Ratliff, 1981) are often employed. DSM-III criteria have been used for both patient selection and assessment of outcome in studies of the different therapies. This has been particularly true in studies of cognitive therapy (e.g. Elkin *et al.*, 1985). However, behavior therapists have been showing increasing interest in the use of these criteria and measures (e.g., Nathan, 1981). Outcome studies of short-term psychodynamic therapies have employed DSM-III criteria as well (e.g., Steuer *et al.*, 1984).

In addition to the use of DSM-III criteria, there has been a tendency for studies of the different therapies to use some of the same self-report instruments, such as the Beck Depression Inventory and the Hamilton Rating Scale for Depression (e.g., Elkin *et al.*, 1985; Lewinsohn & Arconad, 1981; Steuer *et al.*, 1984). The trend toward the use of similar screening and assessment procedures in studies of the different therapies is a small but encouraging one that facilitates comparisons across the studies. However, beyond such molar similarities as those discussed before, there remain some real differences among the therapies as to *what* to assess and *how* to assess it.

The question of *what* to assess, beyond the broad assessment of symptoms discussed before, is closely linked to differing views about the important causal factors and most appropriate targets for change in psychotherapy. Behavior therapy places a very strong emphasis on environmental determinants of behavior and the importance of behavior–environment interactions. Given this view, assessment tends to be more situation-specific than in the other approaches, with an emphasis upon how people respond in particular situations. Assessment tends to focus on behaviors and their covariations with antecedents and consequences (O'Leary & Wilson, 1987). Although behavior therapy has acquired a somewhat more cognitive emphasis, it still places considerably greater emphasis on overt behaviors and their interaction with environmental factors than do the other approaches. As such, behavioral assessment is less likely than the other approaches to make assumptions about cross-situational generality.

In both cognitive and psychodynamic therapies, the more important causal factors are seen as dispositions within the individual rather than in the individual's transactions with the environment. Although cognitive and psychodynamic therapies differ as to how they conceptualize and measure these dispositions, they do share a common dispositional assumption that distinguishes them from the behavioral approach. In cognitive and psychodynamic therapies, these inner dispositions are major targets for both assessment and change.

In cognitive therapy, the presumed causal mediators are the cognitive distortions that are associated with different types of psychopathology. This notion is nowhere better illustrated than in the present *Handbook* in Beck and Weishaar's chapter (Chapter 2, this volume). It is the automatic thoughts and schemata underlying the problem that need to be assessed and changed (e.g., Goldberg & Shaw, Chapter 3, this volume), because they are assumed to cause the other symptoms of the problem.

In time-limited dynamic therapy, the main focus for assessment is also an inner dispositional one. However, the nature of the presumed causal mediator is quite different across the two approaches. In TLDP, assessment centers around the formulation of a *dynamic focus*. As discussed by Strupp and Binder (1984), the dynamic focus is a working model or theory of the patient's problems that is developed over the course of treatment. It is a narrative description rather than a quantitative measure, and it is changing rather than fixed. The purpose of the dynamic focus as discussed by Strupp and Binder (1984) is to serve as a ''heuristic guide to inquiry'' (p. 66).

The dynamic focus is a model of the central or more salient interpersonal roles in which patients unconsciously cast themselves, the complementary roles in which they cast others, and the related maladaptive interaction sequences that result, as well as the negative and self-defeating cognitions that accompany this pattern. Following is an abbreviated example of a dynamic focus, adapted from Strupp & Binder (p. 83): (1) *Acts of self:* Arnold seeks acceptance and avoids rejection from others by behaving in a gregarious manner that conceals his anxiety; (2) *Expectations of others:* He believes others will want to control and direct him and that they expect him to live up to expectations which he cannot meet. As a result, he expects to be rejected; (3) *Observations of others:* He recognizes the support and encouragement that others give him but construes it as concealing a veiled threat of rejection and humiliation if he fails to live up to their expectations; (4) *Introject:* He berates himself for his inadequacy and feels depressed and unloved.

As is evident from the foregoing there are considerable differences in the *what* and *how* of assessment across the three approaches, despite some superficial similarities. Assessments in behavioral and cognitive therapy attempt to be more quantitative than the more qualitative assessment of a dynamic focus in psychodynamic therapy. The behavioral focus for assessment is still largely external, with its emphasis upon the interactions between antecedents, behaviors, and consequences. The focus in cognitive and psychodynamic therapy is more internal and dispositional. Although there may be some overlap between the concept of schema in cognitive therapy and dynamic focus in psychoanalytic therapy, there are still differences between them in their approach to assessment.

## THE ROLE OF THE RELATIONSHIP

All three orientations acknowledge the importance of rapport and a good trusting relationship but differ substantially in their views on the role of the relationship in effecting change.

In one of the few reviews of the relationship in behavior therapy, Morris and Magrath (1983) conclude that relationship factors do not appear to significantly influence the outcome of behavioral treatments. From their review, however, it is clear that relatively little has been written about the role of the relationship in behavior therapy. What has been written (e.g., Goldfried & Davison, 1976; O'Leary & Wilson, 1987) views the relationship as a setting for the implementation of the behavioral techniques, requiring cooperation and collaboration.

However, the relationship in behavior therapy is not seen as a significant source, in itself, of therapeutic relearning. The relationship becomes important only when there is noncompliance with the behavior therapy regimen.

Behavior therapists' view of "resistance" illustrates their position well. In general, behavior therapists (e.g., Goldfried & Davison, 1976; O'Leary & Wilson, 1987) see resistance as noncompliance, which must be overcome in order to implement the behavioral techniques. O'Leary and Wilson (1987) argue that such noncompliance may take the form of failure to complete homework assignments and ambivalence about participating in therapy. It may occur because the task (i.e., homework assignment) was not sufficiently explained to the patient, was too anxiety-arousing, or was too time-consuming. Noncompliance might also stem from active interference by the patient's significant others who oppose the changes. Regardless of the source, resistance is conceptualized as an obstacle to be overcome in therapy rather than as a major vehicle in itself for important interpersonal learning. More recent behavioral writings on resistance (see, for example, Goldfried, 1982b) have been somewhat broader in scope, but the basic conclusion remains the same.*

Cognitive therapy (Beck *et al.*, 1979) generally views the role of the relationship in a light somewhat similar to that of behavior therapy. Here, too, a collaborative relationship is a prerequisite to effective therapy. However, the collaborative empiricism that is so central in cognitive therapy gives some additional emphasis to the importance of relationship factors. Although in cognitive therapy, as in behavior therapy, resistance is primarily an obstacle to be overcome, it can also be used as a context for examining distorted assumptions. Thus the relationship in cognitive therapy plays a somewhat more salient role than it does in behavior therapy.

Most psychodynamic therapies, in general, and TLDP, in particular, regard the therapeutic relationship as both a necessary prerequisite to, *and* the major vehicle for, change. The occurrence of troublesome behavior patterns within the transference relationship permits the patient and therapist to examine them, understand them, and facilitate their change. Far from being an obstacle, resistance is seen as a necessary part of the process of change in psychodynamic therapy.

In TLDP, the rules of technique and the therapeutic relationship are inextricable. Strupp and Binder (1984) argue that "the meaning and function of any given technical intervention is determined by the context of the therapeutic relationship" (p. 36). Underscoring the importance of this union between relationship and technique is the assumption that the patient's maladaptive styles will eventually be enacted in the patient–therapist relationship (transference). Within the context of the therapeutic relationship, the therapist will provide corrective emotional experiences to facilitate change in the patient's dysfunctional patterns. As Strupp and Binder put it,

> The therapist's actions either provide patients with a new and direct experience in adult relatedness, or they are a step in the direction of helping patients understand symbolic meanings that are hypothesized to govern their maladaptive patterns of behavior. (p. 138)

As these authors emphasize, the learning that takes place is relationship-based rather than cognitively based. In TLDP, as troublesome patterns become activated within the context of the patient–therapist relationship, the patient can explore and correct the erroneous assumptions underlying his or her maladaptive behavior. An important corollary to this is that patient resistance is an important element of the interpersonal transaction between patient and thera-

---

*Beutler (personal communication) has pointed out that the three approaches differ not only in the general view of resistance but also in terms of what patients are seen as "resisting," e.g., the therapist, the homework assignment, personal change in general, or insight. A more detailed treatment of resistance in the three therapies would be interesting but is beyond the scope of the present paper.

pist. Resistance is seen as one aspect of the maladaptive style, and insight into its nature and meaning serves as a central focus to facilitate change.

Some of the major differences among the three approaches regarding the role of the relationship fall along a continuum that is based upon the centrality of the relationship to the change process. At one end of this continuum is the notion that a good therapeutic relationship is merely a necessary prerequisite for change. At the other end, the relationship is not just a prerequisite but also an *integral part* of the change process. Behavior therapists see the therapy relationship as a necessary prerequisite; psychodynamic therapists view the relationship as the main vehicle by which change occurs; and the outlook of cognitive therapists falls somewhere between these two.

## THE ROLE OF TECHNIQUE

The role played by technique depends upon the extent to which a given method views therapy as a process in which the therapist directly influences the patient to change. The importance of technique is also inversely related to the degree of importance attributed to the therapeutic relationship.

Behavior therapists are the strongest advocates of technique. In fact, behavior therapy has been frequently characterized as a "technology" of behavior change (e.g., London, 1972). The therapist's main task is to induce the patient to change problem behaviors. To accomplish this, the therapist might set incentives, help the patient change environmental factors that maintain the behaviors, train the patient in social skills, or teach the patient behavioral techniques for self-application. Behavior therapists pay little attention to factors not directly related to technique.

In cognitive therapy, techniques are important devices to effect change. However, Beck *et al.* (1979) have cautioned cognitive therapists not to become so enamored of technique that they lose sight of the therapeutic relationship.

Cognitive therapy is more of a general approach or strategy than a collection of therapeutic techniques. It relies heavily upon the inductive method and a Socratic style of questioning to help patients identify and change the fallacies in their thinking and perception. A variety of behavioral and cognitive techniques might be utilized to accomplish cognitive change. Therapists frequently design specific and structured learning experiences to teach patients to identify and monitor dysfunctional thoughts, recognize the connections between thoughts, moods, and behavior, examine the evidence supporting erroneous beliefs, and substitute more realistic interpretations of their experience. Behavioral techniques such as role playing and graded tasks may also be used. The purpose of behavioral assignments, however, is to elicit and collect information about the patient's cognitions, rather than to change the behavior itself. Thus it is clear that, although cognitive therapy is by no means a technology, there is still considerable emphasis on particular techniques and strategies for change, although there is not nearly as strong an emphasis on these factors as there is in behavior therapy.

Last, TLDP and most psychodynamic approaches that emphasize transference see technique and the therapeutic relationship as inseparable. Because the relationship is part of the technique, specific interventions (i.e., interpretations, advice, support) are less important than the nature and quality of the therapist–patient relationship. A crucial goal of therapy is to use this relationship as a forum to help the patient learn about him or herself. Whereas a behavior therapy guidebook reads a bit like a cookbook of techniques (Goldfried & Davison, 1976), a corresponding manual of psychodynamic therapy (e.g., Strupp & Binder, 1984) is more like a set of guidelines for the therapist and a description of the therapist's attitude towards the patient.

In a series of fascinating papers, Messer and Winokur (1980, 1984, 1986) have discussed the idea that the various psychotherapy approaches subscribe to different outlooks on human nature. The approaches themselves, however, rarely make their underlying views of human nature explicit; instead, one must abstract this information from the writings of the orientation's major advocates.

Behavior therapy views the person as being engaged in an ongoing transaction with the environment; people influence as well as react to stimulation from their environment. Even Skinner (1953), the most vocal proponent of environmental control over behavior, acknowledges the existence of "self-control." More recently, Bandura (1977) has developed the concept of "reciprocal determinism" in which the person affects the environment that in turn affects the person in an interactive loop.

Messer and Winokur (1980) characterized behavior therapy's vision of human nature as one in which people face outer-directed obstacles and struggles. Overcoming these difficulties results in a reconciliation between the person and his or her social world.

The outer directedness of behavior therapy stands in contrast to the inner conflict so central to psychoanalytic therapies, particularly the Freudian version. This internal struggle is waged against impulses that threaten to overwhelm the person and that, therefore, must be controlled. According to Messer and Winokur (1986), the psychoanalytic approach also emphasizes that which is unknown, mysterious, and irrational within the person.

This characterization of the psychoanalytic outlook is more accurate for formal (Freudian) approaches than for the newer short-term psychodynamic therapies. In TLDP, the journey into the unknown is curtailed for the purpose of pursuing a central focus (i.e., the dynamic focus). However, TLDP does retain the traditional psychoanalytic search for hidden meanings underlying behavior.

Cognitive therapy's outlook on human nature resembles George Kelly's (1955) image of the "personal scientist." Here, the individual is constantly extracting personally relevant information from the environment, using it to develop theories about oneself and the world, and acting and feeling in accordance with those beliefs. Psychopathology involves the development of inaccurate or distorted theories, which then distort incoming information and ultimately the person's view of him or herself and the world. To cognitive therapists, the individual's central need is for logical consistency. When faced with inconsistencies between their own views of themselves and contrary evidence, people will accept the evidence and change their self-perceptions. The personal scientist is governed by a search for truth and for logical consistency; therefore, behavioral and emotional changes occur as an outgrowth of attempts to resolve inaccuracies and inconsistencies.

According to Messer and Winokur (1986), the cognitive orientation shares with the psychoanalytic approach a focus upon subjective experience and an acceptance of personal imperfections. These two approaches necessarily emphasize inner reflection, whereas behavior therapy is more action-oriented. Both cognitive and psychodynamic therapy stress inner experience as opposed to the individual's transactions with the environment. In psychodynamic therapy, however, discovering the meaning of inner experience is the key to effecting change; in cognitive therapy, it is not the meaning but the presumed accuracy of the person's perceptions that is crucial. The psychodynamic and cognitive models also diverge in the degree to which they see human functioning as determined by rational and logical processes. Psychodynamic thinkers emphasize the irrationality of experience and behavior, as is illustrated by the person's resistance to corrective information about the self. The personal scientist model in cognitive therapy reflects the individual's search for rationality and logical consistency. Behavior therapy's image of the person emphasizes action and responsivity to the environment.

In summary, although the cognitive and psychodynamic perspectives on human nature differ, each has more in common with the other than with behavior therapy.

## MECHANISMS OF CHANGE

Debates about the underlying mechanisms of change in psychotherapy have long been prominent in the psychotherapy literature (e.g., Goldfried, 1980). In recent years, behavioral and cognitive therapists have been embroiled in a controversy over the role of cognition in behavior change and psychotherapy. A number of books and articles have addressed this issue (e.g., Bandura, 1977; Beck, 1985; Beidel & Turner, 1986; Coyne & Gotlib, 1983; Mahoney, 1974, 1977; Schwartz, 1982), and the controversy continues (see Coyne, Chapter 12, this volume).

Early explanations of change in behavior therapy were distinctly noncognitive (e.g., Skinner, 1953; Wolpe, 1958), relying primarily on nonmediational interpretations of classical and operant conditioning to generate techniques and explain changes in psychotherapy.

The work of Bandura (1969, 1977, 1986) illustrates an influential trend in the expansion of behavior therapy from a nonmediational and mechanistic basis to one involving higher order constructs such as expectancies, cognitions, and symbolic processes. Bandura's social learning theory continues to serve as one of the strongest theoretical foundations of modern behavior therapy.

Bandura (1977) argues for the notion of reciprocal determinism, which refers to an ongoing interaction between the person and the environment. Bandura contends that there is a continual interaction among behavioral, cognitive, and environmental factors, all of which must be considered to gain a full understanding of human behavior. Unlike earlier models of behavior therapy, Bandura's view holds that experiences influence our behavior by providing information that contribute to our expectancies. We structure our behavior in accordance with the information we have learned from associations among stimuli (i.e., classical conditioning) or the association of responses with particular outcomes (i.e., operant conditioning). Bandura further emphasizes that such learning may occur through vicarious as well as direct experiences. Learning takes place, then, because of the information we acquire from our experience, rather than through any automatic connections created by experience.

Bandura's views on change in therapy are nicely illustrated by the following statement:

> On the one hand, explanations of change processes are becoming more cognitive. On the other hand, it is the performance-based treatments that are proving more powerful in effecting psychological changes. This apparent discrepancy is reconciled by recognizing that change is mediated through cognitive processes, but that cognitive events are induced and altered most readily by experiences of mastery arising from successful performance. (1977, p. 79).

Both Beck and Bandura see cognitive change as implicated in therapeutic change. However, Bandura (1977) has argued that purely cognitive techniques that provide contradictory information are rarely effective. In his view, behavioral demonstrations that provide people with disconfirmatory experiences form the basis for change in psychotherapy. At a very general level, both Bandura and Beck might agree about the importance of cognitive change in psychotherapy (although they differ considerably on the precise nature of the important cognitive processes), and both would recommend the use of behavioral techniques or "experiments" for such change. However, cognitive and social learning explanations of change differ substantially on the primacy of cognition. Whereas the cognitive therapist believes that cognitions are primarily responsible for subsequent emotion and behavior, social learning theorists consider cognition as but one link in a behavior–cognition–environment loop that gives primacy to none of these components. This difference leads cognitive therapists to be very concerned with the development and implementation of cognitive techniques (e.g., reattribution) whereas it leads behavior therapists toward more performance-based behavioral interventions.

In social learning theory, cognitions are mediators, whereas in cognitive therapy, they are causes as well (Schwartz, 1982). A number of writers (e.g., Beidel & Turner, 1986; Coyne, Chapter 12, this volume; Coyne & Gotlib, 1983; Schwartz, 1982) have challenged many of cognitive therapy's contentions, particularly its attribution of a causal role to cognition in the development of psychopathology and in behavior change. They argue that, although studies have illustrated the association of depressive cognition with depressive affect, there is not as yet any evidence that cognitions play a causal role in the development and amelioration of the depressive syndrome. In fact, studies of depression have found that measures of cognitive style do not predict the onset of clinical depression (Lewinsohn, Steinmetz, Larsen, & Franklin, 1981), whereas others have demonstrated that various measures of depressive cognitions return to normal or near normal after remission of a depressive episode (see Coyne, Chapter 12, this volume). Thus the available evidence suggests that cognitive distortions may be more of an epiphenomenon than a primary cause of depression. Until there is evidence to the contrary, the unidirectional emphasis on cognition in cognitive therapy must be seriously questioned.

In psychodynamic therapy, any discussion of cognition must be closely linked to a discussion of affect. Psychodynamic therapy relies on a form of experiential and affectively based learning that occurs in the context of the patient–therapist relationship. Learning is relationship-based rather than cognitively based. The therapeutic task is to create conditions in which the patient can reexperience the maladaptive behaviors and defensive interpersonal styles that once served self-protective purposes but that are now self-defeating and inappropriate. The purpose of this reexperiencing is to allow the patient and therapist to identify and understand the underlying meaning of the behavior pattern. This reexperiencing takes place along with the affective arousal (e.g., fear or anger) that accompanied such behavior in the past. This affective reexperiencing of maladaptive patterns in the therapy relationship forms the basis for change in psychodynamic therapy. As Strupp and Binder write:

> One changes as one lives through affectively painful but ingrained scenarios, and as the therapeutic relationship gives them outcomes different from those expected, anticipated, feared, and sometimes hoped for (1984, p. 35).

From this brief discussion of change in psychodynamic therapy, it is clear that this approach places much more emphasis on affective arousal and relationship-based learning than do either cognitive or behavior therapies. However, it is interesting to note that a recent discussion of the theory of cognitive therapy by Beck and Weishaar (Chapter 2, this volume) has underscored the role of emotion in cognitive and behavior change. Beck and Weishaar have argued that change can occur only if the patient is engaged in the problematic situation *and* experiences affective arousal. It is when arousal makes cognitions more accessible, and thus testable, that the stage is set for lasting therapeutic change to occur. This focus on affective arousal in cognitive therapy brings it one step closer to the psychodynamic view of change in therapy. Although behavior therapy also deals with affective arousal, its role is as more of a behavior to be modified than a mediator of behavior change.

In addition to affective reexperiencing in the therapy relationship, a crucial aspect of the change process in psychodynamic therapy is insight. Once the maladaptive patterns are enacted along with affective arousal, the therapist provides disconfirming experiences to the patient's expectancies. Insight into how present behavior and reactions are unduly influenced by the past is a critical component of psychodynamic therapy. Such insight is reinforced by the disconfirming experiences provided during therapy. An awareness of the symbolic and historical meaning of one's maladaptive behaviors are presumed to decrease the effects of the past on the present. TLDP does not attempt to create an entire historical reconstruction of the past but focuses instead on those aspects that occur in the therapy relationship and that become part of the dynamic focus. The elements of enactment with arousal, disconfirmation, and insight occur repeatedly during the course of therapy and are the important components of the model of change in psychodynamic therapy.

In summary, then, social learning and cognitive theories point to the importance of cognitive changes in therapy. Such change is ascribed a primary and causal role in cognitive therapy, whereas it is part of a network of interrelated changes in behavior therapy. Behavior therapy still emphasizes the primary importance of direct experiences to create change, whereas cognitive therapists rely more heavily on cognitive techniques. Affective arousal plays an important role in all three approaches but is most central in the psychodynamic approach.

## SUMMARY AND SYNTHESIS

Our comparative analysis has revealed some similarities and differences at both the applied and theoretical levels. In general, behavioral and psychodynamic therapies differ most, with cognitive therapy falling between the two on the different dimensions. A summary of the main findings of our comparative analysis appears in Table 1.

In psychodynamic therapy, the requirement that the disorder be embedded in a long-standing interpersonal style is not shared by the other two approaches. Although there are some commonalities in patient selection and assessment of outcome, there are also substantial differences in the nature of assessment and the most important targets for change in therapy. Behavior therapy places most emphasis on the assessment of external (environmental) determinants of behavior. Although social learning theory has brought cognitive mediating variables into behavior therapy, the emphasis on external determinants of behavior is still the strongest in the behavioral approach. By contrast, cognitive and psychodynamic therapies are more interested in the assessment of internal variables that take the form of inner dispositions and conflicts. However, even cognitive and psychodynamic theories diverge regarding the nature of the internal focus. In cognitive therapy, the dysfunctional thoughts, cognitions, and schemata are most important, whereas in psychodynamic therapy, the conflicts and expectancies that form the basis of the dynamic focus are the most central for assessment and change.

In both behavioral and cognitive therapies, the relationship is primarily a vehicle for the implementation of the techniques and strategies. Resistance is viewed as noncompliance and is a problem to be overcome. In psychodynamic therapy, the relationship itself is the most important source of therapeutic relearning, and resistance is viewed as an aspect of the relationship to be understood and worked through, rather than simply as an obstacle. Technique and relationship seem inversely related. The more the therapy emphasizes the importance of techniques, the less it stresses the centrality of the relationship. Behavior therapy falls at one end of this continuum, psychodynamic therapy at the other, with cognitive therapy once again falling between the two. However, cognitive therapy does seem more similar to behavior therapy than psychodynamic therapy in its view of technique and relationship factors. In its view of human nature, behavior therapy tends to have a more action-oriented view, whereas cognitive and psychodynamic therapies have a more reflective and inner-directed vision.

Some of the most intriguing results of our analysis emerged from the consideration of mechanisms of change. Behavioral and cognitive therapies agree about the importance of cognitive change but differ regarding its causal role in therapy and how to best effect such change. Cognitive therapy sees cognition as primary and tries to change cognitions through providing new experiences in the form of "experiments" and through the use of more purely cognitive techniques. Behavior therapists who rely on a social learning perspective see cognition as one mediating factor in a continuous behavior–cognition–environment loop and emphasize providing the patient with new experiences as the main way to change cognitions.

| Dimension | Behavior therapy | Cognitive therapy | Time-limited psychodynamic psychotherapy |
|---|---|---|---|
| 1. Patient selection criteria | None specified | None specified | Patients whose problems are embedded in a long-term interpersonal style |
| 2. Assessment and targets for change | Uses standardized objective measures of outcome | Uses standardized objective measures of outcome | Uses standardized objective measures of outcome |
| | May use DSM-III criteria | May use DSM-III criteria | May use DSM-III criteria |
| | Focus on external situational variables (antecedents, consequences, and behaviors) | Focus on internal and dispositional variables (cognitive style) | Focus on internal and dispositional variables (the dynamic focus) |
| 3. Role of the therapy relationship | A prerequisite for the implementation of behavioral techniques | A prerequisite for the implementation of cognitive and behavioral techniques | Not seen as primarily a prerequisite for the implementation of specific techniques |
| | Not a major source of therapeutic relearning in itself | A partial source of therapeutic relearning in which relationship-based cognitive distortions may be examined | The major source of therapeutic relearning |
| 4. Role of techniques | Specific techniques are central in therapy | Specific techniques are important but only as part of a more general cognitive strategy | Specific techniques are less important than the therapist–patient relationship |
| 5. Views of human nature | Outer-directed toward actions to overcome obstacles in the environment | Inner-directed toward information processing about the self and world, emphasizing logical consistency | Inner-directed toward subjective experience and the search for hidden meanings, emphasizing the irrationality of experience and behavior |
| 6. Mechanisms of change | Emphasizes the importance of extratherapy new experiences | Emphasizes the importance of extratherapy new experiences | Emphasizes the importance of within-therapy new experiences |
| | Affective arousal accompanying the new experiences of some value for therapeutic change | Affective arousal accompanying the new experiences of some value for therapeutic change | Affective arousal accompanying the experiences are essential for therapeutic change |
| | Little emphasis on insight/awareness for change | Emphasis on awareness of dysfunctional schemata for change | Insight/awareness of connections between past and present are central for change |
| | Cognitions are mediators that are part of a behavior–cognition–environment loop | Cognitions are primarily responsible for our mood and behavior | Cognitions are inextricably linked to affect |
| | The important cognitions are expectancies about oneself and one's performance. | The important cognitions are distorted views about the self, the future, and the world. | The important cognitions relate to one's history as it affects present functioning. |

HAL ARKOWITZ and
MO THERESE
HANNAH

Psychodynamic therapy also sees the importance of providing patients with new experiences to change dysfunctional expectancies but does so primarily in the context of the therapeutic relationship rather than through the provision of extratherapy experiences. Finally, although psychodynamic therapy stresses the need for relevant affective arousal to accompany the new experiences, cognitive therapy and behavior therapy do so to a lesser degree. In psychodynamic therapy, new experiences lead to insight which mediates subsequent behavior change. In cognitive therapy and behavior therapy, new experiences lead to cognitive changes that mediate subsequent behavior changes. Thus at a certain level of abstraction, all three approaches emphasize providing patients with new experiences (which may be accompanied by affective arousal), disconfirmation of dysfunctional expectancies through those experiences, and a corresponding change in behavior in relevant situations outside of therapy. This conclusion forms the basis for the model of change presented in the next section.

## PROCESSES OF CHANGE IN PSYCHOTHERAPY

Our analysis has revealed some possible common elements that may cut across the three therapies. In the remainder of the chapter, we will explore the possibility that, to an important degree, these therapies may effect change through a common set of processes or pathways that are reached through rather different techniques and styles. The argument for a common factors approach has a foundation in empirical research as well as in conceptual analyses. The empirical basis comes from the numerous comparative outcome studies of psychotherapy that have continued to demonstrate that, in general, therapy works better than no therapy, but that different therapies have not been shown to have substantially different outcomes. Luborsky, Singer, and Luborsky (1975) drew this conclusion from their review of outcome studies and stated that, similar to the Dodo bird in Alice in Wonderland: "Everyone has won and all must have the prizes."

Lack of differential treatment outcome appears to be the rule rather than the exception in comparative therapy outcome studies (e.g., Elkin *et al.*, 1986; Lambert, Shapiro, Bergin, 1986; Steuer *et al.*, 1984) and continues to be the case despite the finding that therapists of different orientations do appear to engage in detectably different behaviors in therapy (DeRubeis, Hollon, Evans, & Bemis, 1982; Luborsky *et al.*, 1982). Thus, although therapists of different orientations are indeed engaging in different behaviors, such differences may not be generating different outcomes. The lack of differential outcome has even been found using more recent meta-analytic procedures (e.g., Smith, Glass, & Miller, 1980). In one of the most recent and comprehensive reviews of outcome in psychotherapy, Lambert *et al.* (1986) concluded that

> Research carried out with the intent of contrasting two or more bona fide treatments shows surprisingly small differences between the outcomes for patients who undergo a treatment that is fully intended to be therapeutic. (p. 167)

Our conclusion regarding the relative lack of differential outcome for the different psychotherapies is not meant to rule out any possibilities of individual differences in response to different treatments. Instead, it is intended to underline the distinct possibility that different therapies may share common elements that may account for a significant amount of the change that they effect.

Our discussion of common factors will be directed toward a level of explanation that Goldfried (1980) has termed *clinical strategies,* which, if empirically validated, could be considered "principles of change." Goldfried conceptualized the therapeutic enterprise as involving different levels of abstraction from what is directly observable. Clinical techniques constitute the lowest level of abstraction, whereas the highest level consists of theories of change and philosophies of human nature. Goldfried suggested that similarities might be found at the level of technique but that these would be only trivial. Further, he concluded that differences in the level of theory and philosophy were so great that it was unlikely that analysis at this level would reveal any meaningful commonalities. It is at the level of "clinical strategies" and possible principles of change that he had the most hope for a meaningful analysis of common factors. The analysis presented here is one that attempts this level of abstraction.

The history of the search for common factors in psychotherapy is a long and honorable one and includes such writers as Dollard and Miller (1950), Frank (1961), Goldfried (1980), Kazdin (1979), London (1964, 1986), and Rosenzweig (1936), to name just a few. Many of the seminal papers in the area have been included in Goldfried's (1982b) edited book entitled *Converging Themes in Psychotherapy*. Interest in the discovery of common factors is even stronger today (e.g., Goldfried & Newman 1986; Prochaska & DiClemente, 1986), given the recent trends toward eclecticism and psychotherapy integration discussed earlier in this chapter.

The present analysis draws from earlier conceptualizations by Alexander and French (1946) and Goldfried (1980). In their book, Alexander and French coined the phrase *corrective emotional experience*. They wrote:

> In all forms of etiological psychotherapy, the basic therapeutic principle is the same: to re-expose the patient, under more favorable circumstances, to emotional situations which he could not handle in the past. The patient, in order to be helped, must undergo a corrective emotional experience suitable to repair the traumatic influence of previous experiences. It is of secondary importance whether this corrective experience takes place during treatment in the transference relationship, or parallel with the treatment in the daily life of the patient. (p. 66)

The fact that this was written before either cognitive therapy and behavior therapy were developed is truly remarkable. The convergence of their conclusions, writing from a psycho-analytic vantage point, and ours, which are based on modern-day behavioral, cognitive, and psychodynamic therapies, is quite striking.

Brady *et al.* (1980) underlined the basic idea that providing persons with new experiences, either inside or outside of the therapy relationship, is a key element in psychotherapy. For this paper, therapists of different orientations (including cognitive, behavioral, psychodynamic, and humanistic) were asked to respond to the question: "What is the role played by new experiences provided to the patient/client in facilitating change?" There was a strong consensus about the central importance of such new experiences but considerable differences about how to provide such experiences (the level of technique) or how to conceptualize their role in the change process (the level of theory).

Goldfried (1980) has suggested that the clinical strategies that cut across the different therapy approaches might be broken down into two major types. The first involves having the patient engage in new corrective experiences. The second involves offering the patient direct feedback through which he or she is helped to become more aware of what he or she is (or is not) doing, thinking, and feeling in various situations. The proposals of both Alexander and French (1946) and Goldfried (1980) are important precursors to the present analysis.

Our proposal is that a common pathway to change in psychotherapy consists of providing patients with new experiences relating to their problem, which are accompanied by relevant affective arousal and which result in the disconfirmation of expectancies that previously mediated that problem. The remainder of this chapter will be devoted toward the delineation and specification of the components of this model.

A central concept in our analysis is that of *behavioral enactment*, a term that we believe captures the spirit of our model more so than "new experiences" or even "corrective emotional experiences.'' We would like to express our debt to Strupp and Binder (1984), whose use of the term *enactment* stimulated our thinking in this direction. Strupp and Binder refer to ''enactments'' of the patient's neurotic conflicts in the context of the therapy relationship. In our more generalized use of the term *behavioral enactment,* we refer to a particular interaction of the patient with his or her environment. This interaction is related to an important problem of the patient and may be *problem-congruent* or *problem-incongruent.* An example of a problem-congruent behavioral enactment in psychodynamic therapy is the case of an unassertive patient who begins to act submissively toward the therapist. In behavior therapy, self-monitoring of problem behaviors is another example of a problem-congruent behavioral enactment. An unassertive patient may be asked to observe and record his or her assertive behavior during the week, without trying to make any changes in his or her assertiveness. In cognitive therapy, the therapist might suggest an experiment to depressed persons in which they are to act more depressed than they really feel, in order to collect data about their own reactions and the reactions from others (Beck *et al.,* 1979).

In general, psychodynamic therapy implicitly encourages *problem-congruent enactments* by the patient in the therapy relationship as part of the process of change. Behavioral and cognitive therapies most often encourage *problem-incongruent* enactments in their homework prescriptions to try out *new* behaviors in the direction of therapeutic change. This distinction parallels one in the literature on paradoxical interventions between prescription of symptoms versus prescription of change (Shoham-Salomon & Rosenthal, 1987).

The use of problem-incongruent behavioral enactments is more characteristic of behavior therapy and cognitive therapy than of psychodynamic therapy, although they do play some role in the latter as well. A patient in behavior therapy might be asked to expose him- or herself to increasingly fearful situations. Similarly, a depressed and withdrawn patient might be asked to increase his or her activity level in behavior therapy for depression. In cognitive therapy, depressed patients might be asked to *act* less depressed or to increase their activity in previously enjoyable events to see how such enactments affect their mood and thinking. In psychodynamic therapy, the patient who had previously acted submissively might try out more assertive behavior toward the therapist and others as therapy progressed. Behavioral enactments are interactions that are relevant to some problem in the patient's life. They cut across homework assignments in behavior therapy, experiments in cognitive therapy, and transference enactments in psychodynamic therapy.

In the model proposed here, specific elements of the corrective emotional experience, as we conceptualize it, will be described so that their possible contributions to the change process can be examined. It should be noted that the elements really represent a process in psychotherapy that must be repeated many times for change to occur. The main elements of the model are as follows: (1) selection of the behavioral enactments; (2) staging of the behavioral enactments; (3) behavioral enactments with emotional arousal; (4) self-observation; and (5) disconfirmation of expectancies and cognitive restructuring.

## SELECTION OF BEHAVIORAL ENACTMENTS

It is obvious that not just any new experience will facilitate therapeutic change. It is the relevance of the enactment to some problem behaviors, cognitions, or reactions that make it an active element in therapeutic change. How, then, are behavioral enactments selected? Much of this decision seems to be largely determined by the therapist's judgment rather than by clear guidelines from any of the three therapy approaches. However, each therapy has some guidelines for the selection of relevant behavioral enactments.

In behavior therapy, the behavioral enactment or homework assignment is usually an operationally defined component of the problem behaviors and is usually problem-incongruent. The therapist, in collaboration with the client, arrives at a definition of the problem and attempts to operationalize it in the enactments. Such operational enactments might include a height phobic going up to the first floor of an office building, an unassertive patient being asked to return an item to a store, a couple being instructed to exchange positive rather than negative behaviors, a depressed person being asked to increase his or her activity level, or an agoraphobic asked to spend a few minutes outside of his or her house. Although self-report inventories, self-monitoring strategies, and direct observation techniques might be employed to operationalize the problem behavior, the *choice* and definition of the general problem area is still largely determined by interview and involves a degree of subjective judgment. Behaviorists such as Bandura (1969) and Nelson and Barlow (1981) acknowledge that the selection of targets for change might involve value judgments by the client and/or therapist. However, once the targets are selected, operationalization can proceed more readily, and such operationalizations form the basis for behavioral enactments in behavior therapy.

In cognitive therapy, the choice of the behavioral enactment is determined in collaboration with the patient. The basis for choosing the homework assignments or experiments in cognitive therapy resides in an earlier assessment of the automatic thoughts and dysfunctional assumptions that are believed to mediate the problem behavior. For example, Beck *et al.* (1979) describe an attractive young woman who became depressed after her boyfriend left her. She had numerous ''automatic thoughts'' that she was ugly. When the patient was questioned about the evidence to support this thinking, she suggested that the main evidence for her ugliness was that men were not asking her out (p. 253). The therapist suggested an alternative hypothesis—that she was not being asked out on dates because she spent most of the time alone and did not give herself opportunities to meet men. Experiments (behavioral enactments) were structured in which she became more socially active and stopped turning down invitations to parties. After the patient tried these and had more opportunities to meet men, she started to date. At this point, she no longer believed that she was ugly. The behavioral enactment (becoming more socially active) was based on an earlier assessment of her assumptions about herself that were believed to be mediating the problem. Thus, in cognitive therapy, the main basis for the choice of the behavioral enactment is specifically to test out a previously identified assumption thought to mediate the broader problem.

As we shall see, one important difference between behavioral and cognitive therapies, on the one hand, and psychodynamic therapy, on the other, is that, in the former, new experiences are structured and assigned as part of the therapy, whereas in the latter, the significant new experiences *emerge* in the context of the therapist–patient interaction. Thus for psychodynamic therapy, the question is not which new experiences to select or assign the patient as homework but which new behaviors and experiences to watch for and focus on in the therapist–patient relationship. In this context, it is the dynamic focus that serves as a guide. Thus the basis for selecting behavioral enactments is an operationalization in behavior therapy, identification of maladaptive assumptions in cognitive therapy, and the dynamic focus in psychodynamic therapy.

## STAGING OF BEHAVIORAL ENACTMENTS

Behavioral enactments take different forms across the different therapies and may be ''staged'' in different ways. Whether one way of going about this is more effective than another remains to be determined.

First, staging involves the issue of whether the patient is given a *rationale* for the behavioral enactment. In behavioral and cognitive therapies, the patient is usually given a clear rationale, although the rationale obviously differs between these two frameworks. For example, a phobic patient might be asked to expose him- or herself to fearful situations. The rationale for this enactment is usually based on some kind of extinction model in which repeated exposure to feared situations can reduce the phobic anxiety. Patients in cognitive therapy are asked to adopt a "personal scientist" model and use the behavioral enactments to test out the accuracy of certain thoughts or assumptions.

In contrast to the behavioral and cognitive approaches, the psychodynamic approach does not present any explicit rationale for the enactment, nor is the enactment discretely different from the transaction between the patient and therapist. In psychodynamic therapy, the relevant behavioral enactments *emerge* within the therapy relationship rather than being structured outside of the therapy relationship as they are in behavioral and cognitive therapies. For example, a patient with a strong fear of being abandoned may begin to fear that the therapist will abandon him or her by terminating therapy. In psychodynamic therapy, enactments around this theme will gradually emerge in the relationship. The patient may become suddenly reluctant to talk about personal feelings with the therapist (a problem-congruent enactment), in fearing that closeness may result in their being hurt. Later in therapy, such a patient may discover that he or she can express him- or herself openly to the therapist (a problem-incongruent enactment) without any fear of abandonment. Both the problem-congruent and problem-incongruent enactments *emerge* during therapy and are labeled and discussed. They are not structured and planned as they are in the other two therapies.

An important element of the staging involves the degree of personal responsibility and choice given to the patient in the behavioral enactment. As we shall see in the next section, personal responsibility and choice (Cooper & Axsom, 1982) as well as self-attributions for the behavioral enactment (Kopel & Arkowitz, 1975) may be important dimensions that bear on the cognitive change accompanying the behavioral enactment. The greater the degree of personal choice, responsibility, and self-attribution in the enactment, the more likely it is that corresonding cognitive changes will occur that will facilitate maintenance of behavior change. From the discussion presented here, the behavioral enactments in behavior therapy potentially involve the least perceived choice, responsibility, and self-attribution, although this is not necessarily the case (Kopel & Arkowitz, 1975). The collaborative emphasis in cognitive therapy seems to invoke these factors to a greater extent than does behavior therapy. Finally, the complete lack of rationale and structuring for the behavioral enactments in psychodynamic therapy and the fact that such enactments emerge naturally in the therapy relationship rather than being structured outside of the therapy all suggest that perceived choice, responsibility, and self-attribution will likely be highest for enactments in psychodynamic therapy.

## BEHAVIORAL ENACTMENT WITH EMOTIONAL AROUSAL

In many ways, the heart of our model lies in the importance of providing patients with new experiences or enactments that are relevant to some problem area in their lives. In behavioral and cognitive therapy, the new experiences are structured jointly by patient and therapist for implementation outside of therapy. In psychodynamic therapy, the important enactments presumably occur within the therapy relationship, with minimal structuring and staging. In all three therapy approaches, the enactments are typically accompanied by emotional arousal.* The exposure of the phobic patient to anxiety-arousing situations, the experiments in cognitive therapy to demonstrate how thoughts affect mood and behavior, and the affect associated with the relationship enactment of the patient in psychodynamic therapy all illustrate this point and suggest that enactments accompanied by emotional arousal occur frequently in all three therapies. We know that therapists of very different orientations agree

---

*However, there are also examples of homework assignments in behavior therapy (e.g., self-monitoring of smoking behavior) and cognitive therapy (e.g., play tennis and evaluate your performance) that do not seem to be particularly emotionally arousing.

about the centrality of new experiences in therapy (Brady *et al.,* 1980) and that such new experiences are often emotional in nature. However, we are still left with questions about the precise nature of such experiences and their role in the change process.

We will consider two possible sources of learning that may underlie the importance of behavioral enactments in psychotherapy. One of these relates to the connection between attitude change and behavior change. The other relates to the possibility that emotional arousal may facilitate the accessibility of cognitions, attitudes, thoughts, memories, or expectancies that were previously outside of awareness. Such increased awareness may make them more amenable to change.

Repeatedly engaging in new behaviors that are discrepant with dysfunctional attitudes or expectancies may lead people to question and ultimately change these cognitions. Phobic patients who are now approaching their feared situations may begin to question their previous efficacy and outcome expectations (Bandura, 1977). Patients in cognitive therapy who try out activities that they had previously avoided may find that they are more capable than they previously believed. Patients in psychodynamic therapy who relate to their therapists in characteristic dysfunctional ways may eventually question these attitudes and expectations when the therapist does not react as they had expected. In all of these cases, it is not the enactments or new experiences themselves that may lead to change but the possibility that such enactments may lead people to question, and ultimately abandon, previously held attitudes and expectancies that mediate the problem.

Why might behavioral enactments lead us to question our attitudes and expectancies? An interesting lead comes from research and theory on cognitive dissonance in social psychology. Cognitive dissonance theory (Festinger, 1957, 1964) addressed the relationship of behavior change and attitude change to a greater degree than most other theories. Dissonance theory is still a strong and viable theory in social psychology, despite many modifications that have been made in the light of research findings (e.g., Wicklund & Brehm, 1976; Worchel, Cooper, & Goethals, 1988).

According to this theory, cognitive dissonance is a psychological state that is experienced as an unpleasant tension and that has drivelike properties leading to attempts to reduce this tension. It arises in situations where there is a discrepancy between one's attitudes and one's behaviors. Thus a person who acts in ways counter to his or her beliefs may be in a dissonance-producing situation.

There is one paradigm in dissonance research that we believe is of particular relevance to the present discussion—the paradigm of induced compliance. In this procedure, individuals are induced to behave in ways that are inconsistent with their attitudes. The dependent variables in such studies are typically the cognitive changes that result from such a procedure, and the conditions under which this procedure may affect cognitive change are also examined (Worchel *et al.,* 1988). Although there has been relatively little research on cognitive dissonance that is of direct relevance to psychotherapy (Cooper & Axsom, 1982, is a noteworthy exception), we will make a speculative leap from this laboratory research to clinical situations involving strongly held personal attitudes.

The dissonance created by induced compliance can be reduced in a number of ways that include changing the relevant cognitions, adding cognitions, or altering the importance of the behavior. The amount of attitude change that results increases as inducement for performing the behavior decreases (Festinger & Carlsmith, 1959). However, recent research has suggested other factors that may mediate this effect. In reviewing this literature, Worchel *et al.* (1988) concluded that induced compliance leads to dissonance-produced attitude change when there is perceived choice and personal responsibility for engaging in the behavior, when a degree of public commitment is involved in the counterattitudinal behavior and when the attitude-discrepant behavior is associated with the expectation that some aversive or unpleasant consequences might result.

Behavioral enactments in psychotherapy fit many of these elements fairly well. There is usually little or no external coercion for the patient to engage in the behavioral enactment (although the degree of such external coercion might vary across the therapies). Most therapies emphasize perceived choice and personal responsibility for the behavioral enactment (most notably the cognitive and psychodynamic therapies). The behavioral enactment involves a degree of public commitment to the counterattitudinal behavior. For example, the patient makes a commitment with the therapist to try out the new behaviors in behavior therapy and cognitive therapy. The degree of public commitment is somewhat lower in psychodynamic therapy because the enactment is less discrete and salient. Finally, in most cases, the behavioral enactment involves the expectation of aversive or unpleasant consequences. In fact, it is this expectation that the therapists of all three orientations seek to modify.

Based on these findings, we suggest that behavioral enactments in psychotherapy might be most effective in leading one to question relevant assumptions when there is minimal external inducement for engaging in the enactment along with a correspondingly high degree of perceived choice and responsibility. In addition, the greater the public commitment to the enactment and the more the enactment involves the anticipation of aversive consequences, the greater the likelihood that it may mediate therapeutic change.

From this brief and speculative discussion, it is possible that cognitive dissonance theory can provide one framework for understanding the role of behavioral enactments in therapeutic change. Behavioral enactments may provide new information, thus leading people to question attitudes toward the self and others that may be mediating the problems they are experiencing. Behavioral enactment might, under particular conditions, serve as a source of evidence that the individual finds discrepant with previously held beliefs. Such a discrepancy leads to the possibility of subsequent change in either attitudes, behaviors, or both.

More than a decade ago, Kopel and Arkowitz (1975) arrived at similar conclusions about change in psychotherapy, although using rather different sources. They reviewed the social-psychological research on attributions and self-perceptions, extrapolating from this literature to behavior therapy. They argued that this literature supports the view that "homework assignments" provide a source of self-observation from which patients derive new information about themselves. These new cognitions then lead to subsequent change in therapy and may ultimately mediate the maintenance and generalization of behavior change.

Thus far we have centered our disussion around the link between behavior enactments and cognitive change. It is also possible that, when emotional arousal accompanies such enactments, previously inaccessible cognitive mediators may become more accessible and hence modifiable.

This suggestion regarding the role of affective arousal is consistent with the behavioral, cognitive, and psychodynamic emphases on such arousal, although each therapy has different reasons for such an emphasis. In behavior therapy, the affective arousal is elicited primarily so that it can be extinguished through the disconfirmation of expectancies (Bandura, 1977). In psychodynamic therapy, therapeutic change is brought about by insight that is "the affective experiencing and cognitive understanding of the current maladaptive patterns of behavior that repeat childhood patterns of interpersonal conflict" (Strupp & Binder, 1984, pp. 24–25). Change occurs when an affective and cognitive connection is made between the current enactments and their childhood precursors. Beck and Weishaar (Chapter 2, this volume) write that "Change can only occur if the patient is involved in the problematic situation and experiences affective arousal" (p. 29). Consistent with this statement, Beck and Weishaar further argue that the cognitive constellations that underlie the problem become accessible and modifiable only with affective arousal.

These suggestions about the role of affective arousal in the retrieval of previously inaccessible material are also consistent with recent neurobiological and cognitive research. For example, Jacobs and Nadel (1985) reviewed literature that suggested that we may not have conscious access to specific early memories because such autobiographical memory may depend on a late-maturing hippocampal brain system. They review research that suggests that stress may suppress this late-maturing system, providing unusual access to information stored in the early maturing brain systems prior to the onset of hippocampal functioning. Tataryn, Nadel, and Jacobs (Chapter 5, this volume) have further elaborated this possibility and its clinical applications.

Another relevant line of research deals with the phenomenon of mood-dependent recall. There is a considerable body of research that suggests that retrieval of material is enhanced by reinstating the same mood that the individual was in when the material was originally learned (Blaney, 1986; Bower, 1981; Tobias, 1988). Taken together, it appears possible that affective arousal may be a facilitator in the recall of cognitive material that may be mediating the immediate problem. Problem-incongruent behavioral enactments may lead one to question the underlying assumptions. Enactments with affective arousal may make cognitive material that is relevant to those assumptions more accessible to awareness and modification. This suggests that when behavioral enactments are associated with emotional arousal, the likelihood of cognitive change as well as related behavior change may be greatest.

## SELF-OBSERVATION

In all three therapies, the foregoing processes are accompanied by some form of self-observation during and after the behavioral enactments. The behavior therapist may specifically instruct the client to self-monitor in order to direct his or her attention to some relevant external behavior or otherwise inaccessible internal fantasy behaviors during the course of the behavioral enactments (O'Leary & Wilson, 1987). In cognitive therapy, the patient is also instructed to self-observe, but the self-observation is centered on gathering behavioral data for the hypothesis being tested in the "experiment" or enactment. It is not just the behavior that is being observed but the behavior as it relates to an underlying assumption. The self-observation may be of one's own reactions or of the reactions of others to oneself, and its goal is to determine whether an assumption or belief of the patient is supported or invalidated by the experiment and ensuing observation. In psychodynamic therapy, the self-observation relates to the patient's enactment of problematic styles with the therapist. The therapist, by questions or observations, calls attention to conflicts and issues in the patient's life. In a sense, self-observation in behavioral and cognitive therapy may not be that far removed from insight in psychodynamic therapy.

Consistent with our earlier analysis, we would suggest that, as the emotional arousal makes earlier cognitive material accessible, self-monitoring should focus on that material to the extent that it is mediating the problematic pattern of behavior. However, there is some question as to whether the important material is, in fact, historical in nature as suggested by psychodynamic theory and recent versions of cognitive theory or may be more present-based. In any case, the material elicited by the affective behavioral enactments needs to become part of the individual's awareness so that he or she can examine the appropriateness of these cognitions in his or her present life. As people are able to see that their cognitions are not really appropriate to their current circumstances, they may be more willing to modify them.

## DISCONFIRMATION AND COGNITIVE RESTRUCTURING

Behavioral theorists such as Bandura (1977, 1986) speak of expectancies, cognitive theorists speak of schemata, and psychodynamic therapists speak of dynamic themes and a dynamic focus. To what extent may all of these be referring to previously learned expectancies about oneself and the world that no longer apply? If so, the more these expectancies can be brought to conscious awareness *in* the behavioral enactments, the greater is the possibility that the patient will have evidence from his or her own observations that these expectancies no longer apply. We would suggest that it is the eliciting of these expectancies in relevant behavioral enactments with the affective arousal that best sets the stage for the disconfirmation and restructuring of the expectancies. Cognitive restructuring may take the form of different "languages" for each of the different schools of therapies, but all involve a new way to view oneself and the world that replaces the previous expectancies. Persons may learn that they are more capable than they previously believed or that they do not need to succeed in everything in order to be loved. Whether these new conclusions about oneself are couched in the relatively nonmentalistic language of behavior therapy, the rational language of cognitive therapy, or the historical and conflict-based language of psychodynamic therapy, each provides some way of reconceptualizing oneself and the world after disconfirmation occurs.

## CONCLUSIONS

The essence of the model that we have presented here includes selection and staging of behavioral enactments in therapy. Such behavioral enactments may be problem-congruent or problem-incongruent. The enactments provide a behavioral basis for questioning previously held cognitions and assumptions that are potentially relevant to the problem. Further, emotional arousal accompanying the enactments may facilitate the accessibility to consciousness of previously inaccessible cognitive material that can then be examined and modified in therapy. Self-observation, disconfirmation, and cognitive restructuring complete the process. Repetitions of this process are needed before change is effected.

The model we have presented here is obviously a highly speculative one. It is based on a conceptual analysis of commonalities among the three therapies, rather than on any solid evidence of its own. It is presented to stimulate research in common factors in psychotherapy and not as a finalized proposal.

If our analysis is correct, it appears that cognitive therapy may come somewhat closer to capturing the most important components of the model than either behavioral or psychodynamic therapy. Behavior therapy has only a limited theory of cognitive mediation, and the role of affect is one of a target for change rather than as part of the change process. Psychodynamic therapy involves much less clear and structured behavioral enactments than do the other two approaches and may be limited for this reason. However, the emphasis on affect and the importance of awareness of cognitive material from the past is a possible strength of the psychodynamic approach, when viewed from the perspective of our model.

More recent versions of cognitive theory and therapy, as represented by the writings of Beck and Weishaar (Chapter 2, this volume), have clarified the role of behavioral enactments and have emphasized the importance of choice and personal responsibility in these enactments. Their view sees affect as playing an important role in accessing relevant cognitive mediators and uses behavioral enactments to elicit and correct the mediating cognitions. Thus cognitive therapy seems to operationalize the elements we have discussed to a somewhat greater extent than the other therapies and is more explicit about them.

There are many issues we have not considered here due to space limitations. The nature and role of resistance in therapy is an important one that merits more extensive consideration. The place of experiential therapy in our analysis is another.* In addition, the model is by no

---

*Although we have omitted experiential therapy from our consideration, its mechanisms of change are generally consistent with those outlined here. Greenberg, Safran, and Rice (Chapter 9, this volume) write that "in experiential therapy, schema-inconsistent evidence is generated not by homework designed to provide contradictory information but by the stimulation of previously unsymbolized aspects of internal processing into awareness and the creation of new experience in therapy."

means meant to be a comprehensive model of change in psychotherapy. Instead, we have tried to elucidate what we believe is *one* component of the processes of change that may be common to many different therapies.

Whether the model presented here will stimulate new research and useful clinical applications remains to be seen. A number of empirical questions emerge directly from the model. For example, do enactments that arise naturally within the context of therapy facilitate change more so than do those that are structured and carried out outside of therapy? Do problem-congruent enactments have different effects than problem-incongruent ones? Is affective arousal necessary for change to result from behavioral enactments? How vital is a reconceptualization of the patient's past to therapeutic change? We hope that our analysis will stimulate research on these and other questions and that it will also encourage practitioners of different schools of therapies to persist in the search for common factors in psychotherapy.

ACKNOWLEDGMENTS. The authors would like to express their appreciation to Larry Beutler, Dick Bootzin, Jeff Greenberg, and Carl Ridley for helpful feedback on an earlier draft of this paper.

# REFERENCES

Alexander, F. (1963). The dynamics of psychotherapy in light of learning theory. *American Journal of Psychiatry, 120,* 440–448.

Alexander, F., & French, T. M. (1946). *Psychoanalytic therapy.* New York: Ronald.

Arkowitz, H. (1984). Historical perspective on the integration of psychoanalytic and behavioral therapy. In H. Arkowitz & S. Messer (Eds.), *Psychoanalytic therapy and behavior therapy: Is integration possible?* (pp. 1–31). New York: Plenum Press.

Arkowitz, H., & Messer, S. M. (Eds.). (1984). *Psychoanalytic therapy and behavior therapy: Is integration possible?* New York: Plenum Press.

Bandura, A. (1969). *Principles of behavior modification.* New York: Holt, Rinehart & Winston.

Bandura, A. (1977). *Social learning theory.* Englewood Cliffs, NJ: Prentice-Hall.

Bandura, A. (1986). *Social foundations of thought and action: A social cognitive theory.* Englewood Cliffs, NJ: Prentice-Hall.

Beck, A. T. (1976). *Cognitive therapy and the emotional disorders.* New York: International Universities Press.

Beck, A. T. (1985). Cognitive therapy, behavior therapy, psychoanalysis, and pharmacotherapy: A cognitive continuum. In M. M. Mahoney & A. Freeman (Eds.), *Cognition and psychotherapy* (pp. 325–347). New York: Plenum Press.

Beck, A. T., Rush, A. J., Shaw, B. F., & Emery, G. (1979). *Cognitive therapy of depression.* New York: Guilford.

Beck, A. T., Emery, G., & Greenberg, R. (1985). *Anxiety and phobias: A cognitive approach.* New York: Basic Books.

Beidel, D. C., & Turner, S. M. (1986). A critique of the theoretical bases of cognitive-behavioral theories and therapy. *Clinical Psychology Review, 6,* 177–197.

Blaney, P. H. (1986). Affect and memory: A review. *Psychological Bulletin, 99,* 229–246.

Bower, G. H. (1981). Mood and memory. *American Psychologist, 36,* 129–148.

Brady, J. P. et al. (1980). Some views on effective principles of psychotherapy. *Cognitive Therapy & Research, 4,* 271–306.

Cohen, A. R. (1962). An experiment on small rewards for discrepant compliance and attitude change. In J. W. Brehm & A. R. Cohen (Eds.), *Explorations in cognitive dissonance* (pp. 97–104). New York: Wiley.

Cooper, J., & Axsom, D. (1982). Effect justification in psychotherapy. In G. Weary & H. T. Mirels (Eds.), *Integrations of clinical and social psychology* (pp. 214–230). New York: Oxford.

Coyne, J. C., & Gotlib, I. H. (1983). The role of cognition in depression: A critical appraisal. *Psychological Bulletin, 94,* 472–505.

DeRubeis, R. J., Hollon, S. D., Evans, M. D., & Bemis, K. M. (1982). Can psychotherapies for depression be discriminated? A systematic investigation of cognitive therapy and interpersonal therapy. *Journal of Consulting and Clinical Psychology, 50,* 744–756.

Dollard, J., & Miller, N. E. (1950). *Personality and psychotherapy.* New York: McGraw-Hill.

Elkin, I., Parloff, M. J., Hadley, S. W., & Autry, J. H. (1985). NIMH Treatment of Depression Collaborative Research Program: Background and research plan. *Archives of General Psychiatry, 42,* 305–316.

Elkin, I., Shea, T., Watkins, J., & Collins, J. (1986, May). *NIMH Treatment of Depression Collaborative Research Program: Comparative treatment outcome findings.* Paper presented at the meeting of the American Psychiatric Association, Washington, DC.

Ellis, A. (1962). *Reason and emotion in psychotherapy.* New York: Lyle Stuart.

Endicott, J. and Spitzer, R. L. (1978). A diagnostic interview: The schedule for affective disorders and schizophrenia. *Archives of General Psychiatry, 35,* 837–844.

Festinger, L. (1957). A theory of cognitive dissonance. Evanston, IL: Row, Peterson.

Festinger, L. (1964). *Conflict, decision, and dissonance.* Stanford, CA.: Stanford University Press.

Festinger, L., & Carlsmith, M. (1959). Cognitive consequences of forced compliance. *Journal of Abnormal and Social Psychology, 58,* 203–210.

Frank, J. D. (1961). *Persuasion and healing.* New York: Schocken.

French, T. M. (1933). Interrelations between psychoanalysis and the experimental work of Pavlov. *American Journal of Psychiatry, 89,* 1165–1203.

Goldfried, M. R. (1980). Toward the delineation of therapeutic change principles. *American Psychologist, 35,* 991–999.

Goldfried, M. R. (1982a). On the history of therapeutic integration. *Behavior Therapy, 13,* 572–593.

Goldfried, M. R. (1982b). Resistance and clinical behavior therapy. In P. L. Wachtel (Ed.), *Resistance: Psychodynamic and behavioral approaches* (pp. 95–113). New York: Plenum Press.

Goldfried, M. R. (Ed.). (1982c). *Converging themes in psychotherapy: Trends in psychodynamic, humanistic, and behavioral practice.* New York: Springer.

Goldfried, M. R., & Davison, G. C. (1976). *Clinical behavior therapy.* New York: Holt, Rinehart & Winston.

Goldfried, M. R., & Newman, C. (1986). Psychotherapy integration: An historical perspective. In J. Norcross (Ed.), *Handbook of eclectic psychotherapy* (pp. 25–61). New York: Brunner/Mazel.

Hollon, S. D., & Beck, A. T. (1986). Cognitive and cognitive-behavioral therapies. In S. L. Garfield & A. E. Bergin (Eds.), *Handbook of psychotherapy and behavior change* (3rd ed.; pp. 443–482). New York: Wiley.

Jacobs, W. J., & Nadel, L. (1985). Stress-induced recovery of fears and phobias. *Psychological Review, 92,* 512–531.

Kazdin, A. E. (1978). *History of behavior modification.* Baltimore: University Park Press.

Kazdin, A. E. (1979). Nonspecific treatment factors in psychotherapy outcome research. *Journal of Consulting and Clinical Psychology, 47,* 846–851.

Kelly, G. A. (1955). *The psychology of personal constructs.* New York: Norton.

Kiesler, D. J. (1966). Some myths of psychotherapy research and the search for a paradigm. In A. P. Goldstein & N. Stein (Eds.), *Prescriptive psychotherapies* (pp. 102–126). New York: Pergamon.

Kopel, S., & Arkowitz, H. (1975). The role of attribution and self-perception in behavior modification. *Genetic Psychology Monographs, 92,* 175–212.

Koss, M. P., & Butcher, J. N. (1986). Research on brief psychotherapy. In S. L. Garfied & A. E. Bergin, (Eds.), *Handbook of psychotherapy and behavior change* (3rd ed; pp. 627–670). New York: Wiley.

Lambert, M. J., Shapiro, D. A., & Bergin, A. E. (1986). The effectiveness of psychotherapy. In S. L. Garfield & A. E. Bergin (Eds), *Handbook of psychotherapy and behavior change* (3rd ed.; pp. 157–212). New York: Wiley.

Lewinsohn, P. M. (1974). A behavioral approach to depression. In R. J. Friedman & M. M. Katz (Eds.), *The psychology of depression: Contemporary theory and research.* New York: Wiley.

Lazarus, A. A. (1981). *The practice of multimodal therapy.* New York: McGraw-Hill.

Lewinsohn, P. M., & Arconad, M. (1981). Behavioral treatment of depression: A social learning approach. In J. F. Clarkin & H. I. Glazer (Eds.), *Depression: Behavioral and directive intervention strategies* (pp. 33–67). New York: Garland Press.

Lewinsohn, P. M., Steinmetz, J. L., Larson, D. W., and Franklin, J. (1981). Depression-related cognitions: Antecedents or consequence? *Journal of Abnormal Psychology, 90,* 213–219.

London, P. (1964). *The modes and morals of psychotherapy.* New York: Holt, Rinehart and Winston.

London, P. (1972). The end of ideology in behavior modification. *American Psychologist, 27,* 913–920.

London, P. (1986). *The modes and morals of psychotherapy* (2nd ed.). New York: Hemisphere.

Luborsky, L. (1984). *Principles of psychoanalytic therapy: A manual for supportive-expressive treatment.* New York: Basic Books.

Luborsky, L., Singer, B., & Luborsky, L. (1975). Comparative studies of psychotherapies: Is it true that everybody has won and all must have prizes? *Archives of General Psychiatry, 32,* 995–1008.

Luborsky, L., Woody, G., Lellan, A. T., O'Brien, C. P., & Rosenzweig, J. (1982). Can independent judges recognize different psychotherapies? *Journal of Consulting and Clinical Psychology, 50,* 49–62.

Mahoney, M. (1974). *Cognition and behavior modification.* Cambridge, MA: Ballinger.

Mahoney, M. J. (1977). On the continuing resistance to thoughtful therapy. *Behavior Therapy, 8,* 673–677.

Malan, D. H. (1979). *Individual psychotherapy and the science of psychodynamics.* London: Butterworth.

Mann, J. (1973). *Time-limited psychotherapy.* Cambridge: Harvard University Press.

Meichenbaum, D. (1977). *Cognitive behavior modification: An integrated approach.* New York: Plenum Press.

Messer, S. B., & Winokur, M. (1980). Some limits to the integration of psychoanalytic and behavior therapy. *American Psychologist, 35,* 818–827.

Messer, S. B., & Winokur, M. (1984). Ways of knowing and visions of reality in psychoanalytic therapy and behavior therapy. In H. Arkowitz & S. B. Messer (Eds.), *Psychoanalytic therapy and behavior therapy: Is integration possible?* (pp. 63–100). New York: Plenum Press.

Messer, S. B., & Winokur, M. (1986). Eclecticism and the shifting visions of reality in three systems of psychotherapy. *International Journal of Ecclectic Psychotherapy, 5,* 115–124.

Morris, R. J., & Magrath, K. H. (1983). The therapeutic relationship in behavior therapy. In M. J. Lambert (Ed.), *Psychotherapy and patient relationships* (pp. 154–188). Homewood, IL: Dorsey-Jones, Irwin.

Nathan, P. E. (1981). Symptomatic diagnosis and behavioral assessment: A synthesis. In D. Barlow (Ed.), *Behavioral assessment of adult disorders* (pp. 1–11). New York: Guilford.

Nelson, R. O., & Barlow, D. H. (1981). Behavioral assessment: Basic strategies and initial procedures. In D. H. Barlow (Ed.), *Behavioral assessment of adult disorders* (pp. 13–44). New York: Guilford.

O'Leary, K. D., & Wilson, G. T. (1987). *Behavior therapy: Applications and outcome* (2nd Ed.). Englewood Cliffs, NJ: Prentice-Hall.

Prochaska, J., & DiClemente, C. C. (1986). The transtheoretical approach. In J. C. Norcross (Ed.), *Handbook of eclectic psychotherapy* (pp. 163–200). New York: Brunner/Mazel.

Robins, L. N., Helzer, J. E., Croughan, J., and Ratcliff, K. S. (1981). National Institute of Mental Health Diagnostic Interview Schedule. *Archives of General Psychiatry, 38,* 381–389.

Rosenzweig, S. (1936). Some implicit common factors in diverse methods in psychotherapy. *American Journal of Orthopsychiatry, 6,* 412–415.

Schwartz, R. M. (1982). Cognitive-behavior modification: A conceptual review. *Clinical Psychology Review, 2,* 267–294.

Shoham-Salomon, V., and Rosenthal, R. (1987). Paradoxical interventions: A meta-analysis. *Journal of Consulting and Clinical Psychology, 55,* 22–28.

Sifneos, P. (1979). *Short-term dynamic psychotherapy: Evaluation and technique.* New York: Plenum Press.

Skinner, B. F. (1953). *Science and human behavior.* New York: Macmillan.

Smith, M. L., Glass, G. V., & Miller, T. I. (1980). *The benefits of psychotherapy.* Baltimore: Johns Hopkins University Press.

Steuer, J. L., Mintz, J., Hammen, C. L., Hill, M. A., Jarvik, L. F., McCarley, T., Motoike, P., & Rosen, R. (1984). Cognitive-behavioral and psychodynamic group psychotherapy in the treatment of geriatric depression. *Journal of Consulting & Clinical Psychology, 52,* 180–189.

Strupp, H. H., & Binder, J. (1984). *Psychotherapy in a new key.* New York: Basic Books.

Tobias, B. A. (1988). *Mood-dependent recall: A review.* Unpublished manuscript, University of Arizona, Tucson, Arizona.

Wachtel, P. L. (1977). *Psychoanalysis and behavior therapy: Toward an integration.* New York: Basic Books.

Wachtel, P. L. (1987). *Action and insight.* New York: Guilford.

Weiss, R. L. (1980). Strategic behavioral marital therapy. In J. P. Vincent (Ed.), *Advances in family intervention, assessment, and theory* (Vol. 1, pp. 229–271). New York: Academic.

Weiss, R. L., Hops, H., & Patterson, G. R. (1973). A framework for conceptualizing marital conflict, a technology for altering it, same data for evaluating it. In F. W. Clark & L. A. Hammerlynck (Eds.), *Proceedings of the fourth Banff international conference on behavior modification* (pp. 309–342). Champaign, IL: Research Press.

Wicklund, R. A., & Brehm, J. W. (Eds.) (1976). *Perspectives on cognitive dissonance.* Hillsdale, NJ: Lawrence Erlbaum.

Wolpe, J. 1958). *Psychotherapy by reciprocal inhibition.* Stanford: Stanford University Press.

Wolpe, J. (1973). *The practice of behavior therapy.* New York: Pergamon.

Worchel, S., Cooper, J., & Goethals, G. (1988). *Understanding social psychology* (4th ed.). Homewood, IL: Dorsey Press.

# 9

# Experiential Therapy

## Its Relation to Cognitive Therapy

LESLIE S. GREENBERG, JEREMY SAFRAN, AND LAURA RICE

*Experiential therapy* refers to the broad class of humanistic and phenomenological therapies that emerged in the 1940s and were developed thereafter as an alternative to behavioral and psychoanalytic perspectives. The experiential psychotherapy tradition is best exemplified by the work of Carl Rogers and Fritz Perls, the founders of client-centered and gestalt therapy, respectively. Other writers in the client-centered tradition such as Eugene Gendlin, who has extensively used the term experiential therapy, have made important contributions to the theory and practice of experiential psychotherapy as have others from humanistic and existential traditions (Frankl, 1959; Jourard, 1971; Laing, 1975; Mahrer, 1978, 1983, 1986; Whittaker, 1975). Although there are important differences between gestalt therapy and client-centered therapy just as there are differences between different cognitive theorists such as Beck and Meichenbaum, for the purposes of this chapter we will be looking at the common, core aspects of these approaches that define them as experiential.

Experiential therapies focus on the client's current feelings, perceptions, and bodily sensations and emphasize the formation of an accepting person-to-person relationship between client and therapist. The client is seen as final arbiter of his or her own experience, and therapy is designed to promote the client's ability to make his or her own choices. In experiential therapy, the therapist works actively with clients, often using special techniques to enhance awareness and to promote experience and expression of emotionally laden material. Becoming aware of and integrating disowned aspects of experience or aspects that are in conflict is an important theme. The goal in experiential therapy is to discover and explore what one is experiencing and use this to inform choice and action. The therapist is reflective or experimental in style, guiding the client's attentional focus and making suggestions to stimulate new experience. The therapist refrains from being an expert on the client's experience and from

LESLIE S. GREENBERG AND LAURA RICE • Department of Psychology, York University, Downsview, Ontario M3J 1P3, Canada    JEREMY SAFRAN • Clarke Institute of Psychiatry, Toronto, Ontario M5T 1R8, Canada.

interpreting the client's reasons for his or her experience or advising him or her on how to solve problems.

At the core of experiential therapy is the emphasis on working with a person's moment-by-moment construction of reality through the medium of current awareness and current experiencing. Expanded awareness of inner and outer reality is seen as providing both new information and a new way of processing information that ultimately leads to improved orientation in the world and increased ability to choose and act constructively. This process, of increased awareness leading to choice, is a key process in experiential therapy.

## EXPERIENTIAL THERAPY AND INFORMATION PROCESSING

A central organizing principle in an experiential view of human functioning is that perception determines behavior. Reality is not objective but rather that which subjectively appears to us, and peoples' perceptions of reality are regarded as influencing their actions. Experiential therapies are phenomenological in method, dealing with peoples' view of the world as it is revealed to them in the moment. Rogers emphasizes the determining nature of the perceptual field and claims that behavior depends on how the self and the situation are viewed. Perls refers to the significance of the gestalt figure/background formation process, claiming that people organize their reality into meaningful wholes, and it is these wholistic meaning configurations that determine behavior. Perception, however, is regarded as being influenced by information processing that is occurring out of awareness.

In experiential therapy, the therapist works with the client's ongoing stream of awareness. The therapist focuses on that which is in the client's conscious awareness and that which is in peripheral awareness, that is, at the edge of awareness, in order to get at that which is not currently in awareness but is influencing perception. Information not in awareness is regarded as capable of being brought to awareness by attentional allocation or concentration and by explication of implicit meaning by the client. Client-centered therapy has emphasized reflecting to clients only those aspects of their experience that are in awareness or peripherally available to awareness. Gestalt therapy is more likely to actively pursue material currently out of awareness and to focus on avoidance processes occurring in the moment.

## UNCONSCIOUS PROCESSING

The unconscious is viewed, in experiential therapy, as that which is currently not in awareness but is potentially available to awareness. Experiential therapy believes that certain information not currently in awareness may be influencing conscious perception, experience, and behavior and that not attending to, and processing, certain information leaves the organism impaired. New information can be brought to awareness by focused attending, concentration, and differentiation of new meaning to produce improved functioning. Experiential therapy involves the use of experiments of deliberate awareness, to revive in people the sense of what it is they are experiencing and the sense that it is they who are experiencing, thinking, feeling, or sensing.

Unlike psychoanalysts, neither client-centered nor gestalt therapists view the unconscious as a dynamic system in which unconscious information is forcefully pressing to come into consciousness and needs to be defended against. Rather, unconscious information is viewed as information potentially available to awareness but not currently being attended to. Freud was concerned predominantly with experience that was thrust out of awareness but that actively pushed to gain access to consciousness and manifested itself in symptom formation, dreams, and slips of the tongue. In the contrasting view of unconscious processing from an experiential view, there are no special motive forces driving the contents of the unconscious toward the threshold of consciousness. In fact, rather than referring to the unconscious as though it is a portion of the mind as is often done in psychoanalytic writing, it is more appropriate in experiential therapy to refer to *unconscious processing* because what is being referred to is not a unitary or actual entity, ''the unconscious,'' but rather a way of processing information. Experiential therapy thus ascribes to the notion of a cognitive rather than a dynamic unconscious in which the way information is processed and organized determines what is available to consciousness. It is how information is processed and organized that then becomes the focus of the therapy, not what is *in* the unconscious.

In the practice of client-centered therapy, there is in fact no view of dynamic forces pushing information toward or away from the threshold of consciousness, and there is no view of a duality between what is in the client's awareness and what is actually occurring for the person outside of awareness (Zimring, 1974). All that exists and is responded to by the therapist is what is in the client's awareness. This is the hallmark of client-centered practice—reflection back to the client of his or her intended meaning. Although Rogers's early theory suggests a type of duality between what the organism experiences and what is consciously acceptable, this has been a problem in client-centered theorizing, and client-centered practice does not reflect this duality. In gestalt therapy, however, there is a view of the organism engaging in active attempts to keep information out of awareness. People are viewed as actively avoiding aspects of inner and outer realities. In this view, people are seen as either deliberately or automatically avoiding paying attention to, and becoming aware of, certain information. The avoided information is not, however, seen as dynamically pushing to come into awareness. The focus in gestalt therapy is on bringing the avoidance process into awareness and giving the client the opportunity to experience previously avoided experience.

The focus in experiential therapy, on working with clients' conscious awareness in order to access aspects of automatic information processing that are influencing their functioning, bears a striking similarity to the focus in cognitive therapy on working with conscious cognition and the attempts to access automatic thoughts and underlying beliefs and modify internal representations that influence functioning.

How people process information and create meaning is thus of central importance in both experiential and cognitive approaches. In fact, experiential therapy may be thought of as essentially working with enhancing and modifying different ways of processing information by means of a set of interventions that target different internal operations such as encoding, attention allocation, and appraisal, which are involved in the perception of reality. Both therapies are thus interested in internal cognitive operations.

## FEELINGS

The experiential approach, in addition to focusing on the current functioning of different types of mental operations and how they influence present reality construction, has also emphasized particular types of information as being central in understanding human functioning. Rather than emphasizing what people think, or conceptual-level processing, as being the primary determinant of meaning and reality construction, experientialists have emphasized the central role of feelings in therapy and change. Although feelings have never been clearly defined in operational terms (Greenberg & Safran, 1987), it has always been made clear that a certain set of inner experiences, referred to as *feelings,* are different from another set of internal phenomena, referred to as *thinking*. Client-centered writers have conceptualized feelings as including a broad spectrum of experiential components, including emotions, attitudes, sensations, and motives as well as the client's felt meanings of events and experiences. Gestalt therapists have defined emotion as unifying tendencies that integrate bodily sensations with field events to provide indispensable knowledge of the objects appropriate to their needs, indicating the combination of motivational and cognitive components in emotion (Greenberg & Safran, 1987).

An important difference between cognitive and experiential approaches is that cognitive therapists have traditionally tended to focus on undesirable feelings and to view them as by-products of dysfunctional thinking. In contract, experiential therapists emphasize the adaptive role that feelings can play in the change process and regard feelings as a type of preconceptual form of information that can correct inaccurate or incomplete representations at the conceptual level. We will elaborate on this theme in greater detail later in the chapter. For now, however, it is important to point out that, although the distinction between feeling and thinking has an important meaning and is of heuristic value to the practice of experiential therapy, it has never been that clear at a theoretical level how to distinguish between emotion and cognition. The clinical distinction between rationally and emotionally focused intervention unfortunately has tended to be concretized into a distinction between emotion and cognition and into construing feeling as an aspect of an emotional system, independent of cognition, and cognition as that system that produces thinking independent of feeling. This dichotomy has been responsible for the separation of therapeutic endeavors into the rationally oriented cognitive therapies and the feeling-oriented experiential therapies as seperate entities (Greenberg & Safran, 1987b).

Although separation into opposites in this fashion can be productive in that each pole becomes clearly articulated and more differentiated, as has happened in the polarization between cognitive and experiential therapies, a synthesis of opposites can also lead to greater progress in true dialectical fashion. Cognitive therapies, in specifying and developing different rationally oriented intervention procedures designed to modify beliefs, self-statements, and automatic thoughts and experiential therapies in specifying and developing different feeling-oriented interventions such as focusing, evocative reflection, and two-chair dialogue, designed to generate new information, have mapped out therapeutic methods that at the operational level look quite different. Even though these methods are different, involving different targets of change, different therapeutic procedures and different client processes, the claim that cognitive therapies deal only with cognition and not affect and the claim that experiential therapies do not deal with cognition because they are emotionally focused has been one of the greater errors of selective attention in current therapy theorizing.

Clearly, experiential therapy, with major constructs such as awareness and meaning, is centrally concerned with cognitive information processing, whereas recent interest in cognitive therapy in state-dependent cognitions deals with the influences of affect on thought, and the influence of mood on memory. In fact, the more constructive view in the cognitive approach (Guidano & Liotti, 1983) explicitly recognizes the role of emotion in cognitive process.

We have been involved in an enterprise of attempting to demonstrate that the view that cognition and affect are independent and causally related in a linear fashion is better replaced by a view in which cognition and emotion are viewed as more fused than separate (Greenberg & Safran, 1984, 1987a,b; Safran & Greenberg, 1986). Emotion is best viewed as a constructive synthesis of different levels of information processing involving expressive motor, schematic, and conceptual levels. This view has led us to focus on the role of affective change processes in therapy regardless of the therapeutic school. In so doing, we have been impressed with the importance on the one hand of "hot cognitions," that is, affect-laden appraisals, thoughts, and beliefs in cognitive therapy (Safran & Greenberg 1986) and with the importance of meaning-laden feelings in experiential therapy. Cognitive therapy involves affective change as well as cognitive change, whereas experiential therapy involves conceptual change as well as emotional change. In the remainder of this chapter, we will outline some of the similarities and differences in the two therapeutic approaches and discuss the role of conceptual change in experiential therapy and the role of affective change in cognitive therapy.

TARGETS OF CHANGE

An important similarity between cognitive and experiential therapies can be found in some of their targets of change. Both experiential therapy and cognitive therapies are involved in changing clients' perceptions of self and others. Although the different cognitive therapy approaches have identified a variety of different targets, such as irrational beliefs, automatic thoughts, self-statements and attributions, the schema is rapidly becoming seen both in cognitive psychology and cognitive therapy as an important underlying construct in attempting to explain perception, experience, and performance (Goldfried & Robins, 1984). The schema is a key target of change in both cognitive and experiential therapy. A schema was defined initially by Bartlett (1932) as "an active organisation of past reactions, or of past experiences, which must always be supposed to be operating in any well-adapted organic response" (p. 201). Later, Piaget and Morf (1958, p. 6) described a schema as "an organized set of reactions susceptible to being transferred from one situation to another by assimilation of the second to the first." Generaly speaking, schemata are currently viewed as "unconscious cognitive structures and processes that underlie human knowledge and skills (Brewer & Nakumura, 1984, p. 136).

In cognitive therapy, Beck described the functioning of schemata in depression as early as 1967, pointing out that, under normal circumstances, the schema that is used to interpret a situation is one whose content and structure closely matches that of the stimulus input but that in depression this function breaks down (Beck, 1967). He argued that when a nondepressed person is exposed to stimulus input, an appropriate schema with which to interpret the information is activated and that this leads to an accurate construction of the input. When a person is depressed, this matching process between the stimulus input and schemata is upset by "hyperactive" depressogenic schemata. As these depressogenic schemata become more active, less of a match is needed between them and the stimulus input in order for the latter to be encoded by these schemata. This leads to an inaccurate construction of the input. Beck expresses this in the following passage:

> As these schemas become more active they are capable of being evoked by stimuli less congruent with them ("stimulus generalization"). Only those details of the stimulus situation compatible with the schema are abstracted, and these are reorganized in such a way as to make them congruent with the schema. In other words, instead of a schema being selected to fit the external details, the details are selectively abstracted and molded to fit the schema (Beck, 1967 p. 286).

Thus, when a person becomes depressed, depressogenic schemata replace more appropriate ones in encoding stimulus input. In effect, these schemata are evoked by a wider range of situations as they become more active. When used to interpret events, depressogenic schemata lead to "chronic misconceptions, distorted, invalid premises, and unrealistic goals and expectations" (Beck, 1967). Out of this view, modifying dysfunctional schema grew to be a central aim of cognitive therapy.

In client-centered therapy, the notion of schema has similarly received increasing attention (Wexler & Rice 1974) in discussions of the process of change. Rice (1974) suggested that problems arise because people react in inappropriate and unsatisfying ways to certain classes of stimulus situations because of the relatively enduring schemata that are brought to bear on the construing of each new situation. Clients continue to behave maladaptively because they have built up over time schemata that are faulty, in the sense that they fail to take account of the reality structure of the situations to which they are relevant. She further suggested that the way to change such faulty constructions was to explore fully the client's reaction in any one such situation and thus to reprocess the experience in such a way as to force reorganization of the relevant schemes. The term *scheme* was used by her to refer to "the relatively enduring clusters of cognitive and affective structures that serve to assimilate input and organize output" (Rice, 1974, p. 295).

In her view, clients' schemes have been built up over time often in situations under high drive conditions. In each situation, a person perceives a mass of extremely complex, idiosyncratic, and often contradictory data. In order to act efficiently, the person must organize this complex flow into units and must group together, into a single class, data that are similar but not identical. In order to form efficient categories of this sort, there is a loss of differentiation and complexity in the information processed. When a person's schemes are relatively adequate in relation to the actual structure of the situations encountered, the result is adaptive, but when the schemes involve distortion or simplification, they tend to lead to maladaptive reactions.

According to this formulation, the problem of change in psychotherapy is therefore the problem of changing inadequate and distorting schemes. Thus we see that schema change is an important goal in Rice's approach to client-centered therapy. A number of other client-centered authors have also taken on information-processing and schema views of change in client-centered therapy (Anderson, 1974; Wexler, 1974; Zimring, 1974). Schema change has also been proposed as central to working with a number of different affective change processes from experiential therapy (Greenberg & Safran, 1987), ranging from allowing and accepting emotion to completing emotional expression. Conflict resolution in gestalt therapy has also been construed as involving the integration of conflicting schemes (Greenberg, 1984). Schema change is thus a common goal in a number of experiential approaches.

The adoption of the schema concept by both cognitive therapists and experiential therapists should not, however, be taken as indicating a greater degree of commonality than exists in reality. A closer look at the fashion in which Beck (1967) actually employs the concept of depressogenic schema suggests that he tends to equate it with the notion of dysfunctional attitude that colors everything, the person's view of self, other, and the world. Rice (1974) and Rice and Sapiera (1984), on the other hand, refers to schemes as idiosyncratic representations of the self in specific situations that are not nearly as enduring as depressogenic schemata. Thus, although the employment of the schema concept can potentially provide an important conceptual bridge between cognitive and experiential therapies, first some important conceptual and definitional clarification will have to take place.

## RELATIONSHIP STANCES AND CHANGE PROCESSES

One of the interesting and important distinguishing characteristics of different theoretical approaches is their general model of the role the therapist should play in promoting change and the relationship stance he or she should adopt. Certain therapies involve a change agent model in which the therapist is seen as creator of change. The therapist actively intervenes and provides the impetus for change. These therapies fall into modification traditions. Cognitive therapy that targets core cognitions for change and challenges these or uses homework to provide new evidence falls into the modification tradition. Other therapeutic traditions, of which experiential therapy is one, believe that the force for change should come from within the client and not from the therapist and that the role of the therapist is to raise awareness of what is blocking change. In this view, change comes about by people becoming aware of and accepting what they do and how they do it. Once they acknowledge and accept their experience, they are free to develop further. These are the facilitation traditions where the therapist does not work toward actively or directly modifying specific behaviors but rather works toward helping people become more aware. Identification of blocks to change and acceptance and understanding of disclaimed action tendencies are seen as providing people with new options.

As pointed out before, both experiential therapy and cognitive therapy are involved in the process of schema change, but the two therapies postulate different sources of this change. In cognitive therapy, the therapist uses influence and reason to challenge faulty beliefs, uses homework to generate schema-inconsistent evidence, and uses training to modify self-statements. In all these cases, the forces of change are external to the client. In experiential therapy, the focus is on discovery of unacknowledged experience and the creation of new meaning. Schema-inconsistent information is generated by accessing previously unacknowledged feeling that acts as an internal challenge to faulty schema. The therapist works to stimulate inner experience and vivid situational memories in order to access information that was available in the experience but not symbolized. In addition, the therapist raises awareness of how the person is organizing experience or avoiding certain areas of experiences in order to provide him or her with a meta-cognitive perspective (awareness) of personal functioning. This provides people with the possibility of greater conscious control of their own processing. The therapist role is not that of an active change agent or a fixer who modifies the person's behavior but more of a facilitator or a consultant who helps the person discover obstacles to growth.

The role relationship occupied by the therapists and the change processes induced in the two traditions are therefore somewhat different. In cognitive therapy, the client/therapist relationship is somewhat more like a collaborative student–teacher role relationship, whereas in experiential therapy, the relationship is more like a leader of an expedition and a consultant. In experiential therapy, the client, as leader of the expedition, consults an experienced explorer who understands the processes involved in productive search. The client chooses the content to be explored and will be the one who recognizes when his or her destination has been reached. The consultant is sensitive to ''markers'' and signs that indicate when the client is stuck or is ready for vigorous search and uses these to help discover that for which he or she is searching. The consultant makes suggestions as to when and how to go, is directive in process, suggesting ways of getting information, but does not suggest what content should be explored, and even at the process level, takes only as much influence as the client is willing to give. Although gestalt and client-centered approaches differ in the degree to which the therapist leads and follows, both aspire to a role relationship in which clients are respected as experts on their own experience.

In cognitive therapy, the therapist takes greater control, is more directive concerning the content being dealt with, and does not regard the client's experience as the final reference for what is true. Rather, the therapist attempts to provide evidence to disconfirm experience. The therapist has explicit material to teach about cognitive errors and uses this to help the client change in agreed-upon and clearly stated directions. Beck suggests that the therapist and client collaborate as two scientists searching for evidence to confirm or disconfirm certain hypotheses, but, even in this process, the therapist is still the senior scientist leading the questioning process, pointing out what hypotheses should be investigated and suggesting what evidence should be collected. The therapist points out errors and gives homework to help clients learn about their mistakes and provides training and practice to enhance correct ways of reasoning.

The two therapeutic approaches thus tend to utilize different role relationship stances and associated models of therapeutic change. In cognitive therapy, the teacher helps clients identify dysfunctional cognitions and then uses different active methods to modify the cognitions. The approach to change is one of direct influence in which clients are encouraged to think of or view self or situation in a specific way. The therapist determines what is faulty in the client's view of reality and works to help the client generate new information, of a specific nature, which is discrepant from the therapist-determined, faulty view of reality. The new evidence that is sought after is designed to lead to changes of the client's negative views of self, world, and future and to the modification of what the therapist assesses as the client's cognitive errors, such as overgeneralization, magnification, or arbitrary inference. The mechanisms of change in cognitive therapy involve people in becoming more logical and assume that more rational thinking and accurate representation will lead to improved functioning.

In experiential therapy, a different role relationship model is suggested. The consultant helps clients explore their inner worlds rather than teaching specific ways of being and helps them access and identify previously unsymbolized aspects of their experience. The experiential approach to change involves stimulation of inner experience, focusing of attention to help the client discover new information that comes from within, and symbolization of this experiential information (Gendlin, 1980). The client's memory of an experience is regarded as fuller than his or her construction of it (Rice, 1974). As clients talk about their experience, their accounts will convey a mixture of their levels of processing, including their conceptual view, emotional memory, and sensorimotor responses. Both their conceptual construction of the experience and also other more schematic and sensorimotor material that is not encompassed by the construction but is much closer to the original experience will be conveyed. Thus clients know more than they can say, and the therapist is helping them to capture what it is they know but have not symbolized. The extra material may or may not be inconsistent with the construction. It has been left outside the original scheme, either displaced by other materials that were more salient at the time the original experience took place, or actively avoided at the time because it was too threatening to process. If the therapist listens freshly in the therapy hour to the totality of the client's description, including how it is said and watches the nonverbal expression as it is being said, rather than listening just to the client's conceptualization, he or she will receive a variety of sensory impressions that go beyond the client's conceptual scheme. The therapist can then either synthesize these impressions into a whole that more closely approximates the client's original experience than does the client's own conceptual construction or help the client use awareness experiments to generate more information for the creation of a new, more encompassing construction. The client can thereby construct a new view that more closely resembles both the external and internal features of the original situation.

It is important in this process for the therapists to avoid placing their interpretations on the clients' constructions, and experiential therapists disciplinedly leave clients free to explore their total experience in the situation and to symbolize it uniquely for themselves in their own way. It is important for clients to construct their own realities in this way because, although the therapist can pick up and synthesize impressions that are fuller than the client's construction, the client is the only one who can fully know what it was like for him or her in that situation. By helping clients to further and further differentiate their own experience and by encouraging them to check each newly synthesized construction against their primary experience, the therapist is less likely to build in therapist bias or oversimplifications. There is thus a true element of discovery in this process, for neither client nor therapist knows beforehand where the exploration will lead.

We see from the foregoing that, in general terms, cognitive and experiential therapies share certain similarities but that they differ in the role relationship stances adopted by client and therapist and in the type of therapeutic change processes induced by their general styles of intervention. When, however, one takes a closer look at specific therapeutic tasks in experiential therapy, as we will do later, a much more differentiated view of similarities and differences will arise. In fact, the outstanding observation is that most therapeutic tasks, be they experiential or cognitive, involve both important cognitive and important affective change processes, which the use of different languages in the traditions has tended to obscure.

We will first explore the general role cognition plays in experiential therapy. This is followed by a discussion of the role of cognitive and affective change processes in four experiential interventions; evocative responding for resolving problematic reactions, two-chair work for resolving conflict, focusing for generating new meaning, and empty-chair work for completing emotional expression.

Gestalt therapy works with cognition in a number of general ways. First by virtue of working with awareness, it is essentially interested in how people perceive and organize their reality and how they process information. The gestalt therapist in fact attempts to train people to process specific types of information to the exclusion of others. The information processing and attentional allocation of the client is modified to focus the client's attention on current sensory and affective information, as opposed to automatically attending to future expectations or past memories. The assumption here is that much maladaptive thinking involves either the generation of catastrophic expectation about the future that produces anxiety or the dwelling on memories of past events that produces emotions that are not useful in orienting to the present situation. Optimal functioning is seen as occurring by attending to internal and external realities in the present, uncluttered by future expectations or past memories. The assumption of the superiority of present-centered processing is based on the notion that neurotic functioning is characterized by an excess of catastrophizing and ruminating. Rather than denying the importance of thinking, planning, and remembering as appropriate at the right time for goal-directed activity, gestalt therapy emphasizes the importance of present contact with sensory reality as providing an important fundamental source of information for appropriate orientation and action.

Training clients to attend to and be aware of what is currently occurring within the boundary of their skin and to discriminate between direct sensory reality and self-created, and often catastrophic, fantasies is a central process in gestalt therapy. Once this has occurred, gestalt therapists are particularly interested in identifying coercive and evaluative self-statements or automatic thoughts. The identification and awareness of "shoulds" or "oughts" and of self-criticisms and evaluations that interrupt spontaneity and block experience is a cornerstone of gestalt practice. How these are dealt with once they have been brought to awareness differs somewhat from a cognitive approach. Although there is a component of cognitive modification in gestalt therapy, through the therapists conveying the attitude that "shoulds" and self-criticisms are dysfunctional, by far the major processes for modifying shoulds involve awareness of these internal injunctions and gaining control over them by doing intentionally what was previously being done automatically (Greenberg & Safran, 1987). In accordance with the dictum of changing to "be what you are rather than what you are not," clients are encouraged to become aware of the shoulds, to make them explicit, to practice saying them to themselves, and to "own" them as their own. This is encouraged both in the session and as homework, until such time as clients decide on their own accord to incorporate the injunctions as integrated personal values, to give them up, or contest them. It can be seen from the practice of gestalt therapy that persistent and continuous awareness and repetition of negative self-statements, regarded by the therapist and client as dysfunctional, eventually leads the client to choose to identify with the statements and change behavior or to stop or reduce the frequency of these negative cognitions.

In addition to modification of negative self-statements involved in self-criticism, gestalt therapy works with identifying maladaptive cognitions in many other areas of dysfunction. Maladaptive thoughts are also focused on as central in the maintenance of fears and avoidances. As mentioned previously, the experiment is the major tool of gestalt intervention, and it is used extensively in working with fears. For example, in working with avoidance, clients are instructed to try doing, in the safety of the therapeutic situation, what they fear or avoid, such as being assertive or getting close to someone, and then the automatic thoughts and negative self-statements that impede the process are identified. Thus the client is asked to experiment *in vivo* with attempting an actual behavior, in a therapy group with another member of the group, or in individual therapy with the therapist or by means of the gestalt dramatic techniques of dialogue with people in an empty chair. This behavioral experiment leads to an activation, in the present, of interruptive cognitions that impede the desired performance. Once these cognitions have been identified, the client takes responsibility for and becomes the agent of the negative cognition using the dramatic method of dialogue. In this drama, clients sit in one chair and express verbally and nonverbally, to themselves, imaged as sitting in an empty chair, the negative self-statements and attitudes that produce the fear reaction. In other words, they engage in a dialogue in which the process of frightening themselves is enacted. Clients for example, speak to themselves, saying out loud such things as ''be careful, you'll mess up'' or ''be rejected'' or whatever it is that they say to themselves that results in the fear. The therapist does not attempt directly to challenge these statements as illogical or irrational but rather encourages clients to become aware of and take responsibility for how they do these things to themselves. Thus an important change process, one encouraged by the therapist, is for clients to see themselves as agents in the process of construction of their negative experience. In instances in which fear is the problem, clients come to see themselves as doing something to themselves that creates and maintains the fear. This is done with the idea that awareness of what they are doing makes it more possible for them to stop. A context of choice is created. Rather than attempting to directly modify the statement, an opportunity for change is created by making a client aware that it is he or she who is doing something to him- or herself. It is important to note that clients' responsibility for their experience is not communicated with a sense of blame or implication attached to it that they could change if they wished but are just stubborn. On the contrary, the process is engaged in with a perspective of discovery, to find out what they do to themselves and to accept this as an aspect of who they are. Only then can this ''self-statement'' process be seen as a part of their functioning, rather than as something happening to them. In addition, it is important to note that awareness of functioning is not intended here to mean insight, which once seen leads to change. Rather, awareness means the disciplined ongoing process of being aware of what one is doing. It involves practice and is more of a skill than simply a new perception.

Gestalt can thus be seen to work extensively with identifying interruptive automatic thoughts and negative self-statements, but these cognitions are generally seen as dysfunctional not only because they are negative but also because they interrupt some other aspect of functioning of a growth-oriented organismic process. This view of self-interruptive cognitions often leads gestalt therapists to focus on a different set of dysfunctional cognitions than would cognitive therapists. Although gestalt therapy, like cognitive therapy, does focus strongly on self-criticisms, as one set of negative statements, it also regards as dysfunctional those self-statements that impede or interrupt the expression of biologically adaptive underlying feelings (Greenberg & Safran, 1987). In addition, many expectations on the self, such as expectations of perfection, excellence, success, are viewed as self-coercive, as impeding spontaneity and creativity, and as interrupting a more natural self-forming process based on interest. Thus *shoulds* and *oughts* are often seen as being attempts to pull or push the organism away from a more self-motivated and natural, interest-driven process. These introjects are regarded as being foreign or unhealthy standards or injunctions taken in from the environment rather than as integral values of the person.

In addition to working with negative self-statements, gestalt therapy also works extensively with clients' attributions, of meaning, referred to in gestalt as *projection,* but meaning essentially the clients' construction and interpretation of reality (Greenberg, 1982). Gestalt is particularly interested in identifying clients' hypersensitivity (i.e., selective attention) to aspects of the environment and behavior of others that confirm dysfunctional views of self. Clients are seen as being their own worst enemies and as overattributing hostility, criticism, and negative evaluation to the environment as a function of their own negative views of themselves. Again, this attribution process is worked with, not by challenging or disputing this view, but rather by helping clients become aware that it is they who are their worst enemies and are the source of the negative views that they attribute to the environment. Identification with, and enactment of, the attributed views are key methods to help clients recognize that it is they who are attributing meanings to environmental events. The client is asked to become the person or people in the environment who are experienced as denigrating, critical, or persecuting and enact their role. Clients, by becoming this construction and speaking as this person or persons, begin to realize that it is they who are doing these things to themselves. Again an experiment is used to create the context for discovery of a dysfunctional process.

As can be seen from the preceding procedures, key elements of the gestalt approach to working with cognitions involve identification of the negative cognition, increased awareness of when and how thought impedes functioning, and, what is most important, the recognition by the client of the self as an agent in an experinece in which the self was previously experienced as being a victim. There is a cognitive shift from a position of helpless passivity, ''It is happening to me,'' be it feeling depressed, worthless, or incompetent to a position of ''I am doing it to myself.'' It is important to note that this agency must be discovered by the person and experienced fully not just thought to be true (i.e., it must become known by a process of knowledge by acquaintance rather than knowledge by association). This shift to seeing the self as an agent of experience is a key aspect of the change process in experiential therapy.

Gestalt therapists, however, unlike cognitive therapists such as Beck (1967), do not systematically categorize different types of dysfunctional thinking styles. The dysfunctional cognitive processes that would appear to be emphasized most in gestalt therapy are catastrophic expectations, *shoulds,* or *introjects,* and projections or attributions. These can be seen as corresponding roughly to catastrophizing, *shoulds,* and arbitrary inferences in Beck's (1976) system. The emphasis on these areas in gestalt therapy can be understood in terms of three fundamentally important themes in Gestalt therapy. The emphasis on catastrophizing reflects the gestalt view that anxiety is produced by catastrophic expectations about future events. The concern with introjects reflects the gestalt emphasis on learning not to allow dysfunctional thoughts to interfere with adaptive organismic tendencies and needs. The focus on projection or attribution can be understood in terms of the gestalt theoretical assertion that self-evaluations and the disowning of parts of the self as a function of this are major sources of dysfunction. Here the gestalt theoretical understanding of what underlies what Beck (1974) would refer to as arbitrary inference is radically different than the cognitive-behavioral perspective. In gestalt therapy, how one perceives the world or attributes meaning to events is a function of internal processes of self-criticism and the disowning of aspects of experience.

Another theme in experiential therapy involves the importance of changing not only the content of perception but also the manner of processing information (Toukmanian, 1986). In therapy, the emphasis is not only on the content of clients' perceptions and experience but also on the process and manner of organizing experiencing and perception. The content of clients' communications is primarily important in terms of what it conveys about *how* the client is perceiving or construing a particular situation. The goal of therapy ultimately is one of effecting change in the way clients' construe and encode. The focus in experiential therapy is on clients' encoding of reality, and the aim is having the clients discover how they are construing themselves and the world, recognizing that these are their constructs, and changing them from automatic to more controlled processing (Greenberg & Safran, 1981). This creates the opportunity for changing the manner of construal.

This change in manner from rigid to flexible, vigilant to relaxed, is definitely a change in cognitive information processing, but it differs from approaches that emphasize a change in content of cognition alone or change in type of cognition, such as changing irrational to rational beliefs, negative to positive self-statements, or illogical to logical thoughts. Rather the focus is on clients' discovering that they are the agents of their construal, how they are construing, and then bringing this under deliberate control. They can then themselves, after time, change the manner in which they construe themselves, others, and the world if they so choose. Specific maladaptive cognitions are therefore seen as a product of a dysfunctional system in which encoding and construal of reality are the dysfunctional elements. It is change by clients themselves of the processes of encoding and construing, that is, in the manner of processing information and representing reality, that is the ultimate goal of experiential therapy, not direct modification by the therapist of cognitions which are the products of this process (Greenberg & Safran, 1981).

In experiential therapy, awareness of one's own dysfunctional style or manner of processing is seen as leading to the possibility of self-generated change. Once clients are aware of how they are constructing their reality and experience, they become free to change. In the experiential view, what makes clients able to change is not primarily the therapist's instruction or direction but rather the client's adaptive motivation and the client's desire to cope with and master situations.

Similar to the gestalt approach, the client-centered approach also operates by bringing new information to awareness. Although it uses less active and experimental means of intervention to raise awareness, its use of reflection of attitudes, feelings, and experience, at the edge of clients' awareness is designed to help clients expand their awareness. The ultimate goal in client-centered therapy is also one of achieving a change in the client's manner of processing information. Rogers referred to the process of change as involving a loosening of rigid constructs and the change to a less rigid and more fluid manner of processing information. Rogers (1961), in his stages-of-growth conception, saw the process of change as involving, among other things, a discovery of one's own personal constructs. He claims that, in change, there is a definite recognition of these as constructs and that there is a beginning questioning of their validity. Rogers's views a healthy functioning person as an optimal information processor who is freely allocating attention to internal information, abstracting what is new in the situation, differentiating new meaning and thereby creating new options.

A number of client-centered therapists have focused on the process of therapy as one in which information processing is altered (Wexler & Rice, 1974). Anderson (1974) suggests that refocusing or retraining of attentive capacity is an important factor contributing to change in psychotherapy. He suggested that refocusing of attention brings neglected aspects of information into focus. This leads to the elaboration and articulation of information processing rules, that is, to awareness of how one is constructing reality and to the realization of new options inherent in situations that are freshly perceived. Wexler, on the other hand, sees clients in therapy as actively differentiating and integrating meaning and learning that they can be their own source for creating new experience and change via their own cognitive functioning. He sees the therapist as a surrogate information processor who, in delivering an optimal empathic response, is helping to provide a new organization of information that more fully captures and better organizes the meaning of the information in the client's field than the structures the client had previously generated to organize this information. Zimring (1974) suggests that, in client-centered therapy, the therapist selects and organizes information provided by the client in order to provide the client with new ways of processing and symbolizing internal emotional information. Therapy, in this view, is thus a process of creation of new meaning rather than a revealing or uncovering of material kept out of awareness. This view, that empathic interaction leads to the creation of meaning, captures an important aspect of the change process in client centered therapy.

Finally, Rice (1974) and Rice and Sapiera (1984) has focused on the change process as involving the bringing into awareness of new information, available to the client in memory, but not symbolized in the clients' conscious construction of the situation. This new information is brought to awareness by a process of evocative responding in which the therapist stimulates the clients' exploration using vivid imagery, sensory, and connotative language and helps to reevoke the situational memory as vividly as possible. This provides the best opportunity for accessing information available but not symbolized. Once the new information is available, it is seen as forcing reorganization of the old schema or organization.

Thus client-centered therapists, in this information-processing view, have focused on important cognitive processes involved in organizing information and constructing reality. Client-centered therapy is seen as enabling the client to change the manner of organizing information, new organizations for symbolizing internal information, and generating new information that leads to change in schematic organization.

At the core of experiential processes for changing cognition is the process of discovery, which has been contrasted to the process of influence engendered by interpretation, or challenge. These latter processes are seen as providing preformed ways of organizing client experiential information from the therapist's theoretical or personal frame of reference. In contrast, experiential therapy emphasizes the crucial importance of the client organizing the material for him- or herself. An externally supplied organization such as ''you are avoiding your anger'' or a challenge such as ''it's irrational to believe one rejection means you're unlovable'' is not seen as the best means for the client of creating a new internal organization. Creation of a stable, enduring new cognitive organization is seen as requiring the construction of the internal structure by the client him- or herself from subjectively generated experiential information. Formation of new cognitive structures involves processes of attending, selecting, encoding, and representing this experiential information. These are processes that only the client can engage in, and it is crucial if the organization is to endure that it be based on information from the client's own experience and be his or her own active construction, not just the adoption of a construct, even if it is correct, from an external source. If a new structure is taken on through influence, then the adopted construct is seen as simply overlaying the original construction, as possibly modifying conceptual-level processing, but not as modifying the constitutive processes of attending, selecting, and encoding involved in the construction of the new and destruction of the old structure.

Beck's (1974) cognitive therapy, in its use of homework to generate schema-inconsistent evidence, appears sensitive to the need for experiential evidence to change schemata. The difference is that, in experiential therapy, schema-inconsistent evidence is generated not by homework designed to provide contradictory information but by the stimulation of previously unsymbolized aspects of internal processing into awareness and the creation of new experience in therapy. Attending to this new information leads to coding situations and self-experience in new ways. Thus new self-generated cognitive organizations of experience and reality are the desired products of experiential therapy. In addition to these self-formed organizations being regarded as more stable and enduring because of their self-created nature, they are seen as being more valid for the client in that they were self-determined and less open to distortion or influence from therapists' implicit values or views.

Experiential therapy thus can be seen to concern itself directly with client information processing and with cognition. Once we adopt a common information-processing language, both experiential and cognitive therapies can be seen to be concerned with changes in cognition and information processing. As we have attempted to show, the types of cognitive change in the two approaches overlap in part and also differ in part. One common goal is schema change, although, as we have seen, the multiplicity of meanings associated with this concept is problematic. One basic difference is experiential therapy's view of the organism as an active information processor, curious and mastery oriented, motivated by interest, and by biologically adaptive tendencies. The tendencies promote the organism's self-directed cognitive change, inclining the person to construct more and more accurate and more adaptive representations of self and reality when given access to how he or she is construing situations and to new information from his or her experience.

A fundamental difference between experiential and cognitive therapies thus lies in their view of the self. At the heart of experiential therapy is the belief that the path to therapeutic change lies in the discovery of the nature and experience of an essential "self," which is fundamentally growth-oriented, and that it is the disowning of aspects of this self that causes pathology. In contrast, cognitive therapy has no articulated self-theory and sees pathology as resulting from dysfunctional thinking. Cognitive therapy thus emphasizes the correction of distorted perceptions of reality as the path to health.

Given the general comparisons previously mentioned, we will proceed to analyze next, some specific experiential interventions, highlighting the information-processing and cognitive operations involved in the different interventions.

## EXPERIENTIAL INTERVENTIONS

### Two-Chair Dialogue

Gestalt two-chair dialogue for resolving conflict involves a complex set of cognitive and affective change processes (Greenberg, 1979, 1980, 1984). Certain components that discriminated resolution performances from nonresolution performances have been identified by means of a task analysis of conflict resolution performances. A number of resolution components, the primary of which is a softening from harsh self-criticism toward a more self-accepting attitude, have been shown to relate to therapeutic outcomes (Greenberg & Webster, 1982). Intensive analysis of conflict resolution performances across a number of clients and therapists has revealed a number of steps on the path to resolution. The essential steps to resolution are outlined later. The two aspects of the self in the two-chair dialogue are referred to as the "other chair" and the "experiencing chair" (Greenberg, 1984). The other chair contains the person's negative self-statements, automatic thoughts plus the views of others as the person construes them. The experiencing chair involves the person's organismic response and biologically adaptive affects (see Figure 1).

In this model, we see the critic move from global negative cognitions to more specific concrete ones and then to cognitions that are less negative, less blaming, and less directed against the self. In this process, criticisms are transformed to statements of internal values of the self rather than negative injunctions. The progression that the self-criticisms follow to this point is from global, negative accusations to specific, concrete criticisms to nonhostile statements of core values. The experiencing chair, in which more primary affect resides, moves from an affective reaction of depression, withdrawl, or rebellion against the attack, to a differentiation of underlying feelings in order to access and symbolize inner experience and internal resources. It is here that the growth-oriented organismic response emerges. From the information that is produced by the differentiation process, the client forms a new construct for organizing inner material, and a new sense of emotionally based self-experience emerges. The action tendency (Arnold, 1960; Greenberg & Safran, 1987) associated with the new emotional

| Other chair | Experiencing chair |
|---|---|
| 1. Harsh criticisms | 1. Affective reaction |
| 2. Specific criticism | 2. Differentiation of feelings |
| 3. Statement of values and standards | 3. Emerging new experience |
| 4. Softening | 4. Wants and needs |
| 5. Integration of opposing views | |

FIGURE 1. Gestalt two-chair dialogue for conflict resolution.

experience is then symbolized as a need or want. The experience in this chair thus moves from an affective reaction, to the accessing of underlying feelings through differentiation and integration of meaning, to the emergence of a new affective experience and the assertion of a want in opposition to the value. In the other-chair, resolution occurs when the person reexamines and reevaluates both values and wants and finds a way of reducing the opposition between these. The process repeatedly involves the emergence of a more self-acepting or "softened" stance. Thus the core cognitions of the more critical aspect of the personality are softened, and a newfound self-organization and sense of direction in the experiencing chair is affirmed. These combined internal operations result in a new more self-accepting stance in the internal dialogue. This essentially represents the formation of a new view of self in the situation. This process, although it involves a lot of work with emotion, predominantly in the "experiencing chair," also involves a number of processes found in cognitive therapy such as identifying negative, self-critical thoughts and the modification of negative self-statements. This latter modification process, however, occurs in experiential therapy by a process of self-confrontation rather than by therapist confrontation. It challenges their own thoughts from their newly emerged self-experience. Schema change thus occurs by being confronted with new inner experience from the experiencing chair. Thus self-criticisms are challenged by an inner sense of worth. In addition to the modification of dysfunctional cognitions, other important cognitive processes also occur in two-chair work. Processes such as the generation of new meaning by differentiation, integration, and symbolization, and the construction of new perceptions by the modification of attentional allocation to focus on different features of inner experience are other essential cognitive change processes.

### EVOCATIVE UNFOLDING

Rice and Saperia (1984) have identified by means of task analysis the steps in the resolution of problematic reactions. A "problematic reaction" is a point in therapy at which a client expresses, directly or indirectly, that his or her own reaction in a particular situation was puzzling and problematic. Once it is confirmed that the client sees his or her *own* reaction as puzzling, the client is encouraged to describe the incident as vividly as possible, thus reevoking the sights, sounds, and feelings experienced during the incident, including those not consciously processed at that time. Thus the clients reenter the scene and are able to recognize which aspects (external or internal) felt salient at the time. This in turn can lead to a new awareness of how they were construing the potential impact (demand characteristics) of the stimulus situation at that time. That is, clients become aware not only of the nature of their own construals but also of themselves as agents in their own construals. Some clients seem especially to be well able to access the particular quality of their own affective reaction aroused by the stimulus and thus to become freshly aware of their own idiosyncratic construal of impact. Others focus more on the salient qualities of the stimulus situation and thus become aware of the nature of their subjective construal. For most clients, accessing both the affective qualities of their reaction and the salient qualities of the stimulus are involved in the exploration.

Once a client becomes aware of the way in which his or her puzzling and problematic reaction was a direct response to his or her own idiosyncratic construal and the aroused affect, this mode of functioning is usually recognized as an example of a more general style, and the client is motivated to explore this personal style and its consequences. Thus the stage is set for the client's "owning" of this problematic mode of functioning more broadly and for exploring in a differentiated way how it relates to his or her own needs, values, and fears. When these explorations are successful and "resolution" is reached, it results in the construction of a new and more personally satisfying sense of self, together with new options and possibilities.

| Stimulus side | Response side |
|---|---|
| 1. Vividly reconstruct stimulus situation | 1. Reenter scene with high arousal and exploratory stance |
| 2. Scan situation for salient features | 2. Focus attention on inner reaction |
| 3. (a) Identify subjective construal | 3. Identify unique quality of reaction, especially that which reflects the demand characteristics of the stimulus as construed. |
|    (b) Identify demand characteristics (potential impact) of the stimulus as construed | |

4. Problematic reaction recognized as response to impact of stimulus as construed
5. Recognize broader personal meaning systems involved in such construals
6. Recognize and explore new options for self

FIGURE 2. Resolution of problematic reactions.

This resolution performance involves a number of internal information-processing operations relating to the perception of the stimulus and to the response to it. These operations are outlined in Figure 2.

Successfully engaging in this process has been shown to lead to successful outcome in therapies involving exploration of problematic reactions (Lowenstein, 1985). This process involves focusing on inner reactions and feelings but also works extensively with clients' information processing, their construals of the situation, and the generation of new meanings. The process of modification of cognitions once again is seen to occur through an exploratory, self-generated modification process in which new evidence is generated from internal sources and serves to force reorganization of schemata.

This process involves focusing on inner reactions and feelings but also works extensively with clients' information processing, their construals of the situation, and the generation of new meanings. The process of modification of cognitions once again is seen to occur through an exploratory, self-generated modification process in which new evidence is generated from internal sources and serves to force reorganization of schemata.

## FOCUSING

In the focusing process (Gendlin 1981), clients who are feeling confused and are describing an experience verbally without really experiencing what they are saying, or who are going around and around trying to say but not really being able to get at what they want to express, are asked to close their eyes and focus in on the bodily felt sense of what it is they are feeling. The steps through which the client proceeds are described next:

1. Attending to the felt sense, that is, directly referring to the bodily felt referent of a personal meaning. This is a definitely felt but conceptually vague referent, and the client pays attention to it silently without thinking or describing it.

2. Symbolizing the referent in an attempt to express in words or images the meaning of the referent.
3. Checking the new words or symbols against the felt referent to see if they fit. This involves comparing the constructed meaning with the feeling to see if they match.
4. Referent movement occurs. A definite change either in the form of a bodily felt release of tension, or a different feel to the bodily referent occurs. The focusing process can then begin again with attending to this new vaguely felt referent.
5. Creation of new meaning. The focusing process involves the creation of a new view of the self in the situation. New connections and associations are made, and new possibilities emerge for resolving what was previously experienced as confused or unclear.

As can be seen from the preceding steps, focusing involves a cognitive process of creating new meanings from an inner felt sense that is initially preverbal and preconceptual. The changes in information processing sought in this process involve the initial limiting of conceptual processing, and the allocation of attention to the preverbal sense that is available to awareness but is as yet undifferentiated and unsymbolized. This is followed by symbolization that gives meaning to the implicit feeling and conceptual elaboration of the symbols to generate new meaning. This is an active constructive information processing task utilizing a combination of both active and passive processes that occur in attentional processing. Broadbent (1977) suggests that attention operates first by means of an early passive and global analysis of information followed by a later active and more detailed analysis of the information. This is what occurs in focusing, wherein the initial act of attending involves the application of a passive receptive attentional stance and the latter step of symbolizing involves a more active detailed analysis of the information. The process of change in this procedure is seen to occur through an exploratory, self-generated modification process in which new evidence is generated from internal sources and serves to force reorganization of schemata.

UNFINISHED BUSINESS

The final experiential process we will discuss here is the emotional restructuring (Greenberg & Safran, 1987) brought about by finishing unfinished business (Perls, Hefferline, & Goodman, 1951). In this type of process, an emotional restructuring of a client's emotional memory of a significant other takes place. Emotional restructuring involves the activation of schematic memory in the session. This process is generally accompanied by high affective arousal and expression. This affective arousal occurs because the sensorimotor components of the scheme representing the emotional experience at the time are now activated and allowed to surface in the safety of the therapeutic situation. A number of steps through which the client proceeds in this type of emotional restructuring have been described (Greenberg & Safran, 1987) and are presented next.

1. Evocation of schematic emotional memory of a significant other representing the negative or troubling view of the other.
2. Arousal of previously unexpressed emotional reactions associated with this view.
3. Differentiation of the emotional reaction into different discrete emotions such as hurt and anger and the expression of each.
4. Development of the capacity to see the world from the viewpoint of the other.
5. Evocation of alternate more positive view of the significant other.
6. Construction of a new schematic representation of the self–other relationship, incorporating and combining features from the earlier good and bad representations.

This process, although it involves the arousal and expression of intense affect, usually anger, hurt, or sadness, is not a cognition-free process. It appears that the therapeutic effect of the arousal of emotion is some form of cognitive reorganization, a change in view of self and other. Affective arousal provides access to underlying schematic structures and core pathogenic beliefs that guide conscious processing and it also allows for a sensorimotor change providing a bodily release of tension. It is not the emotional release alone that leads to change, but rather it is the emotional experience that promotes a cognitive reorganization. Once emotional memories are aroused, they become amenable to restructuring, and the type of emotional restructuring that takes place in finishing unfinished business with significant others that is described in detail elsewhere (Greenberg & Safran, 1987) involves, in addition to an expressive process, a significant cognitive component.

## CONCLUSION

First, we suggest that the utilization of a common information-processing language will help to illuminate the similarities and differences between cognitive and experiential therapies. Both approaches clearly deal with people's internal worlds and their representations of reality. In so doing, they clearly overlap. Further theoretical clarification and research is needed to help determine commonalities and differences in the approaches. Although it is by no means our contention that the therapies are the same, in fact, at the level of practice, they are rather different, it is our view that certain similar processes do occur in the different approaches. Clear identification of the different change processes (Greenberg, 1986) will clarify how they may overlap and how they can complement each other.

Second, we suggest that both traditions will benefit from inspection of the other. Cognitive therapy can be enhanced by focusing more on the role of affective processes, whereas experiential therapy can benefit by clarifying how it works with cognition and by recognizing the role of cognitive processes in change.

## REFERENCES

Anderson, W. (1974). Personal growth and client-centered therapy: An information-processing view. In D. A. Wexler & L. N. Rice, (Eds.), *Innovations in client-centered therapy* (pp. 21–48). New York: Wiley.

Arnold, M. B. (1960). *Emotion and personality* (Vols. 1 & 2). New York: Columbia University.

Bartlett, F. (1932). *Remembering: A study in experimental and social psychology.* Cambridge: Cambridge University Press.

Beck, A. T. (1974). The development of depression: A cognitive model. In R. J. Friedman & M. M. Katz (Eds.), *The psychology of depression* (pp. 118–142). New York: Wiley.

Beck, A. T. (1967). *Depression: Clinical, experimental and theoretical aspects.* New York: Harper & Row.

Brewer, W. F., & Nakamura, G. V. (1984). The nature and function of schemas. In R. W. Wyer, Jr., & T. K. Srull (Eds.), *Handbook of social cognition* (Vol. 1, pp. 173–198). Hillsdale, NJ: Erlbaum.

Frankl, V. (1959). *Man's search for meaning.* New York: Washington Square Press.

Gendlin, E. T. (1981). *Focusing.* New York: Bantam.

Goldfried, M., & Robins, C. (1984). Self schemas, cognitive bias and the processing of therapeutic experiences. In P. Kendall (Ed.), *Advances in cognitive-behavioral research and therapy* (Vol. 2, pp. 221–247). New York: Academic.

Greenberg, L. S. (1979). Resolving splits: The two-chair technique. *Psychotherapy: Theory, Research and Practice, 16,* 310–318.

Greenberg, L. S. (1980). The intensive analysis of recurring events from the practice of Gestalt therapy. *Psychotherapy: Theory Research and Practice, 17,* 143–152.

Greenberg, L. S. (1982). The relationship in gestalt therapy. In M. Lambert (Ed.), *Psychotherapy and patient relationships* (pp. 149–171). New York: Dorsey.

Greenberg, L. S. (1984). A task analysis of intrapersonal conflict resolution. In L. N. Rice & L. S. Greenberg

(Eds.), *Patterns of change: Intensive analysis of psychotherapy process* (pp. 67–123). New York: Guilford Press.

Greenberg, L. S. (1986). Change process research. Journal of Consulting and Clinical Psychology, *54,* 4–9.

Greenberg, L. S., & Safran, J. (1981). Encoding and cognitive therapy: Changing what clients attend to. *Psychotherapy Theory, Research and Practice, 18,* 163–169.

Greenberg, L. S., & Safran, J. (1984). Integrating affect and cognition: A perspective on the process of therapeutic change. *Cognitive Therapy and Research, 8,* 559–578.

Greenberg, L. S., & Safran, J. D. (1987a). *Emotion in psychotherapy: Affect cognition and the process of change.* New York: Guilford Press.

Greenberg, L. S., & Safran, J. D. (1987b). Emotion, cognition and action. In H. Eyesenk & I. Martin (Eds.), *Theoretical foundations of behavior therapy* (pp. 215–311). New York: Plenum.

Greenberg, L. S., & Webster, M. (1982). Resolving decisional conflict by means of two-chair dialogue: Relating process to outcome. *Journal of Counseling Psychology, 29,* 468–477.

Guidano, V. F., & Liotti, G. (1983). *Cognitive processes and emotional disorders.* New York: Guilford.

Jourard, S. (1971). *The transparent self.* New York: Van Nostrand Reinhold.

Laing, R. (1975). *The divided self.* London. Tavistock Publications.

Lowenstein, J. (1985). *A test of a performance model of problematic reaction points.* Unpublished master's thesis, York University, Toronto.

Mahoney, M. (1983). Cognition, consciousness and the process of personal change. In K. D. Craig & R. J. McMahon (Eds.), *Advances in clinical behavior therapy* (pp. 224–249). New York: Brunner/Mazel.

Mahrer, A. R. (1978). *Experiencing: A humanistic theory of psychology and psychiatry.* New York: Brunner/Mazel.

Mahrer, A. R. (1983). *Experiential psychotherapy: Basic practices.* New York: Brunner/Mazel.

Mahrer, A. R. (1986). *Therapeutic experiencing: The process of change.* New York: W. W. Norton.

Perls, F., Hefferline, R., & Goodman, P. (1951). *Gestalt therapy.* New York: Dell.

Piaget, J., & Morf, A. (1958). Les isomorphismes partiels entre les structures logiques et les structures perceptives. In J. S. Bruner, F. Bresson, A. Morf, & J. Piaget (Eds.), *Logiques et perception* (pp. 79–96). Paris: Presses Universitaires de France.

Rogers, C. R.(1961). *On becoming a person.* Boston: Houghton Mifflin.

Rice, L. N. (1974). The evocative function of the therapist. In D. Wexler & L. Rice (Eds.), *Innovations in client-centered therapy.* New York: Interscience.

Rice, L. N., & Sapera, E. (1984). A task analysis of the resolution of problematic reactions. In L. Rice & L. S. Greenberg (Eds.), *Patterns of change: Intensive analysis of psychotherpeutic process* (pp. 29–66). New York: Guilford Press.

Safran, J. D., & Greenberg, L. S. (1986). Hot cognition and psychotherapy process: An information processing/ecological approach. In P. Kendall (Ed.), *Advances in cognitive-behavioural research and therapy* (Vol. 5, pp. 143–177). New York: Academic Press.

Toukmanian, S. G. (1986). A measure of client perceptual processing. In L. Greenberg & W. Pinsof (Eds.), *The psychotherapeutic process: A research handbook* (pp. 107–130). New York: Guilford Press.

Wexler, D. A. (1974). A cognitive theory of experiencing self-actualization and therapeutic process. In D. A. Wexler & L. N. Rice (Eds.), *Innovations in client-centered therapy* (pp. 49–116). New York: Wiley.

Wexler, D. A., & Rice, L. N. (Eds.). (1974). *Innovations in client-centered therapy.* New York: Wiley.

Zimring, F. M. (1974). Theory and practice of client-centered therapy: A cognitive view. In D. A. Wexler & L. N. Rice (Eds.), *Innovations in client-centered therapy* (pp. 117–138). New York: Wiley.

# 10

# Piagetian Theory and Cognitive Therapy

## Hugh Rosen

The Piagetian paradigm holds considerable promise for providing developmental depth to extant cognitive therapy models, as well as for generating clinical guidelines and strategies. It also offers theoretical and empirical support for much of what is already current practice (Rosen, 1985). The primary aim of this chapter is to provide a succinct exposition of Piaget's theory and to examine a leading model of cognitive therapy from its perspective.

## THE PIAGETIAN PARADIGM

### Foundations of Cognitive Development

Piaget is the founder of the science of genetic epistemology. His work spans such fields as biology, psychology, philosophy, and education. Genetic epistemology deals with the acquisition of knowledge in the individual—how it originates and its ontogenesis from infancy to maturity. Although broader in its full sweep, genetic epistemology is often approached as a theory of cognitive development.

A cornerstone of Piaget's theory is that the growth of knowledge involves a process of interaction with and adaptation to the environment. The human organism, interacting with the environment from birth onward, constructs a set of evolving cognitive structures whose growing organization and complexity provide an increasingly greater adaptation of the individual to his or her physical and social surroundings. A cognitive structure provides a generic form or way of knowing and a general set of rules for processing information. These structural forms of knowing are to be found universally among people of all cultures, and they always develop in the same invariant stage sequence. Cognitive development involves an ongoing process of structural differentiation and integration with each successive stage constituting a more hierarchical conceptual reorganization of what preceded. The reasoning strategies of each succeed-

Hugh Rosen • Department of Mental Health Sciences, Hahnemann University, Philadelphia, Pennsylvania 19102.

ing stage become more efficient and effective. Increasingly, the growing youngster develops a greater comprehension of the world and enhanced problem-solving abilities. The child's expanding understanding of the world, however, is not merely a matter of additive pieces of information, as in Lockean epistemology, but instead is characterized by a qualitatively different way of knowing-in-the-world at each new stage.

The heart of Piaget's epistemology resides in its constructionist orientation. For Piaget, structures are not innate categories of mind, as in Kant's philosophy or Chomsky's linguistic theory. At birth, the infant possesses only primitive schemes (early structures), such as grasping, looking, and sucking. Upon interacting with the environment, however, newly encountered demands and challenges lead to the refinement and coordination of these schemes into more complex organizations and to the invention of new structures. This constructionist activity spans all of development to encompass the adolescent's attempt to "grasp" geometry as well as the infant's attempt to grasp a nearby object.

Piaget's theory is correctly conceived of as a stage theory of cognitive development. However, a fuller comprehension of his system comes with the recognition that, for Piaget, knowledge inheres in neither the knower nor the known but is instead a relation between the knowing subject and the object known. The same object is known or understood differently at varying levels of development. A plastic circle hanging by a string above an infant's crib may be known initially by her or him only as something to be swung, later as a round object to be classified accordingly, and finally as a geometric form possessing 360 degress. This evolving relationship, constituting knowledge, between the epistemic subject and that which is known by her or him is characteristic not only of coming to know the physical world but also such varying phenomena as feelings, friendships, justice, and God. Virtually anything that is known is known in relation to one's level of cognitive development. This relation is constitutive of meaning for the individual (Kegan, 1982). Hence, it follows that cognitive structures serve as mediating variables throughout the developmental spectrum. An external stimulus does not make an unvarying imprint upon or elicit a rigid response from the growing individual. Instead, a stimulus is interpreted and understood in different ways according to a person's cognitive-structural level of development. The individual's behavioral repertoire is in turn both influenced and delimited by her or his network of cognitive structures. The nature and significance of these mediating cognitive structures are presented in the next section.

## THE DEVELOPMENT OF NATURAL THOUGHT

### Sensorimotor Intelligence

The origins of intelligence are to be found during the period of infancy (Piaget, 1946/1962a, 1936/1963, 1936/1971). Major categories of knowing such as space, time, causality, relations, classification, and object permanence all have primitive roots in the six developmental substages ranging from birth to 18 to 24 months. Manifestations of intelligence during the sensorimotor period are evident on a practical or behavioral plane but without benefit of conceptual or representational thought.

At the beginning of life, the infant is in a state of radical egocentrism, which renders him or her incapable of differentiating between his or her own body and the world of objects extending beyond his or her own outer skin. As the infant interacts with the environment, refining and coordinating early schemes, as well as inventing new ones, he or she gradually differentiates between himself or herself and objects other than herself or himself. Eventually the child undergoes a "miniature Copernican Revolution," now demonstrating behaviorally that his or her own body is but one in a personal universe of many objects, each existing in relation to one another, none being the center of the others. He or she will comprehend this more than once with greater conceptual complexity each time as knowledge is reflected onto

higher planes of knowing and transformed structurally. This recurring conquest of egocentrism
and achievement of greater objectivity is of singular importance to the fields of psychopathology and clinical treatment.

191

PIAGETIAN THEORY

*Preoperational Thought*

The preoperational period ranges from 18 to 24 months through 6 or 7 years of age. It
begins with the emergence of representational thought. Absent objects can now be represented
to the mind. The child is liberated from her or his rootedness in the immediate present and her
or his newly developing capacity for memory and imagery provides her or him with a greater
flexibility to mentally move through time. It is the ability to think on a symbolic plane that now
enables her or him to engage in mental imagery and to acquire language.

Despite the significant advance of representational thought, the preoperational child is
primarily described by the constraining features of cognition. Egocentrism is a limiting feature
of cognition, which is defined as an inability to differentiate between internal and external,
between subject and object, between knower and known. Although it winds its way throughout
development, its presence during the preoperational period is given special attention by Piaget
(1923/1955, 1926/1960, 1927/1969b). One form it takes is that of the subject's inability to
decenter from his or her own point of view in order to take the perspective of another. A
developmental lag in this area will impede social reasoning and lead to serious interpersonal
difficulties. We will return to this form of egocentrism in another section.

Ontological egocentrism (Piaget, 1926/1960, 1927/1969b) refers to the child's conceptions of the world and physical reality. An adequate understanding of physical causality is not
reached by the child until about 11 or 12 years of age, although by age 7 there has been marked
progress (Piaget, 1971/1974). Before that time, however, the notion of chance to account for
events is not available to the child. Preoperational thought is not predicated upon a grasp of
independent, and sometimes interdependent, causal forces and networks that come into play
objectively irrespective of the child's own whims, desires, and purposes. It is only gradually
that the child distinguishes between self and world on a conceptual plane. Before achieving
that distinction the child ascribes purposes, justifications and motives of a precausal character
to natural events. When rudiments of this type of precausal thinking persist into adulthood and
are applied to one's personal life events, the individual is in for serious trouble. Rather than
seeing a series of unfortunate events that has befallen him or her as the result of chance, a
depressed patient may be convinced that events are somehow conspiring to work against him
or her. Another individual who persistently engages in self-defeating behavior may be failing
to accommodate to reality, being guided by the tacit false belief that reality should accommodate her or his wishes. Ontological egocentrism is elaborated upon by Piaget (1926/1960) and
Rosen (1977, 1985).

Lacking objectivity, the child's thinking is both subjective and absolutistic. He takes his
own subjective point of view as an absolute standard of the way things are. Applied to the
realm of emotion, a feeling may be experienced as a necessarily valid criterion of truth. The
tacit rule is, "Because I feel guilty, it follows that I must necessarily have done something bad
or wrong." The child does not manifest a sense of the relational character of some concepts.
For example, being a "foreigner" is thought to be an absolute trait, and the child never
conceives of herself as being a foreigner. The state of being "in the middle" is thought of in
absolute terms rather than recognizing that, in relational terms, it is simultaneously to the right
of one object and to the left of another. Absolutistic thinking of this sort provides fertile soil for
the dichotomous reasoning that is so prevalent in depressed and other emotionally disturbed
patients (Beck, 1976; Beck & Emery, 1985; Beck, Rush, Shaw, & Emery, 1979).

A major limitation of the preoperational period is that the young child is readily misled by
salient perceptual cues from which she or he draws conclusions without inferential reasoning.

Although she or he may seem to know something correctly on a conceptual level, such knowing is not embraced with certitude in the face of an optical illusion or misleading perceptual cue. Given such circumstances, she or he will abandon her or his conceptual knowledge in favor of the perceptually salient (Cowan, 1978). Without the capacity to make correct inferences on an abstract level, appearance is mistaken for reality. Flavell (1986) provides an excellent illustration of this. A red toy car is placed behind a green filter that makes it appear black. It is taken from behind the filter and shown to a 3-year-old who then inspects the red car. When it is again placed behind the green filter, the 3-year-old insists that it is black when asked what color it "*really* and *truly* is." In contrast, 6-year-old children invariably identify the toy car as being red even after it is placed behind the green filter again, assuming once more the appearance of being black. Flavell and his colleagues have been studying the appearance–reality distinction for several years and have found developmental stages in understanding this distinction ranging from the preconceptual phase through to the college years of some subjects. This distinction is surely of great importance to cognitive therapists given the considerable attention in practice to misattributions, misperceptions, false premises, and disconfirmed expectations. Many patients will vigilantly scan for facial and behavioral cues of significant others from which they automatically conclude that they are being disapproved of and ignored. They do not infer any of the wider varieties of possible interpretations beyond what is most apparent from the perceptual manifestation. Hence, a scowl means disapproval of me, rather than that the scowler might have a severe headache. The combination of egocentrism and the tendency to be misled by perceptual cues makes such an interpretation much more likely than an objective one that would also consider alternative possibilities.

The child lacks a structural organization for hierarchical classification. She or he cannot deal with inclusion relationships between subclasses and superordinate classes (Inhelder & Piaget 1959/1969; Piaget, 1924/1969a; 1946/1962a). In the preconceptual phase (2–4 years) of the preoperational period, the child cannot even conceive of single classes systematically, such as boys, candy, or toys (1946/1962a). This leads to transductive reasoning, which is neither inductive or deductive but rather shifts from particular to particular and is not based on an abstract defining notion or attribute that can consistently cut across all members of a single class. In transductive reasoning, the child links merely customary or accidental associations together as if they were logically related. For example, she or he may conclude that it is not yet afternoon because she or he has not yet had her or his customary afternoon nap. This primitive phase of classification competence imparts an undifferentiated and globular character to the child's thinking. For example, she may fuse all furry animals into the notion of "doggie." During the intuitive phase (4–7), the child does comprehend single classes but not hierarchies of classes. The lack of a mature classification structure lends a certain character of "disorder" to the child's thought. When persisting into adulthood, it is more likely to be considered a "psychological disorder." Not being able to simultaneously coordinate part and whole, an ephemeral outburst of "hate" may be taken as the totality of what one feels toward the other. The intensely experienced negative emotion is not recognized as a subset of a hierarchy of emotions, constituting only a brief and partial aspect of the much more rich set of complex feelings one has toward the other. As Cowan (1982) states

> Children at this age tend to display fluctuating emotional states, to focus on one attribute of the situation at a time, with either-or, love-hate feelings and private, idiosyncratic use of feeling language. (p. 67)

The absence of a maturely organized cognitive-structural classification system will promote not only either–or (dichotomous) thinking but a tendency toward overgeneralization as well. Both dichotomous thinking and overgeneralization will be recognized as two of the major forms of cognitive distortions found by Beck in emotionally disordered patients.

The preoperational youngster lacks the ability to conserve in areas such as amount, weight, volume, number, space, and time. Conservation judgment involves the recognition that, despite changes in certain properties of an object or set of objects, other properties remain invariant. To illustrate, the child who observes a ball-shaped piece of clay being elongated into a sausage shape will believe that there is more clay in the latter. His thinking is centered insofar as he focuses only on the length that has increased but ignores the width. It is static for he does not take into account the transformation that is occurring as decreasing width is compensating for increasing length. Finally, it is irreversible as he does not seem to reason that, because the clay could be returned to its original position where it would be the same amount, it must be the same amount now. The principle of conservation, with some qualifications, may be applied to the social realm, encompassing loyalty, friendship, feelings, and love. Piaget (1954/1981) held that there exists an analog between intelligence and affectivity with respect to conservation. As the child progresses beyond the preoperational period, she experiences more stable and enduring feelings, an increasing sense of regulated duty, and eventually an autonomous set of firm values. During the preoperational period, however, a friendship is more likely to be construed in terms of what is happening at the moment rather than as a bond that is conserved despite disruptions of the moment. Greenspan (1979) makes the same point regarding the conservation of a coherent sense of self under extreme stress. The more cognitively advanced person who has acquired conservation in the physical world will enjoy an increasingly greater parallel capacity to conserve a sense of a stable self despite duress.

*Concrete Operational Knowledge*

It is in the concrete operational period that the child's cognitive-structural organization achieves its systematic character grounded in a developing set of logical operations. Piaget has organized his work pertaining to these accomplishments into nine logico-mathematical models called groupings (Inhelder & Piaget, 1959/1969). This period of development starts at approximately 7 years of age and continues until the beginning of adolescence at about 11 or 12 years of age.

The concrete operational period ushers in a new level of conceptual attainment through the mental operation. An operation is an internal mental action that never exists in isolation but is integrally related to the network of the total cognitive-structural system. Further, an operation is reversible in that thinking can go forward from a starting point and return. Reversible thinking has the flexibility to go in two directions. Thought that is rooted in a cognitive operation promotes a sense of logical certitude. Knowledge that is a logical necessity will be true regardless of application to content and context. For example, the transitive operation, if $A = B$ and $B = C$, then $A = C$ is always true in the physical world no matter where and to what it is applied. In contrast, merely empirical truth is true as a matter of custom and convention. To illustrate, in the United States it is true that one is expected to wear a bathing suit when at a public beach. However, this is not true in all places of the world, nor is it necessarily true for the United States, as the custom could conceivably be changed, albeit unlikely. Patients in therapy often confuse custom and convention with necessity, hence need help in discriminating between the two. Use of the well-known tyrannical *should* is frequently an indicator to this confusion. Alternatively, patients many times do not recognize logical necessity for what it is, acting as if their wish or whim could change an aspect of reality that is immutable. To go beyond this primitive thinking, they must recognize the way they interpret reality.

Concrete operational thought is conceptually, rather then perceptually, grounded. The youngster is not deceived by appearances because she is able to make inferences that go beyond the sensory data before her. Thought is now decentered, transformational, and reversible. In the conservation task, the young person no longer centers on length alone but now decenters to coordinate the transformation taking place, noting that, as length increases, width reciprocally decreases. She also now thinks reversibly, inferring that, because the sausage-shaped clay could be rolled back into the shape of a ball and then have the same amount as originally, it must now have the same amount even though the shape is different. Reversibility can also be seen in the adding and subtracting of classes (girls plus boys equals children; children minus boys equals girls) and the ordering of various-sized objects (stick C is larger than sticks A and B but smaller than sticks D and E; or stick C is larger than B and reciprocally stick B is smaller than C). Repeated experiments demonstrate that the preoperational child does not have this ability, which can be applied to seriating musical tones, emotional intensity, and elements of a value system, as well as many other domains.

The concrete operational child is egocentric in the sense that she or he can apply thinking only to objects known to her or him. The child can reason only about that which is part of her or his own experience and, therefore, familiar to her or him. Although her thinking is no longer centered in many ways, she cannot decenter from her own convictions and assumptions in order to deductively draw conclusions from hypothetical assumptions. The child cannot reason from premises for which she has no available empirical support. For example, the child answers incorrectly when requested to respond hypothetically to the statement, "Elephants are either plants or animals. If they are not animals, then what are they?" (Moshman, 1986). Elkind (1974) has suggested that what is essentially egocentric about concrete operational thought is that the youngster does not sufficiently differentiate between empirical reality and her or his own assumptions. When confronted with evidence that contradicts her or his assumptions, she or he will tend to alter the new information so that it will conform to the assumption. The child does not modify the assumption to accommodate evidence contrary to it. The ensuing beliefs, based on modified evidence blended with personal assumptions, are called "assumptive realities" by Elkind. Clearly, the cognitive therapist who poses the strategic question, "What is the evidence?", must keep in mind that a client thinking in concrete operational terms will not relinquish her or his prior assumptions without a struggle, even when confronted with data opposing them. The theoretical orientation that cognitive therapy draws upon places a great emphasis upon rationality. There is an operating assumption that when confronted with contradictory evidence, the patient will modify or correct maladaptive premises or beliefs. That may be more true when working with a patient at the formal or final stage of cognitive development, which is defined as essentially that of scientific reasoning. However, adopting a developmental perspective enables the therapist to differentiate and classify patients, recognizing that not all of them will be equally receptive to each technique. A fruitful pursuit of inquiry would be to test-out the efficacy of a range of cognitive therapy techniques in relation to the cognitive stage of patients. Recognizing the limitation of a concrete operational patient in the face of information running contrary to what she or he is already familiar with may serve as an impetus to inventing new cognitive therapy techniques. Finally, it is conceivable that one source of failure, when it occurs, in conducting cognitive therapy is that the therapist may be using tactics with a concrete operational thinker that are better suited to a formal operational thinker.

The emergence of concrete operational structures has a profound effect in bringing more order and stability into the young person's emotional and interpersonal life. She or he now has the ability to decenter and coordinate at least two variables at a time, to take the perspective of another person, and to order her or his own feelings into a hierarchical classification. Hesse and Cicchetti (1982), commenting on this achievement, state

> An integration or conservation of conflicting emotional tendencies becomes possible only when children are capable of concrete emotional thinking and feeling, which is characterized by the emergence of logical operations that allow the coordination of different people's social and cognitive perspectives, different physical dimensions, and the formation of higher-order categories. (p. 17)

Operations of the concrete operational period are considered to be first-degree operations because they deal with actual objects in the real world. Transcending this constraint, formal operational thought utilizes second-order operations, which promote hypothetico-deductive reasoning. By adolescence, that which is real or actual is subsumed by the universe of the possible, which is the domain of formal thought. The developing adolescent becomes capable of designing scientific experiments to test her or his hypotheses about what *might possibly* be true (Inhelder & Piaget, 1955/1958). The formal operational thinker has constructed a combinatorial system that enables her or him to arrange a set of elements into all possible combinations and to systematically test-out the effect of any variable or union of variables upon the elements in the set.

The adolescent who achieves formal thought can follow the form of a proposition irrespective of its content. A line of reasoning can be understood on a purely abstract or symbolic level without a necessity for knowing the specific content to which the symbols apply. Take, for example, the assertion "From if A, then B, it follows that if not B, then not A" (Flavell, 1977). It is not necessary to know what A and B refer to in order to conclude that the statement is correct. The reasoning in this example is called interpropositional because it deals with two propositions, an indication of second-degree operations. Concrete operations are intrapropositional, as they constitute single propositions about objects in the real world.

A distinguishing feature of the formal operational period is the epistemic subject's new capacity to think about her or his own thought. She or he is now no longer simply thinking through her or his thought processes but is now able to think self-reflexively about those thought processes. More than just bringing to bear strategies of reasoning upon the environment, she or he is now capable of being aware of those strategies, analyzing them, and even changing them. She or he has attained a level of development where she or he not only has theories about reality, as in the concrete operational period, but now has theories about her or his theories. This capacity for thinking about one's own cognitive processes is known as metacognition. As with all developmental advances, indications of metacognition can be found in less complex forms during earlier stages. The presence of metacognition or its potential for being fostered is of considerable significance to the cognitive therapist who is interested in having her or his clients become aware of and modify cognitive errors.

The adolescent who develops formal thought structures becomes enamored of her or his new found thinking capacity to the point of ascribing boundless powers to it. It is as if her or his thoughts of social reform and utopia can itself bring about the desired change without the resistance of empirical reality and the opposing views of other members of society. Locked into a new form of egocentrism, the adolescent believes that her or his most cherished experiences are unique to her or him. Thus, no one has ever loved as intensely as she or he does. Common human experiences are believed to be unique to her or him. Further, she or he believes that what preoccupies her or his own mind is the very same thing that captures and sustains the attention of others. For example, an almost invisible facial scar that one might believe makes her or him unattractive is taken to be the object of interest on the part of others. Social interaction with peers and assuming adult work responsibilities are critical to the decline of egocentrism. (See Elkind, 1967, 1974, on childhood and adolescent egocentrism.) The more abstract formal reasoning that appears in adolescence not only promotes thinking about thinking, but it also engenders feelings about ideas, values, and moral principles. This is in contrast to the concrete operational thinker whose feelings are confined to a range of specific people, events, places, and things (Cowan, 1978).

Piaget's theory posits that adults normally reach the formal operational stage of development, but there is evidence that not all adults actually do so. Research by Kuhn, Langer,

Kohlberg, and Haan (1977) indicate that the majority of adults remain at a developmental state between the concrete and formal operational periods. Approximately 15% of their subjects failed to evidence any formal operational thought at all, whereas only about 30% had gone beyond the stage mixture of the majority to demonstrate that they had fully entered the formal operational period. Studies of college students suggest that slightly less than 70% are formal operational in their thinking and that no more than 20% are in the late formal stage (Cowan, 1978). Furthermore, Piaget (1972) has acknowledged that being at the formal operational stage does not necessarily mean that the individual will perform at that level of competence in all sectors of his or her life. Aptitude and interest are critical variables, so that a brilliant lawyer who is expert in his field may typically exhibit formal thought in matters of jurisprudence, yet approach music or physics initially as a concrete operational thinker. Also, because not all problems require formal thought for successful resolution, even a formal thinker may use concrete operations when no more than that is called for. Other variables that may lead to cognitive-stage functioning below what one is capable of include stress, anxiety, fatigue, and trauma. There is also the presence of residual acausal or magical thinking, as reflected in such activities as impatiently snapping one's fingers to change a red light in traffic, carrying an umbrella to avert rain, and a spectator's body movement to influence a sports event (Pulaski, 1971). Wason and Johnson-Laird (1972), Tversky and Kahneman (1973), and Nisbett and Ross (1980) have drawn attention to the many illogical errors that pervade the thinking of adults. Last, it is not known for certain why some adults do not reach the period of formal thought, or why many others go no further than to bridge the two last stages of development. Possibly those who have not moved completely into the final period of cognitive development have not had enough exposure to a sufficiently challenging environment to facilitate progression to formal thought (Cowan, 1978).

### Conclusion

Cognitive development can be seen as a series of qualitative advances based on the differentiation, integration, and reorganization of preexisting and newly invented structures. Each new synthesis represents an advance to a new perspective on the world and on the prior stage of development. Upon the advent of each emerging stage, the psychological structures and reasoning strategies of the growing person evidence greater mobility, durability, and range of application. As knowledge becomes increasingly more abstract, the growing person is liberated from both the context and content that form the constraints of the preceding stage.

Before proceeding further, a word on psychopathology is in order. Piaget had studied abnormal psychology as a young man, but, throughout his career, he evidenced an interest in researching and theorizing about normal cognitive development only. He did predict, however, that there will eventually evolve an interdisciplinary science of developmental psychopathology that will incorporate his own science of genetic espistemology. To date, even within the field of cognitive development, there does not as yet exist a coherent and integrated paradigm for explaining psychopathology. Nevertheless, over the years there has been a series of isolated attempts to use Piaget's work in an effort to explore specific domains of psychopathology (Cowan, 1978; Kegan, 1982; Rosen, 1985).

### COGNITIVE DEVELOPMENT, BEHAVIOR, AND EXPERIENCE

Although Piaget places primary emphasis upon the growing person as a self-regulating active organism, the role of the physical and social environments in providing appropriate experience for cognitive growth is a necessary one. Cognitive structures do not develop automatically over the years as if emerging in response to a fixed time schedule. They are constructed by the individual through interaction with the environment. However, as Haroutunian (1983) states,

> While the organism acts directly on the environment, the environment cannot act directly on the organism, nor can it convey effects of the organism's actions except as the organism interprets them. Hence, the organism may act on the environment, but it *interacts* with the environment only insofar as it acquires information about the actual effects of its actions upon the environment. (p. 105)

The nature of this specific type of interaction is the subject of the remainder of this section.

In order to derive cognitive-structural knowledge from the environment, the child must act upon it. Piaget's theory of abstraction (Piaget, 1974/1980a), so crucial to the acquisition of knowledge, depicts this process. In its simplest form, there is empirical abstraction viewed as exogenous knowledge because it is derived from properties that are intrinsic to objects in the environment. To illustrate, when observing and handling an object, we may gain information about its weight, size, and contour. Reflexive abstraction, in contrast, constitutes endogenous knowledge in which emphasis is not upon properties of the external object but upon the knower's internal process of constructing knowledge that is not directly observable. Piaget (1964) illustrates this with an example of a child on the threshhold of the concrete operational period. The child has a row of pebbles before him. He discovers that regardless of whether he counts from left to right or right to left, there are 10 pebbles in the row. He proceeds to reassemble the pebbles into various shapes, discerning that pebbles always add up to 10 irrespective of the shape taken by them. What the child will gradually come to realize is not an attribute of any of the pebbles but something derived from a coordination of his own actions upon the objects: The order that the pebbles are cast in has no bearing on the sum, which remains immutable. Reflecting upon his own activity, he will eventually invent a cognitive structure that operates out of the rule that the sum of any array of objects is independent of the order of its members. The general form of this structure will enable him to apply the rule widely to different objects at varying times, and in new places. The product of knowing in an immediate context has been reflected onto a new plane of abstract knowledge, undergoing a process of endogenous reconstruction. Reflecting abstraction occurs throughout development as knowledge acquired on one level is periodically transposed or reflected to a higher plane where it is reconstructed.

The origins of maladaptive assumptions of patients in cognitive therapy may often be traced to reflexive abstraction carried out within the family matrix. For example, a young child may be raised in a family by parents who are exceptionally inflexible and firm, if not harsh. Over time, the child makes numerous attempts in many different situations to persuade his or her parents to yield to his or her wishes and viewpoints. Despite altering his strategies and tactics, he or she continues to meet with repeated failure. Eventually he or she constructs a schema or rule that states that important people in one's life are unyielding regardless of one's persistent efforts to have them be otherwise. As an adult the rule is now applied to his or her nuclear family and in the workplace, resulting in unassertive behavior, indirect methods for achieving interpersonal goals, a sense of helplessness, and periodic depression. An essential difference between endogenous abstraction in Piaget's system and the hypothetical example offered here, is that in the former, the child's constructed knowledge is adaptive because it brings him or her into correspondence with the actual structure of the physical world, whereas in the latter, the child's constructed knowledge is maladaptive because it provides him or her with a false generalization about the social world. Because of the passive and despairing orientation he or she has adopted by the time of adulthood, he or she does not test-out the rule in new situations but tacitly accepts it as a guide to behavior and reality.

The interaction between environmental experience and cognitive self-regulation can be further amplified by examining Piaget's equilibration model, of which the process of constructing endogenous knowledge is one aspect. The model is offered by Piaget as an explanatory device to account for transitions through developmental stages. Piaget's theory of cognitive growth through stages is rooted in the biological concept of adaptation, comprised of the opposing twin processes of assimilation and accommodation. All cognitive structures both assimilate and accommodate external experiences. Assimilation takes information from the environment and transforms it to fit the cognitive structure as it presently exists. Accommodation changes the structure to meet the demands or contours of the incoming information. Adapted intelligence is a balance of assimilation and accommodation functioning in appropriate proportions. For example, an infant has no conceptual structure for understanding a ball as a geometric object. At first, the infant has only a primitive grasping scheme or structure to which the ball is assimilated. The ball is known on a behavioral plane merely as an object to be grasped. The scheme of grasping, however, is modified and expanded as it acommodates the various shapes of objects grasped, such as a ball, a rattle, and a button. Because of the unique shape of each object, it places a demand for accommodation of the scheme to its contours at the very moment that it is being assimilated to that same grasping scheme. As the child progresses with age, however, she or he develops complex higher order conceptual structures that enable her or him to comprehend the ball as one of many geometric forms. She or he can now assimilate the ball to such cognitive structures as diameter, area, and circumference, far surpassing her or his earlier limited way of knowing the ball merely as something to be grasped. At the same time that the ball is being assimilated now as a geometric form, its specific diameter, area, and circumference must be accommodated by the structure.

Every act of cognitive knowing involves a state of equilibrium in which assimilation and accommodation proceed in harmony. However, frequently, in the course of development, the present stage of cognitive organization proves inadequate to understanding new experiences or solving unfamiliar problems. The existing cognitive structures cannot adequately assimilate the new information or experience. When such an occurrence is perceived by the person as a disturbance or contradiction, a state of disequilibrium is introduced. To resolve the disequilibrium, a major form of accommodation is necessary, calling into play either a radical modification of the existing structure or the invention of a new one. Siegler (1986) gives the example of a typical late preoperational child who believes that only animals are alive. Upon hearing older children and adults referring to plants as alive also, she may be cast into a state of puzzlement and disequilibrium. She cannot assimilate the notion of plants as alive to her current scheme of "alive." Further inquiry and reflection will eventually lead her to discover that growth and reproduction are unifying characteristics of life, hence her cognitive scheme for understanding what it means to be alive becomes more differentiated, complex, and inclusive.

Although Piagetian examples draw upon children and adolescents, we might readily apply the experience and resolution of disequilibrium to adults. Supposing a man has developed a cognitive scheme embodying the rule that all men who express tender feelings are weak and cowardly. This is a belief that can certainly cause him much distress should he find himself with a marital partner who expects her spouse to periodically express tender feelings toward her. Over time, he makes the acquaintance of several men who demonstrate a history of strength and courage. However, these same men are also known to publicly exhibit soft, tender feelings. As in the previous example, this new information cannot be readily assimilated by the existing conceptual scheme. The disequilibrium that ensues is resolved by a major revision of the scheme to accommodate the information that a strong and courageous man can also express tender feelings. From a clinical standpoint, this is an example that could conceivably result in a behavioral change as the hypothetical adult under discussion can now with logical consistency express tender feelings toward others without risk of labeling himself as unmanly.

We have been discussing what Piaget refers to as the equilibrating process. It is this process through which Piaget explains both short-term changes within stages and long-term changes from one major stage to the next. It is important to recognize that the self-regulating process through which the individual goes beyond a state of disequilibrium to a new state of equilibrium always involes a reorganization of cognitive structures to a higher level of conceptual development. Piaget is not talking merely about a homeostatic mechanism leading to the reduction of tension or cognitive dissonance that restores a former balance. Rather, the elimination of inconsistencies produces a new equilibrium characterized by a greater capacity for problem-solving behavior, an increased understanding of some aspects of the world, a widening perspective, and a decreased basis for disequilibrium from new disturbances. This is true to some extent for within-stage changes but even more so for developmental shifts from one complete stage to the next.

Inhelder, Sinclair, and Bovet (1974) and Piaget (1974/1980a) have produced a number of instructive training studies designed to promote their subjects' cognitive understanding and growth based on a contradiction-inducing strategy. The strategy moves the subject to a state of disequilibrium and triggers the self-regulating process.

## SOCIAL-COGNITIVE DEVELOPMENT

The field of social cognition is a burgeoning one (Fiske & Taylor, 1984). It deals with an individual's thinking about other people, her or his own self, social customs and institutions, and moral judgments. A developmental approach to the subject is quite wide-ranging (Damon, 1977, 1978; Flavell and Ross, 1981; Furth, 1980; Overton, 1983; Selman, 1980; Shantz, 1975, 1983; Youmiss, 1980). Development in the area of social cognition mirrors the child's construction of knowledge of the physical world (Flavell, 1985). It proceeds from conceptions based on the surface appearances and behavior of others to making inferences about their feelings, intentions, and motives.

Egocentrism, the inability to take another's point of view, particularly when it differs from one's own, is a serious cognitive flaw that sharply limits an individual's ability to effect good interpersonal relationships and achieve personal goals in a social world. Piaget (1923/1955) observed that the speech of preoperational children is largely egocentric insofar as it does not adequately take into account the informational needs of the listener or exhibit any attempt to verify its assertions. Sociocentric speech, which is listener-adapted, overtakes egocentric speech by 6 or 7 years of age. It is at this time that the child is acquiring the ability to decenter from his or her own viewpoint and to see things from another's perspective. Flavell (1985) suggests that we are ''at risk'' for egocentrism all of our lives. The alert clinician would do well to assess for degrees of egocentric speech in those clients with interpersonal problems and certainly when doing couples therapy.

Working within a Piagetian framework, Selman (1976, 1980) has formulated a model of developmental stages describing interpersonal perspective taking. As he describes it, ''Each advanced level of perspective taking represents a shift, qualitative in nature, in the child's understanding of persons and of the relationship between self's and others' points of view and hence of selves and others'' (1980, p. 49). Selman's cognitive-structural model of perspective taking can be utilized helpfully in clinical practice with the aim of promoting more effective social reasoning. Urbain and Kendall (1980) have presented a review of social-cognitive problem-solving interventions, including perspective-taking training.

Kohlberg (1969, 1971, 1981, 1984), using a Piagetian theoretical orientation, has formulated a major stage theory of moral development, based upon both longitudinal and cross-cultural research. In Kohlberg's theory, the developing ability to take the perspective of another is a critical factor in the individual's evolving conception of justice or fairness, which is at the heart of moral reasoning. Given the centrality of fairness in human relationships, Kohlberg's work merits the attention of all clinicians. Efforts at promoting moral development from a cognitive-structural viewpoint have been successful, utilizing Piaget's equilibration model as a guide to designing interventions (Rosen, 1980).

Cognitive therapy techniques designed to foster objectivity and alternate perspectives (Beck *et al.*, 1979; Beck & Emery, 1985) are related to the social-cognitive developmental field, and a familiarity with it may prove useful to the practicing therapist.

### THE COGNITIVE-AFFECTIVE CONNECTION

The question of the relationship between affect and cognition has received a good deal of attention (Beck, 1976; Ellis, 1962; Izard, 1979; Lazarus, 1982, 1984; Zajonc, 1980, 1984).

Piaget has had very little to say directly about affect, but his main accounting of the subject appears in a book based on a set of lectures he gave at the Sorbonne years ago (Piaget, 1954/1981). Affect can influence the pace of cognitive development, but it cannot have any bearing on the sequence of development or the nature of a cognitive structure. For example, the number structure is a synthesis of classification and relation structures. Because it is a logical necessity that classes and relations be understood before one can organize these two structures into a number structure, then it follows that the order of understanding and development cannot be altered by feeling. Similarly, 2 plus 2 will always equal 4 regardless of how one feels about this fact.

Cognition and affect are conceived of by Piaget as being inseparable but distinct. Affect supplies the energetic component of cognitive activity. It provides the curiosity and interest necessary to start and maintain the cognitive endeavor. It is the source of the satisfaction of a task well-executed or the frustration of a flawed attempt. For Piaget, human cognitive activity never occurs without some element of emotion. On the other hand, there can be no emotion without cognition. Cognitive structures give shape and direction to our emotions. They impart limits to the range across which affect can apply. For example, the emotions of a concrete operational child are confined to the known and familiar, such as her own friends, family, neighborhood, and church. With the advent of formal operations, however, the scope of what the youngster can have feelings about enlarges considerably to include such abstract entities as universal sisterhood, the "Mother Church," political ideologies, and the love of mankind.

Further formulations on affect in relation to Piaget's work can be found in Piaget (1962b, 1964/1968), Greenspan (1979), Cowan (1982), Kegan (1982), Siomopoulos (1983), and Fast (1985).

# PSYCHOTHERAPEUTIC IMPLICATIONS

### OVERVIEW

Cognitive therapy may be defined as that psychotherapeutic approach that intentionally proceeds from a cognitive theoretical orientation with the aim of seeking cognitive change through the use of cognitive strategies and techniques. The cognitive change is believed to yield affective and behavioral changes in areas of problem functioning for the individual. In a similar vein, cognitive-structural change in the Piagetian paradigm is seen to produce adaptive changes in the realms of affective, interpersonal, and problem-solving functioning.

Piagetian theory certainly has an in-depth cognitive orientation, and it has demonstrated a strong interest in the cognitive change process. The equilibration model, based on perceived contradiction and cognitive conflict, has been advanced by Piaget to explain cognitive development. The principle of contradiction creating a disequilibrating experience that fosters development has been adopted by Piagetians as a change strategy in many successful training studies (Cowan, 1978; Inhelder, Sinclair, & Bovet, 1974). Nevertheless, Piaget's theory does not constitute a psychotherapeutic system. The aim of this final section is to illuminate some implications of Piaget's theory for therapy generally and its interlocking relationship to Beck's model of cognitive therapy in particular. I do not regard this effort as translating Beck's model into an alternative language system or frame of reference. Instead, it is my contention that embedded in the model are the Piagetian concepts and principles being addressed. Beck *et al.* (1979) has alluded to this in his own work. The goal here is to make more explicit and to amplify upon that which is already implicit in Beck's formulation of cognitive therapy. Beck's approach has been chosen from among the range of cognitive therapies also because of its combined conceptual sophistication and research grounding. The reader is referred to Guidano and Liotti (1983), Leva (1984), and Ivey (1986) for their comments on integrating Piaget's work with cognitive therapy. Rosen (1985) has also discussed the links between Piaget's work and cognitive therapy. In this exposition, a familiarity with Beck's approach will be presupposed.

## PIAGETIAN IMPLICATIONS FOR PSYCHOTHERAPY

A therapy based upon Piaget's theory would not be neutral or value-free with respect to broad goal setting. It would aim at deep structural change (Arnkoff, 1980), ultimately moving the client toward higher cognitive stage development (Piaget, 1974/1980a), more advanced social reasoning (Selman, 1980), and furthering a self–other balance (Kegan, 1982). The rationale is that later stages of development are more adequate than earlier stages; that some ways of knowing-in-the-world are better than others. Through cognitive development, the client acquires new and wider perspectives, problem-solving competence, capacity for self-awareness, emotional stability and order, interpersonal reasoning, and overall adaptiveness. Thus the achievement of cognitive-structural change imparts greater autonomy and efficacy to the client, whereas the content to which he or she applies these attributes is a matter of his or her own choice. Because many people do not perform fully at the level of competence they have attained, it would be a perfectly legitimate goal to assist clients in the activation and more potent use of cognitive structures at the level of development they have already achieved. Leva (1984), commenting not on major stage shifts but upon short-range goals, states that therapy tends

> toward a higher degree of equilibration in specific problem areas or on specific structural levels. . . . Since the cognitive system normally works self-sufficiently, therapy's goal is to reestablish self-regulation. (pp. 239–240)

The reinstitution of cognitive self-regulation is at the core of her application of Piagetian principles to cognitive-behavioral therapy.

### Matching Communication to Stage

Communication is central to all psychotherapies, and meaning is central to all communications. Therefore, from a Piagetian perspective, it is essential to understand that information transmitted from therapist to client will be transformed in a way that is congruent with the latters cognitive-developmental level. As Jurkovic and Selman (1980) point out, "Structural-development theory may represent a useful paradigm for ordering therapist communication into a developmental hierarchy" (p. 105). The directive to the therapist is that she or he must be familiar with her or his client's epistemology and adjust her or his communications to it. If she or he does otherwise, the client will either ignore it or distort it by assimilating it without accommodation. This phenomenon offers an alternative explanation to the psychoanalytic assumption that an interpretation offered by the therapist is being resisted when it is not readily accepted by the client. The use of metaphors in psychotherapy is receiving increasing attention in modern practice (Barker, 1985; Beck & Emery, 1985; Gordon, 1978). However, the therapist should be cognizant of the fact that analogies and metaphors, particularly extended ones, will require formal thought for full comprehension. After all, is *Moby Dick* a book, a tale of adventure at sea, or an allegory of good and evil? As with communications, treatment interventions of any kind should be designed to take into account the client's level of cognitive development. Examples of doing so can be found in Selman (1980), Kegan (1982), Bobbitt and Keating (1983), Cohen and Schlesser (1984), and Gholson and Rosenthal (1984).

### Role of the Therapist

The role of the therapist in cognitive therapy is an active one with Socratic questioning and the behavioral experiment being two major therapeutic tactics (Weishaar & Beck, 1986). Implicit in Piaget (1974/1976) would be just such a recommendation to the therapist (Tenzer, 1983), with specific similarities to those therapist behaviors advocated by Beck. The Piagetian therapist's role would be analogous to the experimenter who organizes studies that aim to see if children's understanding of new concepts can be accelerated. A secure climate is established in which the subject is invited to explore, predict, look, think, grapple, experiment, recognize, and comprehend. Questions are posed to stimulate the subject's own thinking process with the aim of facilitating the construction of endogenous knowledge. The giving of information and promotion of associationistic learning would have a low priority. Piaget sees the roots of the scientific attitude, with its persistent curiosity and seeking to understand, in infancy. In the same spirit, Beck advocates inducting the client into becoming a "personal scientist," whereas "the task of the therapy is to rekindle curiosity, inquiry, and rationality" (Wright & Beck, 1983, p. 1122).

### Maintenance and Generalization

A critical issue in psychotherapy of any kind is that of maintaining and generalizing gains (Goldstein, Lopez, & Greenleaf, 1979; Kazdin, 1978). All too often, apparent therapeutic improvement does not extend from the office to other contexts or beyond the termination of treatment. The same concern is addressed in Piaget's work from the standpoint of cognitive growth. It is proposed that durability, generalizability, and resistance to extinction can be achieved in cognitive development through structural transformation rather than surface learning (Piaget, 1964; Smedslund, 1961a). Relating this to Beck's model of therapy, successful transformation and reorganization of maladaptive assumptions, which are equivalent to deep structures, are more likely to lead to permanence and transfer of therapeutic gains than working only on the level of automatic thoughts, which are equivalent to surface structures. In one sense, attacking negative automatic thoughts only, is like cutting off the head of the hydra only to see two heads grow in its place. It is necessary to get at its core or heart to stop the heads from growing. However, focusing on negative automatic thoughts does serve as one route to inferring maladaptive assumptions and in doing so also provides an excellent training ground for the client to become aware of and understand the types of cognitive errors he or she engages in. Metacognition, thinking about one's own reasoning strategies, is a growing area within the field of cognitive development (Flavell, 1978, 1979; Flavell & Wellman, 1977; Forrest-Presley, MacKinnon, & Waller, 1985). It is precisely the activity of metacognizing that the cognitive therapist invites the client to pursue when drawing the client's attention to the kinds of cognitive errors that undergird negative automatic thoughts. This higher level cognitive activity enables the client to restrain, modify, and eliminate his or her use of such errors. Skill at thinking about one's own thinking, most fully developed in formal operational thought, is a competence also likely to facilitate the transfer of gains across contexts and beyond treatment termination. As with all developing cognitive competencies, less advanced forms of metacognition are in evidence before the final stage of development (Flavell, 1985; Robinson, 1983; Wellman, 1985). In working with adult clients, the therapist would do well to realize that they will show variation in abilities to metacognize, as not all will possess formal operational capabilities.

### Primitive Cognitions and Preoperational Thought

The cognitions of psychologically disordered patients can be examined from the viewpoint of their resemblance to preoperational thought (Beck *et al.*, 1979; Guidano & Liotti, 1983). Precausal thinking is present, sometimes pervasive, in many patients. Beck and Emery (1985) cite an example of magical thinking: "I sat in this chair at the doctor's office and nothing had happened before, so I always sit in the same chair" (p. 299). This is like the preoperational child who will say that a pebble sank in the water because it is brown. The elements linked together simply have no logical or causal connection. Precausal thinking can also be seen in the cognitive error of misattribution, an example of which might be a depressed patient attributing the blame for being unemployed to his own actions when, in fact, the real cause is the mismanagement of funds by his employer, which led to the downfall of the business. In a word, the preoperational thinker sees relationships where none exist. Much of primitive thought in adults, like the preoperational thought it is rooted in, is globular and absolute. Depressed or anxious patients all too frequently can be found calling themselves "worthless," "stupid," "fearful," and "anxious." They do not differentiate with respect to time, place, or intensity. The anxiety-laden patient is not likely to say, "I have more anxiety when I mix with strangers at parties than when I am with colleagues at work, but less anxiety than when I have to give a report before my boss and his administrative staff." The contextual and relational nature of his anxiety is not recognized. It is one task of therapy to help him recognize it. The individual with a phobia does not ordinarily view his problem with reversible thinking, but, rather, he sees the problem as irreversible. He would have difficulty saying and believing, "There was a time when I was not afraid to cross bridges, and I can return to that unafraid state again." Feelings become indicators of reality for many disturbed people. They reason that if they feel guilty, then they must be guilty of something; if they feel anxious, then there is really something out there to be afraid of. This is very suggestive of the preoperational turn of mind called realism, in which a subjective psychic element, such as a dream or a name, is accorded external, objective existence. Patients distressed by anxiety often use imagery in a way that can be described by realism. For example, someone with an image of driving off a bridge and plunging into the water below may respond as if the image is the precursor of that event as it actually will occur in the future.

People with problems around anger frequently do not decenter from their own point of view to look at the situation from the other's perspective; to reciprocally take into account the feelings, intentions, and motives of the other. The incapacity and, therefore, failure to do this is typical of the preoperational child. The chronically angry adult is likely to have many cognitions such as "He shouldn't have done that," "He's uncaring and insensitive," and "What right does he have to take that," all with little understanding about what the "offender" might have to say in justification of his actions. Suffice it to say at this point that, from a cognitive-developmental perspective, the source of primitive thought in adults is to be found in the preoperational period, characterized by centration, irreversibility, absolutism, precausality, realism, and egocentrism.

Adults who function with primitive cognitions in disturbed areas are not likely to be totally in the preoperational period developmentally. Beck posits that dormant primitive cognitive schemes trigger negative automatic thoughts when areas of the individuals personal domain are impinged upon by events in the environment, especially stressful ones. Autoregulation through rational and causal thought is overriden by the frequency and intensity of negative automatic thoughts. The goal of the therapist is to employ treatment strategies and techniques that will restore objective, decentered thought to the patient's personal domain.

### THE CHANGE MECHANISM IN COGNITIVE THERAPY

The field of psychotherapy is rife with speculation on what produces change. There are theories pertaining to common elements that cut across all therapies (Goldfried, 1982) and others that identify specific mechanisms that are believed to be unique to particular models (Corsini, 1981). Raimy (1975) proposes that regardless of the model or its techniques, cognitive modification is what ultimately accounts for change. By its very nature, Beck's model of cognitive therapy intentionally seeks cognitive change through the use of cognitive techniques. Indeed, research supports the efficacy of this model (Kovacs, Rush, Beck, & Hollon, 1981; Rush, Beck, Kovacs, & Hollon, 1977), particularly in the treatment of depression, although the model has been used to treat other problems as well. However, to suggest that cognitive techniques work because they cause cognitive change does not resolve the more precise question of the nature of the cognitive change.

The equilibration theory of Piaget (1975/1977) and the experimental research supporting it (Inhelder, *et al.* 1974; Piaget 1974/1976, 1974/1980b) point to cognitive conflict (perceived contradictions, inconsistencies, discrepancies, and incongruities) and reflexive abstraction as that which generate change and development. In one way or another, all psychotherapies expose the patient to disequilibrating experiences, which in turn lead to attempts at achieving a more adaptive balance than previously held. Ivey (1986) states,

> Psychotherapy could be defined as the art of effective perturbation—the art of confronting client discrepancies and contradictions wisely and accurately and in a timely fashion. Effective confrontation of client behavior is a major precursor to growth, development, and later integration of new knowledge and skills. (pp. 192–193)

An examination of Beck's cognitive approach readily highlights the primary role of contradiction in its strategies and techniques. The behavioral experiment in cognitive therapy is designed to have the patient test-out a prediction or expectation, based on a belief or cognitive scheme. When disconfirmed, the patient is confronted with a contradiction between prediction (a belief about the world) and outcome (the structure of the world). The subjective sense of disturbance or disequilibrium, accompanied by surprise and curiosity, fuels efforts toward structural accommodation and increased understanding, which in turn will lead to more adaptive beliefs and behavior. Referring to one source of contradiction in Piaget's equilibration model, Gallagher (1978) states:

> A major source is the request for the child to anticipate the outcome of an event. There is no disturbance if the discrepancy is ignored. If there is an awareness of the contradiction between the prediction and the observation, however, such an awareness is the basis for the projection to a new level of understanding and a reordering or reequilibration. (pp. 17–18)

The point made here about the possibility of the discrepancy being ignored is not inconsequential. From a developmental perspective, without the appropriate cognitive-structural framework, the individual will not be in a position to interpret the discrepancy as a contradiction. Therefore, he or she will not experience the disequilibrium and impetus that lead to reequilibration and greater understanding. This is emphasized in the work by Piaget (1974/1976) on the grasp of consciousness in which children who perform correctly on a behavioral plane offer incorrect verbal explanations for what they are doing. Even when, upon observation, it first becomes evident that what they are doing is different from what their "theory" states they are doing, the children reject the contradictory evidence and persist in claiming the validity of their theory. Such mental dynamics are not dissimilar from what adult scientists have been known to engage in when evidence contradicting their fundamental beliefs first becomes manifest (Kuhn, 1972; Mahoney, 1976). The denial and distortion of that which contradicts prior theory may precede the appropriate revision or abandonment of that theory. The cognitive therapist who anticipates and understands such activity as part of the process will be better equipped to maintain her or his own equilibrium when it occurs.

Another major source of contradiction as postulated in Piaget's equilibration model is the incompatibility between two subsystems or schemes. The same mental organization embraces two separate and opposing rules or premises. When these opposing cognitive schemes are brought into direct action against one another (Kuhn, 1972; Inhelder *et al.*, 1974; Smedslund, 1961b; Walker, 1983), the occasion for disequilibrium and cognitive reorganization arises. The cognitive therapist utilizes the Socratic method to help the patient discern the absurdities and incongruencies among many of his or her firmly held assumptions, as well as automatic negative thoughts. Shaw and Beck (1977) observe, "Questioning is a major tool . . . to expose inner contradiction, inconsistencies, and logical flaws in the patient's conclusions. A well-timed properly phrased question may serve to open a closed belief system" (p. 311). Now compare that statement to one by Inhelder *et al.* (1974) on attempting to resolve conflicting schemes: "Questions and discussions at certain crucial points in the learning process can induce an awareness of contradictions, and provide the impetus for higher-level coordinations leading to new cognitive structures" (p. 167).

We have dealt here with two major cognitive therapy strategies, designing a behavioral experiment and logical analysis. However, an inspection of many specific cognitive therapy techniques would reveal that they also serve to highlight discrepancies and inconsistencies in the patient's thought process and belief systems. Piagetian experiments explicitly researching the cognitive dynamics of development lend direct support to those methods employed in the cognitive therapy model.

## PIAGETIAN STRATEGIES OF INTERVENTION

Piaget's theory with its emphasis upon contradiction and disequilibrium offers a guide for designing intervention strategies that are not necessarily linked to any particular system of psychotherapy. The general rule would be to engage the client in experiences that promote perceived discrepancies, leading to active efforts toward constructive resolutions. We have already recognized that all psychotherapies do this to some extent. However, by extrapolating the general principle, the therapist is free to design new tactics that are not wedded to any one school in practice, althought the theoretical explanation remains within a cognitive-structural framework.

Let us explore a hypothetical example of a depressed adult who believes that a person is worthless unless someone loves him. Asked whether he thinks a scientist who has discovered a cure for cancer is worthwhile, he responds in the affirmative. Combining the two features, he is now confronted with what is to him the contradiction of a hypothetical unloved scientist who is, nevertheless, worthwhile. In an adaptation from a Piagetian task with children, the therapist can actually go further by devising 12 little wooden men who are identified as scientists. Ten of them are marked "loved," and 2 of them are marked "unloved." Each is said to have discovered a new cure for a disease that has plagued mankind for years. The patient is now asked to put all the worthwhile scientists on one side and all the unloved ones, who by implication are not worthwhile, on the opposite side. The logical and physical impossibility of performing this very concrete task that contradicts his beliefs creates a disequilibrium that demands resolution. Weiner (1985), using a Piagetian framework, has designed over 200 puzzling tasks that he uses in the therapeutic hour to help the client acquire greater self-understanding and competence. Commenting upon Piaget's theory of cognitive growth, Weiner (1985) states,

> These growth inducing processes have been identified as essential ingredients in therapeutic change. . . . [They] can serve as points of departure for independent development and reformulation of therapeutic method and technique, and leave room for the individual practioner to apply the processes creatively and to develop a unique style. (p. xix)

Inherent in the therapeutic dialogue itself is an infinite potential for the imaginative therapist to play a disequilibrating role, as intuitive therapists of all schools have been doing all along. The point is that a metacognitive knowledge of the change process under discussion expands its utility as it can then be applied not only intuitively, but with intentionality.

Cognitive developmentalists have been actively involved in perspective-taking training. Perspective taking involves the ability to see things from another's viewpoint, to coordinate that viewpoint with one's own, and to recognize that the other is capable of reciprocally taking one's own viewpoint. A developmental deficiency in this skill can lead to serious interpersonal problems in work and love as it greatly impedes the capacity for social reasoning. Most of the training thus far, although successful, has been with children and adolescents (Chandler, 1973; Chandler, Greenspan, & Barenboim, 1974; Ianotti, 1978; Selman, 1980; Silvern, Waterman, Sobesky, & Ryan, 1979). However, this is a potentially fruitful field to extend into work with adults. A departure from effective perspective taking can be seen in the cognitive distortion of "mind reading" in which the client assumes that he knows what it is that the other is thinking. Stages of perspective taking do not involve knowing the content of another's viewpoint but rather represent structural advances that enable one to decenter from his own viewpoint and take increasingly more objective perspectives than one's own. For example, Selman's third-person perspective-taking stage is one in which an individual can assume the role of a hypothetical onlooker observing the role of that individual and another interacting. The hypothetical third-person perspective allows the individual to coordinate his and the other's actions. A therapist working with someone diagnosed as low in perspective taking may want to raise a series of questions designed to facilitate having the patient decenter from his own viewpoint and adopt alternate ones. Such questions as, "How would you feel in his shoes?", "What do you think it might have been like for her?", "What would you need to know about each other to resolve this conflict?", and "How do you think it would look to her, bearing in mind that she doesn't have the information you have about the situation?" would be useful. A great diversity of such questions can be generated and posed over a period of time. A more active method that has been successfully employed has been to have members of a group rotate through the enactment of each role in a skit and then to discuss with one another what it felt like and how they saw things from the perspective of each character portrayed (Chandler *et al.*, 1974). The skit involved can be crafted expressly to encompass the problems and dilemmas participants are experiencing. The most fine-grained clinical work to date on perspective taking has been conducted by Selman (1980).

A particularly important aspect of Selman's work pertains to the fact that, as children move through cognitive stages, their ability to understand emotions in self and others undergoes a progression of increasingly greater complexity. Initially a child has no concept of self-deception. At the next stage, he or she realizes that it is possible to have hidden emotions that are other then what one presents socially. From this, he or she evolves a more abstract conceptualization of a self-reflexive mind; of a mind that seeks to understand itself. In a fourth and final stage, with the aid of formal thought, he or she constructs a schema for understanding the mind, predicated upon a concept of the unconscious. There are alternative ways of conceiving of an unconscious (Bowers & Meichenbaum, 1984), and the schema or silent assumption structural theory in Beck's model is one of them. The therapist need not be wedded to the notion of a dynamic unconscious as formulated by Freud. The significance of Selman's model even in working with adults is that the therapist cannot assume an equal capacity among patients for self-awareness. Cognitive therapists generally attempt to socialize patients into the therapeutic context by explaining the theoretical underpinnings of the cognitive model that guides their work. However, it is dubious that patients who have not developed to the stage of constructing a concept of the unconscious will fully comprehend the role of silent assumptions in emotional disturbances. Psychotherapists have sometimes been too quick to dismiss a "difficult" patient as lacking psychological mindedness. Selman's cognitive-structural developmental portrait offers a more highly differentiated way of looking at this phenomenon. It suggests that, if therapists were to adapt their communications and expectations to the patient's stage-level capacity for self-awareness, then the therapeutic process would be more likely to run smoothly.

The cognitive moral developmental theory of Kohlberg (1969, 1971, 1981, 1984) has generated an enormous amount of research over the last several decades. There has been a practical side to it that has involved promoting stage progression, largely in populations found in schools and prisons. Because of the centrality of issues concerning fairness and respect for persons, which define the moral stages, hierarchical progression through the stages is important to ordinary relationships, family matters, and societal welfare. Turiel (1966), in a laboratory experiment, was successful in facilitating stage growth in subjects by presenting them with two opposing solutions of moral dilemmas; each of the solutions was one stage beyond the moral-stage reasoning capacity of the subjects. He theorized that the disequilibrium induced by the inconsistency created through the strategy led to a more adaptive reorganization of the subjects' moral stage. Presenting opposing solutions that were either one stage below or two stages above subjects in control groups did not lead to any significant changes. In the former case, the subjects' moral stage was already more adequate than the proposed solutions, and, in the latter case, no disequilibrium ensued because the solutions were too far advanced to be comprehended. Because there is always some stage mixture in development, the experimental subjects were able to glimpse the meaning in the solutions one stage beyond their dominant stage and to perceive the inconsistency between the two stages. Attempts to eliminate the inconsistency and emerge with a more adaptive capability led to moral-stage progress.

Hickey and Scharf (1980) have reported on their successful attempts to channel Kohlberg's moral theory and the equilibrating model as a change strategy into the prison system. Their field of operation extended far beyond Turiel's laboratory experiment to encompass the creation of intensive communities of prisoners who engaged in group discussions around moral dilemmas and the democratic forging of just policies. In the words of Hickey and Scharf (1980),

> Instead of seeking to gain insight into the inmates "hang-ups" or changing their "antisocial behavior," we sought to stimulate their conception of their moral relationships with their friends, family, and peers. We hoped to offer a new therapy based on the ideals of the socratic dialogue rather than on those of the "depth" psychology of Freud or the "mechanistic" behaviorism of Watson or Skinner. (p. 46)

In order to arrive at the fourth stage of moral development, an individual must be at least in the early phase of formal thought. However, being in the formal operational period does not necessitate that the individual will be at the fourth or higher stages of moral development. It follows from this that many people will not be at a moral stage that corresponds to their level of cognitive development. Taking this into account, I would suggest that the stimulation of cognitive-structural moral development is a proper sphere of activity for the cognitive therapist to engage in, as it would enhance the quality of interpersonal and familial relationships.

HUGH ROSEN

Piaget's work has proven to possess enormous heuristic value. Even many who are at variance with some or all of his theories are exploring questions and issues that have arisen only because of the Piagetian paradigm. One area to which his work can be extended fruitfully is that of psychotherapy and, in particular, cognitive therapy. The field of cognitive therapy is a robust and evolving one. Perhaps because it has sought to emphasize the present over the past, with the notable exception of Guidano and Liotti (1983), the theoretical foundation of cognitive therapy models has lacked a strong developmental component. However, it is not necessary to abandon a present-centered stance to treatment in order to understand and apply the cognitive dynamics of Piaget's constructionist psychology. It is precisely the patient's present level of cognitive competence and performance, within a developmental framework, to which the therapist will want to be attentive.

In summary, I would like to cite the major contributions of Piaget's paradigm that have been discussed in the present chapter: (1) Therapeutic communications and interventions should be adapted to the client's developmental stage for optimal effectiveness. (2) To maximize generalization and maintenance, it is desirable to foster cognitive-structural change. (3) Piaget's theory provides a fine-grained description of the cognitive developmental stages that are implied and embedded in Beck's cognitive therapy model. (4) The equilibration model offers a guide to understanding effective therapeutic change processes and a strategy for designing new techniques based on its principles of contradiction and conflict. (5) Piaget's theory lends theoretical and empirical support to the major techniques in Beck's model insofar as they are based on disequilibrating tactics.

Despite the strong connections between Piaget's and Beck's work there are limitations that should be recognized. Piaget was primarily a genetic epistemologist. He pursued the nature of knowledge—its origins and development. The focus of his theory and research was exclusively upon infants, children, and adolescents. He disavowed any personal interest in psychopathology and chose instead to study normal development. He had very little to say about affect, and most of his work dealt with the child's construction of the physical world. In contrast, Beck is a clinician who has had a major interest in psychopathology generally and who is a world-renowned expert on depression. His theoretical work and clinical practice focus not upon children but upon adults. Although his theory is cognitively oriented, much of his attention has been devoted to describing affect and its link to cognition. Finally, although Piaget focused upon the study of universal cognitive-structural development, Beck, whether focusing upon content or structure, addressed idiographic features of the individual's cognition. These striking differences impose limits to the extent that Piaget's and Beck's work can be thoroughly integrated. However, those connections that have been drawn are clear and strong. It is worth noting that the lack of emphasis in Piaget's work on affect, social cognition, and psychopathology is being reversed today by many cognitive-developmental researchers, both in the United States and abroad.

If Piaget had been interested in developing a system of psychotherapy, he may well have conceptualized something closely resembling Beck's model of cognitive therapy. Couched in the framework of Piaget's genetic epistemology, cognitive therapy loses none of its vitality and efficacy, yet it acquires even greater theoretical depth and developmental dimensions.

# REFERENCES

Arnkoff, D. B. (1980). Psychotherapy from the perspective of cognitive therapy. In M. J. Mahoney (Ed.), *Psychotherapy process* (pp. 339–361) New York: Plenum Press.

Barker, P. (1985). *Using metaphors in psychotherapy*. New York: Brunner/Mazel.

Beck, A. T. (1976). *Cognitive therapy and the emotional disorders*. New York: International Universities Press.

Beck, A. T., & Emery, G. (1985). *Anxiety disorders and phobias: A cognitive perspective.* New York: Basic Books.

Beck, A. T., Rush, A. J., Shaw, B. F., & Emery, G. (1979). *Cognitive therapy of depression.* New York, Guilford.

Bobbit, B. L., & Keating, D. P. (1983). A cognitive-developmental perspective for clinical research and practice. In P. C. Kendall (Ed.), *Advances in cognitive behavioral research and therapy* (pp. 198–239). New York: Academic Press.

Bowers, K. S., & Meichenbaum, D. (Eds.). (1984). *The unconscious reconsidered.* New York: Wiley.

Chandler, M. J. (1973). Egocentrism and anti-social behavior: The assessment and training of social perspective-taking skills. *Developmental Psychology, 9,* 326–332.

Chandler, M. J., Greenspan, S., & Barenboim, C. (1974). Assessment and training of role-taking and referential communication skills in institutionalized emotionally disturbed children. *Developmental Psychology, 10,* 546–553.

Cohen, R., & Scheleser, R. (1984). Clinical development and clinical interventions. In A. W. Meyers & W. E. Craighead (Eds.), *Cognitive behavior therapy with children* (pp. 45–68). New York: Plenum Press.

Corsini, R. J. (Ed.). (1981). *Handbook of innovative psychotherapies.* New York: Wiley.

Cowan, P. A. (1978). *Piaget with feeling.* New York: Holt, Rinehart & Winston.

Cowan, P. A. (1982). The relationship between emotional and cognitive development. n D. Cicchetti & P. Hesse (Eds.). *New directions for child development: Emotional development,* No. 16 (pp. 49–81). San Francisco: Jossey-Bass.

Damon, W. (1977). *The social world of the child.* San Francisco: Jossey-Bass.

Damon, W. (Ed.). (1978). *New directions for child development: Social cognition,* No. 1. San Francisco: Jossey-Bass.

Elkind, D. (1967). Egocentrism in adolescence. *Child Development, 38,* 1025–1034.

Elkind, D. (1974). *Children and adolescents: Interpretive essays on Jean Piaget.* New York: Oxford University Press.

Ellis, A. (1962). *Reason and emotion in psychotherapy.* New York: Lyle Stuart.

Fast, I. (1985). *Event theory: A Piaget-Freud integration.* Hillsdale, NJ: Erlbaum.

Fiske, S. L., & Taylor, S. E. (1984). *Social cognition.* Reading, MA: Addison-Wesley.

Flavell, J. H. (1977). *Cognitive development.* Englewood Cliffs, NJ: Prentice-Hall.

Flavell, J. H. (1978). Metacognitive development. In J. M. Scandura & C. J. Brainerd (Eds.), *Structural process theories of complex human behavior.* Alphen ad Rign, the Netherlands: Sijtoff & Noordhuff.

Flavell, J. H. (1979). Metacognition and cognitive monitoring. *American Psychologist, 34,* 906–911.

Flavell, J. H. (1985). *Cognitive development* (2nd ed.). Englewood Cliffs, NJ: Prentice-Hall.

Flavell, J. H. (1986). The development of children's knowledge about the appearance-reality distinction. *American Psychologist, 41,* 418–425.

Flavell, J. H., & Ross, L. (Eds.). (1981). *Social cognitive development: Frontiers and possible futures.* New York: Cambridge University Press.

Flavell, J. H., & Wellman, H. M. (1977). Metamemory. In R. V. Kail, Jr., & J. W. Hagen (Eds.), *Perspectives on the development of memory and cognition* (pp. 3–33). Hillsdale, NJ: Lawrence Erlbaum.

Forrest-Pressley, D. L., MacKinnon, G. E., & Waller, T. G. (Eds.). (1985). *Metacognition, cognition, and human performance.* New York: Academic Press.

Furth, H. G. (1980). *The world of grown-ups: Children's conceptions of society.* New York: Elsevier.

Gallagher, J. M. (1978). Reflexive abstraction and education: The meaning of activity in Piaget's theory. In J. M. Gallagher & J. A. Easley (Eds.), *Knowledge and development. Vol 2: Piaget and education* (pp. 1–20). New York: Plenum Press.

Gholson, B., & Rosenthal, T. L. (Eds.). (1984). *Applications of cognitive-developmental theory.* New York: Academic Press.

Goldfried, M. R. (Ed.). (1982). *Converging themes in psychotherapy.* New York: Springer.

Goldstein, A. P., Lopez, M., & Greenleaf, D. O. (1979). Introduction. In A. P. Goldstein & F. H. Kanfer (Eds.), *Maximizing treatment gains: Transfer enhancement in psychotherapy* (pp. 1–22). New York: Academic Press.

Gordon, D. (1978). *Therapeutic metaphors.* Cupertino, CA: META Publications.

Greenspan, S. I. (1979). *Intelligence and adaptation.* New York: International Universities Press.

Guidano, V. F., & Liotti, G. (1983). *Cognitive processes and emotional disorders.* New York: Guilford.

Haroutunian, S. (1983). *Equilibrium in the balance: A study of psychological explanation.* New York: Springer-Verlag.

Hesse, P., & Cicchetti, D. (1982). Perspectives on an integrated theory of emotional development. In D.

Cicchetti & P. Hesse (Eds.), *New Directions for child development: Emotional development*, No. 16 (pp. 3–48). San Francisco: Jossey-Bass.

Hickey, J. E., & Scharf, P. L. (1980). *Toward a just correctional system*. San Francisco: Jossey-Bass.

Ianotti, R. J. (1978). Effects of role-taking experiences on role-taking, empathy, altruism and aggression. *Developmental Psychology, 14*, 119–124.

Inhelder, B., & Piaget, J. (1958). *The growth of logical thinking from childhood to adolescence* (A. Parsons & S. Milgram, Trans.). New York: Basic Books. (Originally published 1955)

Inhelder, B., & Piaget, J. (1969). *The early growth of logic in the child* (E. A. Lunzer & D. Papert, Trans.). New York: Norton. (Originally published 1959)

Inhelder, B., Sinclair, H., & Bovet, M. (1974). *Learning and the development of cognition* (S. Wedgwood, Trans.). Cambridge, MA: Harvard University Press.

Ivey, A. E. (1986). *Developmental therapy*. San Francisco: Jossey-Bass.

Izard, C. E. (Ed.). (1979). *Emotions in personality and psychopathology*. New York: Plenum Press.

Jurkovic, G. J., & Selman, R. L. (1980). A developmental analysis of intrapsychic understanding: Treating emotional disturbances in children. In R. L. Selman & R. Yando (Eds.), *New directions for child development: Clinical-developmental psychology*, No. 7 (pp. 91–112). San Francisco: Jossey-Bass.

Kazdin, A. (1978). *History of behavior modifications: Experimental foundations of contemporary research*. Baltimore: University Park Press.

Kegan, R. (1982). *The evolving self*. Cambridge, MA: Harvard University Press.

Kohlberg, L. (1969). Stage and sequence: The cognitive developmental approach to socialization. In D. A. Goslin (Ed.), *Handbook of socialization theory and research* (pp. 347–480). Chicago: Rand McNally.

Kohlberg, L. (1971). From is to ought: How to commit the naturalistic fallacy and get away with it in the study of moral development. In T. Mischel (Ed.), *Cognitive development and epistemology* (pp. 151–235). New York: Academic Press.

Kohlberg, L. (1981). *Essays on moral development, Vol. 1, The philosophy of moral development*. San Francisco: Harper & Row.

Kohlberg, L. (1984). *Essays on moral development, Vol. 2, The psychology of moral development*. San Francisco: Harper & Row.

Kovacs, M. J., Rush, A. T., & Hollon, S. D. (1981). Depressed outpatients treated with cognitive therapy in pharmacotherapy. *Archives of General Psychiatry, 38*, 33–39.

Kuhn, D. (1972). Mechanisms of change in the development of cognitive structures. *Child Development, 43*, 833–844.

Kuhn, D., Langer, J., Kohlberg, L, & Haan, N. S. (1977). The development of formal operations in logical and moral judgement. *Genetic Psychology Monographs, 95*, 97–188.

Kuhn, T. S. (1972). *The structure of scientific revolutions* (2nd ed.). Chicago: University of Chicago Press.

Lazarus, R. S. (1982). Thoughts on the relations between emotion and cognition. *American Psychologist, 37*, 1019–1024.

Lazarus, R. S. (1984). On the primacy of cognition. *American psychologist, 39*, 124–129.

Leva, L. M. (1984). Cognitive behavioral therapy in the light of Piagetian theory. In M. A. Reda & M. J. Mahoney (Eds.), *Cognitive psychotherapies* (pp. 223–250). Cambridge, MA: Ballinger.

Mahoney, M. J. (1976). *Scientist as subject: The psychological imperative*. Cambridge, MA: Ballinger.

Moshman, D. (1986, May). Discussant of *"Necessity: The Developmental Component in Reasoning,"* by F. Murray. Paper presented at the 16th Annual Jean Piaget Symposium, Philadelphia, PA.

Nisbett, R., & Ross, L. (1980). *Human inference: Strategies and shortcomings of social judgement*. Englewood Cliffs, NJ: Prentice-Hall.

Overton, W. F. (Ed.). (1983). *The relationship between social and cognitive development*. Hillsdale, NJ: Lawrence Erlbaum.

Piaget, J. (1955). *The language and thought of the child* (M. Gabain, Trans.). Cleveland: Meridan Books. (Originally published 1923)

Piaget, J. (1960). *The child's conception of the world*. (J. & A. Tomilson, Trans.). Totowa, NJ: Littlefield, Adams. (Originally published 1926)

Piaget, J. (1962a). *Play, dreams, and imitation in childhood*. (H. Gattegano & F. M. Hodgson, Trans.). New York: Norton. (Originally published 1946)

Piaget, J. (1962b). Three lectures (The stages of the intellectual development in the child; The relation of affectivity to intelligence in the mental development; Will and Action). *Bulletin of the Menninger Clinic, 26*, 120–145.

Piaget, J. (1963). *The origins of intelligence in the child*. (M. Cook, Trans.). New York: Norton. (Originally published 1936)

Piaget, J. (1964). Development and learning. In R. E. Ripple & V. N. Rockcastle (Eds.), *Piaget rediscovered* (pp. 7–20). Ithaca, NY: School of Education, Cornell University.

Piaget, J. (1968). *Six psychological studies* (A. Tenzer, Trans.). New York: Vintage Books. (Originally published 1964)

Piaget, J. (1969a). *Judgement and reasoning in the child* (M. Warden, Trans.). Totowa, NJ: Littlefield, Adams. (Originally published 1924)

Piaget, J. (1969b). *The child's conception of physical causality* (M. Gabain, Trans.). Totowa, NJ: Littlefield, Adams. (Originally published 1927)

Piaget, J. (1971). *The construction of reality in the child* (M. Cook, Trans.). New York: Ballantine. (Originally published 1936)

Piaget, J. (1972). Intellectual evolution from adolescence to adulthood. *Human Development, 15,* 1–12.

Piaget, J. (1974). *Understanding causality* (D. Miles & M. Miles, Trans.). New York: Norton (Originally published 1971)

Piaget, J. (1976). *The grasp of consciousness* (S. W. Wedgwood, Trans.) Cambridge: Harvard University Press. (Originally published 1974)

Piaget, J. (1977). *The development of thought* (A. Rosin, Trans.). New York: Viking. (Originally published 1975)

Piaget, J. (1980a). *Adaptation and intelligence* (S. Eames, Trans.). Chicago: University of Chicago Press. (Originally published 1974)

Piaget, J. (1980b). *Experiments in contradiction* (D. Coltman, Trans.). Chicago: University of Chicago Press. (Originally published 1974)

Piaget, J. (1981). *Intelligence and affectivity: Their relationship during child development* (T. A. Brown & C. E. Kaegi, Trans. and Eds.). Palo Alto, CA: Annual Reviews Monograph. (Originally published 1954, in outline form)

Pulaski, M. A. S. (1971). *Understanding Piaget.* New York: Harper & Row.

Raimy, V. (1975). *Misunderstanding of the self.* San Francisco: Jossey-Bass.

Robinson, E. (1983). Metacognitive development. In S. Meadows (Ed.), *Developing thinking.* New York: Methuen.

Rosen, H. (1977). *Pathway to Piaget.* Cherry Hill, NJ: Post-Graduate International.

Rosen, H. (1980). *The development of socimoral knowledge.* New York: Columbia University Press.

Rosen, H. (1985). *Piagetian dimensions of clinical relevance.* New York: Columbia University Press.

Rush, A. J., Beck, A. T., Kovacs, M., & Hollon, S. (1977). Comparative efficacy of cognitive therapy and pharmacotherapy in the treatment of depressed outpatients. *Cognitive Therapy and Research, 1* (1), 17–37.

Selman, R. L. (1976). Social-cognitive understanding: A guide to educational and clinical practice. In T. Lickona (Ed.), *Moral development and behavior* (pp. 299–316). New York: Holt, Rinehart & Winston.

Selman, R. (1980). *The growth of interpersonal understanding.* New York: Academic Press.

Shantz, C. W. (1975). The development of social cognition. In E. M. Hetherington (Ed.), *Review of development research* (Vol. 5; pp. 257–323). Chicago: University of Chicago Press.

Shantz, C. H. (1983). Social cognition. In J. H. Flavell, & E. M. Markman (Eds.), *Handbook of child psychology: Cognitive development* Vol. 3; pp. 495–555). New York: Wiley.

Shaw, B. F. & Beck, A. T. (1977). The treatment of depression with cognitive therapy. In A. Ellis & R. Grieger (Eds.), *Handbook of rational emotive therapy* (pp. 309–326). New York: Springer.

Siegler, R. S. (1986). *Children's thinking.* Englewood Cliffs, NJ: Prentice-Hall.

Silvern, L. E., Waterman, J. M., Sobesky, W., & Ryan, V. L. (1979). Effects of a developmental model of perspective taking training. *Child Development 50,* 243–246.

Siomopoulos, V. (1983). *The structure of psychopathological experience.* New York: Brunner/Mazel.

Smedslund, J. (1961a). The acquisition of conservation of substance and weight in children. I. Introduction. *Scandinavian Journal of Psychology, 2,* 11–20.

Smedslund, J. (1961b). The acquisition of conservation of substance and weight in children. II. External reinforcement of conservation of weight and of the operations of addition and subtraction. *Scandinavian Journal of Psychology, 2,* 71–84.

Tenzer, A. (1983). Piaget and psychoanalysis. Some reflections on insight. *Contemporary psychoanalysis, 19,* 319–339.

Tversky, A., & Kahnemann, D. (1973). Availability: A heuristic for judging frequency and probability. *Cognitive Psychology, 5,* 207–232.

Tvriel, E. (1966). An experimental test of the sequentiality of developmental stages in the child's moral judgments. *Journal of personality and social psychology, 3,* 611–618.

Urbain, E. S. & Kendall, P. C. (1980). Review of social-cognitive problem-solving interventions with children. *Psychological Bulletin, 88,* 109–143.

Walker, L. J. (1983). Sources of cognitive conflict for stage transition in moral development. *Developmental Psychology, 19,* 103–110.

Wason, P. C., & Johnson-Laird, P. N. (1972). *The psychology of reasoning.* London: Batsford.

Weiner, M. L. (1985). *Cognitive-experiential therapy: An integrative ego psychotherapy.* New York: Brunner/Mazel.

Weishaar, M. E., & Beck, A. T. (1986). Cognitive therapy. In W. Dryden & W. Golden (Eds.), *Cognitive-behavioral approaches to psychotherapy* (pp. 61–91). London: Harper & Row.

Wellman, H. (1985). The origins of metacognition. In D. L. Forrest-Pressley, G. E. MacKinnon, & T. G. Waller (Eds.), *Metacognition, cognition, and human performance* (pp. 1–31). New York: Academic Press.

Wright, J. H., & Beck, A. T. (1983). Cognitive therapy of depression. *Hospital and Community Psychiatry, 34,* 1119–1127.

Youniss, J. (1980). *Parents and peers in social development.* Chicago: University of Chicago Press.

Zajonc, R. B. (1980). Feeling and thinking: Preferences need no inferences. *American Psychologist, 35,* 151–175.

Zajonc, R. B., (1984). On the primacy of affect. *American Psychologist, 39,* 117–123.

# 11

# The Relativity of Reality
## Second-Order Change in Psychotherapy

E. THOMAS DOWD AND TERRY M. PACE

The view that people are active participants in the construction of their own reality is the hallmark of constructivist approaches to psychological theory, which stands in contrast to purely empiricist approaches to psychology. Modern psychology, especially in America, has been dominated by empiricism. Both behaviorism (e.g., Hull, 1943; Skinner, 1974; Watson, 1925) and its chief competitor, information-processing psychology (e.g., Anderson & Bower, 1973; Atkinson & Shiffrin, 1968; Newell & Simon, 1972) are tied to empiricist philosophy that holds that reality exists independently of the perceiver and that knowledge is acquired only through sensory experience. Weimer (1977) has described this common metatheoretical base of both behaviorism and information-processing psychology as a sensory metatheory of the mind.

The focus of theories based on sensory metatheoretical assumptions is on the overt response of the organism to environmental events, as in behaviorism, or on the cognitive processing of environmental information, as in information processing. The commonality is that both behaviorism and information-processing psychology view the flow of influence or information as being from the outside inward. Popper (1972) has described this position as "the bucket theory of the mind." The senses serve as funnels through which information about the external world is poured, whereas the mind is seen as an empty bucket that receives the information from the senses. Behaviorism simply ignores this process and focuses exclusively on what can be seen in the environment and the overt behavior of the organism. Information-processing psychology differs only in that the mind is viewed as an active transformer of information. That is, information from the external world passes through a series of complex filters and processors prior to being poured into the bucket. The metaphor is that of the computer that processes information input from the environment.

As opposed to sensory theories, Weimer (1977) describes motor theories of the mind. Motor theories are based on the metatheoretical assumption that knowledge flows from the

E. THOMAS DOWD • Department of Educational Psychology, Kent State University, Kent, Ohio 44242.
TERRY M. PACE • Department of Educational Psychology, University of Nebraska, Lincoln, Nebraska 68588.

E. THOMAS DOWD
and TERRY M. PACE

inside outward. The mind is viewed as not only active, but constructive. What we know is a product of the structures of the mind acting upon the environment. Human cognition consists of both feedback mechanisms through which the environment activates the cognitive system and feedforward mechanisms through which the cognitive system constructs what is perceived in the environment (Mahoney, 1985). According to constructivist metatheory, reality exists at three levels: (1) in the external world, (2) in the cognitive system, and (3) in the knowledge created through human action (Popper, 1966). In this view, the mind is a motor system, a system of action through which we construct our knowledge and theories of the world and of ourselves (Weimer, 1977).

A key foundation of constructivist psychology is an evolutionary conception of the origin of knowledge (Guidano & Liotti, 1985). Knowledge of the world and of ourselves emerges through the ongoing adaptive activity of the organism in response to environmental pressures. It is in the world of action that knowledge exists. It is in the world of action that our language, beliefs, concepts, and theories develop (Popper & Eccles, 1977). In short, all of the structures that organize and make intelligible the contents of our experiences are constructions developed through the adaptive action of the organism. As Guidano & Liotti have stated:

> Knowledge evolution appears to be an ongoing process, unfolding in its progressive elaboration of environment-modeled templates, able to order and decode incoming experience, since ordering and decoding are the essential devices for effective survival . . . . Knowledge itself appears to be very far from a mere sensorial copy of reality (empiricism), as well as far from a mere unfolding of schemata already performed in the individual (innatism). On the contrary, knowledge appears to be a progressive, hierarchical construction of models of reality where, step by step, the furniture of experience is molded inside knowledge structures by the ordering activity carried out by the knowing subject. (Guidano & Liotti, 1985, p. 102)

Constructivist views have been proposed and elaborated by a number of important psychological theorists. Indeed, constructivism seems to be competing with empiricism for prominence in contemporary psychology. Among the most important constructivist approaches are Piaget's (1970, 1977) views of cognitive development, the various schema theories (e.g., Bartlett, 1932; Bobrow & Norman, 1975; Markus, 1977; Minsky, 1975; Neisser, 1976; Rummelhart, 1980; Schank & Abelson, 1977), and personal construct theory (Kelly, 1955). Within the field of counseling and psychotherapy, a number of other theorists have recently expressed constructivist positions (e.g., Arnkoff, 1980; Beck, 1976; Frank, 1973; Guidano & Liotti, 1982; Mahoney, 1980). The contributions of these constructivist approaches to an understanding of change processes in counseling and psychotherapy will be briefly discussed in the following section.

## CONSTRUCTIVIST APPROACHES TO CHANGE PROCESSES

It is Piaget who most clearly represents the constructivist position. Starting from a view of man as a biological organism, Piaget saw development as a process of adaption to the environment (Piaget, 1970). Beginning in infancy, the child utilizes innate sensory structures and motor responses to interact with the environment. In this sensorimotor stage of development, the child constructs a world that reflects ways of knowing. Thus, to an infant, the world consists of things to suck, grasp, look at, hit, and listen to (Miller, 1983). For the infant, these various actions carried out upon the environment become the knowledge of the world. With continued experience and biological maturation, these activities become organized into behavioral schemes. Schemes stabilize or gain a relative state of equilibrium as the infant is able to act successfully upon the environment, assimilating experiences into organized behavioral patterns. However, as the infant continues to explore and gain increasingly new experiences, the existing schemes begin to fail in being able to adequately organize all of the new information. This failure of existing knowledge structures results in the accommodation of old structures to meet the new demands. Through accommodation, the infant reorganizes the knowledge structures with the result that the world of the infant is known in new ways (Miller, 1983; Piaget, 1954).

The same pattern found in infant development continues across the other developmental stages identified by Piaget. At each stage, the child's knowledge of the world is constructed out of the interaction between the existing knowledge structures and the environmental experience. It is, in this sense, that knowledge is always bound up in human action, be it overt and motoric or covert and cognitive. To know the world is to act upon it.

As long as experience remains consistent with current knowledge structures, the child is in a state of relative equilibrium. Equilibrium is maintained through the adaptive process of assimilating new experience into existing knowledge structures. As experience moves beyond the realm of current knowledge structures and can no longer be easily assimilated, the child adapts through the process of accommodation. The knowledge structures of the child are reorganized to accommodate new experiences. It is the state of disequilibrium between existing knowledge structures and current experience that leads to accommodation and reconstruction of knowledge structures (Piaget, 1977). Extending Piaget's theory of development and cognitive-behavioral change into adulthood may provide a viable framework for understanding change processes in counseling and psychotherapy.

Indeed, within the specialities of cognitive and social psychology, the constructivist framework developed by Piaget has been applied to the study of adult cognition. These approaches have come to be known as schema theories. Although acknowledging the contributions of Piaget, contemporary schema theorists trace their heritage back to the work of Bartlett (1932), whose view of schemata has been described as being very near to current uses of the concept (Brewer & Nakumura, 1984). Bartlett (1932) considered a schema to be ''an active organization of past reactions or of past experiences, which must always be supposed to be operating in any well-adapted organic responses'' (p. 20). According to Brewer and Nakumura (1984), the emergence of contemporary interest in schema theory may be traced to the mid-1970s and the works of such authors as Bobrow and Norman (1975), Minsky (1975), Neisser (1976), Rummelhardt (1975), and Schank and Abelson (1977).

Contemporary schema theories are characterized by a general theoretical perspective that holds that individuals develop organized knowledge structures through interaction with the environment. Brewer and Nakumura (1984) have described schemata as

> unconscious mental structures and processes that underlie the molar aspects of human knowledge and skill. They contain abstract generic knowledge that has been organized to form qualitative new structures. Schemas are modular-different cognitive domains have schemas with different structural characteristics (p. 141).

Schemata serve an adaptive function by organizing experience and reducing the complexity of the environment. By selectively limiting, guiding, and organizing the information-processing activity of the organism, schemata make efficient thinking and action possible (Mandler, 1984; Taylor & Crocker, 1981).

There are many types of schemata that have been identified. Some of these include prototypes (Rosch & Mervis, 1975), frames (Minsky, 1975), and scripts (Schank & Abelson, 1977). Hastie (1981) grouped the various types of schemata into three general categories: central tendency schemata (prototypes), template schemata (frames), and procedural schemata (scripts). Central tendency schemata are abstracted prototypical representations of knowledge. Template schemata are specific structures that serve as cognitive filing systems for organizing and classifying knowledge. Procedural schemata provide rules for activating sequences and patterns of behavioral activity.

Schemata are considered to be interdependent and interactive. Individual schemata range

E. THOMAS DOWD
and TERRY M. PACE

from highly concrete to highly abstract structural units. Schemata may be linked to each other through both hierarchial and lateral networks. In addition, schemata may be embedded within other schemata (Hastie, 1981; Rummelhart & Ortney, 1977; Wyer & Srull, 1981).

Schema theory holds that people are active constructors of their own cognitive-behavioral experience. The constructive nature of schema theories may be seen in their view that schemata actively bias perception and memory processes. Indeed there is considerable evidence that schemata bias the encoding storage and retrieval of information (Brewer & Nakumura, 1984; Hastie 1981; Taylor & Crocker, 1981).

The use of a particular schema that consists of a specified knowledge structure will interact with the information available in the environment to construct the person's subsequent knowledge or memory of the event. Depending on the relationship between the schema and the environmental event, the constructive action may occur as a result of either attention and encoding or storage and retrieval processes (Hastie, 1981). Environmental information may be unattended to, may be rejected from deep processing due to a lack of fit into the processing structure, or may be bypassed during retrieval as a result of schematic influences (Brewer & Nakumura, 1984; Hastie, 1981; Taylor & Crocker, 1981). Schemata may also play a constructive role in knowledge development by filling in missing information with preexisting schemabased information. Events that are highly inconsistent with a schema, are ambiguous or complex, or that are experienced under conditions allowing only brief processing time may be especially subject to schema-based substitutions or inferences (Taylor & Crocker, 1981). Minsky (1975) has referred to these inferences as default values. It is through these processing effects that schemata act to construct the knowledge available to each person.

These constructive biases may be related to many clinical problems as well as to the processes of change in counseling and psychotherapy (Turk & Salovey, 1985). Particular types of schemata with direct implications for counseling are self-schemata (Markus, 1977). Self-schemata are "cognitive generalizations about the self, derived from past experience, that organize and guide social experience" (Markus, 1977, p. 63). Through the processing effects of self-schemata, individuals construct their views of themselves and other people (Markus, 1977; Markus & Smith, 1981; Markus, Smith, & Moreland, 1985). Indeed, there is evidence suggesting that depressive self-schemata may underly clinical depression (Derry & Kuiper, 1981; Kuiper & Derry, 1982; McDonald & Kuiper, 1985). From this perspective, the depressed world view of the depressive client is a world constructed through the processes of schematic influence. This view is consistent with Beck's (1967, 1976) cognitive theory of depression. Kelly's (1955) personal construct theory also views the individual's cognitive constructions as underlying behavior and behavior change.

Kelly's (1955) personal construct theory provides the most complete application of constructivist metatheory to counseling and psychotherapy. Kelly's fundamental postulate states that "a person's processes are psychologically channelized by the way in which he anticipates events (Kelly, 1955, p. 46). In this view, knowledge results from the interaction between the person's active anticipations and the environmental information that is encountered. The individual construes reality based on his or her own structuring of experience (Nystedt & Magnusson, 1982).

Kelly's views closely parallel those of Piaget and the schema theorists (Mancuso & Adams-Webber, 1982). In all of these theories, the person is seen as developing organized knowledge structures that are related in complex and multiple ways. Through the interaction of the person's knowledge structures and environmental information, the person constructs a unique understanding of reality.

Unlike the other theorists discussed here, Kelly was a psychotherapist who applied his theory to the clinical issues he confronted in his clients (Neimeyer, 1986). Through his clinical experience, Kelly identified a number of dysfunctions and breakdowns in the way people construe their experience. He also developed a number of strategies for therapeutic intervention (Neimeyer, 1986).

More recently, a number of other theorists have applied constructivist views to counseling and psychotherapy. For example, Arnkoff (1980) presented a cognitive framework from which to view clinical phenomena and argues for the application of constructivist theory to clinical concerns. She states that

> the basis of the perspective to be presented is that each individual creates a model of the structure of the world. The model is a map, or set of structural relations, which constitute the framework from which the individual interprets events and determines actions to be taken. The model both guides behavior and provides a structure for inferring the meaning of events. In fact, the model creates events, in that it determines what will be perceived in the individual's internal and external environment. (Arnkoff, 1980, p. 340)

Arnkoff further argues that enduring change in psychotherapy results from a change in the structure of the client's cognitive model of the world.

Beck's (1967, 1976) cognitive theory of depression is also consistent with a constructivist position. Beck views emotional disorders as resulting from distorted cognitive structures that bias the person's perception and thinking. Client problems are seen as ''inadequacies in organizing and interpreting reality'' (Beck, 1976, p. 19). As a result, change is seen in terms of changes in the clients cognitive-behavioral construction of reality. This change occurs through the correction and reorganization of faulty cognitive-behavioral structures.

Frank (1973) is another theorist who describes client functioning and change from a constructivist position. Frank describes each person as developing an ''assumptive world'':

> This is a short-hand expression for a highly structured, complex, interacting set of values, expectations, and images of oneself and others, which guide and in turn are guided by a person's perceptions and behavior and which are closely related to his emotional states and feelings of well being. (Frank, 1973, p. 27)

The assumptive world is essentially an organized construction that regulates cognitive-behavioral activity. Change is brought about in psychotherapy by creating new ways from which the client comes to view the world. In this sense, change is again seen as being essentially cognitive and structural.

Guidano and Liotti (1982) have recently elaborated upon the application of constructivist theory to psychopathology and psychotherapy. It is the individual's own construction of events that underlie emotional disorders and that are the targets for therapeutic change. In arguing for the validity of a constructivist framework Guidano and Liotti state:

> The point of view that emerges from this conceptual framework is that of a mind that is no longer a passive container of sensations that form a copy of reality (''naive realism''), but rather a system that constructs its own model of reality, a model comprehending the very basic sensations underlying the construction of itself (''critical or hypothetical realism''). (p. 8)

Finally, Mahoney (1980, 1985) has been an active representative and integrator of constructivist approaches to psychotherapy. Drawing from fields as disparate as philosophy of science, cognitive psychology, and neurology, Mahoney has argued that cognitive-behavioral actions are influenced by underlying structures of knowledge. These knowledge structures are further supported through central nervous system ordering processes.


## THERAPEUTIC SYSTEMS AS CREATORS OF MEANING

Constructivist metatheory as epitomized by schema theories and other theories discussed here share one common assumption: that reality is not invariant but is created by each individual according to his or her self-schemata and tacit rules governing the creation and organization of knowledge. These rules and schemata are organized as a result of the individual's progressive experience over the years. Keeney (1983) has noted that a primary task of individuals is to punctuate and organize into recursive patterns the ongoing and undifferentiated stream of experience. Although the stimuli making up the stream of experience may possess objective reality, the organization of this stream into patterns of organization will be unique to each individual. How we thus organize our experience of the world will thus determine our perception of reality and will in fact create reality for us as we in turn respond to new environmental stimuli. In other words, each of us draws distinctions among phenomena and that act of creating distinctions also creates our reality and our ways of knowing the world. It is instructive to consider that Eskimos have many different words for different kinds of snow (a very important experience for them), whereas we in turn have many different words for automobile (e.g., car, station wagon, sedan, truck), a very important experience for *us*. The fact that different individuals will organize and punctuate the same stream of experience in different ways means that they each have created their own reality.

Such a view is at variance with the assumptions underlying most systems of therapeutic change, which implicitly consider reality to be an independently determined phenomenon. These assumptions lead to a focus on standard outcomes across different individuals; for example, it is widely thought that clients who complain of anxiety or depression require standard therapeutic efforts directed toward the alleviation of these symptoms. Much effort in psychology over the years has been devoted to a search for specific techniques that will possess sufficient power to foster therapeutic change by themselves. It is the task of the therapist to then specify the problem and arrive at a diagnosis and treatment according to a standard nosology. This epistemological view of the therapeutic process does not and cannot consider the particular meaning and function that the symptom has in the client's life, nor its relation to the client's social interactions with others. Nor can it account for the apparent "functional autonomy" (Allport, 1937) of symptoms, in which they seem to acquire a life and meaning of their own long after they have ceased to have any obvious function. In this fashion, both diagnosis and therapeutic outcome are reified and thus assume an independent reality beyond the particular individual client and therapist involved. It would therefore seem that a different epistemological view of symptoms and their meaning and function might be in order.

The search for valid diagnostic systems, such as the DSM-III, and specific therapeutic techniques that are uniquely valuable in the solution of particular clinical problems are both reflective of an empiricist epistemology. Despite the large amount of outcome research purportedly demonstrating the effectiveness of intervention techniques, no strategies have been shown to be clearly more effective than others (e.g., Sloane, Staples, Cristol, Yorkston, & Whipple, 1975) with clients in general. Likewise, diagnostic systems are commonly assumed to reflect reality, rather than simply methods of punctuating and organizing an ongoing stream of experiential phenomena. We assume this to be true despite continuous changes and refinements in diagnostic systems and the lack of specific treatment interventions that follow from differential diagnoses. The inability of psychologists to tie treatment strategies to symptom topology and problem etiology is in fact a major difference between psychological and medical diagnosis.

All therapeutic systems can be seen as creators of meaning for clients, in that their function is to provide an acceptable explanation for the problem or symptom as well as a socially sanctioned treatment. They thus interpret and explain clients' experiences to them and assist them in organizing reality differently. In this regard, it is interesting that research on the function of interpretation (Claiborn, 1982; Claiborn & Dowd, 1985) in therapy has shown that the particular content of the interpretation makes little or no difference. What matters is the discrepancy of the interpretation from the client's existing viewpoint. Apparently providing the client with a different point of view is more useful than the specific point of view that is presented.

Existing therapeutic systems can thus be seen as adhering to a empiricist epistemological world view, which assumes that reality is objective and fixed and that the task of the therapist is to rectify the problem within the confines of this reality. In contrast, a constructivist epistemology assumes that both client and therapist come to the therapeutic encounter with their own unique views of reality. It is the latter's task to modify the former's construction of reality by means of a variety of procedures—both behavioral and cognitive—designed to assist the client in first recognizing that reality is not invariant and second in undergoing experiences that will act to produce different outcomes from previously utilized actions. It is likely that all therapeutic systems are effective insofar as they assist clients in using their new experiences in the creation of new systems of meaning. As Bergin and Lambert (1978) have indicated, perhaps the major source of variance in client change is client variables.

One theory of human change that has especial relevance for a constructivist metatheory is that of second-order change and specifically the usefulness of paradoxical interventions in bringing about that change. It involves not only the performance of the same behavior in a different context designed thereby to force a change in the meaning of that behavior but also involves a shift from one level of meaning to another. It is to a discussion of these concepts and their place within constructivist metatheory that we now turn.

## FIRST-ORDER CHANGE: ATTACKING THE PROBLEM

Most attempts at human change through psychotherapy are in reality attempts at first-order change. Watzlawick, Weakland, and Fisch (1974) have defined first-order change as change that occurs within a system that itself remains unchanged following unchanging rules of operation. This kind of change is usually attempted by applying the opposite of the problem behavior. If this intervention does not result in a decrease in the symptomatic behavior, the therapist generally applies "more of the same" (i.e., more of the original treatment), which often leads to no better results than the initial intervention. This continues until the therapist dismisses the client as "unmotivated" or until the client seeks a new therapist.

An example may illustrate what we mean here. If an individual is depressed, the therapist may attempt, by a variety of change-producing efforts, to cheer him or her up. Whether done by behavioral methods, such as graded activity schedules, or by cognitive methods, such as rational disputation, the therapist is applying the opposite of the problem directly to the problem behavior. What is not changed, however, is the system of relationships in which the individual lives, or the system within which the symptom functions, whether it be a family, a work relationship, or the relationship with the therapist. If, contrary to expectation, the client does not improve, the therapist has no alternative but to do "more of the same" because the therapeutic "rules" dictate that that is the treatment of choice. As one therapist put it, "even if the patient doesn't improve, it's nice to know you're doing the right thing."

A key element in the concept of first-order change is that the rules or assumptions governing the application and choice of therapeutic interventions are themselves not open to change and indeed are often not even known nor able to be articulated. Thus, although each therapeutic system may provide for differences in therapeutic operations and punctuate the stream of experience differently, the basic assumptions governing the nature of human change are not open to question. In Popper's (1966) system, reality exists at the first two levels only. Likewise, the rule system behind the client's self-schema or assumptive world and governing his or her construction of reality, as discussed earlier, is not subject to challenge when first-order change is attempted.

It should be obvious that first-order attempts at change often do result in change occurring, thus accounting for most of the successes reported by the various systems of psychotherapies. Too often, however, first-order change results in one member of a system improving, whereas one or more of the other members deteriorate. An example is improvement in the wife's depression as marriage problems develop. Although elements in the system have changed, the overall system has not. First-order change may be similar to what Mahoney (1980) is referring to when he discusses "peripheral" (as opposed to core) changes in the individual's adaptation paradigm (p. 177). Mahoney suggests that peripheral changes can in fact often be made relatively easily, given a circumscribed problem and a motivated client. Many problems, however, are not amenable to first-order change methods, especially where the individual's core structure or self-schemata are implicated, or where the problem is being maintained by the client's interaction with others. Self-schemata are resistant to change, and the client often acts to defeat the efforts of the therapist. Other interventions are needed.

## SECOND-ORDER CHANGE: ATTACKING THE SOLUTION

The two strategies of "applying the opposite" and "more of the same" often surprisingly do not result in the desired change. Paradoxically, the attempted solution often not only makes the problem worse, but the solution can in fact *become* the problem. This happens as repeated efforts to solve the problem result in repeated failure and a more recalcitrant problem that becomes functionally autonomous. The most obvious examples are entrenched problems such as anxiety or insomnia. In insomnia, for example, applying the opposite, that is, trying harder to fall asleep, only results in an exacerbated problem. The individual, applying first-order change principles, then does more of the same, that is, tries even harder to fall asleep, with predictable results. Repeated attempts to solve the problem only leave the individual with chronic insomnia instead of occasional sleeplessness. The meaning of sleeplessness has thus been changed from an occasional annoyance to a chronic problem. Eventually, as fear of insomnia creates more insomnia, the solution becomes the problem.

Watzlawick *et al.* (1974) have proposed second-order change as a way of extracting oneself from the self-reflexive trap inherent in many first-order attempts at change, that is, the harder one tries the less one succeeds. Second-order change has several characteristics that are worthy of discussion. Change efforts are typically applied to the attempted solution (which by now has often become the problem) rather than to the problem itself. In doing so, it violates not only the rules governing the production change but also changes the meaning that the symptom has for the individual (Dowd & Milne, 1986). Meaning is changed in two ways. Omer (1981) has referred to this process as a decontextualization because the symptom now takes place in a modified context and therefore loses its original meaning or intent. This occurs because a binding and reinforcing relationship exists between a symptom and its context, which is, of necessity, changed when the context changes. Second-order change thus places the problem in a different frame of reference and changes its meaning to the person. This is especially important for the present discussion. By shifting the meaning of the symptom, second-order change fosters a shift in the rules of reality or the assumptive world (Frank, 1973) that the individual uses to organize and punctuate the ongoing stream of experience. Not only is the assumption of the invariant nature of reality challenged, but the person is behaviorally challenged to construct an alternate belief system that may be more facilitative to personal development. It is important to note that this is done, not by attempting to persuade clients to see things differently, but by using the very behavior that is the problem in service of its own change.

As Dowd and Milne (1986) have noted, second-order change is generally seen as confusing and unsettling. People do not easily change their core concepts and rules for organizing and punctuating their experience easily, and the greater the shift in frame of reference required, the greater will be the resistance. Mahoney (1985) has argued that there is long-term survival value for people in homeostasis and that the brain is wired to protect us from sudden threats to equilibrium. Although individuals are resistant to core cognitive changes, when they occur, they are more likely to be associated with profound and enduring changes in thoughts, behavior, and emotion (Mahoney, 1980). Likewise Guidano and Liotti (1983) have referred to a sense of confusion, loss of identity, and cognitive disorientation that are characteristic of individuals undergoing changes in their core cognitive structures. Crisis intervention therapists have long known that people are much more amenable to change when they are confused and disorganized during an emotional crisis.

Second-order change can foster the state of disequilibrium between existing knowledge structures and the individual's current experience that is the hallmark of Piaget's theory of development. The individual is forced to accommodate his or her knowledge structures to new data rather than being able to assimilate the new data in current knowledge structures. Because the symptomatic behavior is now occurring in a modified context, the person's current experience with the symptom no longer matches the existing knowledge structure. If the symptom continues to be performed in the new context, it is more difficult to assimilate it into already existing knowledge structures. Disequilibrium occurs, and the individual is forced to reconstruct his or her knowledge structure regarding the problem. As Bandura (1977) has noted, behavioral changes such as these may be especially efficacious at fostering subsequent cognitive change.

Second-order change also undercuts the linear causal mode of thinking that most of us automatically use and fosters a more circular view of reality (Riedel, 1984; Varela, 1984). When individuals cease looking for the ultimate cause of an event or phenomenon and begin looking at causality as circular in which everything is caused by everything else, they are enabled to do two things (Watzlawick, 1984). First, they can begin to recognize their own responsibilities in the causal linkage. Second, they can begin to recognize that reality is indeed relative and thereby gain tolerance for another's point of view. In doing so, they can implicitly learn to be tolerant of their own point of view as well and begin to see the possibility of making profound changes in their way of constructing reality.

Second-order change also confuses levels of meaning (Watzlawick *et al.*, 1974) and in doing so assists clients in reorganizing their construction of the world. Paradoxical interventions in particular confuse member and class in ways that are unsettling to conventional ways of thinking and thus make it difficult to assimilate the new data into existing cognitive structures. The individual is thus forced to accommodate by reorganizing his or her cognitive schemata. A familiar example of member–class confusion is the statement by Epimenides the Cretan that ''All Cretans are liars.'' Attempts to reconcile this apparent contradiction forces one to engage in new modes of thought.

Second-order change in psychotherapy can thus be seen as a way of helping people to change their frame of reference regarding their problematic situation and thereby reorganize their view of reality. In doing so, many implicit rules for living that derive from the individual's organization of reality are called into question. Because these rules are not directly challenged by the therapist but are implicitly and indirectly challenged by the new actions that the client takes in response to the therapist's directives, the client cannot easily account for these changes. Whenever individuals cannot find external reasons for events (i.e., make external causal attributions), they are more likely to locate the causes for these events within themselves (i.e., make internal causal attributions) that are considered to be more enduring (Kopel & Arkowitz, 1975). Thus, second-order change interventions, precisely because they are confusing and unsettling, may lead to more enduring changes.

## REACTANCE AS A CLIENT VARIABLE

As Mahoney (1980, 1985) has noted, core cognitive changes are generally resisted vigorously by people. Yet most therapists would agree that some individuals appear to resist therapeutic influence considerably more than others. Brehm (1966) has developed the concept

E. THOMAS DOWD
and TERRY M. PACE

of psychological reactance to account for the tendency to resist influence from others when one's free behaviors are perceived as threatened. Although Brehm considered reactance to be a situational variable, others (e.g., Beutler, 1979; Dowd & Swoboda, 1984; Jahn & Lichstein, 1980) have considered reactance to be in part an individual difference variable.

Beutler (1983) has found that reactance is related to locus of control in that individuals with an internal locus of control over personal reinforcement exhibit high reactance and tend to be resistant to external influence. Those with an external locus of control, on the other hand, appear to be low in reactance and therefore more susceptible to external influence. Paradoxically, Beutler notes, one consequence of the persuasion process known as psychotherapy is to make clients more reactant and therefore less persuasible! Apparently successful psychotherapy is its own worst enemy; if successful, it renders it less successful in the future.

It is possible that individual differences in psychological reactance may mediate outcome resulting from different types of psychological treatments. Beutler (1979), in a review of 52 comparative psychotherapy studies, determined the relative efficacy of a variety of therapeutic procedures with three types of clients. He found that cognitive modification (e.g. rational-emotive therapy) was superior to affective insight therapy (e.g., client-centered therapy) but inferior to cognitive insight therapy (e.g., psychoanalytic therapy) with high-reactant clients. Tentatively, he also found that behavior therapy was more effective than cognitive insight therapy for low-reactant clients (i.e., external locus of control), whereas the reverse was true for high-reactant clients (i.e., internal locus of control). Apparently high-reactant clients prefer to retain control of the therapeutic process and are less likely to accept direction from the therapist than are low-reactant clients. Similarly, interventions that are designed to produce second-order change (which are known collectively as defiance-based strategies) are particularly useful in overcoming resistance, because the client changes in the process of attempting to defy the therapist's directive. Other interventions, called compliance-based strategies, produce change as the client attempts to comply with the directive and are appropriate for low-reactant clients.

Second-order change techniques can thus be viewed as especially powerful ways of encouraging core cognitive change. Because they violate many of the implicit rules by which individuals organize reality, they are helpful in encouraging changes in core cognitive structures as the person is forced to consider the possibility of an alternative reality. The characteristics and utility of specific second-order change interventions will now be discussed.

## SECOND-ORDER CHANGE TECHNIQUES

### REFRAMING

This is a widely used technique and is known by other names in different systems of psychotherapies. Reframing is best used with a relatively compliant client and involves shifting the meaning attached to a problem or event. In positive reframing (or positive connotation), the behavior or situation that was once viewed as negative is now viewed as positive, as when a depressed person is told, "you are fortunate to be so aware of your feelings." Many incidents that people encounter in daily life also shift meaning from positive to negative, in a sort of negative reframing (or negative connotation), as when invidious motives are attributed to an ostensibly altruistic act. The cognitive therapy of Beck (1976) as well as the Personal Construct Therapy of Kelly (1955) contains an implicit reframing component as the therapist attempts to help the client in constructing alternative meaning systems for the problem situation. What gives reframing its power is that one cannot easily return to one's former view of reality after reframing, as illustrated by the figure–ground reversal problems familiar to every student of introductory psychology.

This is the most familiar of the second-order change techniques. The therapist directs the client to deliberately perform or exaggerate the problem behavior; for example, an anxious individual is told to deliberately become as anxious as possible in problem situations. This instruction places the client in a double-bind, in that compliance with the directive places the problem more under the client's control, whereas defiance of the directive reduces the problem. Either way, therapeutic gain results. Alternatively, the client may be instructed to schedule his or her symptom at a particular time in order to place it under voluntary control. In addition, the very act of engaging in this type of therapeutic exchange tends to violate the implicit rule that the problem should be reduced and that it is the task of the therapist to reduce it. The meaning of the symptom is also changed from an act or event that is out of one's control to one that is deliberately engaged in, resulting in decontextualization of the problematic behavior (Omer, 1981). The individual is thus forced to accommodate to a new reality. Finally, when changes do occur, they are inexplicable to the client so that internal attributions for change tend to occur. The end result is to change the meaning the symptom in the individual's life and to aid in the construction of an alternative reality.

## Restraining

There are several types of restraining strategies that are particularly useful with reactant clients. In inhibiting change, the therapist encourages the client to change only at a slow pace. In prohibiting change, the therapist actively discourages the client from changing at all or for a specific period of time (e.g., make no changes for a week). Another technique that is especially useful for ambivalent clients is to stress the negative consequences of changing and to urge that they carefully consider all the benefits of remaining just as they are. In predicting or prescribing a relapse, the therapist implicitly redefines the meaning of a relapse from a failure to an expected event on the road to recovery. These strategies have several attributes in common. They encourage a reactant client to resist the therapist by changing, thus reducing the problem behavior. Attempts by the therapist to encourage change might have led the reactant client to resist by remaining the same. In addition, they violate the implicit rule that symptoms are completely nonfunctional and must be eliminated or reduced. They thus shift the meaning of the symptom from an unmitigated problem to a behavior that serves the individual in some capacity. The result is that the client may construct an alternative reality around the changed view of the role of the symptom in his or her life.

## Positioning

This is also a useful technique with reactant clients who hold negative views of themselves in order to elicit positive comments from others (akin to fishing for compliments). The therapist not only agrees with the client's negative view of self but may go on to exaggerate it, thus sabotaging the reciprocal power game implicit in such a communication pattern. To continue to be oppositional, the client must of necessity adopt (or at least verbalize) a more positive view of self. Adlerian therapists have called this technique ''spitting in the client's soup.'' Such interchanges tend to violate the implicit rules governing power games of this nature, thus encouraging the client to try different communication strategies and encouraging him or her to construct an alternative reality of interpersonal communications. This technique is all the more powerful because the client's viewpoint or behavior is never directly challenged, a hallmark of second-order change strategies. Because the old communication pattern is blocked, a new one must be created.

E. THOMAS DOWD
and TERRY M. PACE

The concept of second-order change rests on the assumption that reality is not fixed but is uniquely constructed by each individual. The core assumptions of the individual's unique construction of reality are embodied in what are called schemata. Once defined as reality, these schemata are increasingly resistant to change. First-order change-producing efforts are applied to one element within the social-cognitive system (the symptom) and often are not able to modify the total social-cognitive system. Instead, other aspects of the individual's social and intrapsychic realities are modified so as to cancel out the efforts at change. Thus, first-order attempts at change often have difficulty challenging long-term and implicit schemata. The result is change within the system that leads to no change in the system.

Second-order change is a metachange, or change of change, theory. By modifying the attempts at change and violating the usual rules governing change-producing efforts, it forces the individual to redefine the nature of reality and provides an implicit message that reality is indeed relative. By encouraging the individual to react to the environment in qualitatively different ways, it provides for an evolutionary development of knowledge as described by Guidano and Liotti (1985). The person is required to modify his or her knowledge structure in response to the symptomatic behavior performed in a different context and with a different meaning. This shift in meaning, which is at the heart of second-order change, requires the core schemata, especially, those organized around the symptomatic behavior, to be modified. By thus constructing alternative models of reality, the individual is assisted on the path of increasing differentiation and integration.

At this point, it is an empirical question as to whether the unusual character of second-order change interventions or the double-binding character of these interventions are primarily responsible for their power. Certainly both seem to be important. The history of psychotherapy shows that new techniques tend to achieve the greatest successes. Perhaps they are able to be more successful precisely because their newness enables them to more powerfully challenge existing schemata. However, the double-binding nature of second-order change strategies do provide a powerful stimulus to encourage clients to modify their core schemata, especially resistant clients. Perhaps future research will clarify these issues. Meanwhile, it is apparent, as Dowd and Milne (1986) have demonstrated, that second-order change efforts have proved efficacious.

# REFERENCES

Allport, G. W. (1937). *Personality: A psychological interpretation.* New York: Henry Holt & Co.

Anderson, J. R., & Bower, G. H. (1973). *Human associative memory.* Washington, DC: V. H. Winston.

Arnkoff, D. B. (1980). Psychotherapy from the perspective of cognitive theory. In M. J. Mahoney (Ed.), *Psychotherapy process* (pp. 339–362). New York: Plenum Press.

Atkinson, R. C., & Shiffrin, R. M. (1968). Human memory: A proposed system and its control processes. In K. W. Spence & J. T. Spence (Eds.), *The psychology of learning and motivation: Advances in theory and research* (Vol. 2, pp. 89–195). New York: Academic Press.

Bandura, A. (1977). *Social learning theory.* Englewood Cliffs, NJ: Prentice-Hall.

Bartlett, F. C. (1932). *Remembering: A study in experimental and social psychology.* Cambridge, England: Cambridge University Press.

Beck, A. T. (1967). *Depression: Clinical, experimental and theoretical aspects.* New York: Harper & Row.

Beck, A. T. (1976). *Cognitive therapy and the emotional disorders.* New York: International University Press.

Bergin, A. E., & Lambert, M. J. (1978). The evaluation of therapeutic outcomes. In S. L. Garfield & A. E. Bergin (Eds.), *Handbook of psychotherapy and behavior change* (pp. 139–190). New York: Wiley.

Beutler, L. E. (1979). Toward specific psychological therapies for specific conditions. *Journal of Consulting and Clinical Psychology, 47,* 882–897.

Beutler, L. E. (1983). *Eclectic psychotherapy: A systematic approach.* New York: Pergamon Press.

Bobrow, D. G., & Norman, D. A. (1975). Some principles of memory schemata. In D. G. Bobrow & A. Collins (Eds.), *Representation and understanding* (pp. 1–34). New York: Academic Press.

Brehm, J. W. (1966). *A theory of psychological reactance.* New York: Academic Press.

Brewer, W. F., & Nakumura, G. V. (1984). The nature and function of schemas. In R. S. Wyer, Jr. & T. K. Srull (Eds.), *Handbook of social cognition* (Vol. 1, pp. 119–160). Hillsdale, NJ: Erlbaum.

Claiborn, C. D. (1982). Interpretation and change in counseling. *Journal of Counseling Psychology, 29,* 439–453.

Claiborn, C. D., & Dowd, E. T. (1985). Attributional interpretations in counseling: Content versus discrepancy. *Journal of Counseling Psychology, 32,* 188–196.

Derry, P. A., & Kuiper, N. A. (1981). Schematic processing and self-reference in clinical depressives. *Journal of Abnormal Psychology, 90,* 286–297.

Dowd, E. T., & Milne, C. R. (1986). Paradoxical interventions in counseling psychology. *The Counseling Psychologist, 14,* 237–282.

Dowd, E. T., & Swoboda, J. S. (1984). Paradoxical interventions in behavior therapy. *Journal of Behavior Therapy and Experimental Psychiatry, 15,* 229–234.

Frank, J. D. (1973). (Rev. ed.). *Persuasion and healing.* Baltimore: Johns Hopkins.

Guidano, V. F., & Liotti, G. (1982). *Cognitive processes and emotional disorders: A structural approach to psychotherapy.* New York: Guilford.

Guidano, V. F., & Liotti, G. (1985). A constructionist foundation for cognitive therapy. In M. J. Mahoney & A. E. Freeman (Eds.), *Cognition and psychotherapy* (pp. 101–142). New York: Plenum Press.

Hastie, R. (1981). Schematic principles in human memory. In E. T. Higgins, C. P. Herman, & M. P. Zanna (Eds.), *Social Cognition: The Ontario symposium* (Vol. 1, pp. 39–88). Hillsdale, NJ: Erlbaum.

Hull, C. L. (1943). *Principles of behavior.* New York: Appleton-Century.

Jahn, D. L., & Lichstein, K. L. (1980). The resistive client: A neglected phenomenon in behavior therapy. *Behavior Modification, 4,* 303–320.

Keeney, B. P. (1983). *Aesthetics of change.* New York: The Guilford Press.

Kelly, G. A. (1955). *The psychology of personal constructs.* New York: Norton.

Kopel, S., & Arkowitz, H. (1975). The role of attribution and self-perception in behavior change: Implications for behavior therapy. *Genetic Psychology Monographs, 92,* 175–121.

Kuiper, N., & Derry, P. (1982). Depressed and nondepressed content self-reference in mild depressives. *Journal of Personality, 50,* 62–74.

Mahoney, M. J. (1980). Psychotherapy and the structure of personal revolutions. In M. J. Mahoney (Ed.), *Psychotherapy processes* (pp. 157–180). New York: Plenum Press.

Mahoney, M. J. (Ed.). (1985). Psychotherapy and human change processes. In M. J. Mahoney & A. E. Freeman (Eds.), *Cognition and psychotherapy* (pp. 3–48). New York: Plenum Press.

Mancuso, J. C., & Adams-Weber, J. R. (1982). *The construing person.* New York: Praeger.

Mandler, G. (1984). *Mind and body: Psychology of emotion and stress.* New York: Norton.

Markus, H. (1977). Self-schemata and processing information about the self. *Journal of Personality and Social Psychology, 35,* 63–78.

Markus, H., & Smith, J. (1981). The influence of self-schemata on the perception of others. In N. Cantor & J. F. Kihlstrom (Eds.), *Personality, cognition, and socialization* (pp. 223–262). Hillsdale, NJ: Erlbaum.

Markus, H., Smith, J., & Moreland, R. L. (1985). Role of the self-concept in the perception of others. *Journal of Personality and Social Psychology, 49,* 1494–1512.

McDonald, M. R., & Kuiper, N. A. (1985). Efficiency and automaticity of self-schema processing in clinical depressives. *Motivation and Emotion, 9,* 171–184.

Miller, P. H. (1983). Piaget's cognitive-stage theory. In P. H. Miller (Ed), *Theories of developmental psychology.* San Francisco: Freeman.

Minsky, M. A. (1975). A framework for representing knowledge. In P. H. Winston (Ed.), *The psychology of computer vision* (pp. 211–277). New York: McGraw-Hill.

Neimeyer, R. A. (1986). Personal construct therapy. In W. Dryden & W. L. Golden (Eds.), *Cognitive behavioral approaches to psychotherapy* (pp. 224–260). London: Harper & Row.

Neisser, V. (1976). *Cognition and reality.* San Francisco: Freeman.

Newell, A., & Simon, H. A. (1972). *Human problem solving.* Englewood Cliffs, NJ: Prentice-Hall.

Nystedt, L., & Magnusson, D. (1982). Construction of experience: The construction corallary. In J. C. Mancuro & J. R. Adams-Webber (Eds.), *The construing person* (pp. 33–44). New York: Praeger.

Omer, H. (1981). Paradoxical treatments: A unified concept. *Psychotherapy Theory, Research, and Practice, 18,* 320–324.

Piaget, J. (1954). *The construction of reality in the child.* New York: Basic Books.

Piaget, J. (1970). *Structuralism*. New York: Harper & Row.

Piaget, J. (1977). *The development of thought: Equilibration of cognitive structures*. New York: Viking.

Popper, K. R. (1966). *The open society and its enemies* (5th ed.). Princeton, NJ: Princeton University Press.

Popper, K. R. (1972). *Objective knowledge: An evolutionary approach*. Oxford: Claredon Press.

Popper, K. R., & Eccles, J. C. (1977). *The self and its brain*. New York: Springer International.

Riedel, R. (1984). The consequences of causal thinking. In P. Watzlawick (Ed.), *The invented reality* (pp. 69–94). New York: W. W. Norton.

Rosch, E., & Mervis, C. B. (1975). Family resemblances: Studies in the internal structure of categories. *Cognitive Psychology, 7*, 573–605.

Rummelhardt, D. E. (1975). Notes on a schema for stories. In D. G. Bobrow & A. Collins (Eds.), *Representations and understandings: Studies in cognitive science* (pp. 211–236). New York: Academic.

Rummelhart, D. E. (1980). Schemata: The building blocks of cognition. In R. J. Spiro, B. C. Bruce, & W. F. Brewer (Eds.), *Theoretical issues in reading comprehension: Perspectives from cognitive psychology, linguistics, artificial intelligence, and education* (pp. 33–58). Hillsdale, NJ: Erlbaum.

Rummelhart, D. E., & Ortony, A. (1977). The representation of knowledge in memory. In R. C. Anderson, R. J. Spiro, & W. E. Mortague (Eds.), *Schooling and the acquisition of knowledge*. Hillsdale, NJ: Erlbaum.

Schank, R., & Abelson, R. (1977). *Scripts, plans, goals, and understanding*. Hillsdale, NJ: Erlbaum.

Skinner, B. F. (1974). *About behaviorism*. New York: Alfred A. Knopf.

Sloane, R. B., Staples, F. R., Cristol, A. H., Yorkston, N. J., & Whipple, K. (1975). *Psychotherapy versus behavior therapy*. Cambridge: Harvard University Press.

Taylor, S. E., & Crocker, J. (1981). Schematic bases of social information processing. In E. T. Higgins, C. P. Herman, & M. P. Zanna (Eds.), *Social cognition: The Ontario Symposium* (Vol. 1). Hillsdale, NJ: Erlbaum.

Turk, D. C., & Salovey, P. (1985). Cognitive structures, cognitive processes, and cognitive behavior modification. Client issues. *Cognitive Therapy and Research, 9*, 1–17.

Varela, F. J. (1984). The creative circle: Sketches on the natural history of circularity. In P. Watzlawick (Ed.), *The invented reality* (pp. 309–323). New York: W. W. Norton.

Watzlawick, P. (1984). *The invented reality*. New York: W. W. Norton.

Watzlawick, P., Weakland, J., & Fisch, R. (1974). *Change: Principles of problem formation and problem resolution*. New York: W. W. Norton.

Watson, J. B. (1925). *Behaviorism*. New York: Norton.

Weimar, W. B. (1977). A conceptual framework for cognitive psychology: Motor theories of the mind. In R. Shaw & J. Bransford (Eds.), *Perceiving, acting, and knowing: Toward an ecological psychology* (pp. 267–311). Hillsdale, NJ: Erlbaum.

Wyer, R. S., & Srull, T. K. (1981). Category accessibility: Some theoretical and empirical issues concerning the processing of social stimulus information. In E. T. Higgins, C. P. Herman, & M. P. Zanna (Eds.), *Social cognition: The Ontario symposium* (Vol. 1, pp. 161–197). Hillsdale, NJ: Erlbaum.

# 12

# Thinking Postcognitively about Depression

## James C. Coyne

> Cut the pie any way you like, "meanings" just ain't
> in the head.
>
> Putnam, 1975, p 227

The resurgence of the cognitive perspective in the early 1970s was so strong that it became widely described as the "cognitive revolution" (Dember, 1974). More than a decade later, there still has been little in the way of critical response or sober reevaluation of the enthusiastic claims and polemics that accompanied this shift in perspective. As measured by the continued outpouring of articles, chapters, books, and even new journals, the cognitive perspective is clearly in ascendance in clinical psychology, as well as much of the rest of the discipline. Dissent is muted, and, with the exception of the perennial question of the causal priority of cognition over emotion (Lazarus, 1984; Zajonc, 1984), there is little in the way of spirited theoretical debate. On the rare occasions when theoretical disagreements do occur, they are largely confined to minor issues arising *within* the cognitive perspective, rather than representing any challenge to the basic assumptions *of* the perspective.

Does this state of affairs demonstrate that all is well? Was this the revolution to end all such fundamental shifts in conceptual and theoretical frameworks? Has clinical psychology finally found its long-sought, general, unifying paradigm? Or is this "cognitive revolution" better seen as just another wave, soon to crash on the shore and be followed by yet another such transformation of perspective? Certainly, any suggestion of the crash of the cognitive perspective seems premature, if not grossly exaggerated. Yet, serious problems are accumulating, indicating that even if not imminent, its demise is inevitable. This chapter will explore some of these fundamental problems and suggest why their solutions are likely to prove elusive, as well as what the next wave might look like.

The issue is neither whether we should return to the rigidity and narrowness of behav-

JAMES C. COYNE • University of Michigan Medical School, Ann Arbor, Michigan 48109.

iorism, nor whether what people think might be irrelevant to how they adapt to their circumstances or to how we might modify this adaptation to their benefit. Indeed, the cognitive perspective is not going to succumb to findings that decisively indicate that thinking is irrelevant to adaptation but to the boredom and frustration arising from the limited puzzles that its theory and methods actually solve. The cognitive perspective tends to involve strong inferences about the elaborate deliberations involved in the most mundane of everyday achievements. There is an intuitive appeal and an appearance of richness to the explanations of human adaptation that it offers, but a persistent ambiguity as to the referents for key concepts and an apparently unclosable gap between such strong inferences and characteristically weak methods.

As we will see, one basic problem is that cognitive perspective separates what people say they think from circumstances in which it is said, the conditions of their lives, and how they and those around them cope. What we think is important to how we can lead our lives, but it is not the only, and it is often not the primary, determinant of the outcomes that we achieve. Finally, although cognitive theory was initially a source of great inspiration and innovation in psychotherapy, it is now a constraint on both creative and critical thinking, and the limits of its assumptions deserve careful scrutiny. This chapter will review these issues with particular reference to how the cognitive perspective guides the study and treatment of depression, the disorder that has received the greatest attention and that therefore allows the fairest evaluation of the strengths and weaknesses of the perspective as it has matured.

## THINKING COGNITIVELY ABOUT DEPRESSION

Although differing in how they describe such processes, cognitive theorists regard some form of cognitive disturbance as basic to depression. As Segal and Shaw (1986b) note,

> They agree that "depressed patients view their environments as overwhelming, as presenting insuperable obstacles that can not be overcome . . . resulting in failure and loss" (Beck & Young, 1985, p. 207), but suggest that this view arises from the depressed person's negatively biased evaluations of self, world, and future and their consequent action, which predicated on these beliefs, often leads to confirmatory behavioral outcomes. (p. 711)

Beck's cognitive model of depression postulates three sets of interrelated cognitive concepts to explain the psychological phenomena of depression: the cognitive triad, schemata, and cognitive distortions (Kovacs & Beck, 1978). Taken together, these concepts are intended to explain the misperceptions and misinterpretations that depressed persons voice about themselves, their situations, and their future possibilities; specifically, how they tailor facts to fit their negative conclusions, overgeneralize, selectively abstract negative details out of context, and resist the implications of the more positive features of their circumstances. Further, these concepts are taken to reflect enduring features of depressed persons: "Certain cognitive processes seem chronically atypical among depressed patients and may represent a stable characteristic of their personality" (Kovacs & Beck, 1978, p. 530).

Recent theoretical and empirical work derived from Beck's model has tended to emphasize the importance of either a depressogenic self-schema or automatic thoughts in depression. For instance, Dobson and Shaw (1987) have attempted to utilize a self-referent encoding task to examine the operation of a self-schema presumed to preexist the onset of depression. Similarly, a number of authors have utilized the Dysfunctional Attitudes Scale (DAS; Weissman & Beck, 1978) for this purpose (Ross, Gottfredson, Christensen, & Weaver, 1986). Alternatively, the Autonomic Thoughts Questionnaire (ATQ; Hollon & Kendall, 1980) attempts to measure the actual cognitive ruminations generated by such self-schema.

As first presented, the reformulated learned helplessness model of depression held that the kinds of causal attributions that people make for uncontrollable events determine the onset, intensity, and chronicity of their depressive reactions (Abramson, Seligman, & Teasdale, 1978). A later refinement suggests that it is a negative life event to which the person attaches some degree of importance that results in depression (Halberstadt *et al.*, 1984), although this emphasis does not yet seem to be reflected in any shift in the focus of research.

Depression occurs when an individual makes internal, stable, and global attributions for such a negative event. Attributions of negative events to internal factors cause a reduction in self-esteem; attributions to global factors lead to a generalization of the expectation of noncontigency and the resulting behavioral deficits; and attributions of stable factors lead to a persistence of deficits over time. Recent work has focused on the tendency to make internal, global, and stable factors as a both a correlate of depression and a vulnerability factor, and proponents of the learned helplessness model view such a depressive attributional style as a stable, enduring aspect of personality (Peterson & Seligman, 1984). Thus, Abramson *et al.* (1978) stated earlier that "our model predicts that attributional style will produce depression proneness, perhaps the depressive personality" (p. 68).

Of course, the negativity, pessimism, and self-complaints of depressed persons were not discovered by cognitive theorists, but these theorists proclaimed a new and special significance to them: These complaints were more than an *aspect* of depression; they reflect core and even causal cognitive processes. Discussions of the cognitive perspective on depression rarely include consideration of rival plausible interpretations of these complaints, but it would be useful to note them.

The traditional interpretation of these complaints has been that they are simply features or symptoms of depression. One might go so far as to argue that it is tautological that depressed persons complain about themselves and their situations: Not surprisingly, people who are identified as depressed because they endorse self-complaints on the Beck Depression Inventory (BDI; Beck *et al.*, 1961), for instance, are likely to endorse similar self-complaints when they are given other opportunities to do so, whether it be on an attributional questionnaire or whatever. A variation of this view is that depressed persons' complaints might be seen as reflecting a secondary demoralization and self-blame for their condition, and thus as effects rather than a cause of depression (Klein, 1974). Indeed, one might argue that many moderately and severely depressed persons realize that they are coping badly, and they may attribute this to either a particular symptom of depression such as fatigue or inability to concentrate or to their absorption in their painful feelings of depression that seem as if they will never end. Therefore, depressed persons may be more inclined to endorse internal, stable, and global attributions for negative experiences *because* they are depressed, and when they make such attributions, they may mean something different than when a nondepressed person makes them.

One implication of such a perspective is that the study of the role of cognition in depression is essentially a descriptive exercise, the results of which are largely a foregone conclusion. In an apparent reply to such an argument, Rush and Giles (1982) state that Beck's theory

> makes a clear causal relationship between cognition and behavioral, affective, and physiological disturbances. The theory goes beyond descriptive detailing of the experience of depression and asserts that cognitions cause and maintain the depressive syndrome. (p. 151)

Similarly, Sacco and Beck (1985) stated that "the cognitive theory of depression proposes that depression is primarily a result of the tendency to view the self, the future, and the world in an unrealistically negative manner" (p. 4). This statement accompanied a review of studies "which provide support for the notion that negative perceptions are causally related to the other symptoms of depression" (Sacco & Beck, 1985, p. 21). Thus, the study of cognition in depression has thus been represented as much more than a mere descriptive exercise, but the burden is then assumed of demonstrating such a pivotal role for cognition. As we will see, the effort to do so consists of studies of whether the dysfunctional attitudes or attributional style associated with being depressed endure after recovery.

A *contextual* or *transactional* alternative to the cognitive interpretation of the complaints of depressed persons is that they reflect the nature of the depressed persons' involvement in their everyday lives or that they are in some way aspects of this involvement: They complain because what is happening is depressing. Perhaps they are able to find ample reason to feel unsupported, invalidated, criticized, unloved, powerless, suppressed, or a failure. These experiences may be the result of how they handle a situation that others would not find difficult or depressing, their failure to adapt to changes that require new ways of coping, their simply being in a situation that to most anyone would be devastating, or—more likely—some combination of these possibilities.

One implication of this is that depressed persons' complaints ought to be first examined in terms of their exchanges with their environment, without the presumption that they are distorted in their perceptions of what is happening. How they think is an aspect of these exchanges but hardly the whole picture, and what is happening may have an important constraint on what they think. For instance, the point prevalence of diagnosable clinical depression among female physicians is alarmingly high, perhaps 31% (Welner *et al.*, 1979). They may indeed think differently about themselves than male physicians do, but it would be unconscionable to suggest that their problems lie in their thinking without first carefully examining the differences in the circumstances of female versus male physicians.

A second suggestion of a contextual perspective is that depressed persons' complaints may be seen in part in terms of how they affect or manage their circumstances. The complaints and distress of depressed persons may influence others' behavior and, in the short run at least, afford some respite in a negative situation (Coyne, 1976a,b). Consistent with this, Biglan *et al.* (1985) have shown how depressed women's self-complaints temporarily suppress their husbands' display of hostility toward them, even though the husbands remain negative in their feelings and may even be further annoyed by their behavior. A less frequently considered possibility is that depressive self-complaints may be self-manipulative. If successful, depressive self-complaints and simply being depressed may allow one to reduce one's own expectations for oneself, avoid the implications of potential failures, and serve as a self-handicapping strategy (Snyder & Smith, 1982). Rather than merely reflecting information processing, complaints of being incompetent may represent a strategy of self-indoctrination in a threatening situation. This could be seen as a way of attempting to keep a bad situation from getting worse. Of course, this leaves aside questions of the efficacy of such a strategy.

A contextual perspective suggests that there may be no one essential psychological process or mechanism inherent in depressive self-complaints and statements of pessimism. It further suggests that *before* we focus on the distorted cognitive processes as the core or causal disturbance in depression, we should first examine the readily observable features of the context in which such complaints occur. As a prelude to considering what depressed persons think, we need to know something about the depressed persons' ecological niches, what these provide, and how depressed persons and those around them are responding (Coyne, 1982).

Undoubtedly, no single explanation for the self-complaints of depressed persons will suffice, and the influence of the cognitive perspective in reducing these complaints to a matter of biased and distorted thinking will ultimately be judged as an unfortunate narrowing of the study of depression.

To give a seemingly simple example that quickly becomes complex, suppose that Harry complains that it always rains when he plans a picnic, and Sue is more optimistic. Harry was recently left by his girlfriend, and he has since been having problems at work. His pessimism about a picnic may reflect cognitive processes instigated by his relationship problems. That is the immediate conclusion suggested by the cognitive perspective. He has now over-generalized, and he is pessimistic about anything going well and that may also have led to his problems at work. This of course introduces assumptions about the contingency of his work problems on his thinking and behavior, an assumption that can be checked out. However, before making elaborate inferences about the reasoning involved in the Harry's complaints, it would be helpful to know that he is in Olympia, Washington (average annual rainfall: 50.7 inches). Sue has just arrived from Yuma, Arizona (average annual rainfall: 2.7 inches) and does not know yet what to expect. Certainly we would ascribe different cognitive processes to Harry than if *he* were in Yuma rather than Olympia and had lived there all his life. *Construction of the cognitive processes implicit in a particular judgment always involves making some assumptions about the content of available information.* The environment must be described first because *what* there is to be interpreted has to be stipulated before one can talk about *how* it is interpreted.

Perhaps on reflection, Harry would admit that it does not always rain, but it would be better to assume that it will and thereby not add to the disappointments that his work and love life are already providing. That would be a kind of pessimism but a strategic, defensive pessimism. Perhaps he is hoping for the outside possibility that Sue will get the hint and invite him to dinner at her house instead of going to the office picnic, and maybe she might even improve his love life or at least be more supportive than everyone else seems to be. Maybe he would be reassured if she simply became more adamant that it will not rain and she *really* wants him to go on the picnic. Harry has been annoying people lately, particularly women, with his efforts to elicit such reassurance, but he at least succeeds some of the time before they get annoyed and avoid him.

Perhaps he is *kvetching* as he has been doing lately, and predictably he will go and enjoy himself. He just complains a lot, and one quickly learns not to take him seriously. Thus the "cognition" that one might infer from his verbal complaints is different than the "cognition" one would infer from his other behavior. The cognitive perspective takes for granted the convergence of these ways of inferring cognition, although depressed persons probably have no monopoly on sometimes complaining in ways that are inconsistent with their other behavior. The concept of *kvetching* is potentially quite useful in dealing with the complaints of depressed persons, and introducing it reopens the ignored but crucial question of when and to what extent depressed persons actually act on their complaints in the manner that they and others typically act on self-statements.

Thus, taking verbal complaints at face value and out of context and inferring that they reveal basic cognitive processes—and distorted ones at that—is fraught with difficulty. The meaning or significance of such complaints is not in their semantic content but in their relationship to their context. Explicating the significance of these complaints involves more than "getting in the head." Furthermore, the interpretation of the complaints is much more complex than the question of whether to attribute the complaints to the environment or the depressed person's cognitions.

The cognitive perspective does not deny that there is an environment or that it matters, nor does it deny that depressed persons may be facing difficult circumstances. The perspective, however, greatly simplify matters and closes the considerations that have just been outlined. Although current cognitive theories acknowledge the existence of an environment, there is little elaboration on how it might be connected to cognitive processes. Indeed, cognitive concepts are assigned so much work in explaining depression that there appears to be little reason to consider any complexities of the environment. The primary role of the environment is to yield the life event that activates the biased attributional processes postulated by the learned helplessness model and to provide information that is at least ambiguous enough to allow the negative schematic processing and interpretation postulated by Beck. The problem lies not in what happens to depressed persons but how they interpret it. Empirically, interest in depressed persons' exchanges with their environments is largely limited to their reports of life events, and even here the focus is on their interpretation, not the particulars of the events *per se*.

Further, what depressed persons *do* is also taken to be less interesting than what they *think*. The learned helplessness model assumes that the depressed persons has "behavioral deficits," but these follow "inexorably, rationally" (cf. Abramson *et al.*, 1978, p. 68) from attributional processes and the resulting expectations of noncontingency. Similarly, Beck and his followers refer to unrealistic beliefs producing "confirmatory behavioral outcomes" (Segal & Shaw, 1986b, p. 711). Consistent with these assumptions, recent cognitive theory and research has concentrated on the description of how depressed person's responses to questions about hypothetical, laboratory, and naturalistic events differ from those of non-depressed persons and how interpretations of the depressed person may be biased or distorted. With the passing of interest in anagrams as a way of eliciting "behavioral deficits" (see Buchwald, Coyne, & Cole, 1978, for critique of this work), there has been little attention from cognitive researchers as to what depressed persons actually do and whether what they do is linked to their complaints. The nature of behavioral deficits associated with depression—failure to initiate responses, passivity, lack of aggression (Seligman, 1975)—have been taken for granted, despite evidence that this pattern of deficits does not characterize depressed persons (Depue & Monroe, 1978). The link from "cognition" as it is assessed by attributional questionnaires to behavior is assumed, rather than demonstrated.

## THE AMBIGUITY OF COGNITIVE CONCEPTS

Wittgenstein (1980) has pointed out how erratic and inconsistent our everyday use is of the terms *thinking* and *thought*. In a similar vein, Ryle (1949) has pointed out that "thinking" is an adverbial verb, similar to "trying," "hurrying," and "repeating," in that it is incapable of being consistently specified in terms of one or more concrete ingredients. There may be connections among the various usages of thinking and thought, but that is not to say that there is an essential nature to thinking or that the various usages of the concept converge toward any center. The concept of *cognition* is heir to the same problems as the everyday concept of *thinking,* and seemingly precise cognitive concepts often prove slippery and indeterminate when we attempt to specify singular referents or even common features in their usage.

One reflection of this problem is the existence of two elaborate theories, Beck's and the learned helplessness model, that invoke quite different concepts, and yet that apparently cannot be pitted against each other in any decisive way. Despite the large literatures that have developed around each of the models, one can find little evidence of attempts to identify contrasting predictions and execute decisive empirical tests in a way that would allow an integration or emergence of a single dominant paradigm (Coyne & Gotlib, 1986). Are the two theories offering alternative descriptions of the same processes? Do depressed persons routinely engage in *all* of the deliberations suggested by *both* theories? In attempting to resolve these issues, it quickly becomes apparent that, at least at the present time, key concepts in the study of cognition in depression are no more than loosely metaphorical in nature, despite any appearance of precision.

One basic requirement of a cognitive construct that is not met by either schema or attributional style is that there be some specification of: (1) what information is required for the working of the construct; (2) the range of information that would resist the construct's biasing or distorting tendencies; and (3) what would bring about a change in the subsequent interpretations that are made. Presumably, one might still want to postulate a "depressive attributional style" if depressed persons were making their "depressive" attributions in life circumstances that were rich and stable in their support of such interpretations, but this would be different from the attributional style ascribed to them if there were no such environmental support. Further, the nature of this attributional style would be quite different if depressed persons were observed to shift their attributions readily with a change in what had been a stable negative environment. Under those circumstances, the ascription of an attributional style to them would potentially be trivial or misleading, depending on precisely what was meant by it.

What does it take for a depressed person to make an external, unstable or specific attribution for a negative occurrence, and what would deactivate this style? Given that there are now well over a hundred studies of attributional style (Sweeney, Anderson, & Baily, 1986), one would expect some refinement or explication of the concept, but, at the present time, it appears that attributional style is whatever is measured by an Attributional Style Questionnaire (Peterson *et al.*, 1982). There is a basic circularity of reasoning from which this large literature has yet to escape: Depressed persons make depressive attributions because of the operation of a depressogenic attributional style, and we know this because they make depressive attributions.

One can even ask a more basic question of what does it mean to make an attribution. Surely, from time to time we all stop and ponder a provocative event and deliberate on how it might have come about. Yet, what evidence is there that we do this routinely, or that it guides our behavior and determines our affect? Efforts to establish the routine nature of explicit attributional processes have centered on limited contexts such as sports stories in newspapers and jury deliberations (Weiner, 1985), and the reasoning in these contexts is undoubtedly different from what guides coping and adaptation in everyday life. When we do not deliberate and cannot report any attributions except in a *post hoc* reconstruction of our thought processes, is it the same as if we had taken the time to ponder our situations and ask *Why* questions? If a theorist postulates "implicit attributions," what basis is there for assuming that these are equivalent to "explicit attributions" and to what would be obtained with an attributional questionnaire? "Attribution" is an inherently and unresolvably ambiguous concept.

Other problems are associated with the concept of schema (Fiedler, 1982). Although the concept has a long history in experimental cognitive psychology, it is invoked in discussions of depression in a way that is looser than its original usage, and it now provides a mere label rather than much explanatory power. As typically employed in the study of depression, it is an effort to explain why depressed persons persist in thinking negatively, as seen in their self-complaints. There is an aura of specificity and explanatory power to the suggestion that such self-complaints reflect the "operation of hyperactive schemata" (Segal & Shaw, 1986) or that negative self-schema "eventuate in negatively toned cognitive distortions of the self, world, and future and further lead to depressive emotion and behavior" (Dobson & Shaw, 1987, p. 37). Operationally, however, one can find little suggestion in the current literature as to how that is different from the old-fashioned, common-language explanation that depressed persons have a negative attitude. Indeed, the heavy reliance on the Dysfunctional Attitude Scale to assess negative self-schema adds to the doubts that there is really any difference.

Commitment to schema as an explanation makes it difficult to accomodate the observation that humans (including depressed persons) can readily make changes in their thought processes as a result of their experience (Shaw, 1979). Accepted as an explanation of why depressed persons make negative interpretations of themselves, their circumstances, and their possibilities, the concept of schema makes it less understandable that depressed persons shift these interpretations as other symptoms remit, even in the apparent absence of any effort to alter their thinking (Eaves & Rush, 1984).

Although his interest was in memory and not depression *per se*, Malcolm's (1977) criticisms of cognitive theorists might just as aptly be applied to depression theorists:

> The cognitive theorist makes a useless movement, he invents a . . . process to fill what he thinks
> is a explanatory gap but his own explanation creates his own explanatory gap. He is deceived in

thinking that some progress and explanation has been achieved, a gap offended him and a gap remains. It is as if a man did not like to have paint on the wall so he tried to get rid of it by painting over it. (p. 102)

## THE GAP BETWEEN THEORY AND DATA

Coyne and Gotlib (1983) reviewed the then-available literature concerning the role of cognition in depression. We concluded that there was little progress being made in explicating the role of cognition in depression despite a large and growing literature. What is more important is that we pointed to fundamental conceptual and methodological problems in attempts to establish unambiguously what people think, that depressed persons are distorted or biased in their thinking, or that cognition has the role in depression postulated by Beck and the learned helplessness model. (Segal and Shaw, 1986a, argued that such criticisms were more appropriate to the learned helplessness model than to Beck's model. For a reply, see Coyne & Gotlib, 1986.)

Studies of the role of cognition in depression have continued to accumulate at an impressive rate. Yet, taking an overview of recent work, there appears to be little reason to modify our earlier evaluation of the literature, with one qualification. At the time of the Coyne and Gotlib (1983) review, there had been few studies of self-reported cognitions in recovered depressed persons. Such studies were needed to a provide at least a partial test of the hypothesis that even when not actually depressed, persons who become clinically depressed think differently than persons who do not become depressed. Miller and Norman (1986) have noted:

> The persistence of maladaptive cognitions after remission of other depressive symptoms is a crucial concept in cognitive theories of depression. If maladaptive cognitions only covary with depressive symptoms and do not persist after clinical improvement, then the argument for the enduring and causal nature of these cognitions is weakened. (p. 212)

As we will see, the evidence is now relatively clear that upon full recovery, depressed persons differ little from nondepressed persons on a full range of cognitive measures.

The bulk of the literature concerning the role of cognition in depression—and the main support for the rich and elaborate explanations of the role of cognition in depression—still consists of demonstrations of a cross-sectional relationship between measures of depression and various measures of cognition, the most widely used ones being the Dysfunctional Attitude Scale (DAS; Weissman & Beck, 1978), the Automatic Thoughts Questionnaire (ATQ; Hollon & Kendall, 1980), and the Attributional Style Questionnaire (ASQ; Peterson et al., 1982). Statistically significant relationships are typically found, and these are interpreted as evidence that—consistent with the cognitive models—depressed persons have a set of depressogenic attitudes, engage in more depressive thinking, and have a style of making more depressogenic attributions. In short, findings of significant correlations are taken as confirmations of cognitive hypotheses about depression and, more generally, the models that are the source for these hypotheses.

The largest proportion of these cross-sectional studies examines correlations between measures of attribution and depression. Sweeney et al. (1986) were able to identify 104 such studies, involving nearly 15,000 subjects. Based on their meta-analysis of these studies, they concluded that "attributions are related to depression in the manner predicted via the cognitive models" (Sweeney et al., 1986, p. 987). Across studies employing dimensionalized attribution ratings of negative outcomes, effect sizes of approximately .20 were obtained for internal, stable, and global dimensions. Somewhat lower effect sizes were found for positive events, ranging from $-.06$ for globality to $-.19$ for internality.

Sweeney *et al.* (1986) reviewed a mountain of data, but is there more than a molehill of theoretical significance to be found in it? Tests of statistical significance in both the studies these authors reviewed and the resulting meta-analysis assume a null hypothesis of $r = 0$. Yet one does not need the benefit of a cognitive theory of depression for *a priori* doubts about the plausibility of this null hypothesis. Based on the similarities in the semantic content of depression scales and measures of attributions, one would expect an effect size of at least the magnitude that Sweeney *et al.* calculated. For instance, in a sample of college students, the item-scale correlations for the Beck Depression Inventory are .61 for a self-blame item, .55 for an item tapping feelings of being a failure, .61 for a discouragement item, and .64 for an item tapping disappointment and disgust with the self (Gotlib, 1986). Given how crucial such self-descriptions are for a subject to obtain an elevated depression score, one might ask whether the psychometric limitations of commonly utilized measures of attribution prevented an even larger effect size from being obtained.

Similar objections can be raised about the substantive interpretations that are typically made of correlations between depression scales and other measures of depressive cognitions. For example, the Automatic Thoughts Questionnaire (Hollon & Kendall, 1980) contains such items as ''I'm a loser'' and ''Nothing ever works out for me.'' Questions about semantic overlap aside, there is little evidence that such questionnaires tap the cognitive processes of depressed persons routinely occurring in the absence of such a structured inquiry. The concepts, questions, and dimensions are predetermined by the experimenter, and we cannot be sure if the processes involved in answering the questions are the same as what would occur in the absence of such prompts, or that such thoughts guide the behavior of depressed persons. The parsimonious explanation remains that depressed persons feel badly about themselves and the way they are handling their situation, and that they make inferences from these diffuse feelings in order to address the specific questions asked by the experimenter. What is thus obtained is a matter of semantic structure rather than ongoing cognitive processes. Consistent with this possibility is the acknowledgment by Beck (1976) that many depressed persons have to be trained to report their automatic depressogenic thoughts.

It is relatively easy to conduct a study of the role of cognition in depression that results in a significant correlation. There are further studies possible with yet new measures of depressive cognition that—based on their overlap with the BDI (Beck, Ward, Mendelson, Mock, & Erbaugh, 1961) or other depression scales—can almost be guarranteed to yield a statistically significant correlation. Yet what progress does this represent, and are we learning anything new about depression from such studies?

There have some efforts to develop measures of depressive cognition that do not merely exploit the semantic content of depression scales. The Self-Referent Encoding Task (SRET; Davis, 1979) appeared to allow a measurement of the efficient processing of negative self-relevant adjectives by depressed persons and thus to allow a partial test of Beck's notion of the depressogenic self-schema. However, the results of a well-designed recent study were disappointing: ''Not surprisingly we can reliably conclude that depressed subjects endorse depressed-content adjectives as being self-referential more than do nondepressed subjects. In contrast, the indexes that the SRET provides to document the operation of a consistent self-schema—rating time and recall of adjectives—were not found to distinguish groups reliably'' (Dobson & Shaw, 1987, p. 38). Thus, efforts to demonstrate a relationship between depression and cognition beyond what is predictable from semantic overlap were not successful.

Of course, such cross-sectional relationships would take on new meaning if it could be shown that even when not in a depressive episode, depressed persons think differently from nondepressed persons. Such findings would be evidence of the traitlike nature of cognition postulated by cognitive theories. Yet in a prospective study with clinical diagnosis as the criteria for depression, Lewinsohn, Steinmetz, Larsen, and Franklin (1981) showed that measures of cognitions such as causal attributions, expectancies of positive and negative outcomes, perception of control, and self-esteem did not predict the onset of clinical depression in a community sample.

Other studies utilizing recovering depressed patients have found that various measures of depressive cognitions return to normal or near normal after remission of a depressive episode (Dobson & Shaw, 1987; Hamilton & Abramson, 1983; Hollon, Kendall, & Lumry, 1986; Miller & Norman, 1986; Persons & Rao, 1985; Reda, 1984; Silverman, Silverman, & Eardly, 1984; Simons, Garfield, & Murphy, 1984; Wilkinson & Blackburn, 1986). In an apparent exception to this otherwise consistent pattern of findings, Eaves and Rush (1984) found the DAS and ASQ scores to be still somewhat elevated upon remission of a depressive episode, even though these scores had significantly declined. However, their criteria for remission—a Hamilton Rating Scale for Depression (HSR-D; Hamilton, 1960) score of 10 or less for 2 weeks—were less stringent than in these other studies. Taken together, studies that have attempted to identify a persistent traitlike quality to depressive cognitions have generated considerable evidence to the contrary, that is, these measures are state dependent, perhaps simply representing measurements of a subset of depressive symptoms. Depressed people complain about themselves and evaluate themselves negatively and largely cease to do so when they recover.

We are left then with a theoretical perspective that provides elaborate explanations of the crucial role of cognitive processes in depression. Yet, in the large body of research that it has generated, the measurements that have been made have typically been crude, confounded, and incapable of supporting precise distinctions among possible cognitive concepts. The results that have been obtained are both predictable on the basis of semantic content and interpretable in terms of other hypotheses outlined earlier in this chapter. More important for the development of subsequent models of depression, however, the cognitive perspective has provided an impoverished view of both the environment of depressed persons and how they cope. It has dulled curiosity about how these factors might be relevant and discouraged what will undoubtedly prove to be more productive lines of research.

## TOWARD A POSTCOGNITIVE VIEW OF DEPRESSION

Not all persons who get divorced, lose their jobs, or face some other major life event become depressed. This observation has been taken to support the view that it is not a matter of life events, but the interpretations that depression-prone people make of them that lead to depression. There is now a large body of literature that has grown up around having subjects complete an inventory of life events and then rate some or all of the endorsed events in terms of some attributional scales or other cognitive variable. In most studies, differences in the events giving rise to a set of attributions are ignored, with the focus being the attributions that are made for the events. Differences between depressed and nondepressed persons are then explained in terms of the traitlike attributional style, schema, or other cognitive variable that is presumed to give rise to these differences. As Hammen, Marks, Mayol, and de Mayo (1985) noted,

> Most cognitive mediation theories of depression . . . have paid scant attention to event occurrence or characteristics, focusing nearly exclusively on intraindividual processes such as depressive cognitive styles or ''distortions.'' (p. 317)

An item on a life events scale, ''became divorced,'' for example, is a rather thin description (cf. Geerwitz, 1973) of a complex set of circumstances. A thicker description or a closer look at the situations of two individuals getting divorced may reveal features that adequately explain why one person gets depressed and another is free of depression is not a matter of the depressed person's idiosyncratic interpretations or distortions. One person might have no marketable job skills, difficulty obtaining child care, and an environment in which most people consider a divorce a failure and remarriage unthinkable. Another person might have a PhD, be childless, and in an environment with a surplus of eligible members of the opposite sex. The friends and relatives of one person might voice the opinion that that person's character defects brought ruin to a good relationship, whereas those of another praise that person's courage in getting out of a troubled and undependable relationship. Current methodologies employed by cognitively oriented researchers ignore the possibility that the particulars of some situations compel some interpretations or attributions and rule out others, or that "making an attribution" may be a matter of uncritically accepting a consensual judgment rather than one of personal deliberation. Interpretations of significant events are likely to be less a matter of personal deliberation and more a matter of social processes and the acceptance of an available consensus (cf. Coyne, 1985) than cognitive theories of depression acknowledge.

Consistent with this view, Brown and Harris (1978) have provided an important alternative to relying on thin descriptions of events and strictly cognitive-mediational explanations of the relationship between life events and depression. Adopting a contextual approach, they utilized interviewers to obtain extensive background information about the life events that respondents reported, and this information was rated on various dimensions by people other than the interviewers. Brown and Harris (1978) found that raters who were provided with the details of the circumstances of a life event a person had faced, *but not the person's interpretations or subjective reactions,* were able to identify the events resulting in depression. Essentially, the raters made a judgment about how they thought most people would react given such an event in such a set of circumstances.

For example, a number of the women in Brown and Harris's (1978) study had become clinically depressed postpartum. Ignoring these respondents' subjective reactions to pregnancy and the birth of a child, raters concentrated on the particulars of their circumstances and how it was judged most people would react. In this way, it was found that, for the women who became depressed, the pregnancy had given added significance to already existing problems:

> Pregnancy and birth . . . can bring home to a woman the disappointment and hopelessness of her position—her aspirations are made more distance or she becomes even more dependent on an uncertain relationship. (p. 141)

Overall, it was found that only events that have a long-term threat to a person's well-being resulted in depression. Approximately half of such events resulted in diagnosable depression. "Events threatening only in the short-term, however painful or outrageous, do not seem to bring about depression" (p. 100). Brown and Harris's (1978) findings concerning the concordance of contextual ratings and self-ratings are of particular interest in our reevaluation of cognitive interpretations of the relationship between life events and depression. The concordance was remarkable; 84% for patients and 95% for depressed persons drawn from the community. In only a small minority of cases were higher ratings by depressed persons of the threat of events judged to be a matter of their depression or some long-term "neurotic" trait. Thus, rather than being biased and idiosyncratic, the judgments that depressed persons make about events in their life fit well with raters' independent judgments about how most people would react. Given this, one might even reverse the usual emphasis of the cognitive perspective and inquire what personal and social resources allow a person to resist what are consensually depressing circumstances and what allows him or her to persist in an idiosyncratic interpretation that is not associated with depression.

Brown and Harris (1978) examined some factors that might influence the relationship between severe life events and depression, and the availability of an intimate relationship with a spouse emerged as a crucial buffer of the relationship between life events and depression.

Overall, they have provided a rich analysis of some limited aspects of the relationship between life circumstances and depression. However, they left for future research the question of how depressed persons "get caught up in a crisis or difficulty, try to cope with it, and the resources that they have for it" (p. 293). If we begin to examine the circumstances of depressed persons, what they are attempting to do about them, and with what effect, we soon find that the cognitive perspective's emphasis on negative distortion and bias in explaining the persistence of depression is overstated, if not misplaced.

Depressed persons are often dealing with distressing circumstances that do not yield to their efforts, although their ineffectiveness may be in part a matter of the response they receive from others. That depressed persons get rejected in even fleeting encounters with naive strangers is now established as a robust finding in the experimental literature (Coyne, 1976a; Strack & Coyne, 1983; for a review, see Gurtman, 1986). Three minutes into an interaction, the effects of being with a depressed person are already detectable in the nonverbal behavior of a partner (Gotlib & Robinson, 1982). Whereas by themselves, such findings lend support to the view that the sense of rejection of some depressed persons is not just a matter of cognitive distortion (Coyne, 1976b), other findings suggest that the close relationships of depressed persons are implicated in more complex ways in depressive self-complaints.

The assumption of cognitive models of depression, particularly the learned helplessness model (Abramson et al., 1978; Seligman, 1975), that depressed persons behave in a passive and helpless manner may be overly simplistic. In stressful encounters with others, depressed persons are characterized by confrontative strategies, ineffective support seeking, wishful thinking, and efforts at escape and avoidance (Coyne, Aldwin, & Lazarus, 1981; Folkman & Lazarus, 1986). Anger is a key feature of their close relationships with others (Kahn, Coyne, & Margolin, 1985). The family relationships of depressed persons are hostile and conflictful (see Coyne & DeLongis, 1988, and Coyne, Kahn, & Gotlib, 1987, for reviews), and the hostility between depressed persons and their spouses is secondary only to what occurs between depressed persons and their children (Weissman & Paykel, 1974). In problem-solving interactions, depressed persons and their spouses are quite similar in being hostile and even aggressive, low in constructive problem solving, and high in withdrawal and avoidance, and this similarity may part of what keeps their situation intractible (Kahn, et al., 1985).

Vaughn and Leff (1985) found that the majority of depressed patients, particularly women, were fearful of loss and rejection and desirous of continual comfort and support. By itself, such an observation is not inconsistent with the portrayal of depressed persons by cognitive theorists. Yet, contextualizing this observation, Vaughn and Leff suggest some very different processes by which depressed persons may be maintained in such fears and perceptions. Namely,

> few depressed patients described as chronically insecure or lacking in self-confidence were living with supportive or sympathetic spouses . . . when this was the case, the patients were well at followup. (p. 95)

Vaughn and Leff (1985) found that the majority of the spouses of depressed persons were critical of them and that spousal criticism at the time of a depressed patient's hospitalization was highly predictive of subsequent relapse. This relationship held independent of the patient's level of symptoms at the time of hospitalization, and it has been replicated in another study (Hooley, Orley, & Teasdale, 1986). Such a hostile, critical environment can be the origin of depressed person's self-complaints and hopelessness, a means of validating and expanding upon existing self-criticism, and a buffer against change. Experimental studies suggest that hostile, critical intimates can effectively insulate depressed persons from positive experiences that might otherwise challenge their negative view of themselves (Swann & Predmore, 1985). Further, the poor quality of the relationships of some depressed persons tends to persist beyond their episode (Rounsaville, Weissman, Prusoff, & Herceg-Baron, 1979) and remains a source of vulnerability to recurrent depression (Rounsaville, Prusoff, & Weissman, 1980).

In short, the more one admits such data into discussion and the more one becomes open to an ecologically complex view of depression, the less adequate cognitive accounts of the disorder become. The challenge is not one of simply linking the processes assumed by cognitive models to the environment. Rather, it is a matter of ceasing to look exclusively to idiosyncratic cognitive processes for explanations of what can better be understood in terms of the observable exchanges of depressed persons with their everyday environments. It is a matter of rekindling curiosity about what the lives of depressed persons are like and ceasing to ignore obvious problems that are not just in their thinking. It is a matter of no longer trivializing the distress of depressed person and of no longer doing them the injustice of assuming that it is their thinking that is responsible for their predicament.

Or are such considerations unnecessary? A lack of accomplishment in efforts to explain depression in terms of cognitive processes does not detract from clear evidence that cognitive therapy for depression is effective. Does this effectiveness establish the basic soundness of the cognitive perspective, if not as a basis for understanding the etiology of depression, then at least for guiding the treatment of depression?

## COGNITIVE THERAPY AND COGNITIVE THEORY

In a seminal study, Rush, Beck, Kovacs, and Hollon (1977) showed that, with outpatients, cognitive therapy is a more effective treatment for depression than medication is. Subsequent research has furnished additional support for the efficacy of cognitive therapy (Blackburn, Bishop, Glen, Whalley & Christie, 1986; Murphy, Simons, Wetzel, & Lustman, 1984). However, the relevance of this to cognitive theory is less clear than it first appears.

As I have discussed, cognitive theories readily explain why depression might persist in a benign environment and how depressed persons might fail to benefit from positive, antidepressant experiences. In contrast, cognitive therapy utilizes behavioral task assignments to exploit the ability of depressed persons to benefit from such experiences. Beck *et al.* (1979) state:

> The role of the therapist is clear. There is no easy way to ''talk the patient out'' of his conclusion that he is weak, inept, or vacuous. He can see for himself that he is not doing those things that once were relatively easy and important to him. By helping the patient change certain behaviors, the therapist may *demonstrate* to the patient that his negative, overgeneralized conclusions were incorrect. (p. 118)

From this account, it appears that change comes about as a result of the patient engaging the environment differently. Apparently the patient's depression has persisted up until the time of therapeutic intervention because the patient has not spontaneously engaged the environment in a way that counters such negative self-perceptions. In contrast to the *explicit* cognitive models of depression, the theory of depression *implicit* in such methods is that depression persists because of the manner in which the depressed person typically engages the environment. If these ways of coping can be interdicted or redirected, depression is alleviated. Rather than illuminating the mechanism by which the behavioral tasks of cognitive therapy produce change, the cognitive concepts of schema and attributional style suggest that the patient's depression should persist in the face of such interventions. Such concepts are better able to accomodate resistance to change than its occurrence. In the decade since the report of the Rush *et al.* (1977) study, evidence has accumulated that behavioral (McLean & Hakstian, 1979) and interpersonal therapies (Elkin, Shea, Watkins, & Colloins, 1986) are similarly effective in the treatment of depression. The theoretical rationales for these approaches differ, and, taken at face, they seem to suggest that these approaches act upon different, specific aspects of depression. Yet they share some common features. All are relatively brief, goal-oriented, and highly structured, and they emphasize constructive changes in behavior, rather than the attainment of insight. Apparently, more narrowly insight-oriented therapies are less effective (Covi et al., 1974; McLean & Hakstian, 1979).

Cognitive therapy is thus not uniquely efficacious for the treatment of depression. It is somewhat surprising that it does not appear that it is different from other effective approaches in its impact on cognition as measured by self-report measures. Effective treatments seem to be nonspecific in their impact, and the remission of symptoms in successfully treated depression appears to be global, rather than delimited by the content or focus of intervention. Zeiss, Lewinsohn, and Munoz (1979) compared the differential impact of social skills training, the scheduling of pleasant activities, and cognitive therapy. As well as being equally effective, the treatments has similar effects, with, for instance, cognitive therapy increasing pleasant activities as much as the explicit scheduling of them did, and scheduling of activities having as much impact on cognition as cognitive therapy. Simons et al., (1984) found that tricylic antidepressant medication and cognitive therapy had similar effects on self-report cognitive measures. This led Simons et al. (1984) to conclude that

> the cognitive distortions that are the focus of cognitive therapy appear to behave more as *symptoms* of depression than as causes. . . . [Cognitive therapy] is effective in alleviating the signs and symptoms of depression. Assigning *causality* to cognitive change, however, appears to be unjustified. (pp. 49–50)

The availability of a variety of effective treatments does not mean that the problem of depression has been solved. The effects of intervention, whether pharmacological or psychotherapeutic are often not long-lasting, and resolution of an acute depressive episode is apparently an easier matter than freeing someone from the threat of relapse. Over half of the patients receiving cognitive therapy in the Rush et al. (1977) study were depressed or had sought further treatment within a year. Apparently, even the provision of subsequent booster sesions does not reduce relapse (Baker & Wilson, 1985). Treatment with tricyclics involves similar difficulties. Over 80% of the patients who received medication in the Rush et al. (1977) study were classified as having relapsed or were unrecovered at the end of one year by the same criteria (Kovacs et al., 1981).

At least some of the solution to the problem of freeing depressed person from the burden of further problems may lie in their social environments. Perhaps because of the stressful nature of the close relationships of many, if not most depressed persons, those who have recently ended their intimate relationship fare somewhat better than those who remain in an enduring relationship (Keller et al., 1984; Parker & Blignant, 1985; Parker, Tennant, & Blignault, 1985; Parker, Holmes, & Manicavagar, 1986).

Further, depressed patients with marital problems derive considerably less benefit from individual psychotherapy (Courney, 1984) or antidepressants (Rounsaville et al., 1979) than do those in supportive relationships. Preliminary results from a study comparing cognitive therapy and marital therapy, alone and in combination, suggest that cognitive therapy alone may be ineffective for depressed persons with marital problems (Jacobson, Schmelling, Salsalusky, & Follette, 1987). Overall, depressed persons in troubled relationships benefit less from intervention and are more vulnerable to subsequent problems and depression. Apparently, assessments of marital problems or spousal criticism (Hooley et al., 1986; Vaughn & Leff, 1985) are better indicators of prognosis than are measures of cognition. Further work is needed to develop ways of helping depressed patients who derive less benefit from currently available treatments. The field needs to come to terms with the recurrent nature of depression and the relative ineffectiveness of therapy and medication in preventing relapse and residual problems. Taking a closer look at how depressed persons are involved in their environments, particularly their close relationships, may be an important first step in developing appropriate interventions. Creative ways of intervening directly in these relationships and of enlisting significant others in the process of change need to be considered (Coyne, 1984, 1988). In pursuing these possibilities, the notions that depression can be reduced to a problem of biased and distorted thinking and that therapeutic change is fundamentally a matter of changing cognition are likely to prove handicaps. An explicit focus on the changing of cognitions is not an essential feature of effective intervention, and the mistaken belief that it is may cause us to reject prematurely interventions based on direct manipulation of either how depressed persons are involved in their environments or how significant others respond (Watzlawick & Coyne, 1980).

## CONCLUSIONS

Theoretical models rarely disappear as a direct result of negative or null findings, even though specific hypotheses are sometimes discarded after contact with disconfirming data. Rather than being discarded, theoretical models are likely to be qualified in order to discount the embarrassment of such data. Thus proponents of Ptolemaic astronomy defended it against discrepant observations of planetary positions and the precession of the equinoxes by continually adjusting Ptolemy's system of compounded circles with the addition of new circles. Similarly, in the face of an apparent inability to demonstrate traitlike qualities to cognitive measures of depression, proponents of the cognitive perspective have begun to argue for latent and deep processes (Beck, 1984; Riskind & Steer, 1984; Segal & Shaw, 1986) and beliefs that are held but not thought (Hollon et al., 1986). In a parallel fashion, Hollon et al. (1987) have argued for a distinction between the nonspecificity of observed changes in cognition in treatment with medication or psychotherapy and the underlying causal status of cognition in such changes. Although effective in the short-run, such strategies weaken the tie between theory and data. Ultimately, they rob a theoretical framework of whatever clarity and parsimony it possesses. At some point, theorists and researchers without vested interests in a perspective discard it and begin to look toward the development of new models and the identification of more interesting and resolvable puzzles. For their part, practitioners can be expected at some point to discard dogma and look for better ways to explain what is effective and what is not in what they do, and they will look for a framework that is more capable of stimulating the development of innovative techniques of intervention. In the case of the cognitive perspective on depression, that point may have not yet arrived, but it is coming into sight.

ACKNOWLEDGMENT. Special thanks are due Bruce Denner for his stimulating discussions of some of the issues explored in this chapter.

## REFERENCES

Abramson, L. Y., Seligman, M. E. P., & Teasdale, J. D. (1978). Learned helplessness in humans: Critique and reformulation. *Journal of Abnormal Psychology, 87,* 49–74.

Beck, A. T. (1976). *Cognitive therapy and emotional disorders.* New York: Guilford Press.

Beck, A. T., & Young, J. E. (1985). Depression. In D. H. Barlow (Ed.), *Clinical handbook of psychological disorders: A step-by-step treatment manual* (pp. 206–244). New York: Guilford Press.

Beck, A. T., Ward, C. H., Mendelson, N., Mock, J., & Erbaugh, J. (1961). An inventory for measuring depression. *Archives of General Psychiatry, 4,* 53–63.

Beck, A. T., Rush, A. J., Shaw, B. F., & Emery, G. (1979). *Cognitive therapy of depression: A treatment manual.* New York: Guilford.

Biglan, A., Hops, H., Sherman, L., Friedman, L. S., Arthur, J., & Osteen, V. (1985). Problem-solving interactions of depressed women and their husbands. *Behavior Therapy, 16,* 431–451.

Blackburn, I. M., Bishop, S., Glen, A. I. M., Whalley, L. J., & Christie, J. E. (1981). The efficacy of cognitive therapy in depression: A treatment trial using cognitive therapy and pharmacotherapy, each alone and in combination. *British Journal of Psychiatry, 139,* 181–189.

Brown, G. W., & Harris, T. (1978). *Social origins of depression: A study of psychiatric disorder in women.* New York: Free Press.

Buchwald, A. M., Coyne, J. C., & Cole, C. S. (1978). A critique of the learned helplessness model of depression. *Journal of Abnormal Psychology, 87,* 180–193.

Courney, R. H. (1984). The effectiveness of social workers in the management of depressed female patients in general practice. *Psychological Medicine 14,* (Monograph Suppl. 6).

Covi, L., Lipman, R. S., Derogatis, L. R., Smith, J. E., & Patterson, J. H. (1974). Drugs and group psychotherapy in neurotic depression. *American Journal of Psychiatry, 131,* 191–198.

Coyne, J. C. (1976a). Toward an interactional description of depression. *Psychiatry, 39,* 28–40.

Coyne, J. C. (1976b). Depression and the response of others. *Journal of Abnormal Psychology, 2,* 186–193.

Coyne, J. C. (1982). A critique of cognitions as causal entities with particular reference to depression. *Cognitive Therapy and Research, 6,* 3–13.

Coyne, J. C. (1984). Strategic therapy with married depressed persons: Agenda, themes, and interventions. *Journal of Marital and Family Therapy, 10,* 53–62.

Coyne, J. C. (1985). Toward a theory of frames and reframing: The social nature of frames. *Journal of marital and family therapy, 11,* 337–344.

Coyne, J. C. (1988). Strategic therapy with couples having a depressed spouse. In G. Haas, I. Glick, & J. Clarkin (Eds.), *Family intervention in affective illness* (pp. 89–113). New York: Guilford.

Coyne, J. C., & DeLongis, A. (1988). The spouses of depressed persons. *Psychological Bulletin.*

Coyne, J. C., & Gotlib, I. H. (1983). The role of cognition in depression: A critical appraisal. *Psychological Bulletin, 94,* 472–505.

Coyne, J. C., & Gotlib, I. H. (1986). Studying the role of cognition in depression: Well-trodden paths and cul-de-sacs. *Cognitive Therapy and Research, 10,* 695–705.

Coyne, J. C., Aldwin, C., & Lazarus, R. S. (1981). Depression and coping in stressful episodes. *Journal of Abnormal Psychology, 90,* 439–447.

Coyne, J. C., Kahn, J., & Gotlib, I. H. (1987). Depression. In T. Jacob (Ed.), *Family interaction and psychotherapy* (pp. 509–534). New York: Plenum.

Davis, H. (1979). Self-reference and the encoding of personal information in depression. *Cognitive Therapy and Research, 3,* 97–110.

Dember, W. N. (1974). Motivation and the cognitive revolution. *American Psychologist, 29,* 161–168.

Depue, R. A., & Monroe, S. M. (1978) Learned helplessness in the perspective of the depressive disorders: Conceptual and definitional issues. *Journal of Abnormal Psychology, 87,* 3–20.

Dobson, K. W., & Shaw, B. F. (1987). Specificity and stability of self-referent encoding in clinical depression, *Journal of Abnormal Psychology, 96,* 34–40.

Eaves, G., & Rush, A. J. (1984). Cognitive patterns in symptomatic and remitted unipolar major depression. *Journal of Abnormal Psychology, 93,* 31–40.

Elkin, I., Shea, T., Watkins, J., & Colloins, J. (1986). *Comparative treatment findings: Presentation of the National Institute of Mental Health Treatment of Depression Collaborative Research Program.* Paper presented at the annual meeting of the American Psychiatric Association, Washington, DC.

Fiedler, K. (1982). Causal schemata: Review and criticism of research on a popular construct. *Journal of Personality and Social Psychology, 42,* 1001–1013.

Folkman, S., & Lazarus, R. S. (1986). Stress processes and depressive symptomatology. *Journal of Abnormal Psychology, 95,* 107–113.

Geerwitz, C. (1973). *The interpretation of culture.* New York: Basic Books.

Gotlib, I. H. (1986). *A factor analysis of the Beck Depression Inventory.* Unpublished study.

Gotlib, I. H., & Robinson, A. (1982). Responses to depressed individuals: Discrepancies between self-report and observer-rated behavior. *Journal of Abnormal Psychology, 91,* 231–240.

Gurtman, M. (1986). Depression and the response of others: Reevaluating the reevaluation. *Journal of Abnormal Psychology 95,* 99–101.

Halberstadt, L. J., Andrews, D., Metalsky, G. I., & Abramson, L. Y. (1984). Helplessness, hopelessness, and depression: A review of progress and future directions. In N. S. Endler & J. McV. Hunt (Eds.), *Personality and the behavioral disorders* (Vol. 1, 2nd Ed., pp. 373–412), New York: Wiley.

Hamilton, E. W., & Abramson, L. Y. (1983). Cognitive patterns and major depressive disorder: A longitudinal study in a hospital setting. *Journal of Abnormal Psychology, 92,* 173–184.

Hamilton, S. D. (1960). A rating scale for depression. *Journal of Neurology, 23,* 56–61.

Hammen, C., Marks, T., Mayol, A., & de Mayo, R. (1985). Depressive self-schemas, life stress, and vulnerability to depression. *Journal of Abnormal Psychology, 94,* 308–319.

Hollon, S. D., & Kendall, P. C. (1980). Cognitive self-statements in depression: Development of an automatic thoughts questionnaire. *Cognitive Therapy and Research, 4,* 383–397.

Hollon, S. D., Kendall, P. C., & Lumry, A. (1986). Specificity of depressotypic cognitions in clinical depression. *Journal of Abnormal Psychology, 95,* 52–59.

Hollon, S. D., DeRubeis, R. J., & Evans, M. D. (1987). Causal mediation of change in treatment for depression: Discriminating between nonspecificity and noncausality. *Psychological Bulletin, 102,* 139–149.

Hooley, J. M., Orley, J., & Teasdale, J. D. (1986). Levels of expressed emotion and relapse in depressed patients. *British Journal of Psychiatry, 148,* 642–647.

Jacobson, N. S., Schmelling, K. B., Salsalusky, S., Follette, V., & Dobson, K. (1987). *Marital therapy as an adjunct treatment of depression.* Paper presented at the annual meeting of Association for the Advancement of Behavior Therapy, Boston.

Kahn, J., Coyne, J. C., & Margolin, G. (1985). Depression and marital conflict: The social construction of despair. *Journal of Social and Personal Relationships, 2,* 447–462.

Keller, M. B., Klerman, G. L., Lavori, P. W., Coryell, W., Endicott, J., & Taylor, J. (1984). Long-term outcome of episodes of major depression: Clinical and public health significance. *Journal of the American Medical Association, 252,* 788–792.

Klein, D. F. (1974). Endogenomorphic depression. *Archives of General Psychiatry, 31,* 447–454.

Kovacs, M., & Beck, A. T. (1978). Maladaptive cognitive structures in depression. *American Journal of Psychiatry, 135,* 525–533.

Kovacs, M., Rush, A. J., Beck, A. T., & Hollon, S. D. (1981). Depressed outpatients treated with cognitive therapy of pharmacotherapy. *Archives of General Psychiatry, 38,* 33–39.

Lazarus, R. S. (1984). On the primacy of cognition. *American Psychologist, 39,* 124–129

Lewinsohn, P. M., Steinmetz, J. L., Larsen, D. W., & Franklin, J. (1981). Depression-related cognitions: Antecedents or consequence? *Journal of Abnormal Psychology, 90,* 213–219.

McLean, P. D., & Hakstian, A. R. (1979). Clinical depression: Comparative efficacy of outpatient treatment. *Journal of Consulting and Clinical Psychology, 47,* 818–836.

Malcolm, N. (1977). *Memory and mind.* Ithaca: Cornell University Press.

Miller, I. W., & Norman, W. H. (1986). Persistence of depressive cognitions within a subgroup of depressed inpatients. *Cognitive Therapy and Research, 10,* 211–224.

Murphy, G. E., Simons, A. D., Wetzel, R. D., & Lustman, P. J. (1984). Cognitive therapy and pharmacotherapy, singly and together in the treatment of depression. *Archives of General Psychiatry, 41,* 33–41.

Parker, G., & Blignault, I. (1985). Psychosocial predictors of outcomes in subjects with untreated depressive disorder. *Journal of Affective Disorders, 8,* 73–81.

Parker, G., Holmes, S., & Manicavagar, V. (1986). Depression in general practice attenders: Caseness, natural history, and predictors of outcome. *Journal of Affective Disorders, 10,* 27–35.

Parker, G., Tennant, C., & Blignault, I., (1985). Predicting improvement in patients with non-endogenous depression. *British Journal of Psychiatry, 146,* 132–139.

Persons, J. B., & Rao, P. A. (1985). Longitudinal study of cognitions, life events, and depression in psychiatric inpatients. *Journal of Abnormal Psychology, 94,* 51–61.

Peterson, C., & Seligman, M. E. P. (1984). Causal explanations as a risk factor for depression: Theory and evidence. *Psychological Review, 91,* 347–374.

Peterson, C., Semmel, A., von Baeyer, C., Abramson, L. H., Metalsky, G., & Seligman, M. E. P. (1982). The Attributional Style Questionnaire. *Cognitive Therapy and Research, 6,* 287–300.

Putnam, H. (1975). *Mind, language, and reality.* Cambridge: Cambridge University Press.

Reda, (1984). Cognitive organization and antidepressants: Attitude modification during amitriptyline treatment in severely depressed individuals. In M. A. Reda & M. J. Mahoney (Eds.), *Cognitive psychotherapies* (pp. 124–139). Cambridge, MA: Ballinger.

Riskind, J. H., & Steer, R. E. (1984). Do maladaptive attitudes "cause" depression?: Misconception of cognitive theory. *Archives of General Psychiatry, 41,* 1111.

Ross, S. M., Gottfredson, D. K., Christensen, P., & Weaver, R. (1986). Cognitive self-statements in depression: Findings across clinical populations. *Cognitive Therapy and Research, 10,* 159–166.

Rounsaville, B. J., Weissman, M. M., Prusoff, B. A., & Herceg-Baron, R. L. (1979). Marital disputes and treatment outcome in depressed women. *Comprehensive Psychiatry, 20,* 483–490.

Rounsaville, B. J., Prusoff, B. A., & Weissman, M. M. (1980). The course of marital disputes in depressed women: A 48-month follow-up study. *Comprehensive Psychiatry, 21,* 111–118.

Rush, A. J., & Giles, D. E. (1982). Cognitive therapy: Theory and research. In A. J. Rush (Ed.), *Short-term psychotherapies for depression* (pp. 143–181). New York: Guilford Press.

Rush, A. J., Beck, A. T., Kovacs, M., & Hollon, S. (1977). Comparative efficacy of cognitive therapy and pharmacotherapy in the treatment of depressed outpatients. *Cognitive Therapy and Research, 1,* 17–37.

Ryle, G. (1949). *The concept of mind.* New York: Hutchinson University Library.

Sacco, W. P., & Beck, A. T. (1985). Cognitive therapy of depression. In E. E. Beckham & W. R. Leber (Eds.), *Handbook of depression: Treatment, assessment, and research* (pp. 3–38). Homewood, IL: The Dorsey Press.

Segal, Z. V., & Shaw, B. F. (1986a). Cognition and depression: A reappraisal of Coyne and Gotlib's critique. *Cognitive Therapy and Research, 10,* 671–693.

Segal, Z. V., & Shaw, B. F. (1986b). When cul-de-sacs are more mentality than reality: A rejoinder to Coyne and Gotlib. *Cognitive Therapy and Research, 10,* 707–714.

Seligman, M. E. P. (1975). *Helplessness: On depression, development and death.* San Francisco: W. H. Freeman.

Shaw, B. F. (1979). The theoretical and empirical foundations of a cognitive model of depression. In P. Pliner, I. Spigel, & K. Blankstein (Eds.), *Perception of emotion in self and others* (pp. 137–164). New York: Plenum Press.

Silverman, J. S., Silverman, J. A., & Eardley, D. A. (1984). Do maladaptive attitudes cause depression? *Archives of General Psychiatry, 41,* 28–30.

Simons, A. D., Garfield, S. L., & Murphy, G. E. (1984). The process of change in cognitive therapy and pharmacotherapy of depression: Changes in mood and cognition. *Archives of General Psychiatry, 41,* 45–51.

Snyder, C. L., & Smith, T. W. (1982). Symptoms as self-handicapping strategies: The virtue of old wine in a new bottle. In G. Weary & H. Mirels (Eds.), *Integration of clinical and social psychology* (pp. 104–127). New York: Oxford University Press.

Strack, S., & Coyne, J. C. (1983). Social confirmation of dysphoria: Shared and private reactions to depression. *Journal of Personality and Social Psychology, 44,* 806–814.

Swann, W. B., Jr., & Predmore, S. C. (1985). Intimates as agents of social support: Sources of consolation or despair? *Journal of Personality and Social Psychology, 49,* 1609–1617.

Sweeney, P. D., Anderson, A., & Bailey, S. (1986). Attributional style in depression: A meta-analytic review. *Journal of Personality and Social Psychology, 50,* 974–99.

Vaughn, C. E., & Leff, J. (1985). *Expressed emotion in families: Its significance for mental illness.* New York: Guilford.

Watzlawick, P. W., & Coyne, J. C. (1980). Depression following stroke: Brief problem-focused family treatment. *Family Process, 19,* 13–18.

Weiner, B. (1985). Spontaneous causal thinking. *Psychological Bulletin, 97,* 74–84.

Weissman, A. N., & Beck, A. T. (1978). *Development and validation of the Dysfunctional Attitude Scale: A preliminary investigation.* Paper presented at the meeting of the American Educational Research Association, Toronto, Canada.

Weissman, M. M., & Paykel, E. S. (1974). *The depressed woman.* Chicago: University of Chicago Press.

Welner, A., Marten, S., Wochnick, Davis, M. A., Fishman, R., & Clayton, P. J. (1979). Psychiatric disorders among professional women. *Archives of General Psychiatry, 36,* 169–173.

Wilkinson, I. M., & Blackburn, I. M. (1986). Do thinking patterns predict depressive symptoms? *Cognitive Therapy and Research, 10,* 225–236.

Wittgenstein, L. (1980). *Remarks on the philosophy of psychology* (Vol. 1). Oxford: Blackwell.

Zajonc, R. B. (1984). Feeling and thinking: Preferences need no inferences. *American Psychologist, 35,* 151–175.

Zeiss, A. M., Lewinsohn, P. M., & Munoz, R. F. (1979). Nonspecific improvement effects in depression using interpersonal skills training, pleasant activity schedules, or cognitive training. *Journal of Consulting and Clinical Psychology, 47,* 427–439.

# II

# Clinical Applications of Cognitive Therapy

In order to practice any form of psychotherapy well, the therapist must master a variety of "nonspecific" relationship skills, and this is also true for cognitive therapy. Thus, in order to be effective, the cognitive therapist must be able to facilitate rapport, a strong working alliance, trust, mutual respect, an expectation of improvement, an environment conducive to learning and practice, an enhancement of mastery and personal efficacy, all in an atmosphere that encourages honest and open communication (Frank, 1985). However, none of these skills is likely to be sufficient for therapeutic change to occur. These relationship skills must be coupled with mastery of the various technical skills that are specific to cognitive therapy. The mastery of one set of skills without the other leaves the therapy process incomplete and ineffective for most patients.

In spite of this, there are therapists who see psychotherapy as a scientific collection of validated techniques. Having mastered the technique of therapy, they become skilled "technicians." And in fact, the judicious application of techniques may be effective with certain patients. There are also therapists who are relationship experts. They possess the skills, both intuitive and learned, that serve to offer support to others. They see the therapeutic process as more art and magical than scientific. They seem to assume that for patients to spend 50 minutes per week in the therapist's presence will be, in and of itself, therapeutic. These are the "magicians." A third group has mastered techniques within a framework of supportive interpersonal interaction. They offer a combination of the science and art of psychotherapy. These are the "clinicians."

In our opinion, good cognitive therapy requires a clinician rather than a technician or magician. We presume that our clinical readers have mastered therapy's "nonspecific" skills and therefore do not discuss them further (but see Truax & Carkhuff, 1967). However, we also do not provide a cognitive therapy "cookbook" either. We believe that effective cognitive therapy requires the ability to adapt techniques to particular patients based upon accurate conceptualizations of their problems and the subsequent development of personalized treatment strategies. For this reason, we encourage a strong grounding in the theory of the cognitive therapy model as well as providing specific treatment information.

In Part I of this volume, we focused on the history, theory, and research that underlie the cognitive therapy model. Having mastered the basic structure and theory of the model, the clinician is now in a position to integrate the techniques and applications of cognitive therapy into a comprehensive therapeutic approach. Part II of the *Comprehensive Handbook of Cog-*

245

*nitive Therapy* focuses on the various clinical applications of cognitive therapy. Throughout the chapters of Part II, similar intervention techniques will be discussed as they are creatively applied to different clinical populations and with the broad range of clinical syndromes. This portion of the *Handbook* has been designed with the practicing clinician in mind. We asked the authors to proceed by outlining and describing the treatment strategies, adaptations, techniques, and programs developed in many centers around the world. We have endeavored to offer the "front-line troops," the therapists in the consulting rooms, the information to help them start to apply cognitive therapy to the myriad patient problems and patient populations that are part of everyday clinical practice.

Part II of this book is informally divided into three groups of chapters. The initial group of chapters discusses general issues of technique that could apply to any problem or population. The second group of chapters discusses adaptations of cognitive therapy for some very common and difficult clinical syndromes. The final group of chapters demonstrates how cognitive therapy can be applied to some special populations and settings.

The initial group of chapters begins with an in-depth look at cognitive assessment. In Chapter 13, Merluzzi and Boltwood offer the reader a structure for understanding the process of cognitive assessment. Although not providing step-by-step directions, Merluzzi and Boltwood give the reader the background needed for generating an effective assessment procedure. In doing so, they focus on depression and social anxiety, two of the most widely researched problem areas. This chapter complements and expands upon issues raised by Beckham and Watkins (Chapter 4) in Part I.

In Chapter 14, Wright and Schrodt discuss the combined use of pharmacotherapy and cognitive therapy. One of the myths of cognitive therapy is that the therapist eschews the use of medication (Freeman, 1987). Nothing could be further from the actual practice of the therapy. The results of studies that compared cognitive therapy to medication in the treatment of unipolar depression have shown that cognitive therapy is as effective as medication (Blackburn, Bishop, Glen, Whalley, & Christie, 1981; Kovacs, Rush, Beck, & Hollon, 1981; Murphy, Simons, & Wetzel, 1984; Rush, Beck, Kovacs, & Hollon, 1977). In fact, as Wright and Schrodt delineate, pharmacotherapy and cognitive therapy are not mutually exclusive or contraindicated, and the combined effect may be found to be more effective than either treatment alone.

In Chapter 15, Edwards discusses the application of imagery techniques derived from gestalt therapy to cognitive therapy. John Donne's assertion that "no man is an island" is especially apt when applied to psychotherapy. No school of therapy can be so isolated that it ignores the findings, technical advances, and clinical observations of other therapies. Edwards offers the reader specific guidelines and techniques for integrating imagery work into the clinical armamentarium of the cognitive therapist. His chapter does not espouse a clinical electicism but rather a reformulation of the gestalt techniques within a cognitive therapy framework. His transcript from an actual therapy session enables the reader to see exactly how this is done.

The second section of this portion of the book consists of eight chapters dealing with the cognitive therapy of specific diagnostic groups. Each of the authors was asked to present brief reviews of the relevant research, describe the particular syndrome, and then to describe the cognitive therapy approach to treating the particular syndrome. We were especially fortunate in being able to gather chapters on so many of the disorders and populations that clinicians normally encounter in their practices.

Beck's cognitive therapy started from the findings of his research into depression. In Chapter 16, Perris, one of the most noted teachers, writers, and supervisors of cognitive therapy in Scandinavia, describes the treatment of depression, reviewing the most recent research literature and extracting from the studies the elements that contribute to an effective treatment for this common clinical problem. The general and specific techniques are described and explicated.

The threat of suicide is a frightening prospect for the families, significant others, and therapists of the suicidal patient; often, it is more frightening for them than it is for the patient him- or herself. Given the finality of the completed suicide, it is imperative that the therapist be prepared to deal with this clinical problem with a high level of confidence, along with a battery of effective intervention tools. In Chapter 17, Freeman and White describe the myths and realities of suicide, along with a cognitive conceptualization of the suicidal act. The key to treatment, Freeman points out, is an extensive assessment of suicidal ideation and preparations. By identifying the type of suicider and the best interventions for that type, a treatment model is developed. A summary of the cognitive therapy of suicide offers the clinician specific guidelines for intervention.

Anxiety may be a necessary part of the human condition. However, when it actually interferes with functioning, it becomes a clinical problem. Anxiety may occur alone or as a clinical concommitant to depression and other clinical problems. In Chapter 18, Freeman and Simon address the treatment of anxiety from an assessment perspective, with the diagnostic data leading to a treatment conceptualization, strategies, and specific intervention techniques. After laying out a simple assessment scheme, the authors explicate the basic cognitive therapy model, with several clinical examples to illustrate the model.

In Chapter 19 and 20, two sides of eating disorders are discussed. The treatment of eating disorders has, until fairly recently, received only scanty attention in the cognitive therapy literature. The most effective treatment programs must deal with cognitive, affective, and behavioral aspects of this potentially life-threatening problem. Edgette and Prout offer to the reader both cognitive and behavioral treatments for anorexia nervosa. For some manifestations of this disorder, the treatment must be cognitive behavioral. Although for others, the effective treatment will be more heavily behavioral cognitive. In this chapter, the authors describe the perceptual-cognitive and behavioral work necessary to help these patients.

Although excessive loss of weight is a central part of the diagnostic picture in anorexia, the converse, excessive weight gains, can also be threaten life and health. Cognitive-behavioral approaches to the treatment of obesity are the focus of the chapter by Kramer and Stalker. After describing the problem, they go on to discuss the treatment program for obesity developed at the University of Pennsylvania. Along with the elements of the treatment program, they include the many recording and assessment tools that have been utilized in the obesity treatment program. As with the treatment for anorexia, the most effective therapy may be either cognitive behavioral or behavioral cognitive. These two chapters on eating disorders offer the clinician straightforward treatment tools that can be applied very directly.

Perhaps the most difficult patient group seen in clinical practice is the patients diagnosed on Axis II (DSM-III-R). The patient with one or more personality disorders, described in Chapter 21, may present with any of the clinical problems described in this volume. The therapist must be aware of the diagnostic signs, cognitive conceptualizations, treatment possibilities, and the issues involved in therapeutic noncompliance. Freeman and Leaf offer the reader a theoretical framework for understanding the personality disorders from a cognitive perspective, along with treatment foci and clinical examples.

In Chapter 22, McCarthy examines interventions for the most commonly encountered problems in male and female sexual functioning. By the skillful interweaving of cognitive and behavioral interventions, the clinician can develop large numbers of treatment possibilities. McCarthy demonstrates that good cognitive therapy involves the appropriate clinical use of both types of interventions.

The final paper in this section addresses the difficult problem of chronic pain. In Chapter 23, Eimer illustrates the need for an especially strong working relationship and collaborative set when working with this population. He also emphasizes that the cognitive therapist working with pain patients needs to work closely with the appropriate medical therapists in establishing a comprehensive pain-reduction program. The author points out the importance of the therapeutic relationship in maintaining the patient in therapy despite the experience of the pain.

Chapters 24 through 29 focus on cognitive therapy with specific clinical populations. With the population becoming skewed toward older adults, Glantz's chapter on therapy with the elderly is most timely. The cognitive techniques described elsewhere in this volume require modification and alteration in the therapy of the elderly. In Chapter 24, the author highlights the treatment approach and describes the necessary modifications with emphasis on the older person's special beliefs and assumptions that lead to refusal of therapy and noncompliance. The result is that the reader can clearly see the appropriateness of the elderly as candidates for cognitive therapy.

Epstein and Baucom apply cognitive interventions to marital therapy in Chapter 25. Whereas patients may come for individual therapy with mild symptoms of depression or anxiety, a couple often comes for therapy when the negative interaction has reached a fever pitch. This is especially the case when couples are referred by attorneys prior to the instigation of divorce proceedings. The work that the authors discuss focuses on the negative interaction, dysfunctional behavior, and faulty information processing that increases the aversiveness that each member of the couple experiences.

Although there is little experimental evidence demonstrating the effectiveness of child psychotherapy, DiGiuseppe's chapter on the treatment of children offers the clinician heuristic guidelines for the application of cognitive therapy with this patient group. The author points out that among the difficulties encountered in working with children is the therapist's underestimation of the patient's ability to reason and to think more functionally. Chapter 26 will help the therapist working with children to adapt standard cognitive therapy to these patients.

Davis and Padesky offer the reader an essential perspective for working with women as patients in cognitive therapy in Chapter 27. The authors examine the gender variable and cultural socialization in the establishment of particular schema that manifest themselves in problems specific to women. This important contribution outlines the problems and pitfalls encountered in the therapy of women and is essential information for both female and male therapists.

In Chapter 28, Wessler and Hankin-Wessler describe applications of the cognitive model to group therapy. Treatment in the group context is qualitatively different from individual therapy and provides many opportunities that individual therapy cannot. The authors see the group experience as having the potential of enhancing the therapy in manifold ways. By offering simple guidelines for the formation of the group, ways of starting the group, and problems and solutions, this chapter will be useful for any clinician wishing to enhance his or her therapeutic repertoire.

The final chapter of the section and of this portion of the volume discusses the application of cognitive therapy to inpatient populations. In Chapter 29, Bowers describes several different treatment programs designed for inpatient application. In addition to the theoretical work, he discusses the applications, modifications, and problems encountered with the treatment of the inpatient.

It is our hope that this section of the *Handbook* will provide the practicing clinician with education regarding the role of conceptualization in cognitive therapy as well as with practical information that can be used in his or her actual clinical work. Beyond this, we hope that these chapters will serve as inspiration to the reader in expanding the application of cognitive therapy to previously unserved populations and problems.

# 13

# Cognitive Assessment

## Thomas V. Merluzzi and Michael D. Boltwood

### INTRODUCTION

The focus of this chapter is on the clinical assessment of cognition. In order to provide a conceptual framework for cognitive assessment methods, Kendall and Ingram (1987) have proposed a taxonomic system that includes four major components: (1) cognitive structure, (2) cognitive propositions, (3) cognitive operations, and (4) cognitive products (pp. 91–92). After a brief exposition of these components and a discussion of the validity of self-reports, the remaining portions of the chapter will contain a review of prevalent methods and present examples of cognitive assessment.

#### Conceptual Framework for Cognitive Assessment

As noted, Kendall and Ingram (1987) include four domains in their taxonomic system. First, cognitive structure refers to the organization of information or how the client represents information internally. Second, cognitive propositions refer to the content that is stored in those cognitive structures. The combination of structure and content form a construct called a schema. Interest in the schema construct has fostered both research and theory in a variety of areas in social, clinical, and cognitive psychology (Merluzzi, Rudy, & Glass, 1981). The reader is encouraged to consult Kendall and Ingram (1987), Landau and Goldfried (1981), and Winfrey and Goldfried (1987) for more information on schemas and the assessment of schemas. Also, of particular interest to clinicians is the work of Markus (Markus & Wurf, 1987) on self-schemas.

The third domain, cognitive operations, refers to the processes by which information is encoded, stored, and retrieved. Based on the information-processing paradigm and cognitive science methodologies, research on cognitive operations or processes has included studies on selective attention, perceptual distortion, and selective encoding and retrieval. A volume edited by Ingram (1987) and, in particular, a chapter by Nasby and Kihlstrom (1987) in that

Thomas V. Merluzzi • Department of Psychology, University of Notre Dame, Notre Dame, Indiana 46556.   Michael D. Boltwood • Counseling Psychology Program, School of Education, Stanford University, Stanford, California 94305.

THOMAS V.
MERLUZZI and
MICHAEL D.
BOLTWOOD

volume present an information-processing perspective on psychopathology. In addition, Goldberg and Shaw (Chapter 3, this volume) present research on cognitive processes.

The final category in Kendall and Ingram's taxonomy is cognitive products that refer to the ''by-products'' of cognitive schemas and operations. These products may be the thoughts, self-evaluations, ideas, and feelings that a person experiences and, in many instances, is able to consciously recollect and report. From a strictly clinical perspective, cognitive products are the easiest cognitive data to collect and evaluate and the most clinically useful for treatment planning.

Although the majority of the assessment devices to be reviewed in this chapter are cognitive products, the clinician should not be discouraged from assessing schemas or studying cognitive processes. However, those approaches have been primarily used in research and not in clinical practice. Consequently, most of what is reviewed in this chapter will be subsumed under the category of cognitive products.

## Validity of Self-Reports of Cognitions

Cognitive products are obtained through the verbal reports of clients. However, approaches to the collection of cognitive data in this manner are not uncontroversial. The major issue concerning the validity of self-reported data, articulated by Nisbett and Wilson (1977), is that subjects or clients are not able to report accurately causal explanations of their behaviors. Furthermore, they state that if subjects are accurate in causal explanations, it is because they are responding as an observer of their own behavior or they have a predictive model that would be accurate regardless of the specific data.

In a discussion of the Nisbett and Wilson argument, Genest and Turk (1981) note that

> it is important to distinguish between the situations in which it does and does not make sense to use subjective cognitive accounts as data. (p. 239)

The experiments reported in Nisbett and Wilson tended to include judgments that required subjects to arrive at causal explanations of their behavior rather than simply report thoughts.

Genest and Turk (1981) also note that it is important to distinguish between data and causality. If one considers cognitive reports as data rather than as veridical causal explanations, then the analysis of the data is the work of the clinician or researcher. Furthermore, if collected, the subject's causal explanation would be viewed merely as data about the subject's causal explanation for that situation (Peterson, Luborsky, & Seligman, 1983). Also, although their work did not focus on the self-report of thoughts, the work of Howard and colleagues (Howard, 1982) suggests that self-reports are better measures of constructs such as assertiveness and depression than behavioral measures. Finally, Mischel (1981) notes that the predictions possible from simple direct self-ratings and self-reports generally have not been exceeded by those from more indirect, costly, and sophisticated personality tests, from test batteries, and from expert clinical judges (p. 481).

The methods of collecting data greatly affect the accuracy of self-report data. In an attempt to improve validity, Meichenbaum and Cameron (1981) offer the following guidelines for the collection of self-report data.

1. The inquiry should be conducted as soon as possible following the cognitive events of interest, assessing directly for information in short-term memory whenever possible.
2. The amount of probing should be minimized in order to decrease the likelihood that client or subject will engage in inferential processes about his or her own cognitive experience or about the expectancies of the clinician or experimenter.
3. Analysis of the internal consistency of such reports should be included in order to assess the validity of the verbal report.

4. Clients or subjects should be asked to describe verbally their cognitive experience. They should not be asked to explain why they behaved as they did or provide motives for their behavior.
5. Clients or subjects should be given a set that motivates them to provide honest and full accounts. In providing such a set, the assessor might emphasize that his or her ability to study the target experience depends entirely upon honest, careful reporting.
6. It may be helpful to provide a set that legitimizes disclosure of cognitions. For example, clients or subjects might be asked to provide their ''impressions'' or descriptions of their experience during the experimental task, as opposed to being asked to ''recollect'' what occurred or to the tell what they ''did.''
7. Providing the client or subject with retrieval cues immediately after performance may also foster full and veridical reporting.

These guidelines are offered to acquaint the reader with optimal assessment conditions. Although in clinical practice the adherence to these guidelines may be impractical, knowledge of these conditions may allow the clinician to plan better cognitive assessments and to evaluate the compromises one has to make in clinical assessment compared to the more ideal conditions in a research setting.

## ASSESSMENT OF COGNITIVE PRODUCTS IN ANXIETY AND DEPRESSION

The following sections contain approaches to the assessment of cognitive products. Two problem areas, anxiety and depression, have been chosen to illustrate the assessment methods because of the prevalent use of cognitive therapies to treat these disorders and also the current cognitive conceptualizations of them (Beck, Rush, Shaw, & Emery, 1979; Beck & Emery, 1985). The discussion of cognitive assessment of anxiety will focus on the assessment of self-statements, and cognitive assessment of depression will focus primarily on automatic thoughts and attributions.

### ASSESSMENT OF SELF-STATEMENTS AS COGNITIVE PRODUCTS OF ANXIETY

One of the most popular approaches to the cognitive assessment of anxiety is the assessment of self-statements. Glass and Merluzzi (1981) developed a taxonomy for classifying methods of self-statement assessment that includes: (1) recognition methods, (2) recall methods, (3) prompted-recall methods, (4) expressive methods, and (5) projective methods.

#### Recognition Method of Self-Statement Assessment

This approach to self-statement assessment involves presenting the client with a series of statements or thoughts and asking how frequently he or she might had have had each thought. These statements are usually contained in questionnaires that are designed for a specific problem such as nonassertiveness or social anxiety and typically include positive and negative subscales. In general, they are easy to administer and score; however, they require a great deal of work to devise and validate.

*Social Interaction Self-Statement Test.* The Social Interaction Self-Statement Test (SISST; Glass, Merluzzi, Biever, & Larsen, 1982) is a 30-item measure that contains 15 positive (facilitating) and 15 negative (inhibiting) thoughts that relate to initial heterosocial encounters.

The client rates on a 5-point scale the frequency of occurrence of each thought. The SISST may be given after a real or imagined social encounter or in anticipation of a social encounter. The authors reported split half-reliabilities of .73 and .86 for the positive and negative scales, respectively. Concurrent validity coefficients with measures such as the Social Avoidance and Distress Scale, the Fear of Negative Evaluation Scale, and the Survey of Heterosocial Interactions ranged from .45 to .77. Also, judges' ratings of skill and anxiety were significantly correlated with the negative subscale of the SISST but not the positive subscale. Also, Merluzzi, Burgio, and Glass (1984) found that the negative but not the positive subscale of the SISST was a significant predictor of self- and clinician's ratings of shyness problems in an outpatient clinic population. Those authors also found that a Difference score (i.e., SISST-Positive minus SISST-Negative) was a better predictor of shyness ratings than the negative SISST score. Segal and Marshall (1985) and Heimberg, Nyman, & O'Brien (1987) and also found that the SISST-Negative subscale was more highly correlated with behavioral ratings and self-report data on social skills than the SISST-Positive. Finally, Beidel, Turner, and Dancu (1985) found that socially anxious individuals endorse more negative and fewer positive statements on the SISST than nonsocially anxious persons.

*Assertive Self-Statement Test.* The first and most well known of the self-statement tests is the Assertive Self-Statement Test (ASST; Schwartz & Gottman, 1976). The ASST has 34 items, 17 positive (facilitating assertion) and 17 negative self-statements (inhibiting assertion). Like the SISST the client indicates on a 1 to 5 scale how frequently each thought had occurred in a particular situation. Schwartz and Gottman (1976) found that highly and moderately assertive subjects had more positive than negative thoughts, and those who were low in assertion tended to have an equal amount of positive and negative thoughts.

A factor analysis of the ASST (Bruch, Haase, & Purcell, 1984) revealed that the negative scale consists of two factors, one dealing with the consequences of assertion and the other concerned with moral values such as hurting others. The former but not the later factor was a significant predictor of assertiveness scores. Bruch *et al.* (1984) also report an internal consistency value of .78.

*Cognitive Interference Questionnaire.* A measure similar to the ones presented before is the Cognitive Interference Questionnaire (CIQ; Sarason & Stoops, 1978). It is a measure of negative interfering thoughts. The CIQ consists of eleven 5-point scales to which the client responds as to how often each thought occurred during a task. In addition, there is one 7-point scale assessing "the degree to which your mind wandered." In studies that contrasted high versus low test-anxious groups, Sarason and Stoops (1978) and Hollandsworth, Glazeski, Kirkland, Jones, and Van Norman (1979) found the high-anxious groups endorsed more negative interference thoughts than low-anxious groups. Also, in an outcome study, Kirkland and Hollandsworth (1980) reported that both a relaxation training group and a "test taking attentional skills training" group showed lower CIQ scores than a practice control group.

Other recognition methods have been developed but have not been used extensively enough to assess their strengths and weaknesses. For example, Kendall and Hollon (1987) have developed an Anxious Self-Statement Questionnaire. An interesting aspect of that measure is its use of what the authors have termed *automatic questioning* (e.g., What will they think of me?). The excessive use of automatic questions by anxious persons appears to be related to a disproportional emphasis on the future (Ingram & Kendall, 1987), and perhaps the anticipation of negative outcomes.

Recognition methods are easy to administer, score, and are quite versatile. However, a disadvantage is that the statements contained in these questionnaires may not be the actual thoughts that the client has had in a particular situation but are prototypical statements that the client can identify as typifying his or her thoughts. From a clinical perspective, this is not that problematic because the goal of assessment is to uncover anxiety-promoting thoughts and to foster the monitoring of those types of thoughts. The fact that the items in self-statement questionnaires are not precisely the thoughts of the client or that they represent prototypical thoughts probably will not affect the quality of treatment. Finally, by selecting statements from the client's responses on the questionnaire, the therapist can probe into the idiosyncratic meaning of each statement.

*Recall Methods of Self-Statement Assessment*

This method of self-statement assessment is also known as the "thought-listing" approach (Cacioppo & Petty, 1981). The client is asked to list thoughts he or she might have had during a specific time (e.g., prior to, during, or after an event). Usually a certain amount of time (typically 2 to 3 minutes) is allowed for the client to list all the thoughts that might have occurred. For example, a clinician may have a socially anxious client recall a recent social encounter that was particularly troublesome. After imagining the encounter the clinician asks the client either to verbalize or to write each thought. The client is instructed to "list thoughts that went through your head, whether about yourself, the other person or the situation; whether positive, negative, or neutral" (Cacioppo, Glass, & Merluzzi, 1979).

To facilitate scoring, the thoughts should be separate and distinct from one another. The form typically used for a written thought listing contains a series of separate boxes, and only one thought is written in each box. However, if the thoughts are not written in separate boxes, judges or the clinician may segment the information into thought units. With minimal prompting, judges are able to separate this information into scorable thought units. If the thought listing is done orally, subjects should be instructed to give concise thoughts and pause or signal between thoughts. However, if that procedure is not feasible, the division into thought units can be performed on the oral thought listing after the material has been transcribed.

The protocols generated from thought listing are scored by the clinician or judges. In research on social anxiety, the thoughts are usually scored on a valence dimension—that is, positive (facilitating) versus negative (inhibiting). In addition, the clinician may have the client score or categorize his or her statements as a method of assessing the client's subjective evaluation of his or her thoughts and to teach the client to monitor the quality of his or her thoughts in anxious situations.

Another approach to scoring thoughts takes into account the subjective importance of each statement as well as the valence. Huber and Altmaier (1983) had phobic subjects rate (on a 3-point scale) the salience of each thought they had generated. Judges then rated each thought on the degree of threat expressed after each thought was cast into a bipolar format. The subjects' salience values and the judges' threat values were then used as weights to determine the subjects' score. Phobics had higher overall threat value scores (salience multiplied by judged threat) than nonphobics. By taking into account the subjective judgments of the subject and the objective threat value of the thought, the authors were able to make a more finely tuned analysis of the thoughts of the subjects.

Cacioppo *et al.* (1979) and Malkiewich and Merluzzi (1980) have shown, in the former study, that high-versus low-anxiety groups differ on negative self-statements elicited by the recall method and, in the latter study, that negative statements change as a function of treatment. It is highly likely that anxiety states facilitate the recall of thoughts that are consistent with previous thoughts in those situations. This retrieval process then reinforces the anxiety and dread, thus perpetuating the anxiety (Ingram, 1987; Ingram & Kendall, 1987) and emphasizes the negatively valenced thoughts. Finally, the thought-listing approach appears to tap certain types of cognitions that are more oriented toward self-evaluation rather than problem solving (Blackwell, Galassi, Galassi, & Watson, 1985).

The advantage of this approach is that it is easy to administer and is applicable to a variety of problems and situations. The disadvantages are: (1) that the thought-listing protocols must be scored and, therefore, the reliability question is one that must be confronted, and (2) clients or subjects may produce fewer thoughts with this method (Blackwell *et al.*, 1985) than with other methods such as the expressive method.

### Prompted Recall Method of Self-Statement Assessment

The prompted recall method involves the elicitation of self-statements with cues to aid recall. This approach has also been called "thought dubbing" in that subjects view a videotape of their performance and are asked to "dub" or verbalize their thoughts as the performance progresses. Smye and Wine (1980) had male and female high-school students view a videotape of their responses to assertive situations and recall their thoughts. Results indicated that, whereas women were less aggressive than men behaviorally, they also tended to evaluate others more negatively and to deny the impact of others on them. Thus, the cognitive data seem to indicate that, although the women may be less aggressive, they had a "cognitive" buffer to lessen the impact of others on them. Using similar methodology, Hollandsworth *et al.* (1979) found that low-test-anxious subjects had a greater proportion of task-facilitating statements than high-test-anxious subjects.

The advantage of the prompted method is that a large quantity of thoughts is collected, and the sequential nature of these thoughts can be analyzed. The disadvantage is that the client or subject may be reporting thoughts that are unlike those he or she actually had in the situation. The "dubbed" thoughts may represent a *post-hoc* reevaluation of their performance in the situation.

### Expressive or Concurrent Methods of Self-Statement Assessment

Based on the criteria offered by Meichenbaum and Cameron (1981) that were presented earlier in this chapter, the expressive approach appears to be the best overall method. In this approach, the client is asked to "think aloud" while performing the task. The clinician is able to obtain a large sample of thoughts and thus is able to check consistency. Although this approach may be useful in certain situations, it has limited utility in social skills assessment because it is impossible to interact and, at the same time, report your thoughts. Also, Kendall and Hollon (1981) indicate that reactivity may affect the actual flow of self-talk in that subjects who are asked to think aloud spend more time on individual thoughts than those who do not think aloud.

In an adaptation of this method, Goldfried and Sobocinski (1975) and Craighead, Kimball, and Rehak (1979) asked subjects to imagine social situations and to report their thoughts during the imagined interaction. In both studies, negative thoughts were significantly correlated with anxiety. In a variation of this method, Hurlburt (Hurlburt & Melancon, 1987) and Singer (Pope & Singer, 1977) have used a sampling approach to generate thought data. This sampling method could be adapted for research on social interaction by having clients carry a sound generator that beeps at random intervals. That signal would prompt clients to fill out a brief questionnaire (or list thoughts) and indicate the setting (i.e., alone or with someone, etc.).

*Projective Method of Self-Statement Assessment.* In a manner consistent with the traditional approach to projective assessment, this method requires the client not to state his or her own thoughts but those of a character in a picture or vignette. For example, for the assessment of social anxiety, a series of pictures could be presented to the client that depicted social encounters or situations, and he or she would be asked to tell what the person(s) in the picture is thinking. The protocols from the clients would then be scored. Sobel (1981) presents an overview of the uses of this techniques and an example of the methods. His Cancer Problem-Solving Projective Test (CPSPT) was designed to assess self-statements, coping behavior, defense mechanisms, and self-instructional patterns. The CPSPT has a series of cancer dilemmas that consist of two cards. The first is the problem card that presents a problematic situation, and the second is the resolution card showing that the problem has been solved. Because there is no attempt to suggest a particular resolution, thoughts can be elicited about the problem as well as the patient's problem-solving knowledge. This approach has a great deal of potential; however, validation is critical in the development of these types of projective assessment procedures.

INTERPRETATION OF SELF-STATEMENT DATA

There are a variety of approaches to interpreting client's self-statement data. A clinician may attempt to determine the idiosyncratic meaning of a client's self-statements. For example, in Beck's approach to cognitive therapy, he elicits "automatic thoughts," inquires about the meaning of the each thought and how the thoughts promote depression. In fact, the exact meaning of a thought is somewhat less important than its function. Thus, the depression or anxiety-producing function of the thoughts could be explained to the client, and his or her subjective meaning could be used to refine the analysis of those thoughts.

The most prevalent scoring scheme used on self-statement data has been valence, that is, positive versus negative. For example, in the Assertive Self-Statement Test and the Social Interaction Self-Statement Test there are two scales: Positive (facilitating assertion or social interaction) and Negative (inhibiting assertion or social interaction). Interpretation of the scores from these instruments involves evaluating the levels of positive and negative self-statements using appropriate norm groups as reference points.

An alternative to using the positive and negative scales separately is to use a difference score: the positive score minus the negative score. Merluzzi *et al.* (1984) have asserted that this difference score may be a better measure than either of the scales used separately. Schwartz and Garamoni (1986) have offered an explanation concerning why the difference score (positive minus negative) may be a better measure. They have presented a model based on the polarity of thoughts in which they conceptualize the positive–negative dichotomy as an important feature of what they have termed "internal dialogue." They propose a *states of mind model* that includes five states of mind and is based "on the relative balance between positive and negative cognitions" (p. 17).

Those five states are *positive dialogue, negative dialogue, internal dialogue of conflict, positive monologue, and negative monologue*. Each state of mind (SOM) is associated with a different proportion of positive to negative cognitions. Schwartz and Garamoni suggest that the optimal state, positive dialogue, is characterized by 62% (± 6%) positive self-statements and 38% (± 6%) negative self-statements. They propose that this asymmetry promotes a positive, facilitating approach to life while having a sufficient amount of negative thoughts to remain sensitive to problems and to threatening information. Also, because the dominant state of mind is positive, negative information may stand out when it arises and, thus, contributes significantly to the cognitive appraisal of a situation. For example, a person who exhibits the positive dialogue (i.e., 62% positive and 38% negative) on a measure such as the Social Interaction Self Statement Test, has positive cognitions that should facilitate social interaction but also has sufficient negative cognitions to remain interpersonally sensitive.

In contrast to positive dialogue, the negative dialogue pattern is approximately 62% negative and 38% positive self-statements. The dominance of negative cognitions would promote inhibition and a tendency to discount positive events, even though they may stand out against a backdrop of negative thoughts. The internal dialogue of conflict represents approximately 50% negative and 50% positive self-statements. Finally, the positive and negative monologues have predominantly positive (greater than 62% positive) statements in the former and predominantly negative (greater that 62% negative) in the latter.

In their review of cognitive assessment literature covering a variety of assessment methods and problem areas, Schwartz and Garamoni (1986) present convincing evidence supporting the states of mind model. The consistency of the findings across these studies is impressive. Essentially, one finds optimal adjustment in the positive dialogue state, mild psychopathology in the negative dialogue state, and severe pathology in the negative monologue state. The advantage of the states of mind model is that it provides an interpretive framework for the assessment of self-statements. The reader is strongly encouraged to read Schwartz and Garamoni for an extended treatment of the model.

## COGNITIVE ASSESSMENT OF DEPRESSION

This discussion of the cognitive assessment of depression will focus on selected assessment questionnaires that have been psychometrically developed and evaluated. Primary attention will be given to measures that operationalize the central components of two cognitive theories of depression currently dominant in the psychological literature; Beck's cognitive model of depression (Beck *et al.* 1979) and the depressive attributional style hypothesized by the reformulated learned helplessness model (Abramson, Seligman, & Teasdale, 1978).

### Cognitive Model of Depression

Beck's cognitive model of depression (Beck *et al.*, 1979) makes an important distinction between automatic thoughts or self-statements and underlying schemata or belief systems. Negative automatic thoughts are spontaneous self-statements or ruminations characterized by the cognitive triad of negative view of self, negative interpretation of ongoing experiences, and negative view of the future. This model postulates that automatic or spontaneous thoughts will covary with the symptoms of the depressive syndrome. In contrast, cognitive schemata are seen as relatively stable, enduring, traitlike cognitive patterns. Depressive schemata or attitudes are characterized by the negative cognitive triad as well as a number of cognitive errors typically associated with the beliefs of depressed individuals (Beck *et al.*, 1979).

*Automatic Thoughts Questionnaire.* The Automatic Thoughts Questionnaire (ATQ) was developed by Hollon and Kendall (1980) to measure the frequency of negative spontaneous ruminations or automatic thoughts. The questionnaire consists of 30 negative statements such as "I'm no good," "I can't finish anything," and "My life is not going the way I want it to." Subjects are asked to indicate how frequently each thought has occurred to them over the previous week on a 5-point Likert scale ranging from 1 (*not at all*), to 5 (*all the time*). A total score is obtained by summing all item responses, with possible scores ranging from 30 to 150.

The 30 statements were derived from a list of 100 negative cognitions that a pool of male and female undergraduate reported as typically associated with depressing experiences they were able to recall. The initial 100 statements were used in a preliminary questionnaire (ATQ-100) that was completed by a sample of 348 male and female undergraduates. These subjects also completed the Beck Depression Inventory (BDI; Beck, 1978), and the Minnesota Multiphasic Personality Inventory Depression Scale (MMPI-D; Hathaway & McKinley, 1940) that were used to select depressed and nondepressed criterion groups. The final 30 items were selected based on their ability to significantly ($p < .01$) discriminate between the depressed and nondepressed criterion groups identified by the BDI and MMPI-D.

The ATQ was then cross-validated by computing total scores for the depressed (mean = 79.64, SD = 22.29) and nondepressed (mean = 48.57, SD = 10.89) groups. Statistical comparison showed significantly higher scores for the depressed group [$t(17) = 4.85$, $p$

< .001]. Excellent reliability figures were obtained with a split-half reliability coefficient of .97 and a Cronbach's alpha of .96 and item-to-total correlations significant at the .001 level or better.

The validity and reliability of the ATQ has also been examined with a variety of populations. In a large sample of undergraduate subjects, Dobson and Breiter (1983) correlated depression, as measured by the BDI, with several measures of depressive cognitions. These cognitive measures included the ATQ, the Dysfunctional Attitude Scale (DAS; Weissman, 1978; Weissman & Beck, 1978), and the Interpretation Inventory (INTL; Stake, Warren, & Rogers, 1979). The ATQ provided the strongest correlation with the BDI ($r = .64$ for males, $r = .62$ for females). The reliability of the ATQ was .96 (Cronbach's alpha) for males and .95 for women. Concurrent validity was demonstrated by positive and significant correlations with the DAS and the INTL.

More recent studies have used the ATQ to assess clinical populations. In a study comparing depressed patients at a mental health center, nondepressed psychiatric patients, and a control group, Harrell and Ryan (1984) found a significant correlation between the ATQ and depression (as measured by the BDI and the MMPI-D). Eaves and Rush (1984) studied a sample of women diagnosed as having either endogenous of nonendogenous depression based on research diagnostic criteria for definite unipolar, nonpsychotic major depressive disorder (MDD; Spitzer, Endicott, & Robbins, 1978). Subjects were also evaluated with the Schedule for Affective Disorders and Schizophrenia-Lifetime Version (SADS-L; Endicott & Spitzer, 1978). A matched control group of nondepressed women was also included in the study. All depressed subjects were initially evaluated while acutely symptomatic (T1). They were then followed until it was determined clinically that their depression had remitted, at which time they were retested (T2). A subset of subjects who did not recover from their depression during the course of the study were included as an "unremitted" comparison group. At T1, the depressed groups had equivalent mean ATQ scores that were significantly higher than the mean for the control group. Upon remission of their depression (T2), the mean ATQ scores of the initially depressed patients were equivalent to the control group mean scores.

Dobson and Shaw (1986) compared a battery of measures of depressive cognitions in a study involving three hospitalized samples, depressed psychiatric patients, nondepressed psychiatric patients, and nonpsychiatric (control) patients. Upon initial evaluation, the ATQ, when compared to other cognitive measures, provided the strongest differentiation among subject groups. Convergent and discriminant validity was supported by significant correlations between the ATQ and other measures of depressive cognitions but not with those assessing nondepressive cognitions. Retesting of the depressed group while they were still depressed revealed that ATQ scores were quite stable.

Ross, Gottfredson, Christensen, and Weaver (1986) compared depressive symptoms with ATQ scores across a variety of inpatient clinical populations including depressives, schizophrenics, substance abusers, and depressed substance abusers. Depressive symptoms, as measured by the BDI and the MMPI-D, were present in each group but varied significantly across disorders. ATQ scores covaried with measures of depression across each of the groups. Hollon, Kendall, and Lumry (1986) administered the ATQ to a number of subject groups identified as bipolar disorder, depressed; unipolar disorder depressed; substance abuse disorder, depressed; substance abuse disorder, nondepressed; general psychiatric disorder, medical patient control; remitted, bipolar; remitted, unipolar; and normal (nonpatient) control. Similar to Ross *et al.* (1986), they found that ATQ scores covaried with BDI and the MMPI-D scores across a variety of psychiatric diagnoses.

In summary, the ATQ has been used with a variety of depressed and control populations. It has strong internal reliability and is significantly correlated with other measures that tap similar cognitive aspects of depression as well as multiple clinical indexes of depression. Studies that have assessed a variety of clinical populations that often manifest depressive symptoms, such as schizophrenics and substance abusers, indicate that the ATQ is correlated with depression as a syndrome rather than as a nosologic disorder. Most importantly, the ATQ's strong correlations with the BDI and other clinical indexes of depression demonstrate that it is sensitive to variations in levels of depressive symptomatology. These findings are consistent with the cognitive theory (Beck *et al.*, 1979) that describes the automatic negative thoughts associated with depression as being state dependent.

Rule-of-thumb guidelines for clinical interpretation can be estimated based on ATQ scores reported for different populations. Mean scores for "normal" control groups have ranged the 39 to 48 with standard deviations from 10 to 17. Mean scores for major depression groups have been generally in the high 80s and the 90s but have ranged as high as 126. Standard deviations for samples with major depression have ranged from the low to high 20s.

*Dysfunctional Attitude Scale.* The Dysfunctional Attitude Scale (DAS; Weissman, 1978; Weissman & Beck, 1978) is a self-report questionnaire developed to assess negative attitudes or schemata associated with depression as described by Beck (Beck *et al.*, 1979). Each item presents a negative attitude or belief such as "If I do not do well all the time, people will not respect me" or "I cannot be happy unless I know people admire me." Each item is rated on a 7-point Likert scale ranging from 1 (*totally disagree*) to 7 (*totally agree*). Higher scores indicate increasingly dysfunctional attitudes.

Administering the DAS to a volunteer sample of hospital employees, Oliver and Baumgart (1985) reported a Cronbach's alpha of .85. They described item-total correlations as "highly significant but moderate in size" (p. 164). In addition, a 6-week test–retest reliability coefficient of .73 was also reported. When administered to a sample of 234 male and 222 female undergraduate college students (Dobson & Breiter, 1983), DAS items had a Cronbach's alpha of .90 for males and .89 for females. In this "normal" nonclinical sample, the mean DAS score for males was 89.77 with a standard deviation of 29.29. The mean score for females was 88.12 with a standard deviation of 26.76. By way of comparison, the mean BDI scores for this sample were 6.91 for males and 8.39 for females. Correlations between the DAS and BDI were $r = .30$ for females and $r = .36$ for males. Correlations of a similar magnitude were found when the DAS was compared to the ATQ and the INTL.

Dobson and Shaw (1986) administered the DAS to hospital patients with major depression, nondepressed psychiatric patients, and nonpsychiatric hospital patients. Cronbach's alphas ranged from .95 to .94 across the samples. Mean DAS scores for the depressed, psychiatric control, and normal controls were 146.8, 113.5, and 112.35, respectively. Fifteen of the subjects were tested twice while still clinically depressed with an average interval between testing of 14.9 days. For this group, the DAS scores remained quite stable, with means of 138.73 and 136.8. For depressed patients who remitted, (BDI scores at the "low end of 'mild depression,'" p. 21), DAS scores did not show a significant change. The mean DAS at initial testing was 131.4, whereas the mean upon remission was 121.67. Both Dobson and Breiter (1983) and Dobson and Shaw (1986) found support for the validity of the DAS in the form of positive correlations with other concurrently administered measures of depressive cognitions.

In a study of clinically depressed patients, Eaves and Rush (1984) found that endogenous depressives had an mean DAS of 166.7 and nonendogenous depressives a mean of 159.5. When measured again following remission, scores for endogenous and nonendogenous groups both dropped significantly, to 142.2 and 124.1, respectively. However, these improved scores still fell short of the control (nondepressed) group mean scores of 102.6 and 95.5. Scores for a group of depressives who had not shown remission between the first and second DAS completion failed to show a significant change in their scores.

Rush, Weissenburger, and Eaves (1986) have addressed the issue of whether levels of dysfunctional attitudes are predictive of future depressive symptoms. They followed a group of 15 patients from an earlier study (Eaves & Rush, 1984) who had been initially evaluated when clinically depressed and then tested a second time after demonstrating symptomatic remission. These patients were again evaluated 6 months after their evaluation while remitted. A controlled comparison of their DAS scores reported at the time of initial remission with levels of depression 6 months later indicated that the DAS scores accounted for 25% of the variance in subsequent depressive symptoms. The authors report that "these results suggest that the DAS measured shortly after remission relates positively to subsequent depressive symptoms" (p. 232). Results supportive of these findings have been reported by Simons, Murphy, and Levine (1984) who found dysfunctional attitudes (along with social adjustment) to be predictive of recurrence of depression 1-year following initial evaluation.

In the study by Hollon *et al.* (1986) described in the previous discussion of the ATQ, the DAS was completed by a number of sample groups representing a variety of psychiatric diagnoses. As with the ATQ, DAS scores varied across groups according to the level of depression they displayed, indicating that the DAS is sensitive to depression as a syndrome but not as a nosologic disorder.

However, the DAS displayed less specificity than the ATQ, in that the correlation of the DAS with the BDI was .54 compared to a correlation of .83 between the ATQ and BDI. The authors note that the relative nonspecificity of the DAS can be accounted for by the elevated scores among schizophrenics within their sample of nondepressed psychiatric patients. They consider this as evidence that the DAS taps cognitions that are associated with general psychopathology. Two groups of remitted depressed patients were found to have mean DAS scores equivalent to the normal control group. This suggests that the DAS is state-dependent, which is consistent with research by Silverman, Silverman, and Eardley (1984) and Hamilton and Abramson (1983).

Research evaluating the DAS has demonstrated that it has good reliability and that it is a valid measure of depressive cognitions. The notion that specific types of attitudes or beliefs can predict subsequent depression is both clinically and theoretically intriguing. However, as noted before, research in this area has produced conflicting data. The conceptual aspects of this area of research are both complex and controversial and are the subject of lively debate in the current psychological literature (Coyne & Gotlib, 1986; Segal & Shaw, 1986a,b). The possibility of isolating and accurately measuring a marker of depressive vulnerability has obvious and important clinical implications. Unfortunately, there is currently no conclusive evidence supporting the use of the DAS for this purpose in a clinical setting. On the other hand, the DAS can provide useful clinical information on the extent and nature of dysfunctional beliefs held by a depressed patient at the onset and throughout the course of treatment. In addition, an item-by-item analysis of patient responses can be helpful in exploring belief systems and identifying cognitive errors (Beck *et al.*, 1979).

*Depressive Attributional Style*

The reformulation of the learned helplessness hypothesis (Abramson *et al.*, 1978) specifies three attributional dimensions central to helplessness and depression. These dimensions are internal/external, stable/unstable, and global/specific. The reformulated learned helplessness model predicts that persons who are depressed or prone to depression will tend to attribute bad outcomes to internal, stable, and global factors. Based on this hypothesis, it has also been speculated that depressed and depression-prone individuals will tend to attribute positive outcome to external, unstable, and specific factors.

*Attributional Style Questionnaire.* The Attributional Style Questionnaire (ASQ; Peterson *et al.*, 1982) was designed to measure attributional style on the three dimensions noted before. The questionnaire contains 12 situations, 6 positive (e.g., you apply for a position that you want very badly, and you get it; you do a project that is highly praised) and 6 negative (e.g., you give an important talk in front of a group, and the audience reacts negatively; you have been looking for a job unsuccessfully for some time). The 12 items include 6 that involve achievement and 6 concerned with affiliation. For each situation, the respondents are instructed to imagine themselves in that situation and write down the one major cause that they would ascribe to the event if it had occurred to them. They then evaluate the cause on each of the three attributional dimensions. Ratings are made using 7-point Likert scales. Low scores indicate external, unstable, or specific attributions, whereas high scores indicate internal, stable, or global attributions. Scoring yields six subscale scores (bad outcome internality, bad outcome stability, bad outcome globality, good outcome internality, good outcome stability, good outcome globality) and two composite scores (composite bad outcome, composite good outcome).

Seligman, Abramson, Semmel, and von Baeyer (1979) note the following Cronbach's alphas for the subscales; bad outcome internality = .44, bad outcome stability = .63, bad outcome globality = .64, good outcome internality = .39, good outcome stability = .54, good outcome globality = .58. Raps, Peterson, Reinhard, Abramson, and Seligman (1982) have reported Cronbach's alphas of .75 for composite good outcomes, .72 for composite bad outcomes along with coefficients ranging from .44 to .69 on the subscales. For a sample of undergraduate college students, Zautra, Guenther, and Chartier (1985) reported 2-week test–retest reliability correlations of .60 for composite good outcomes, .61 for composite bad outcomes, and subscale correlations ranging from .48 to .57. This study provides support for the validity of the ASQ by finding that ASQ ratings were similar to separate ratings that subjects made for real events. However, the study's finding that attributions for good outcomes were either uncorrelated or positively correlated to attributions for bad outcomes failed to support the hypothesis that a single process underlies both positive and negative attributions.

Among a sample of college students, Seligman et al. (1979) found all three subscales for bad outcomes to be modestly but significantly correlated with BDI scores. Among the good outcome subscales, internality and stability were modestly but significantly correlated with BDI scores, whereas there was very little association found between the BDI and good outcome globality.

Studies with clinically depressed samples have yielded mixed results. Raps et al. (1982) compared hospitalized, unipolar depressed patients with a group of hospitalized schizophrenics and a control group of medical patients. They found that the three bad-outcome subscales and the bad-outcome composite scale all significantly ($p < .001$) differentiated the depressed group. Depressed group scores on the good outcome internality and stability subscales were significantly different from those of the other groups at the level, $p < .01$. In contrast, Miller, Klee, and Norman (1982) found no significant difference between depressed and nondepressed patients using a subset of ASQ items.

In a longitudinal study that included endogenous depressed, nonendogenous depressed patients, and a control group, Eaves and Rush (1984) found that upon recent remission, depressives "continued to display a depressive attributional style to a significantly greater extent than did control subjects" (p. 38). They also noted that, among the ASQ subscales, "the tendency to blame oneself for failure appeared to be the most refractory to change with clinical remission" (p. 39). A follow-up study of these same subjects by Rush et al., (1986) suggests that these findings may be short lived. They found that 6 months after initial remission "biased attributions did not relate either to the course of depressive disorder or to symptom severity" (p. 225). However, it should be noted that this study used only the composite failure score rather than the complete ASQ. Golin, Sweeney, and Schaeffer (1981) used a cross-lagged panel correlation design to measure the impact of a depressive attributional style on subsequent levels of depression. Their results support the hypothesis that "stability and global attributions for bad outcomes might be causes of depression." Such support was not found for the hypothesis that internal attributions for bad outcomes lead to later depression.

Numerous recent studies using the ASQ support the general reliability of the ASQ. As suggested by the limited review provided here, the research in the current literature has produced mixed results regarding the ASQ. In a review of such inconsistencies, Peterson, Villanova, and Raps (1985) examined 61 published tests of the reformulated learned help-lessness model of depression. They conclude that studies that had "a large sample, a large number of events about which attributions were made, and [used] hypothetical events" (p. 165) tended to support the reformulated learned helplessness model of depression. Unfortunately their review did not identify or separately analyze those studies that used the ASQ. Based on the brief review presented, it appears that negative findings may be related to use of part of rather than the complete ASQ.

In general, the ASQ appears to be a valid measure of depressive cognitions. As noted with the case of the DAS, the theoretical and clinical implications of the ASQ are currently the subject of spirited debate. The clinical use of the ASQ as an established marker of vulnerability to depression will have to await further research exploration and testing.

## Other Measures of Depressive Cognitions

Although much of the most recent clinical literature on the cognitive assessment of depression has been devoted to the ATQ, DAS, and ASQ, a number of other clinically applicable measures of the cognitive aspects of depression have been recently developed and tested. A sample of other cognitive assessment measure is briefly presented next.

The Cognitive Bias Questionnaire (CBQ; Krantz & Hammen, 1979) was developed to assess the distorted or biased quality of depressive cognitions described by Beck et al. (1979). The CBQ consists of several short stories that describe problematic situations. After the presentation of each situation, respondents are asked to assume the role of the person described in the story and answer several multiple-choice questions concerning the situation described. Each possible answer reflects either depressed-distorted, depressed-nondistorted, non-depressed-distorted, or nondepressed-nondistorted response options. When tested with several depressed and nondepressed samples, the CBQ has demonstrated moderate psychometric properties and has been shown to reliably distinguish between depressed and nondepressed groups (Krantz & Hammen, 1979).

The Cognitive Response Test (CRT; Watkins & Rush, 1983) consists of 36 scenarios of life situations that are each presented to a subject. After each presentation, the subject's verbal responses to the situation are rated as rational, irrational-depressed, irrational-other, or non-scorable. Reported interrater reliabilities among trained raters has been good (Watkins & Rush, 1983). Watkins and Rush (1983) and Simons, Garfield, and Murphy (1984) have reported the CRT is sensitive to changes in levels of depression over the course of therapy. In contrast, Dobson and Shaw (1986) found little change over time in the CRT among a sample that simultaneously demonstrated a clear improvement in depressive symptoms.

The Cognition Checklist (CCL; Beck, Brown, Steer, Eidelsen, and Riskind, 1987) has recently been developed to differentiate anxious and depressed automatic thoughts. Respondents rate a number of dysfunctional thoughts on a 5-point Likert scale, indicating how often each though has occurred to them. The CCL yields separate scores for depressive and anxious thoughts. Although there is a substantial correlation between the subscales, the CCL has been shown to effectively differentiate between groups of depressed and anxious individuals (Beck et al., 1987).

The cognitive assessment of depression is an active and rapidly evolving area of psychological research. Among the measures discussed here, the ATQ is currently the most clearly suited for use in clinical practice. It has demonstrated excellent reliability and has been shown to be strongly correlated with depressive symptoms across a variety of populations. Like the other instruments described, the ATQ measures depression as a syndrome rather than as a nosologic disorder.

The DAS and ASQ have also demonstrated good psychometric properties. As noted earlier, the relationships of the DAS and ASQ to depression are currently being explored and debated in the psychological literature. If either or both of these measures can be conclusively shown to reliably assess cognitions that serve as a marker for depressive vulnerability, they will be of enormous clinical usefulness.

# CONCLUSION

## PRODUCTS VERSUS PROCESSES REVISITED

Although the focus of the chapter has been on the assessment of products as the most clinically useful domain of cognitive assessment, that information represents only a fraction of the information on cognitive assessment. That is, cognitive products give little information about how the mind actually encodes and processes information. In essence, cognitive products are really "by-products" of information processing. Because cognitive treatments have emphasized changing these cognitive products (Meichenbaum, 1977), the focus of assessment has been on assessing those same entities. The advantage of pursuing assessment based on information processing is that assessment may be based more on the actually processes and mechanisms of the mind and less on the intervention strategies that have been used to treat emotional disorders. Hopefully, the use of computer-assisted assessment will enhance the clinical utility of cognitive processes.

## CORE VERSUS PERIPHERAL COGNITIONS

Several authors have made a distinction between core and peripheral cognitive processes (Arnkoff, 1980; Guidano & Liotti, 1983; Safran, Vallis, Segal, & Shaw, 1986). Safran *et al.* (1986) acknowledge the work of Kelly (1955) whose organization corollary defined the hierarchical nature of constructs and the concept of the core construct. The latter is an overarching construct that is somewhat stable, whereas peripheral constructs are those that can change with little effect on the core constructs. Arnkoff (1980) has referred to these core constructs or processes as *deep structure*. The tacit nature of this information may make it more difficult to assess these core processes; however, advances in the assessment of these core processes should ultimately enhance treatment and treatment maintenance.

According to Kelly's organization corollary, changes in peripheral cognitions that have little salience for the individual would have little impact on core cognitions. However, changes in peripheral cognitions that are salient can ultimately have an impact on core cognitions as the deep structure changes as a function of changes in the surface structure. However, one can also posit that changes in salient surface structure or peripheral cognitions do not necessarily imply changes in deep structure or core cognitions. For example, one may use positive or coping self-statements to effectively handle a difficult social situation and yet maintain dysfunction or irrational beliefs about social situations or themselves.

In the depression literature, this core-versus-peripheral distinction may characterize the difference between automatic thoughts and dysfunctional attitudes. The former may represent surface structure or peripheral cognitions, and the latter may represent deep structure or core cognitions. However, both the peripheral and core cognitions are hierarchically ordered.

It would be interesting to use methodology familiar to personal construct theorists wherein the client is asked to hierarchically order self-statements or irrational beliefs such that items lower in the hierarchy have little impact on the other items. Conversely, items near the top of the hierarchy represent more core cognitions that, if changed, have a major impact on all of the other items. Thus, one would assume that if the clinician were to work on a dysfunctional thought that was not a core cognition that the impact on core cognitive change would be minimal.

Safran *et al.* (1986) suggest that clinicians become adept at targeting core cognitions, and they give some markers for those cognitions. They tend to be self-referent, represented by common themes (e.g., irrational beliefs, dysfunctional attitudes), consistent across situations, and emotionally laden. Cognitive assessment would benefit greatly from research in this area. Research strategies such as multidimensional scaling (Goldfried, Padawer, & Robins, 1984; Robins, 1987; Rudy & Merluzzi, 1984) may be useful in the discovery and classification of core cognitions.

### RELIABILITY, VALIDITY, AND BEYOND

In addition to the larger conceptual issues noted before, there are a number of practical issues that deserve attention. First, in general, compared to behavioral assessment, cognitive assessment methods have not been thoroughly studied. As a result, few studies have compared approaches to cognitive assessment (Blackwell *et al.,* 1985) or have assessed cognitions in natural settings (Hurlburt & Melancon, 1987). Moreover, large-scale validity studies, in particular ecological validity, are not plentiful. Well-planned psychometric studies and studies that assess the impact of contextual and demand characteristics (Merluzzi, McNamara, & Rudy, 1983) are essential for the advancement of cognitive assessment.

## SUMMARY

In this chapter, we presented an overview of Kendall and Ingram's (1987) taxonomy of domains of cognitive assessment with an emphasis on the assessment of cognitive products of anxiety and depression. Nisbett and Wilson's (1977) critique of the validity of self-reports was reviewed. A rebuttal to their argument was presented, and practical suggestions were made to enhance the quality of self-reports. Approaches to the cognitive assessment of anxiety and depression were presented as well as the Schwartz and Garamoni (1986) states of mind model. Conclusions focused on the need for advances in the assessment of cognitive processes, the clinical importance of the organization of cognitive information, and the need for basic research in cognitive assessment.

## REFERENCES

Abramson, L. Y., Seligman, M. E. P., & Teasdale, J. D. (1978). Learned helplessness in humans: Critique and reformulation. *Journal of Abnormal Psychology, 87,* 49–74.

Arnkoff, D. B. (1980). Psychotherapy from the perspective of cognitive theory. In M. Mahoney (Ed.), *Psychotherapy process: Current issues and future directions* (pp. 339–361). New York: Plenum Press.

Beck, A. T. (1978). *Depression inventory.* Philadelphia: Center for Cognitive Therapy.

Beck, A. T., & Emery, G. (1985). *Anxiety disorders and phobias: A cognitive perspective.* New York: Basic Books.

Beck, A. T., Rush, A. J., Shaw, B. F., & Emery, G. (1979). *Cognitive therapy of depression.* New York: Guilford Press.

Beck, A. T., Brown, G., Steer, R. A., Eidelsen, J. I., & Riskind, J. H. (1987). Differentiating anxiety and depression: A test of the cognitive content-specificity hypothesis. *Journal of Abnormal Psychology, 96,* 179–183.

Beidel, D. C., Turner, S. M., & Dancu, C. V. (1985). Physiological, cognitive and behavioral aspect of social anxiety. *Behavior Research and Therapy, 23,* 109–117.

Blackwell, R. T., Galassi, J. P., Galassi, M. D., & Watson, T. E. (1985). Are all cognitive assessment methods created equal? A comparison of think aloud and thought listing. *Cognitive Therapy and Research, 9,* 399–414.

Bruch, M. A., Haase, R. F., & Purcell, M. I. (1984). Content dimensions of self-statements in assertive situations: A factor analysis of two measures. *Cognitive Therapy and Research, 8,* 173–186.

Cacioppo, J. T., & Petty, R. E. (1981). Social psychological procedures for cognitive response analysis: The thought-listing technique. In T. V. Merluzzi, C. R. Glass, M. Genest (Eds.), *Cognitive assessment* (pp. 309–342). New York: Guilford Press.

Cacioppo, J. T., Glass, C. R., & Merluzzi, T. V. (1979). Self-statements and self-evaluations: A cognitive response analysis of heterosocial anxiety. *Cognitive Therapy and Research, 3,* 249–262.

Coyne, J. C., & Gotlib, I. (1986). Studying the role of cognition in depression: Well-trodden paths and cul-de-sacs. *Cognitive Therapy and Research, 10,* 695–705.

Craighead, W. E., Kimball, W. H., & Rehak, P. J. (1979). Mood changes, physiological responses, and self-statements during social rejection imagery. *Journal of Consulting and Clinical Psychology, 47,* 385–396.

Dobson, K. S., & Brieter, H. J. (1983). Cognitive assessment of depression: Reliability and validity of three measures. *Journal of Abnormal Psychology, 92,* 107–109.

Dobson, K. S., & Shaw, B. F. (1986). Cognitive assessment of major depressive disorders. *Cognitive Therapy and Research, 10,* 13–29.

Dodge, C. E., Heimberg, R. G., Hope, D. A., & Becker, R. E. (1986). *Evaluation of the Social Interaction Self-Statement Test with a social phobic population.* Unpublished manuscript, State University of New York at Albany.

Eaves, G., & Rush, A. J. (1984). Cognitive patterns in symptomatic and remitted unipolar major depression. *Journal of Abnormal Psychology, 93,* 31–40.

Endicott, J., & Spitzer, R. L. (1978). A diagnostic interview: The schedule for affective disorders and schizophrenia. *Archives of General Psychiatry, 35,* 107–109.

Genest, M., & Turk, D. C. (1981). Think aloud approaches to cognitive assessment. In T. V. Merluzzi, C. R. Glass, & M. Genest (Eds.), *Cognitive assessment* (pp. 233–269). New York: Guilford Press.

Glass, C. R., & Merluzzi, T. V. (1981). Cognitive assessment of social-evaluative anxiety. In T. V. Merluzzi, C. R. Glass, M. Genest (Eds.), *Cognitive assessment* (pp. 388–438). New York: Guilford Press.

Glass, C. R., Merluzzi, T. V., Biever, J. L., & Larsen, K. H. (1982). Cognitive assessment of social anxiety: Development and validation of a self-statement questionnaire. *Cognitive Therapy and Research, 6,* 37–55.

Goldfried, M. R., & Sobocinski, D. (1975). Effects of irrational beliefs on emotional arousal. *Journal of Consulting and Clinical Psychology, 43,* 504–510.

Goldfried, M. R., Padawer, W., & Robins, C. (1984). Social anxiety and the semantic structure of heterosocial interactions. *Journal of Abnormal Psychology, 93,* 87–97.

Golin, S. Sweeney, P. D., & Schaffer, D. E. (1981). The causality of causal attributions in depression: A cross-lagged panel analysis. *Journal of Abnormal Psychology, 90,* 14–22.

Guidano, V. F., & Liotti, G. (1983). *Cognitive processes and emotional disorders: A structural approach to psychotherapy.* New York: Guilford Press.

Hamilton, E. W., & Abramson, L. Y. (1983). Cognitive patterns and major depressive disorders: A longitudinal study in a hospital setting. *Journal of Abnormal Psychology, 92,* 173–184.

Harrel, T. H., & Ryan, N. B. (1983). Cognitive-behavioral assessment of depression: Clinical validation of the Automatic Thoughts Questionnaire. *Journal of Consulting and Clinical Psychology, 51,* 721–725.

Hathaway, S. R., & McKinley, J. C. (1940). The measurement of symptomatic depression with the Minnesota Multiphasic Personality Schedule. *Psychological Bulletin, 27,* 425.

Heimberg, R. G., Nyman, D., & O'Brien, G. T. (1987). Assessing variations of the thought-listing technique: Effects of instructions, stimulus intensity, stimulus modality, and scoring procedures. *Cognitive Therapy and Research, 11,* 13–24.

Heimberg, R. G., Vermilyea, J. A., Dodge, C. S., Becker, R. E., & Barlow, D. H. (1987). Attribution style, depression, and anxiety: An evaluation of the specificity of depressive attributions. *Cognitive Therapy and Research, 11,* 537–550.

Hollandsworth, J. G., Jr., Galezeski, R. C., Kirkland, K., Jones, G. E., & Van Norman, L. R. (1979). An analysis of the nature and effects of test anxiety: Cognitive, behavioral, and physiological components. *Cognitive Therapy and Research, 3,* 165–180.

Hollon, S. D., & Kendall, P. C. (1980). Cognitive self-statements in depression: Clinical validation of an automatic thoughts questionnaire. *Cognitive Therapy and Research, 4,* 383–395.

Hollon, S. D., Kendall, P. C., & Lumry, A. (1986). Specificity of depressotypic cognitions in clinical depression. *Journal of Abnormal Psychology, 95,* 52–59.

Howard, G. S. (1982). Improving methodology via research on research methods. *Journal of Counseling Psychology, 29,* 318–326.

Huber, J. W., & Altmaier, E. M. (1983). An investigation of the self-statement systems of phobic and nonphobic individuals. *Cognitive Therapy and Research, 7,* 355–362.

Hurlburt, R. T., & Melancon, S. M. (1987). How are questionnaire data similar to, and different from, thought sampling data? Five studies manipulating retrospectiveness, single-moment focus, and indeterminacy. *Cognitive Therapy and Research, 11,* 681–704.

Ingram, R. (Ed.). (1987). *Information processing approaches to clinical psychology.* New York: Academic Press.

Ingram, R., & Kendall, P. C. (1987). The cognitive side of anxiety. *Cognitive Therapy and Research, 11,* 523–536.

Kelly, G. A. (1955). *The psychology of personal constructs.* New York: Norton Press.

Kendall, P. C., & Hollon, S. D. (1987). *Development and validation of the Anxious Self-Statement Questionnaire (ASSQ).* Unpublished manuscript, Temple University.

Kendall, P. C., & Ingram, R. (1987). The future for cognitive assessment of anxiety. In L. Michelson & L. M. Ascher (Eds.), *Anxiety and stress disorders* (pp. 89–104). New York: Guilford Press.

Kirkland, K., & Hollandsworth, J. G., Jr. (1980). Effective test taking: Skills acquisition versus anxiety reduction techniques. *Journal of Consulting and Clinical Psychology, 48,* 431–439.

Krantz, S., & Hammen, C. (1979). The assessment of cognitive bias in depression. *Journal of Abnormal Psychology, 88,* 611–619.

Landau, R. J., & Goldfried, M. R. (1981). The assessment of schemata: Unifying framework for cognitive, behavioral, and traditional assessment. In P. C. Kendall & S. D. Hollon (Eds.), *Assessment strategies for cognitive behavioral interventions* (pp. 363–400). New York: Academic Press.

Malkiewich, L. E., & Merluzzi, T. V. (1980). Rational restructuring versus desensitization with clients of diverse conceptual levels: A test of a client-treatment matching model. *Journal of Counseling Psychology, 27,* 453–461.

Markus, H., & Wurf, E. (1987). The dynamic self concept: A social psychological perspective. *Annual review of psychology, 38,* 299 377.

Meichenbaum, D. H. (1977). *Cognitive-behavior modification.* New York: Plenum Press.

Meichenbaum, D., & Cameron, R. (1981). Issues in cognitive assessment. In T. V. Merluzzi, C. R. Glass, & M. Genest (Eds.), *Cognitive assessment* (pp. 3–15). New York: Guilford Press.

Merluzzi, T. V., Rudy, T. E., & Glass, C. R. (1981). The information processing paradigm: Implications for clinical science. In T. V. Merluzzi, C. R. Glass, & M. Genest (Eds.), *Cognitive assessment* (pp. 77–126). New York: Guilford Press.

Merluzzi, T. V., McNamara, M., & Rudy, T. E. (1983, November). *The effects of demand on the cognitive and behavioral assessment of social skill.* Paper presented at the meeting of the Association for the Advancement of Behavior Therapy, Washington DC.

Merluzzi, T. V., Burgio, K. L., & Glass, C. R. (1984). Cognitions and psychopathology: An analysis of social introversion and self-statements. *Journal of Consulting and Clinical Psychology, 52,* 1102–1103.

Miller, I., Klee, S., & Norman, W. (1982). Depressed and nondepressed inpatient's cognitions of hypothetical events, experimental tasks, and stressful life events. *Journal of Abnormal Psychology, 87,* 78–81.

Mischel, W. (1981). A cognitive-social learning approach to assessment. In T. V. Merluzzi, C. R. Glass, & M. Genest (Eds.), *Cognitive assessment* (pp. 479–502). New York: Guilford Press.

Nasby, W., & Kihlstrom, J. F. (1987). Cognitive assessment of personality and psychopathology. In R. Ingram (Ed.), *Information processing approaches to clinical psychology* (pp. 217–239). New York: Academic Press.

Nisbett, R. E., & Wilson, T. P. (1977). Telling more than we can know: Verbal reports on mental processes. *Psychological Review, 84,* 231–259.

Oliver, J. M., & Baumgart, E. P. (1985). The dysfunctional attitude scale: Psychometric properties and relation to depression in an unselected adult population. *Cognitive Therapy and Research, 9,* 161–167.

Peterson, C., Semmel, A., von Baeyer, C., Abramson, L. Y., Metalsky, G. I., & Seligman, M. E. P. (1982). The attribution style questionnaire. *Cognitive Therapy and Research, 6,* 287–299.

Peterson, C., Luborsky, L., & Seligman, M. E. P. (1983). Attributions and depressive mood shifts: A case study using the symptom-context method. *Journal of Abnormal Psychology, 92,* 96–103.

Peterson, C., Villanova, P., & Raps C. S. (1985). Depression and attribution: Factors responsible for inconsistent results in the literature. *Journal of Abnormal Psychology, 94,* 165–168.

Pope, K. H., & Singer, J. L. (Eds.). (1978). *The stream of consciousness: Scientific investigation onto the flow of human experience.* New York: Plenum Press.

Raps, C. S., Peterson, C., Reinhard, K. E., Abramson, L. Y., & Seligman, M. E. P. (1982). Attribution style among depressed patients. *Journal of Abnormal Psychology, 91,* 102–108.

Robins, C. J. (1987). Social perception and heterosocial self-efficacy: A multidimensional scaling analysis. *Cognitive Therapy and Research, 11,* 197–214.

Ross, S. M., Gottfredson, D. K., Christensen, P., & Weaver, R. (1986). Cognitive self-statements in depression: Findings across clinical populations. *Cognitive Therapy and Research, 10,* 159–166.

Rudy, T. E., & Merluzzi, T. V. (1984). Recovering social cognitive schemas. In P. C. Kendall (Ed.), *Advances in cognitive behavioral research and therapy* (Vol. 3, pp. 61–102). New York: Academic Press.

Rush, J. A., Weissenburger, J., & Eaves, G. (1986). Do thinking patterns predict depressive symptoms? *Cognitive Therapy and Research, 10,* 225–236.

Safran, J. D., Vallis, T. M., & Segal, Z. V., & Shaw, B. F. (1986). Assessment of core cognitive processes in cognitive therapy. *Cognitive therapy and Research, 10,* 509–526.

Sarason, I. G., & Stoops, R. (1978). Test anxiety and the passage of time. *Journal of Consulting and Clinical Psychology, 46,* 102–109.

Schwartz, R. M., & Garamoni, G. L. (1986). A structural model of positive and negative states of mind: Asymmetry in the internal dialogue. In P. C. Kendall (Ed.), *Advances in cognitive behavioral research and therapy* (Vol. 5, pp. 1–62). New York: Academic Press.

Schwartz, R. M., & Gottman, J. M. (1976). Toward a task analysis of assertive behavior. *Journal of Consulting and Clinical Psychology, 44,* 910–920.

Segal, Z. V., & Marshall, W. L. (1985). Heterosocial skill in a population of rapists and child molesters. *Journal of Consulting and Clinical Psychology, 53,* 55–63.

Segal, Z. V., & Shaw, B. F. (1986a). Cognition in depression: A reappraisal of Coyne and Gotlib's critique. *Cognitive Therapy and Research, 10,* 671–693.

Segal, Z. V., & Shaw, B. F. (1986b). When cul-de-sacs are more mentality than reality: A rejoinder to Coyne and Gotlib. *Cognitive Therapy and Research, 10,* 707–714.

Seligman, M. E. P., Abramson, L. Y., Semmel, A., & von Baeyer, C. (1979). Depressive attributional style. *Journal of Abnormal Psychology, 88,* 242–247.

Silverman, J. S., Silverman, J. A., & Eardley, D. A. (1984). Do maladaptive attitudes cause depression? *Archives of General Psychiatry, 41,* 28–32.

Simons, A. D., Garfield, S. L., & Murphy, G. E. (1984). The process of change in cognitive therapy and pharmacotherapy and depression: Changes in mood and cognition. *Archives of General Psychiatry, 41,* 28–30.

Simons, A. D., Murphy, G. E., & Levine, J. C. (1984). *Relapse after treatment with cognitive therapy and/or pharmacotherapy: Results after one year.* Paper presented at the 15th annual meeting of the Society for Psychotherapy Research, Lake Louise, Alberta, Canada.

Smye, M. D., & Wine, J. D. (1980). A comparison of female and male adolescents' social behavior and cognitions. *Sex Roles, 6,* 213–130.

Sobel, H. J. (1981). Projective methods of cognitive analysis. In T. V. Merluzzi, C. R. Glass, & M. Genest (Eds.), *Cognitive assessment* (pp. 127–148). New York: Guilford Press.

Spitzer, R., Endicott, J., & Robbins, E. (1978). Research diagnostic criteria: Rationale and reliability. *Archives of General Psychiatry, 35,* 773–782.

Stake, J. E., Warren, N. J., & Rogers, H. E. (1979). *Coping strategies as mediators in the relationship between cognitive distortions and depression.* Unpublished manuscript, University of Missouri.

Watkins, J., & Rush, A. J. (1983). The cognitive response test. *Cognitive Therapy and Research, 7,* 425–436.

Weissman, A. N. (1978). *Development and validation of the Dysfunctional Attitudes Scale.* Paper presented at the annual meeting of the Association for the Advancement of Behavior Therapy, Chicago.

Weissman, A. N., & Beck, A. T. (1978). *Development and validation of the dysfunctional attitudes scale: A preliminary investigation.* Paper presented at the annual meeting of the American Education Association, Toronto.

Winfrey, L. L., & Goldfried, M. R. (1987). Information processing and human change processes. In R. Ingram (Ed.), *Information processing approaches to clinical psychology* (pp. 241–258). New York: Academic Press.

Zautra, A. J., Guenther, R. T., & Chartier, G. M. (1985). Attributions for real and hypothetical events: Their relation to self-esteem and depression. *Journal of Abnormal Psychology, 94,* 530–540.

# 14

# Combined Cognitive Therapy and Pharmacotherapy

JESSE H. WRIGHT AND G. RANDOLPH SCHRODT, JR.

> *The clashing point of two subjects, two disciplines,*
> *two cultures , , , ought to produce creative chances.*
> C. P. Snow (1959)

Cognitive therapy and pharmacotherapy have developed as separate, and at times, competitive entities. Theoretical constructs and treatment strategies of the two approaches are quite different. Cognitive therapists seek to correct faulty patterns of thinking and behavior with psychological procedures, whereas pharmacotherapists attempt to regulate brain biochemistry with medication. Cognitive therapy has found its largest audience among professionals who are not licensed to prescribe drugs. Pharmacotherapy is largely the province of the physician.

Despite this trend for divisiveness, other forces have encouraged a joining of the two approaches. A movement toward pragmatism is one of these factors. Driven by such pressures as efforts to contain the cost of medical care, clinicians are encouraged to do "what works" in the most expeditious manner possible. Therefore, they may elect to use more than one treatment if they believe this will speed recovery and reduce the risk of relapse.

The demand for combined treatment is also influenced by the patient. Weissman, Prusoff, DiMascio, Neu, Goklaney, & Klerman (1979) noted that patients who dropped out of their controlled outcome study of pharmacotherapy versus psychotherapy and who entered treatment elsewhere, most commonly sought out therapists who would provide both therapies. It is not surprising that patients want the benefits of advances in the biological sciences as well as the understanding and guidance that can be provided by a meaningful psychotherapeutic relationship.

Theoretical arguments that support combined therapy have been made by several authors (Akiskal & McKinney, 1975; Beck, 1985; Group for the Advancement of Psychiatry, 1975;

---

JESSE H. WRIGHT AND G. RANDOLPH SCHRODT, JR. • Department of Psychiatry and Behavioral Sciences, University of Louisville School of Medicine, and Norton Psychiatric Clinic, Louisville, Kentucky 40232-5070.

Wright & Beck, 1983; Wright, 1987). They have noted that it is unlikely that complex mental disorders have a single cause or only one effective method of treatment. Hypotheses concerning potential treatment interactions have been advanced (Group for Advancement of Psychiatry, 1975), and controlled research has begun on combined therapy (Blackburn, Bishop, Glen, Whalby, & Christie, 1981; Murphy, Simons, & Wetzel, 1984; Wright, 1986).

Our main emphasis in this chapter will be on practical aspects of combining treatments. However, theoretical concepts will be discussed first because we think that a model for interactions between treatments is needed to direct therapeutic efforts. General guidelines for combined cognitive therapy and pharmacotherapy will then be offered. Finally, treatment procedures for common psychiatric syndromes will be illustrated.

## COMBINED THERAPY: A THEORETICAL PERSPECTIVE

There are at least three major integrative theories for psychiatric disorders that could be used to justify combining treatments: general systems theory (Chase, Wright, & Ragade, 1981; Miller, 1978), the biopsychosocial model (Engel, 1977), and the psychobiological final common pathway hypothesis (Akiskal & McKinney, 1975; Whybrow, Akiskal, & McKinney, 1984). The latter model has dealt more specifically and systematically with research findings that are familiar to most clinicians. Using depression as an example, Akiskal and McKinney (1975) assessed the validity and relevance of findings from diverse fields of investigation (e.g., cognitive, neurobiological, behavioral, psychodynamic, social, etc.) and concluded that many etiological factors may coalesce to cause development of symptoms. Interactions between these factors are thought to occur through a basic neurophysiological substrate. Thus expressions of symptomatology are much the same regardless of the particular blend of contributing elements.

Mechanisms of interaction are still poorly understood, but there have been numerous reports of influences of one system upon another (Engel, 1977; Miller, 1978; Mohl, 1987). These have ranged from large-scale epidemiologic studies that have demonstrated an association between social factors and physical disease (Schwab & Schwab, 1978), to research on environmentally induced structural changes in the neuronal mechanisms involved in learning and memory (Kandel & Schwartz, 1982). The reader is referred to a recent review and commentary by Mohl (1987) for a synthesis of research data that support integrative models of causality and treatment.

Several general types of possible interactions between psychotherapy and pharmacotherapy have been proposed. Uhlenhuth et al. (1969) suggested that combining the two treatments might lead to (1) *addition*—the effect of the combined treatment is equal to the sum of the individual contributions; (2) *potentiation*—combined effects are greater than the sum of the individual components; (3) *inhibition*—results of combined therapy are less than the contributions from each individual treatment; or (4) *reciprocation*—the result of the two therapies combined is equal to the influence of the most potent treatment.

These observations stimulated several large outcome studies that compared pharmacotherapy with various psychotherapies (e.g., interpersonal, marital, group) in the treatment of outpatients with depression (Hollon & Beck, 1978). Little evidence was found for either positive or negative interactions. After a comprehensive review of this research, Hollon and Beck (1978) concluded that these studies were better at comparing drugs to psychotherapy than they were at assessing interactions between treatments.

Subsequent controlled studies that compared outcome of cognitive therapy alone, pharmacotherapy alone, and combined treatment (Blackburn et al., 1981; Murphy et al., 1984) had design problems similar to earlier studies reviewed by Hollon and Beck (1978). These investigations were directed primarily at measuring the overall effect of the different treatments on symptom reduction, not on detecting or assessing interactions. Specific hypotheses about methods of interaction were not made.

Murphy *et al.* (1984) found no evidence for superiority of combined treatment (combined therapy plus amitriptyline) over either treatment alone. However, Blackburn *et al.* (1981) noted that depressed outpatients treated with cognitive therapy and an antidepressant of the doctor's choice improved to a greater extent than those who received only one of the treatments. In a follow-up to their original report, Murphy's group (Simons, Murphy, Levine, & Wetzel, 1986) observed that the best results 1 year after treatment were achieved by patients who received either cognitive therapy or combined treatment.

More research concerning efficacy of combined treatment is clearly needed. However, common design problems of outcome studies make it unlikely that firm conclusions will be reached. The strict requirements of controlled studies make the treatment conditions considerably different from those usually encountered in clinical practice. For example, in controlled studies, patients usually receive medication and psychotherapy from different therapists who are required to follow a set course of treatment and who do not communicate with each other. In clinical practice, an integrated and flexible approach can be utilized in which therapy decisions can be altered, depending upon the progress of treatment (Wright, 1987). Another limitation of outcome studies is that they have been performed with homogeneous groups of patients with relatively mild or uncomplicated disorders. Most patients encountered in routine practice do not meet the inclusion criteria required by these studies.

The authors' view of interaction between treatments is based on a belief in integrative models of causality, an awareness of research findings from multiple areas of investigation, and clinical experience in using both pharmacotherapy and psychotherapy. During the course of our work, we have developed several assumptions that influence our decisions about treatment. These assumptions are as follows:

1. It is valuable to search for all possible etiological factors for a psychiatric syndrome.
2. Therapy should be customized to meet the unique problems and needs of each patient.
3. For conditions in which both pharmacotherapy and psychotherapy have been shown to be effective, it is advantageous to use both treatments unless there are strong reasons not to do so (e.g., medical contraindications to drug, patient unable to participate in psychotherapy).
4. Medication should be the primary treatment for disorders that have been proven to be responsive to pharmacotherapy, but for which the effectiveness of psychotherapy has not been documented (e.g., bipolar disorder, acute psychosis).
5. Pharmacotherapy and psychotherapy usually facilitate one another if the treatments are applied expertly as an integrated treatment package.

Assumptions 1 to 3 are rather straightforward derivatives of the comprehensive models of causality and treatment discussed earlier. The fourth principle is based upon an assessment of outcome research with disorders (schizophrenia, bipolar disorder, major depression, etc.) for which there have been many replications of basic findings regarding efficacy of pharmacotherapy and/or psychotherapy. The last assumption is the most speculative because of the paucity of research on treatment interaction. However, several proposed mechanisms of interaction are generally accepted by clinicians who use pharmacotherapy together with psychotherapy. Table 1 contains a list of such possibilities (Adapted from Group for Advancement of Psychiatry, 1975).

A full discussion of research concerning these hypothetical interactions is beyond the scope of this chapter. However, a few observations will be made that may have clinical relevance. The positive placebo effect of medication has been well established. The total activity of a medication is the sum of its direct biochemical actions plus the placebo response

(Barrett & Wright, 1984). It should be quite possible to heighten (or diminish) the placebo response through psychotherapy. For example, a therapist's positive attitude toward medication, coupled with encouraging statements about the chances for recovery, should be associated with a better response to the medication than would a disparaging attitude and communications that emphasize problems with drugs. Studies of therapist behaviors have found that this is the case (Barrett & Wright, 1984). Frank (1978) has observed that remoralization is the uniting element in all successful treatment approaches. Cognitive therapy and pharmacotherapy are each capable of inducing increased hopefulness. We would suggest that the two treatments presented together can stimulate hope, in both patient and therapist, at least as much as either treatment alone.

Hypotheses that medications can improve concentration, decrease painful affect, or remove irrational thoughts (and thereby facilitate therapy) were proposed early in the history of psychopharmacology. There is hardly any doubt that medications such as antidepressants or major tranquilizers do indeed diminish such symptoms (Wright, 1986). For example, there has been extensive research on the stimulating effects of antidepressants on learning and memory (Wright, 1985, 1986), and antipsychotic drugs have been repeatedly shown to diminish delusional thinking (Baldessarini, 1977). However, the influence of medication on the process of psychotherapy has, for the most part, gone unexplored (Wright, 1986).

The ability of psychotherapy to enhance drug compliance has also been widely accepted but has been an infrequent subject of controlled investigations. We are aware of only one research study that assessed the influence of cognitive therapy on adherence to pharmacotherapy. Cochran (1982) compared bipolar patients treated with cognitive therapy plus lithium to those treated with lithium alone and found improved compliance in patients who received combined therapy. Regardless of the lack of extensive controlled research, Rush (1988) has made a convincing argument on clinical grounds for the facilitating action of cognitive therapy on medication compliance. Cognitive techniques that can increase adherence to pharmacotherapy will be discussed later in this chapter.

It has been suggested that several types of adverse interactions between pharmacotherapy and psychotherapy may occur (Group for Advancement of Psychiatry, 1975). These include the negative placebo response (drug makes the patient believe he or she is devalued by the therapist), a disruptive effect of psychotherapy (cognitive procedures overwhelm the patient and interfere with symptom-reducing actions of medication), and reduced motivation for psychotherapy due to early symptom relief. Controlled research studies have found no evidence that pharmacotherapy and psychotherapy have deleterious effects on one another (Hollon & Beck, 1978; Murphy *et al.*, 1984). These studies, however, reported on mean values from large groups of patients. Individual negative (or positive) reactions may have been obscured.

TABLE 1. Pharmacotherapy and Psychotherapy: Possible Mechanisms of Interaction

Medications have a positive placebo effect
Medications improve concentration and thus facilitate psychotherapy
Medications reduce painful affect and/or psychophysiological arousal, thereby increasing accessibility to psychotherapy
Medications can decrease distorted or irrational thinking, thus adding to the effect of cognitive therapy
Psychotherapy has a positive placebo effect
Psychotherapy improves drug compliance
Psychotherapy has biological effects and can work in concert with medication to alter chemical abnormalities

In our clinical experience, severe or lasting negative interactions between treatments have been rare. Commonly encountered problems such as maladaptive attitudes about medication usually respond to therapeutic interventions. Our overall strategy for combined therapy is to minimize the possibility of negative interactions, while promoting, where possible, the positive effects of cognitive therapy and pharmacotherapy on one another. The following section will discuss procedures for accomplishing these objectives.

## TREATMENT WITH COMBINED COGNITIVE THERAPY AND PHARMACOTHERAPY

### THE THERAPEUTIC RELATIONSHIP

A good working relationship between patient and therapist is an essential component of all effective psychotherapies (Frank, 1978; Marmor, 1976). Although the therapeutic relationship has been an infrequent subject of research studies in psychopharmacology, it also appears to be an important element of this treatment approach. Attitudes of doctors toward their patients and biases about prescription drugs have been shown to influence response to pharmacotherapy (Barrett & Wright, 1984).

At the present time, most combined cognitive therapy and pharmacotherapy is provided by teams of physicians and other therapists (e.g., psychologists, social workers, nurses) because few psychiatrists have been trained in cognitive therapy. There has been a growing trend to include cognitive therapy education in psychiatry residency programs. However, it is anticipated that combined therapy will continue to be provided in many instances by dual therapists.

The therapeutic relationship is less complicated when one therapist serves as both pharmacotherapist and cognitive therapist. The two approaches can be presented as a cohesive treatment, and the therapist roles can be combined so that one facilitates the other. Dual therapists have a somewhat more challenging treatment situation. The patient may develop intense thoughts and feelings about each of the therapists as individuals and about the relationship between the therapists, so there are at least three possible directions for positive and negative distortions about therapy (Wright, 1987). Problems such as competition between therapists or inadequate communication are readily perceived by patients. Decreased respect for the therapists and damaged rapport can result. An example of an impaired therapeutic relationship will be used to illustrate this point.

> Mrs. A., a 35-year-old woman with a history of recurrent depression and alcoholism, was admitted to the hospital after developing suicidal ideation. She had been in treatment as an outpatient with a psychologist who used cognitive therapy procedures and who encouraged participation in Alcoholics Anonymous. The psychiatrist who treated Mrs. A. believed that her relapse indicated that aggressive pharmacotherapy was needed. The two therapists discussed the treatment plan and agreed to use both cognitive therapy and medication. However, the treatment did not go as smoothly as expected.
>
> The physician believed that Mrs. A. should have been treated with medication before admission and that the "antidrug" attitudes of her outpatient therapist and Alcoholics Anonymous may have increased the chances of recurrence. On the other hand, the psychologist feared that the psychiatrist would "push" drugs and reinforce a pattern of dependency. Although they agreed superficially to cooperate, important underlying attitudes were not communicated openly.
>
> Within the first 72 hours of hospitalization, Mrs. A. had recognized the conflict between the therapists and had reacted to it. She interpreted this as meaning that

JESSE H. WRIGHT and
G. RANDOLPH
SCHRODT, JR.

neither therapist was sure of what he was doing or whether he could help her. Hopelessness and suicidal thoughts intensified after she concluded that there was no solution to her problem.

Wright (1987) has observed previously that teams of therapists need to develop mutual trust, knowledge of the basic principles of both pharmacotherapy and psychotherapy, and a shared model for how the treatments can be used together. The formation of an effective liaison between therapists requires a significant investment of time and energy. Ideally, therapists should work together on a regular basis, get to know one another personally, talk about what information will be given to the patient, and regularly discuss progress during the course of the therapy.

The therapeutic relationship in cognitive therapy has been described as "collaborative empiricism" (Wright & Beck, 1983). Patient and therapist work together as an investigative team. Accurate information processing is encouraged and modeled within the therapeutic relationship. We attempt to develop this type of relationship not only with patients but with other therapists who may help with combined treatment. The objective is to form a well-functioning work group that can coordinate its efforts toward reaching common goals.

## STRUCTURE OF COMBINED THERAPY

Structuring techniques such as agenda setting are used routinely in cognitive therapy (Wright & Beck, 1983). These procedures are most helpful for patients who have problems with learning and memory functioning. Depressed patients, in particular, commonly have deficits in their ability to concentrate, exert sustained effort, or learn material that is abstract or complex (Wright, 1985, 1987). Problems in this area can intensify the patients' sense of helplessness and hopelessness.

When two treatments are used, there are additional demands for time in therapy, and important decisions must be made about prioritization of topics for discussion. Patients for whom medication is prescribed usually have some degree of difficulty with attention and concentration. Thus therapists are encouraged to set appropriate agendas, keep sessions organized, and use directive questions when necessary. Stopping at frequent intervals to give and elicit feedback can also help to avoid misunderstandings.

When one therapist provides both treatments, the agenda will often include problems for which cognitive therapy will be the main approach, in addition to issues such as side effects, plasma levels, and dosage adjustments. A typical agenda for a combined therapy session might include: (1) symptom review, (2) reaction to problems at work, (3) homework assignment (thought record), (4) questions about medication, and (5) plasma-level results.

If dual therapists are used, agenda setting can offer a similar structure for both treatment situations. Pharmacotherapists are encouraged to set agendas with the patient and to use other structuring procedures that promote efficient information processing. Although the main focus will be on pharmacotherapy, the agenda also might include interface issues such as attitudes about medication, effects of medication on concentration, and a report on how the psychotherapy is going. Similarly, it would be profitable for cognitive therapy agendas to contain items related to cognitions about medication.

## PSYCHOEDUCATION

The patient's beliefs and expectations regarding medication may influence compliance, severity of side effects, and overall treatment outcome. Psychoeducational procedures that communicate the indications, risks, and benefits of pharmacotherapy can correct erroneous conclusions, thereby enhancing chances of recovery. Techniques used for this purpose include: (1) verbal presentation of information, (2) answering questions, (3) written instructions, (4) reading pamphlets or books, (5) checking for understanding, and (6) repetition of Steps 1 through 5 if needed.

We usually begin to educate patients about medications by presenting a brief summary of expected benefits and common side effects and then asking for their questions. Extensive lecturing or other purely didactic techniques should be avoided for at least two reasons. It is doubtful that the patient will be able to absorb and retain large amounts of information presented in this manner, and furthermore, such techniques can undermine the development of a collaborative working relationship. An interactive educational process, tailored to the individual patient's cognitive capabilities, biases, and levels of understanding, is most likely to help the patient acquire accurate information about medication.

Although patients may appear to be absorbing information about treatment procedures, this material may be quickly forgotten after they return to the home environment. One of the major reasons for noncompliance is confusion about when to take drugs or how to manage side effects. A written instruction sheet can reinforce material learned in the therapy session and can serve as a reminder of actions that the patient should take to maximize effectiveness of the drug. Printed pamphlets or other handout materials can also help with this process. Table 2 contains a list of publications that we have found useful for instructing patients about medication.

Educational material should be accurate, up to date, and consistent with the combined therapy approach. Certain publications, such as pamphlets from the pharmaceutical industry that present a unitary biological view, may cause confusion. One of the most common sources of information, the *Physician's Desk Reference* (PDR), often leads to exaggerated views about risks of medication. The extensive listing of every side effect that has ever been recorded may lead to unfounded fear about the dangers of pharmacotherapy.

The psychoeducational process continues throughout therapy. Checking frequently for understanding about the effects of medication reinforces learning and helps to avoid memory slippage. Regular questioning about medications can also help to identify new issues (e.g., additional side effects, conflicting information from other sources, questions from family members) that may require further psychoeducational efforts.

TABLE 2. Educational Materials for Combined Therapy[a]

---

Books
    Andreason, Nancy C., *The Broken Brain*
    Burns, David D., *Feeling Good*
    Fieve, Ronald R., *Moodswing*
    Pope, Harrison G., and Hudson, James I., *New Hope for Binge Eaters*
    Sheehan, David V., *The Anxiety Disease*
Articles
    Alper, Joseph, "Depression at an early age."
    Gallagher, Winifred, "The dark affliction of mind and body."
    Murphy, D. L., Sunderland, T., and Cohen, R. M., "Monamine oxidase-inhibiting antidepressants: A clinical update."
    Tavris, Carol, "Coping with anxiety."
Pamphlets
    American Medical Association, *Patient Medication Instruction Sheets*
    Goodwin, Frederick K., *Depression and Manic-depressive Illness*
    National Institute of Mental Health, *Information on Lithium*

---

[a]Full citations found in the references.

JESSE H. WRIGHT and
G. RANDOLPH
SCHRODT, JR.

Although intensive efforts are made to provide rational information about treatment, it is still not uncommon for patients to develop distorted thoughts about combined therapy. These cognitions may be either positive or negative and may act toward the betterment or detriment of treatment. Distortions can occur at two main levels of cognitive processing: automatic thinking and schemata (Wright, 1988). Standard cognitive therapy techniques such as guided discovery, thought recording, imagery, and homework can be used to identify and change maladaptive cognitions (Beck, Rush, Shaw, & Emery, 1979).

In our experience, cognitive responses to medication frequently center on characteristic themes. These themes are usually related to underlying schemata about personal worth and competence:

1. *Themes of personal weakness.* Patients frequently think "I should be able to get better on my own without medication" or "medications are a crutch." Providing information on the biological aspects of psychiatric disorders can often assist patients to develop a more balanced perspective of themselves and their therapy. Analogies can be useful in this regard. For example, the therapist might compare psychotropic drugs to medications used to treat peptic ulcer or migraine headache. These treatments may provide symptomatic improvement and promote healing, but alterations in life-style and other psychological changes are usually necessary for long-term improvement. Cognitive therapy interventions, directed at problems such as low self-esteem, excessive guilt, and negative attributions can also help to change distorted thoughts about the relationship between medication and personal strength or weakness.

2. *Fear of medication effects.* There often may be misunderstandings about what to expect from medication. Patients can even confuse psychotropic medications with substances of abuse. Negative automatic thoughts may ensue, such as, "I'll get dependent on the drug" or "I'll never get off medication." Patients who have a high frequency of cognitive errors (e.g., personalization, magnification, absolutistic thinking) may greatly exaggerate their estimates of the likelihood of experiencing serious side effects. Typical automatic thoughts of these patients might include "I'm always the one to get the side effects"; "nothing ever works right for me"; or "I won't be able to function." Unless such thoughts are altered, there will probably be poor medication compliance and a decreased hopefulness about treatment outcome.

3. *Fear of others' opinions.* At times, patients may believe that their own attitudes about psychotropic medication are shared by others. Fears that taking medication may lead to being treated differently by peers or even losing a job are not always without substance. However, it is extremely rare to find that the prescription of a medication, in itself, will lead to a strongly negative event. Often patients are excessively concerned about the adverse effects of discussing their treatment with their employers. We have found many instances in which employers have been highly supportive of appropriate treatment. Another cognitive distortion centers on the idea of "credit" for improvement. Patients may complain that "If I get better, then my family will credit the medication." Automatic thoughts of this type are related to the themes of personal weakness discussed earlier. Family therapy sessions can be very useful methods of exploring the validity of cognitions about the attitudes of significant others.

4. *Problems with the therapeutic alliance.* The prescription of medication is a powerful intervention that often elicits significant reactions about the therapeutic relationship. Thoughts such as "doctors don't know what they're doing with all these drugs" or "I'm just a guinea pig" are not unusual. Seeing the psychopharmacologist as a "pill pusher" who is not interested in feelings can lead to significant difficulties in providing effective therapy. Developing a good collaborative relationship, in which the therapist is seen as concerned about the whole person, can help to avoid negative distortions about the therapist's intentions.

5. *Misunderstandings about the illness.* "How can drugs help when I have a real-life problem?" Questions such as this are generated when patients have accepted complete personal responsibility for their emotional distress. Beliefs that depression is caused solely by "bad" thinking or that anxiety is due to unconscious conflicts can undermine the use of medication as an important component of treatment. Explaining integrative models of causality, such as the psychobiological final common pathway, usually helps clarify misunderstandings about the nature of psychiatric illnesses.

Positive distortions should also be explored and corrected when they appear to be maladaptive. For example, a patient who believes that medication is virtually a magical cure may have little interest in participating in therapy activities. He or she may expect the medication to "do all the work." However, other positive distortions may enhance recovery. These include somewhat exaggerated beliefs in the therapist's power to relieve symptoms through prescription of medication or through use of specific cognitive therapy techniques. We would generally not address mildly positive distortions that support the placebo component of the response to treatment because this is viewed as a genuine component of effective therapy. On the other hand, distorted positive cognitions that grossly overinflate the powers of the therapist or the medication would be identified and altered.

## BEHAVIORAL STRATEGIES FOR MEDICATION COMPLIANCE

Noncompliance can remain a problem despite the patient being willing to take medication and having reasonably healthy attitudes about pharmacotherapy. Patients with the best intentions have difficulty taking all their medication doses, even for short courses of treatment. When long-term therapy is required, compliance rates decline further. During the acute phase of the illness, painful symptoms such as dysphoria, sleep disturbance, or anxiety serve as powerful reasons to take medication. Relief of these symptoms positively reinforces adherence to the pharmacotherapy regimen. However, after symptoms have largely disappeared, these reinforcers become much weaker. There is still a perceived threat of the symptoms returning, but these concerns usually fade as time passes.

There are at least three major areas (patient, therapist, and family) in which behavioral contingencies may shape medication compliance. A search for reinforcers in each of these areas can provide valuable clues for building adherence to medication. Assessment of the patient could begin with detailed questioning about the behaviors that surround medication taking. This would include time(s) of day, association with other activities (e.g., food, brushing teeth, going to bed), and events that are typically related to "forgetting" medication. A homework assignment to record all daily activities on a written schedule might be used to collect additional information. After completing the behavioral analysis, the therapist would help the patient devise a reinforcement system that emphasizes the positive aspects of taking medication. Specific examples of interventions might include development of reminder systems (e.g., medication logs, checklists, divided pill boxes), pairing the time of medication dose with reinforcing activities (e.g., listening to morning news, a snack at bedtime), and self-reward for meeting compliance objectives.

It also may be useful for therapists to assess their own behaviors pertaining to medication. How often does the therapist ask about medication response, side effects, and compliance? What is the affective tone associated with discussions about medication? Does the therapist show more animation and interest when psychotherapy strategies are being employed? Is the therapist bored with repeating information about medication, and does it show? The underlying attitudes that determine these behaviors should also be examined.

A high level of genuine interest in the pharmacotherapy aspects of treatment will encourage the patient to continue medication. Techniques that convey this attitude include placing medication issues on the agenda of every therapy session, as well as asking frequent questions about drug effects. The therapist's reaction to reports of noncompliance may be especially critical. Stern or angry responses may discourage further communication about adherence problems. On the other hand, if the therapist shows understanding and respect for difficulties in complying with medication, the patient is likely to want to work with the therapist on ways of improving adherence. For example, in a situation where there is intense anxiety about side effects, the therapist might first recognize that fears about adverse effects are very common and that the therapist does not especially like to take drugs either. They could then perhaps develop a graded exposure plan that starts with very low doses of medication. Dosage would be increased gradually while both cognitive and behavioral procedures would be used to gradually desensitize the patient to anxiety about medication.

At times, poor medication compliance may be a product of negative (or insufficient positive) reinforcement from the family or other environmental sources. A patient's spouse might complain about the cost of medication, make negative comments about being "dependent on a drug," and discourage visits to the doctor. Situations such as these may erode the patient's resolve to take medication. Conversely, another patient's spouse might encourage medication compliance by making statements such as "the medication really seems to be helping; I'm glad you got started on it" or offering to go along to the doctor to find out how to manage side effects. Family therapy sessions can be used to identify attitudes and behaviors that can either diminish or increase the chances of medication compliance.

## COMBINED THERAPY ILLUSTRATIONS

### ANXIETY DISORDER

Research on cognitive therapy and pharmacotherapy has shown both to be effective treatments for anxiety disorders (Ballenger, 1984; Beck & Emery, 1985). Other studies have demonstrated the benefits of combined therapy approaches, although debate continues as to the relative contribution of each treatment (Klein, Ross, & Cohen, 1987; Marks, 1987). The following case illustrates how medication can decrease psychophysiological hyperarousal and thereby facilitate cognitive-behavioral procedures in mastering a phobic situation.

> Mrs. C. is a 37-year-old woman who was referred by her family doctor for evaluation of severe anxiety symptoms. She had made multiple visits both to his office and to the emergency room for episodes of intense apprehension, lightheadedness, diaphoresis, palpitations, and chest pain. She believed these were symptoms of a "heart attack."
>
> The first anxiety attack had occurred 3 months previously when she had visited her dentist for minor oral surgery. Subsequently, the episodes increased in frequency to a rate of five to six times per week. She described herself as generally tense and "jumpy." Most nights she had difficulty falling asleep. Mrs. C. had become preoccupied with her health and had dramatically restricted her activities, only leaving the house when absolutely necessary. Attempts by her family physician and a consulting cardiologist to reassure her that she had no evidence of cardiac disease were only mildly effective in decreasing her anxiety.
>
> Cognitive therapy initially focused on Mrs. C.'s tendency to overgeneralize the danger of situations and to engage in catastrophic, anticipatory thinking. By testing her automatic thoughts, she was able to gain a more realistic perspective of her fears of losing control and being the subject of social embarrassment. She left her first appointment with a behavioral assignment and reported she was greatly relieved to have an explanation of what was happening.

The next week she reported significant lessening of generalized anxiety and somatic preoccupation. However, she had experienced panic attacks while starting her car and had been unable to drive. Reviewing her automatic thoughts while starting the car revealed that she had experienced the sensation of diaphoresis and tachycardia and had thought, "If I pass out or have an attack while I'm driving, I'll lose control and innocent people will be killed." Mrs. C. recognized that this idea seemed irrational because she had never passed out or lost control even during previous severe panic attacks. However, when she tried to start the car the next day she again became extremely anxious, got out of the car and called a cab, thinking "better be safe than sorry."

Pharmacotherapy was begun with alprazolam 0.25 mg., three times daily. Alprazolam, a triazalobenzodiazepine, has been shown to be effective in alleviating panic as well as the generalized anxiety that often develops between attacks (Ballenger, 1984). Mrs. C.'s somatic symptoms were significantly reduced after starting medication. The lowering of autonomic arousal appeared to help her master the steps of the following graded task assignment: (1) sit in the car, (2) start the engine but do not drive, (3) pull out of the driveway and go around the block, and (4) drive to the next appointment. Although she continued to occasionally experience palpitations and tachycardia, she was able to reassure herself that this represented a harmless activation of her nervous system.

## BIPOLAR DISORDER

There has been growing evidence that bipolar disorder is a genetically determined illness that usually responds favorably to lithium carbonate or carbamazepine (Goodwin & Roy-Byrne, 1987). In contrast, there has been no substantive controlled research that has documented the effectiveness of any psychotherapy for bipolar disorder. Fuchs and Himmelhoch (1980) have described a single case of treatment of bipolar disorder with cognitive therapy. Although we rely primarily on pharmacotherapy for treatment of bipolar patients, cognitive therapy can help with compliance and be quite useful for the patient who does not have a complete response to medication. The following case illustrates the adjunctive use of cognitive therapy with a patient with bipolar disorder.

Mrs. E., a 44-year-old housewife, has a well-documented history of both depressive and manic episodes. Her father and his brother had also suffered from bipolar disorder. Both had committed suicide. Mrs. E. was admitted to the hospital because severe depression had returned. Relapse had occurred even though she was maintained on acceptable levels of lithium carbonate plus tranylcypromine, a monoamine oxidase inhibitor. After hospitalization, tranylcypromine was discontinued, and treatment with carbamazepine was initiated. However, Mrs. E. continued to have significant symptoms of depression, including intense suicidal ideation. On two occasions, she broke plastic eating utensils and used them in an attempt to cut her wrists.

One of the suicide attempts followed a phone call from Mrs. E.'s husband. He had asked her if he could stop by the hospital to obtain her signature to sell a rental property. Later that day, Mrs. E. was found in her room with superficial lacerations on her wrists. She told her doctor that the phone call had "devastated" her and that she was "ready to die." The doctor responded by attempting to elicit automatic thoughts that occurred during and after the phone call. A series of negative automatic thoughts was uncovered: "He never asks for my advice; all he needs from me is my signature; I don't have any say in what happens; he doesn't care; they would be better off with me dead."

A good collaborative relationship had previously been established, and the patient had some experience in using cognitive therapy techniques. Thus, Mrs. E. was able to

JESSE H. WRIGHT and
G. RANDOLPH
SCHRODT, JR.

respond when the therapist asked her to consider that the depression had twisted her thinking. Cognitive errors such as absolutistic thinking, magnification, and personalization were identified. Furthermore, data were generated that contradicted her negative conclusions: "I manage all the finances when I'm well, and I'm really good at it; we've been trying to sell that property for a long time; he tried to discuss this with me last week, but I really couldn't concentrate on it; this illness has been tough on both of us; he's stuck by me through it all."

The therapist then attempted to solidify gains from the treatment session by devising a homework assignment. Mrs. E. was asked to call her husband back to check the validity of her thinking and also to invite him to a treatment session the next day at the hospital. She reported later that her husband had been very supportive during the phone call. He had readily agreed to see the doctor with her for therapy. Further sessions were used to work on distortions in communication that appeared to aggravate the bipolar disorder.

### Unipolar Nonpsychotic Depression

The following example demonstrates how pharmacotherapy can facilitate accessibility to psychotherapy when these two effective treatments for depression are combined.

Mr. G., a 40-year-old man, had been in cognitive therapy as an outpatient for 2 months because of chronic dysphoria and problems with impaired work performance. Cognitive therapy sessions focused on his tendency to castigate himself about his performance in social situations and at work. Mr. G. appeared to be adapting well to the cognitive therapy approach. He routinely used a Daily Record of Dysfunctional Thoughts (DRDT) (Wright & Beck, 1983) to check for distorted cognitions and had completed several behavioral assignments that were designed to improve the situation at work. An important underlying schema, "I must be better than the rest to survive," was uncovered.

Although there had been some improvement in self-esteem and depressed mood after 2 months of treatment, Mr. G. continued to experience fatigue, insomnia, anorexia, and impaired concentration. This latter problem had contributed to several serious oversights at his job, for which he had been reprimanded by his boss. Mr. G. viewed these errors as evidence of personal inadequacy, and he experienced an intensified sense of worthlessness and hopelessness.

Previously, Mr. G. had been adamantly opposed to the idea of taking medication. He believed that medications were "a crutch" and that "people who take drugs are weak." However, after reading an article his therapist provided on biological aspects of depression, he agreed to a trial of antidepressants.

After a thorough medical evaluation, he was started on nortriptyline. The dosage was gradually increased to 75 mg a day, given in a single bedtime dose. Cognitive therapy sessions continued to focus on the work situation. Mr. G. began to recognize that his job performance had suffered only since he had become depressed. The hope that medication would make him feel better physically and restore his cognitive functioning led to a significant improvement in self-esteem. Within 3 weeks, he was sleeping well, was more energetic, and had improved concentration. Mr. G. was able to complete more complex cognitive and behavioral assignments in therapy, and his job performance noticeably improved.

### Psychoses

There has been little or no evidence gathered for the effectiveness of psychotherapy as a primary treatment for psychotic conditions (Group for Advancement of Psychiatry, 1975).

Pharmacotherapy with an antipsychotic drug plus a tricyclic antidepressant, or electroconvulsive therapy, is recommended for patients who have major depression with psychotic features (Wright & Lippmann, 1988). More severe psychoses, such as schizoaffective disorder and schizophrenia, are usually treated with pharmacotherapy as well.

The use of cognitive therapy as a support to pharmacotherapy for psychotic patients will be illustrated by an excerpt from a session of an aftercare group for chronic schizophrenics. One of the authors (J.H.W.) has led this aftercare group for over 10 years. Patients usually remain as group members for long periods of time. This allows for development of good collaborative relationships and a strong support network among group members. Cognitive therapy techniques are used to help structure sessions, identify and (when possible) change distorted cognitions, provide education about psychiatric illnesses and their treatment, and heighten the chances of medication compliance.

In the following portion of a group session, the members were trying to help a young woman who was having increased paranoia. She had recently stopped work on an assembly line because of delusional thinking.

Ms. K.: I'm having a real hard time. Everybody's throwing signs at me. I just can't get it out of my mind.

Mr. M.: That sounds paranoid to me. I know what that's like.

Mrs. O.: We've all been through that sort of thing. It's really tough, but it gets better. [Group nods in agreement.]

Dr. W.: I can see that most of you have had some experience with this kind of problem. Perhaps we could help by first trying to understand what it is and then talking about ways that you can cope with it.

Mr. R.: I'll start off. I've been paranoid off and on since I first got sick. Sometimes it seems just as real as can be, but I guess I've learned to recognize what it is and to see it as part of my illness. Dr. W. has told us about a chemical imbalance that causes these things, and that makes a lot of sense to me.

Mr. S.: I've sort of gotten used to it, I guess. After a while you get to know what thoughts are unrealistic and you just ignore them. You put a big brick wall up around them and you don't let them out.

Ms. K.: But they seem real to me!

Dr. W.: It sounds like some of the group members have learned how to not let paranoid thoughts bother them. They can recognize them as distorted thoughts and they don't let these ideas affect how they feel or act, but what do you do when they seem real?

Ms. V.: When I get more nervous and get scary thoughts, I usually call Dr. Wright and get more medication. That usually helps.

Mr. Y. (to Ms. K.): Are you taking your medication?

Ms. K.: Well, sort of.

Mr. Y.: That could be part of the problem.

Dr. W.: You've brought up an important issue. Having increased anxiety and more troubling thoughts can be related to problems with medication, either not taking what is prescribed or needing an adjustment in dosage.

Mrs. O.: It's hard to take medication every day, but it's really important. It's kept me out of the hospital.

Ms. K.: I know you're right, but even when I take medication it still seems like people are sending me messages. I just can't get it out of my mind.

Dr. W.: Let's try to summarize what we've learned so far and then try to figure out a way to help Ms. K. cope with her problem. [Goes to blackboard]

During the rest of this exchange the group reviewed what they understood about paranoid thoughts and developed a list of coping strategies. This list included: (1) think of paranoia as a biochemical abnormality just like diabetes or high blood pressure; (2) do not act on paranoid thoughts, because nobody is really trying to hurt you; (3) put a wall in your mind around the thoughts; (4) try to keep active and get involved in things you enjoy; (5) check out thoughts you are not sure about by asking someone you trust; (6) talk about it in group sessions; (7) take medication regularly; (8) develop reminder systems so you will not miss doses; and (9) tell Dr. W. if you feel worse so medication adjustments can be made.

This vignette illustrates how cognitive therapy procedures can be adapted to work with psychotic patients. The therapist's goal was to help the group derive a cognitive-behavioral framework that would help manage paranoid thoughts and improve medication compliance. In our experience, patients with chronic psychosis appear to benefit from the hopeful therapeutic attitude and the pragmatic, problem-oriented strategies that are hallmarks of the cognitive therapy approach.

## SUMMARY

Cognitive therapy and pharmacotherapy have been derived from different theoretical perspectives. Nonetheless, they can complement one another if they are applied as a combined therapeutic approach. The psychobiological final common pathway model is suggested as a broad, integrative theory to guide treatment efforts.

Effective combined therapy is contingent upon the formation of a good working relationship in which the patient and therapist can understand and accept the tenets of both therapies. During the course of treatment, cognitive and behavioral procedures can be used to augment pharmacotherapy in a number of ways. These include enhancing understanding, increasing hope, reducing symptoms not relieved by drug treatment, and managing problems of medication noncompliance. Pharmacotherapy can improve concentration or suppress other symptoms that may interfere with the process of psychotherapy.

As yet, little is known about the precise effects of cognitive therapy and pharmacotherapy on one another. Both seek to alleviate distress by altering the central nervous system activities that control such symptoms as anxiety and depression. We think it unlikely that the two treatments will be found to have independent modes of action. Instead, they may both operate by modulating basic pathways of encoding, learning, and information processing. Studies of the interface between the treatments may eventually add to our understanding of the mechanisms of symptom development and resolution.

## REFERENCES

Akiskal, H. S., & McKinney, W. T. (1975). Overview of recent research in depression: Integration of ten conceptual models into a comprehensive clinical frame. *Archives of General Psychiatry, 32,* 285–305.

Alper, J. (1986, May). Depression at an early age. *Science, 86,* 45–50.

American Medical Association. (n.d.). *Patient medication instruction sheets. Benzodiazepines; Lithium; Monoamine oxidase inhibitors; Neuroleptics; Tricyclic antidepressants.*

Andreason, N. C. (1984). *The broken brain.* New York: Harper & Row.

Baldessarini, R. J. (1977). *Chemotherapy in psychiatry.* Cambridge, MA: Harvard University Press.

Ballenger, J. C. (1984). Psychopharmacology of the anxiety disorders. *Psychiatric Clinics of North America, 7,* 757–771.

Barrett, C. L., Wright, J. H. (1984). Therapist variables. In M. Hersen, L. Michelson, & A. S. Bellack (Eds.), *Issues in psychotherapy research* (pp. 361–391). New York: Plenum Press.

Beck, A. T. (1985). Cognitive therapy, behavior therapy, psychoanalysis, and pharmacotherapy: A cognitive continuum. In M. J. Mahoney & A. Freeman (Eds.), *Cognition and psychotherapy* (pp. 325–347). New York: Plenum Press.

Beck, A. T., & Emery, G. (1985). *Anxiety disorders and phobias*. New York: Basic Books.

Beck, A. T., Rush, A. J., Shaw, B., & Emery, G. (1979). *Cognitive therapy of depression*. New York: Guilford Press.

Blackburn, I. M., Bishop, S., Glen, A. I. M., Whalley, L. J., & Christie, J. E. (1981). The efficacy of cognitive therapy in depression: A treatment using cognitive therapy and pharmacotherapy, each alone and in combination. *British Journal of Psychiatry, 139,* 181–189.

Burns, D. D. (1980). The consumer's guide to antidepressant drug therapy. In *Feeling good* (pp. 375–398). New York: Signet.

Chase, S., Wright, J. H., & Ragade, R. (1981). The inpatient psychiatric unit as a system. *Behavioral Science, 26,* 197–205.

Cochran, S. D. (1982). *Effectiveness of cognitive therapy in preventing noncompliance with lithium regimens.* Paper presented at the annual meeting of the American Psychological Association, Washington, DC.

Engel, G. L. (1977). The need for a new medical model: A challenge for biomedicine. *Science, 196,* 129–136.

Fieve, R. R. (1975). *Moodswing*. Toronto: Bantam Books.

Frank, J. D. (1978). *Psychotherapy and the human predicament: A psychosocial approach.* New York: Schocken Books.

Fuchs, C. Z., & Himmelhoch, J. M. (1980). Pseudomanic-depressive illness and cognitive-behavior therapy. *Journal of Nervous and Mental Disease, 168,* 382–384.

Gallagher, W. (1986, May). The dark affliction of mind and body. *Discover,* pp. 66–76.

Goodwin, F. K. (1982). *Depression and manic-depressive illness.* NIH Publication No. 82-1940. Washington, D.C.: NIH.

Goodwin, F. K., & Roy-Byrne, P. (1987). Treatment of bipolar disorders. In A. J. Francis & R. E. Hales (Eds.), *American Psychiatric Press review of psychiatry* (Vol. 6, pp. 81–107). Washington, DC. American Psychiatric Press.

Group for the Advancement of Psychiatry. (1975). *Pharmacotherapy and psychotherapy: Paradoxes, problems and progress,* Vol. 9, Report No. 93. New York. Mental Health Materials Center.

Hollon, S., & Beck, A. T. (1978). Psychotherapy and drug therapy: Comparisons and combinations. In S. L. Garfield & Bergin (Eds.), *Handbook of psychotherapy and behavior change* (2nd ed.; pp. 437–490). New York: Wiley.

Kandel, E. R., & Schwartz, J. H. (1982). Molecular biology of learning: Modulation of transmitter release. *Science, 218,* 433–443.

Klein, D. F., Ross, D. C., & Cohen, P. (1987). Panic and avoidance in agoraphobia. *Archives of General Psychiatry, 44,* 377–385.

Marks, I. M. (1987). Behavioral aspects of panic disorder. *American Journal of Psychiatry, 144*(9), 1160–1165.

Marmor, J. (1976). Common operational factors in diverse approaches to behavior change. In A. Bunton (Ed.), *What makes behavior change possible?* (pp. 3–12). New York: Brunner/Mazel.

Miller, J. G. (1978). *Living systems*. New York: McGraw-Hill.

Mohl, P. C. (1987). Should psychotherapy be considered a biological treatment? *Psychosomatics, 28*(6), 320–326.

Murphy, D. L., Sunderland, T., & Cohen, R. M. (1984). Monoamine oxidase-inhibiting antidepressants: A clinical update. *Psychiatric Clinics of North America, 3,* 549–562.

Murphy, G. E., Simons, A. D., & Wetzel, R. D. (1984). Cognitive therapy versus tricyclic antidepressants in major depression. *Archives of General Psychiatry, 41,* 33–41.

National Institute of Mental Health. (1981). *Information on Lithium.* DHHS Publication No. (ADM) 81-1078. Washington, DC: Author.

Pope, H. G., Harrison, G., Hudson, J. I. (1984). *New hope for binge eaters.* New York: Harper & Row.

Rush, A. J. (1988). Cognitive approaches to adherence. In A. J. Francis & R. E. Hales (Eds.), American Psychiatric Press review of psychiatry (Vol. 7, pp. 627–642). Washington, DC: American Psychiatric Press.

Schwab, J. J., & Schwab, M. E. (1978). *Sociocultural roots of mental illness.* New York City: Plenum Medical Book Co.

Sheehan, D. V. (1983). *The anxiety disease.* Toronto: Bantam Books.

Simons, A. D., Murphy, G. E., Levine, J. L., & Wetzel, R. D. (1986). Cognitive therapy and pharmacotherapy for depression. *Archives of General Psychiatry, 43,* 43–48.

Snow, C. P. (1959). *The two cultures: And a second look*. London: Cambridge University Press.

Tavris, C. (1946, February). Coping with anxiety. *Science Digest, 46,* 46–81.

Uhlenhuth, E. H., Lipman, R. S., & Covi, L. (1969). Combined pharmacotherapy and psychotherapy. *Journal of Nervous and Mental Disease, 148,* 52–64.

Weissman, M. M., Prusoff, B. A., DiMascio, A., Neu, C., Goklaney, M., & Klerman, G. L. (1979). The efficacy of drugs and psychotherapy in the treatment of acute depressive episodes. *American Journal of Psychiatry, 136,* 555–558.

Whybrow, P. C., Akiskal, H. S., & McKinney, W. T. (1984). *Mood disorders: Toward a New Psychobiology.* New York: Plenum Press.

Wright, J. H. (1985). The cognitive paradigm for treatment of depression. P. Pichot, P. Eenner, R. Wolf, & K. Thau (Eds.), in *Psychiatry* (Vol. 4, pp. 31–36). New York: Plenum Press.

Wright, J. H. (1986). Nortriptyline effects on cognition in depression. *Dissertation Abstracts International, 47* (6), 2667b.

Wright, J. H. (1987). Cognitive therapy and medication as combined treatment. In A. Freeman & V. Greenwood (Eds.), *Cognitive therapy* (pp. 36–50). New York: Human Sciences Press.

Wright, J. H. (1988). Cognitive therapy of depression. In A. J. Francis & R. E. Hales (Eds.), *American Psychiatric Press review of psychiatry* (Vol. 7, pp. 554–570). Washington, DC: American Psychiatric Press.

Wright, J. H., & Beck, A. T. (1983). Cognitive therapy of depression: Theory and practice. *Hospital Community Psychiatry, 34,* 1119–1127.

Wright, J. H., & Lippmann, S. B. (1988). Use of antipsychotic drugs in depression: Problems and opportunities. *Postgraduate Medical Journal, 82,* 61–67.

# 15

# Cognitive Restructuring through Guided Imagery

## Lessons from Gestalt Therapy

Dᴀᴠɪᴅ J. A. Eᴅᴡᴀʀᴅs

> *One picture is worth 10,000 words.*
> Ancient chinese proverb

> *A picture shows me at a glance what it takes dozens of pages of a book to expound.*
> Ivan Turgenev, *Fathers and Sons* (1862)

> *So the soul, being strongly elevated, and inflamed with a strong imagination, sends forth health and sickness.*
> Cornelius Agrippa, 1510, cited by McMahon & Sheikh, 1984, p. 20

Words are powerful tools of thought and communication, but visual imagery has a similar role that is more archaic, powerful, and encompassing. The human infant represents the world to himself or herself in imagery and fantasy long before he or she says his or her first word. The signs of the use of visual imagery still remain in cave paintings that go back thousands of years. In more advanced cultures, the legacy of complex mythologies rich in visual representations of personal and archetypal themes attest to the fact that men and women have used this medium in diverse and sophisticated ways for millennia in their quest for understanding and mastery of self and environment (Samuels & Samuels, 1975).

Although words allow reality to be broken up into a manageable coding of the flow of events in the world, visual imagery has a holistic character that allows it to capture the often intricate relationships between specific facts, beliefs, and assumptions that may be individually

---

Dᴀᴠɪᴅ J. A. Eᴅᴡᴀʀᴅs • Department of Psychology, Rhodes University, Grahamstown 6140, South Africa.

isolated in verbal representation. In therapy, imagery can provide a special type of access to cognitive structures that allows the structures to be worked with in ways that the linear and analytical verbal techniques cannot.

Although Beck (1976; Beck, Rush, Shaw, & Emery, 1979) emphasizes verbal techniques in describing the methods of cognitive therapy, he has related the use of several imagery techniques to the process of cognitive restructuring, both in an important earlier paper (Beck, 1970) and in his application of the therapy to anxiety (Beck & Emery, 1985). He emphasizes the need to elicit information about the client's spontaneous visual imagery and to help him or her to see and restructure the distortions inherent in it, in much the same way as verbally expressed cognitions are tackled. He also recognizes that a person's schematic representations of reality are not fundamentally verbal or visual but can be translated into and restructured through either modality.

Freeman (1981) showed how images from dreams and fantasies provide access to the individual's personal interpretations of reality and the distortions these include. In cases where an individual experiences an emotional reaction to a life situation whose intensity is out of proportion to the facts of the event itself, visual imagery often vividly portrays the distortions that are responsible. This provides a basis for reexamination and restructuring of the relevant beliefs and assumptions.

The use of directed visualization as a route to self-mastery and personal transformation is an ancient practice found in Tibetan Buddhism (Samuels & Samuels, 1975). In modern times, applications of guided imagery to psychotherapy have been Jung's active imagination (Watkins, 1976), Assagioli's (1965) guided fantasy in psychosynthesis, Leuner's (1984) guided affective imagery, and the imagery psychodrama of Perls and the gestalt therapists (Perls, 1969; Polster & Polster, 1974; Stevens, 1971). Imagery techniques have been used to treat depression (Schultz, 1984), and phobias (Habeck & Sheikh, 1984), to increase resistance to cancer (Hall, 1984), and to control pain (Bresler, 1984) (see Sheikh, 1984; Singer, 1974; Watkins, 1976, for descriptions of other applications.) Though on the surface dissimilar, the process of cognitive restructuring through guided imagery has a close affinity to the restructuring that takes place through Socratic questioning and guided discovery in cognitive therapy. Gestalt techniques offer valuable means for identifying key cognitions (Arnkoff, 1981), and in this chapter the imagery psychodrama method of Perls will be described within the framework of the cognitive model.

In one of Perls's best known dreamwork seminars, he worked with "Linda" (Perls, 1971). Linda dreamed of a lake drying up; a group of porpoises were dancing around, sad because they would no longer be able to breed in the dried-up lake. As the water disappeared, she felt a ray of hope that she would find some treasure hidden on the lake bed. But all that appeared was an outdated automobile license plate. This is how Perls (Fritz) worked with her:

> FRITZ: Will you please play the license plate.
>
> LINDA: I am an old license plate, thrown in the bottom of the lake. I have no use because I'm no value—although I'm not rusted I'm outdated so I can't be used as a license plate . . . and I'm just thrown on the rubbish heap. That's what I did with a license plate, I threw it on a rubbish heap.
>
> FRITZ: How do you feel about this?
>
> LINDA: [quietly] I don't like it. I don't like being a license plate—useless.
>
> FRITZ: Could you talk about this. That was such a long dream until you came to the license plate. I'm sure this must be of great importance.
>
> LINDA: [sighs] Useless, outdated . . . The use of a license plate is to allow—give a car permission to go . . . and I can't give anyone permission to do anything because I'm

outdated . . . . In California, they just paste a little—you buy a sticker—and stick it on the car, on the old license plate. [faint attempt at humor] So maybe someone could put me on the car and stick this sticker on me, I don't know.

FRITZ: Okay, now play the lake.

LINDA: I'm a lake . . . I'm drying up, and disappearing, soaking into the earth . . . [with a touch of surprise] *dying*. . . . But when I soak into the earth I become a part of the earth—so maybe I water the surrounding area, so . . . even in the lake, even in my bed, flowers can grow [sighs]. . . . New life can grow . . . from me [cries].

PERLS: You get the existential message?

LINDA: Yes [sadly, but with conviction]. I can paint—I can create—I can create beauty. I can no longer reproduce, I'm like the porpoise . . . but I . . . I'm I . . . keep wanting to say I'm *food* . . . I . . . as water becomes. . . . I water the earth and give life—growing things, the water—they need both the earth and water, and the . . . and the air and the sun, but as the water from the lake I can play a part in something, and producing—feeding.

PERLS: You see the contrast: On the surface you find something, some artifact—the license plate, the artificial you—but then, when you go deeper, you find the apparent death of the lake is actually fertility. . . .

LINDA: And I don't need a license plate, or a permission, a license in order to . . . .

FRITZ: Nature doesn't need a license plate to grow. You don't have to [be?] useless if you are organismically creative, which means if you are involved.

LINDA: And I don't need permission to be creative. . . . Thank you. (Perls, 1971, pp. 86–87. reproduced with permission)

This brief vignette is an elegant therapeutic transaction that leads to a sudden and profound restructuring. To the cognitive therapist, used to identifying the content of the beliefs and assumptions and to challenging them with logical analysis, Socratic questioning, and experiment, what happened in this interchange may seem mysterious. It is, however, a process that is completely familiar, once the implicit restructuring work is made explicit. Through the imagery and the subsequent dialogue, some of Linda's key beliefs and assumptions were laid bare. Without direct intervention from Perls, she recognized the inaccuracy of some of these and discovered an avenue for solution that she saw led to a new conceptualization of herself.

Linda was coming to the end of her period as a fertile woman. Up till this time, she had conceptualized her ability to bear children as something that gave her a role and status. Like the license plate, it gave her permission to be a member of society. The unspoken assumption was, "My role as a woman is to feed [in giving birth and child rearing], and that is what makes me useful". An additional assumption was, "If I can't bear children I can't be creative, so I'm useless." When she took the role of the lake and saw herself as dying, she identified with that assumption, but when she saw how the water could provide life for plants beside the lake, she recognized that the focus of the life-giving power of water in the dream could shift from supporting the porpoises to watering the plants. At this point, her fixed belief about her own creativity being limited to childbearing began to change. She realized that she did not have to be biologically useful in order to be a useful member of society but that there were other ways in which she could contribute creatively.

This is a masterful example of guided discovery. Perls skillfully moved Linda toward new insight, while allowing the nature of the restructuring to emerge from her own thinking and exploration. The dreamwork seminars were not like full therapy sessions, and Perls did not draw out the implications of this discovery for her life or discuss with her how she would experiment with participating in new ways, although, in individual therapy, this stage would be made more explicit, and homework assignments might be set (Polster & Polster, 1974).

In standard cognitive therapy, the therapist elicits key thoughts and themes and explores the idiosyncratic meanings of these for the client by questioning. Perls achieved the same end by creating a miniature psychodrama from the visual image by having the symbols (in this case the license plate and lake) speak a soliloquy or, in some cases, dialogue with each other. Once the meanings and assumptions have been identified, the next step is to challenge those that are dysfunctional. Perls did this through the dialogue of the images, using it to question the uncovered assumptions and suggest and experiment with alternatives.

The goal of this chapter is to show how these methods can be integrated into standard cognitive therapy. In the next section, there is an analysis of specific techniques that are components of this guided imagery method. This is followed by two case examples. Finally, there is a discussion of the factors that need to be considered by the therapist who incorporates these techniques into cognitive therapy.

## A REVIEW OF GUIDED IMAGERY TECHNIQUES

### GETTING STARTED

The main techniques for obtaining an image from which to begin are the visualization of a life event or theme, the reinstatement of a dream or daytime image, and feeling focusing. Despite the misconception held by some therapists that guided imagery requires some sort of hypnotically induced trance state, it is not necessary to use any relaxation or other induction. It is best to have the client's eyes closed, although some can work with eyes open and may prefer this at the early stages if the imagery content is threatening.

For *life event visualization,* the client is asked to visualize a specific event that is the focus of attention in therapy. This may be something recent such as a quarrel with a spouse, or a past event such as a childhood memory of being ridiculed by peers or a teacher at school. *In theme visualization,* the client is asked to focus on a specific theme and let an image arise spontaneously. This has the advantage that the obtained image often expresses key assumptions and meanings related to the theme. The second case example, to be discussed later, is an example of this technique. This client was idealizing her ex-husband, and she was asked to picture him in this idealized form.

*Reinstatement of a dream or daytime image* involves asking for a specific image that has arisen before, either in a dream, daydream, fantasy, or previous guided imagery work. For example, one client, a college student, working on test anxiety, reported a vivid image of his mother while taking tests. This disturbed him and contributed to the anxiety, and he was able to reinstate it during the session. Another client who had been working on weight control dreamed she was in her childhood neighborhood walking past a baby elephant being fed with a bottle, and this was used as the initial image.

*Feeling focusing* is analogous to asking for the automatic thought that accompanies a feeling. The client focuses on a specific emotion that he or she is experiencing in the session. Awareness of the feeling can be intensified by having him or her focus on the bodily sensations related to it or to the overall "felt sense" of it (Gendlin, 1978; Gendlin, Grindler, & McGuire, 1984). Then she or he is asked to let an image arise from the feeling, or portray the feeling. Often an image will arise spontaneously that vividly portrays the meaning framework within which the feeling is embedded. For example, one client who experienced overwhelming dread in the morning obtained an image of himself fusing with and separating from an image of his father. This proved to be an important focus for the next stage of therapy. Another client who suddenly felt overwhelming fear of abandonment and a sense of being like a lump of clay in others' hands got an image of herself in her crib watching her alcoholic mother who had passed out on the bed nearby.

Where imagery is vague, *multisensory evocation* can help to sharpen the detail. Here the therapist directs the client to focus on experience through the different senses. The therapist can ask him what he hears and suggest different sounds that might be found in the setting being visualized; then she can focus attention on smell, taste and touch in addition to the visual modality.

It is important for the therapist to follow the principle of collaborativeness and to respect the imagery that arises in the client, even if it is unexpected or does not fit in with initial intentions. The images that emerge can be a vivid portrayal of important aspects of the cognitive structure that was previously not available for scrutiny. They also indicate what the client is ready to work with. Like a dream, the image often presents both a problem and the seeds of a solution, and it is important to be willing to work with what is given, without preconceptions.

### ASSESSMENT TECHNIQUES

Once an image has been elicited, it is important to discover the idiosyncratic meanings that it has for the client. The therapist may have his or her own hypotheses about some of these but should not rely on textbook interpretations of specific symbols. Instead, it is important to check out interpretations by allowing the content of beliefs, assumptions, and interpretations to come from the client himself or herself.

The imagery of a client who reported feeling angry at and deprived by his girlfriend will be used to illustrate several of the techniques. Feeling focusing elicited an image of himself aged about 6, with his mother, during an incident that had happened when he was about 16. His mother seemed cold and dead. Later he noticed that she held a large key in one hand. In the guided imagery that followed, I helped him to identify a number of assumptions that were implicit in the imagined scene and which supported his feelings of helplessness and rage towards his mother. These included the narcissistic assumptions that he was entitled to be perfectly loved by his mother, that she had a duty to love him perfectly, and that he was entitled to revenge if she failed in this. In addition there was the helplessness-inducing assumption that if his mother did not love him no one could. These assumptions left the initiative for resolution of the situation in her hands, thus leaving him impotent. This was symbolized by his mother holding the key.

I guided him to reach out and take the key, to go with his girlfriend toward the door of the room, and to use the key to let them both out. This process, which was accomplished with considerable hesitancy, challenged the assumptions set out before and offered, as an alternative perspective, the assumptions that he was lovable even if his mother was unloving, that he could accept his girlfriend's love, and that he could use his own initiative to take himself out of the impasse.

One of the basic Gestalt techniques can be called *prompted soliloquy*. In the dreamwork example, Linda was asked to "be the lake". This is a direction to identify herself as the lake and deliver a short soliloquy about her existential status and her feelings in that role. If the client can do this well, a great deal of information about the personal meaning of the image emerges.

However, many clients do not possess the skills to explore the image through soliloquy, and the *interview* technique can be used to give specific prompts about the information being sought. The client takes the role of a person or object in the image, and the therapist asks specific questions. In the case example, the therapist might say, "Now I'd like to interview the boy. Tell me how does your mother look to you right now? . . . Tell me what you are feeling? . . . What do you want from her?" Answers to these questions would lead to further questions as the interview proceeded that would yield information about his feelings of anger toward his mother and the cognitions that were associated with them.

*Prompted dialogue* is similar to the soliloquy and interview techniques. The client takes the role of a person or object in the imaged scene but instead of talking to herself or himself or the therapist, she or he addresses some other person or object. In the example, the therapist could say, ''Be the little boy and tell your mother how you feel when she is so cold and uncaring.'' Or, later, ''Be the key and tell the boy what you can open for him''.

It is important for the therapist to track the client's imagery as closely as possible, and to do this, she or he will need to ask for *prompted descriptions* of what is happening. Information about affect is especially important. When there are several people or objects in the image, the therapist will usually want to focus on the emotions of one or two and asks what emotions particular characters are experiencing. Questions about affect may, of course, be included as part of the interview method. For example, if the therapist used prompted dialogue to ask the boy to tell his mother about his feelings, he would then be interested in the emotional reaction of the mother to hearing this. The client would probably be able to tell this by observing her in the image, and the therapist could prompt this information by asking, ''Can you see how your mother is feeling now?'' or ''What do you notice about your mother's reaction to what you have said?''.

It is also important to track the affect experienced by the client herself or himself as the imagery work proceeds, even where it is not directly represented in the image. The therapist must pay attention to nonverbal cues as to what the client is experiencing and may need to ask questions such as, ''What do you feel when you say that?'' or, ''You seem to be sad when you say that?''

Asking for more detailed description of part of the image is another type of prompted description. In the case example, having established that the mother is holding a key, the therapist might ask which hand is holding it and how tightly. Sometimes asking for details allows the image to come into sharper focus, and new details emerge that were not there before. One client described her parents waving at somebody in the distance, and when asked to zoom in on the figure and describe it, she saw that it was an angel. This turned out to be an important positive image, associated with acceptance of her independence and creativity.

As the work proceeds, the images change. Shifts may be small, such as in facial expression, or large, such as a complete change of scene. Any such change will be called a *transformation*. Transformations provide important information about the clients' personal meanings, and it is therefore important to track them closely. The client can be taught to report transformations spontaneously when they occur, or the therapist can ask about them from time to time.

One client, a member of a minority group, believed others were suspicious of her because of her race. She was imaging herself talking to two white Americans and was asked to imagine that one said to the other, ''We'd better be very careful what we say to Jenny. She's quite different from us and she has relatives in the Soviet Union. We can't be too careful'' [directed dialogue technique: see later text]. When asked what happened next, she reported that both Americans appeared to break into uncontrolled laughter, recognizing that the speech was absurd. This spontaneous transformation demonstrated that Jenny could see that none of her friends would be likely to seriously believe that statement.

In *prompted transformation,* the therapist suggests a change of image. This may be because a particular avenue of work has reached an impasse or because further information about the personal meanings that are involved is needed. One client saw herself frantically searching in the ground for a coin. She was asked to transform the image to show the coin. The image of her searching was replaced by the image of a coin in a jewelry box. Use of interview and prompted dialogue showed that the box represented protection and safety but also restriction on freedom and independence. This clarified the first image that had shown the desperate search for freedom and independence that had been thwarted by unrecognized assumptions about her dependency.

RESTRUCTURING TECHNIQUES

The assessment techniques enable the therapist to identify important assumptions and conflicts that underlie the client's psychological problems. The restructuring techniques allow the therapist to guide the client to actively question and challenge these assumptions.

*Summary and reframing* are basic methods here as they are in regular cognitive therapy. In summarizing, the therapist feeds back what he or she has learned so far from the client's descriptions of images, thoughts, or feelings. In the example, he might say, ''So now the little boy is angry with the mother for having the key and not giving it to him and feels hopeless about ever escaping.'' This serves as a check for the therapist but also makes explicit for the client the structure of thoughts and feelings that has been exposed. In reframing, the therapist suggests an alternative formulation of some of the beliefs and assumptions that have been elicited. In this example, he might reframe by saying, ''The key is lying there, waiting for the boy to take it,'' or ''Maybe she's not holding the key so tightly as you think, take a closer look''. Both summary and reframing are useful preparatory steps for the more active restructuring techniques that follow.

*Directed dialogue* is the major method of restructuring dysfunctional beliefs and assumptions. The therapist directs the client to take the role of one of the imagery figures and to speak certain lines which she or he dictates. This can be used to bring a belief sharply into relief. In the example, the therapist might say, ''Take the role of the boy and say to the mother, 'You are so strong and powerful that there is nothing that I can do to get what I want from you.' '' Sometimes in order to enhance the effect, lines can be given that exaggerate the assumption. (See the example where Jenny was asked to imagine her friends speaking suspiciously about her because of her relatives in the Soviet Union.) Simply putting the assumption into the mouth of one of the characters confronts the client more vividly than talking about it and can bring about spontaneous restructuring because the client's reality-testing processes are automatically brought to bear on it.

In another use of directed dialogue, the therapist dictates words that challenge or contradict dysfunctional beliefs that have been brought into focus. In the example, she might say, ''Be the little boy and tell your mother, 'Even if you don't love me that doesn't mean someone else can't love me. I'm not going to continue letting you hold the key to my happines.' '' This speech contradicts two important assumptions. The use of such directed dialogue does not always automatically achieve the desired restructuring. The therapist needs to obtain feedback as to the impact of what is said by using the assessment techniques. For example, if the boy felt even more hopeless or shrank in size, this would indicate the need to detect other thoughts and beliefs that were preventing restructuring and that would need to be dealt with. On the other hand, if the mother shrank in size or appeared to go weak and pale or if the boy felt optimistic and stronger, this would indicate that restructuring was proceeding in the desired direction.

As restructuring begins to take place and the client's thought processes move on their own toward a new set of assumptions, the therapist can use the less directive *prompted dialogue*. Instead of dictating it word for word he or she can say, for example, ''Tell your mother how you are going to live differently in the future,'' or ''Tell your father how you feel about him now you're becoming an independent adult.'' Less directive prompts such as, ''What do you still need to say to your father?'' or, ''Is there something more you still have to say?'' can be used. This enables the client to express the emotions that emerge and to practice and consolidate the restructured beliefs.

*Directed transformation* provides another way of challenging assumptions. Here the therapist instructs the client to effect a change in the image, for example, by directing one of the characters to take some action. In the example, the therapist directed the boy to take the key from his mother and later to use it to unlock a door that gave him access to the outside. This challenged the assumptions that his mother held the key to his happiness and that until she changed he was trapped.

*Prompted transformation* gives more initiative to the client. Instead of directing a specific change in the image, he or she just suggests the general direction of the change. In the example, instead of directing the boy to take the key from his mother, the therapist might have said, "Find a way for the boy to get the key".

This less detailed direction is useful where restructuring is clearly in process and merely requires facilitation. It can also be used where the therapist perceives an impasse. It allows the client's own creativity to provide a solution and is therefore a good collaborative gesture. In the example, the therapist might ask, "Is there anyone who could help the boy get the key?" This might result in the entry onto the scene of a person whom the client feels supported by. This transformation would then arise from the therapist's prompt and the client's own creative use of her resources.

## CASE EXAMPLES OF IMAGERY WORK

### CASE EXAMPLE 1: C. D.

C. D. was a 27-year-old unmarried woman who had suffered recurrent major depression and taken a number of medication overdoses. She responded well to cognitive therapy and used the dysfunctional thought record conscientiously. However in an early session, when suicidal ideation returned, attempts to address the hopelessness verbally met with limited success, and she phoned for another session the next day. The session described here shows the use of imagery work in a crisis. Because the client was suicidal and there was an urgent need to identify and challenge the assumptions underlying the current hopelessness, an active and directive style was used.

The client's self-schema was not well individuated from her schemata representing other family members. For example, when out shopping and trying to decide what to buy, she heard her mother's and sister's voices giving her advice and criticizing her own preferences. Though not hallucinations, they were vivid and disturbing. In the first part of the session, it became clear that she felt hopeless about being able to be separate from her mother. I asked her to obtain an image of herself and her mother together, and I directed an imagery psychodrama as follows:

D. E.: Imagine she says, "C. You're completely untrustworthy." Now reply to her.

C. D.: I can't. I'm like frozen.

D. E.: Can you picture yourself getting frozen. Can you see what you're doing to freeze yourself?

C. D.: . . . Because she doesn't trust me . . .

D. E.: Even though she doesn't trust you, that doesn't mean you have to freeze yourself. She still doesn't trust you, but see if you can unfreeze yourself . . . What's happening?

C. D.: I'm getting mad.

D. E.: Tell your mother that you're mad that she doesn't trust you.

C. D.: I'm mad that you don't trust me. . . . She comes back, "I know you, You've been giving your grandmother trouble and she told me she asked you to do something and you wouldn't do it . . ."

D. E.: Tell your mother what goes on between you and your grandmother is nothing to do with her.

C. D.: That's none of your business . . . . And then she'll say, "She's my mother and she's old, and when she asks you to do something, you do it."

D. E.: Tell her, "It's none of your business."

C. D.: It's none of your business.

D. E.: "I'm going to make the major decisions in my life now."

C. D.: I'm going to make the major decisions in my life now . . . and then she'll say . . .

D. E.: No. "I'm not a child anymore." [She previously reported that her mother dreamed that she was taking C. D., her sick child to the hospital. C. D. said in a later session she could not envisage herself as more than 9 years old.]

C. D.: I'm not a child anymore.

D. E.: "When you try to keep me as a child, you just make me mad."

C. D.: When you try to keep me as a child you just make me mad.

D. E.: How are you feeling now?

C. D.: Scared.

D. E.: What are you scared of?

C. D.: Her reaction. . . . She's saying, " 'Is this the way you treat me? After all I'm your mother?''

D. E.: A classic line. A classic turn of the guilt screw. What could you reply to that?

At this point I gave her more assertive and independent words to experiment with. She was somewhat hesitant about some of the lines but, with encouragement, said them all:

"It's true that you're my mother but I'm not a child anymore. If we're going to relate to each other you're going to have to respect my independence. You've been treating me like a child all these years, but it's going to stop now. I'm going to have my own opinions and make my own decisions."

At this point C. D. reported that her mother was just laughing at her mockingly, and she felt hopeless because these gestures toward independence were not working. It became clear that she believed she could not individuate unless her mother changed, and she did not believe she could change her mother. I summarized and reframed it for her.

D. E.: I get the sense that you believe you have to change her; that unless you can get her to change, to accept you and your independence, it won't be possible for you to have it.

We explored this for a few minutes but continually met with resistance on the part of C. D. to seeing a path toward true independence. This seemed to confirm the idea that her self-schema was cognitively fused with that of her mother. The next step was to test this hypothesis, and what happened confirmed this formulation.

D. E.: I'm going to give you an idea, and that is that you have two mothers. One is sitting there at home, and the other is the one you carry round in your head. Right now it's as if you had this very manipulative, bitter woman sitting behind your shoulder, whispering in your ear. Now you can't change the one who's sitting there at home, perhaps. But you don't have to have this one sitting on your shoulder. That's the one you've created. . . . Get a picture of your mother at home, and you in the city, with this mother you've created for yourself. See where she'd be. Would she be on your shoulder or inside your head? How would you like to picture her . . . How is she related to the image of you? . . .

C. D.: Her head is like, inside mine, but it almost seems larger. There's just like my face, but then her head is larger and that's all I see.

D. E.: Now keep that image clearly. Her head's inside yours? It's like you've let her take you over? . . . Now talk to this mother who's inside your head. . . . What would you like to say to her?

C. D.: You're driving me crazy. Don't you realize all the pressure you've been putting on me. Don't you realize what it's been doing to me this last dozen of years or so?

D. E.: Let her reply.

C. D.: What do you mean? I sent you to college. I sent you on trips. I provide your food, your clothing, free housing . . .

D. E.: Stop and say to her, "You don't do anything. You're just a figment of my imagination. I created you and you're driving me crazy. And I'm not going to let this go on any longer." [C. D. repeats this] Tell me what's happening.

C. D.: She says, "If it weren't for me you'd never do anything. I have to push you to do everything.

D. E.: Tell her "That's bullshit. If it weren't for you, I'd know what I wanted, and I'd be able to make my own decisions."

C. D.: That's bullshit. If it weren't for you I'd know what I wanted and I'd be able to make my own decisions. . . . Now she says, "You're so independent? Yeah, look at you! You don't have a job. You can't hold a job. You don't know what you want. You never knew how to make up your mind."

D. E.: Tell her, "That's because I've kept you in my head like this, but I'm not going to go on like this any more."

C. D.: That's because I've kept you in my head like this, but I'm not going to go on like this any more.

D. E.: What's happening now?

C. D.: She's getting smaller. . . . She's looking at me . . .

D. E.: How do you feel now she's got smaller?

C. D.: A lot calmer.

D. E.: Tell her, "I feel a whole lot better now you've got smaller. I'm going to be careful not to let you get bigger again."

C. D.: I feel a whole lot better now you've got smaller. I'm going to be careful not to let you get bigger again.

D. E.: What's happening?

C. D.: Everything's going dark. She's getting smaller, and I feel a whole lot better.

There were three stages in this session in terms of the assumptions being dealt with. In the first, where I helped to challenge her mother by giving her direct and assertive lines to say, the focus was on assumptions about being a helpless child who needs her mother to tell her what to do. This is a challenging that needed to be done because C. D. had never talked to her mother like that. This part of the work looks like a covert rehearsal that would be done in assertiveness training. However, it is done with a different intention. It is not a formal practice of something she will later say but a way of experimenting with new assumptions about her own independence. At a later stage in therapy, this did lead to her being more assertive with her mother, but at this stage, the aim was to assess whether there were other cognitive factors that stood in the way of an assertiveness project.

This led to the shift to the next assumption that had to be dealt with, which was, "Unless I can get my mother to change, I can't change." The next stage experimented with challenging that assumption. However, this also failed to resolve the hopelessness, partly because she was scared that, if she took a stand, her mother would reject her, but also, more importantly, because her internal representation of her mother was so powerful and so habitually exercized that she would still be subject to the same pressure from her own fantasy as she was before. The next step in the work was to show that to a great extent what she was responding to was her own fantasy and to show that she could exercise control over that. This proved to be the essential discrimination to teach before the other assumptions could be fully tackled, and the discovery that she need not continually recreate the engulfing relationship with her mother in fantasy resolved the immediate hopelessness.

J. T. was a woman who, 15 years after her divorce, was still experiencing feelings of loss and a great deal of conflict in relation to her ex-husband. She described his behavior as irrational, egocentric, and violent, yet maintained a very idealized image of what he was really like or might become. Starting with a conceptualization that she needed to see clearly what her idealized fantasy of him was and then reality-test it, I guided the session as follows.

D. E.: So it seems that you keep alive B as you wanted him to be?

J. T.: And I keep getting disappointed . . . So what do I do?

D. E.: Bury your fantasy. . . . Do you have a picture in your mind of B. as you wanted him to be? . . . Can you picture yourself with him? . . . Can you tell me what you see?

J. T.: The two of us together, walking down the street?

D. E.: Can you picture yourself looking at him really objectively, seeing what he's like? I want · you to keep that image of yourself looking at him, and I want to interview the you in the image. . . . What are you feeling?

J. T.: A little teary . . . elation.

D. E.: And what is it you're elated about?

J. T.: That life can be so beautiful.

D. E.: And what is making life so beautiful?

J. T.: It's just that I feel so happy.

D. E.: And what are you happy about?

J. T.: Being with somebody that I love.

D. E.: And what is it about him that you love?

J. T.: The way that he looks. His caring, sharing.

D. E.: You like that he cares about you? Shares things with you? . . . What I'd like you to do is to walk along the street with him and come to meet B. as he really is. So the three of you will be together. . . . Tell me what you see.

J. T.: A guy that looks out of place, disheveled.

D. E.: And the B. that you were with just now? Where is he in the picture?

J. T.: Vague . . . [inaudible word] . . . but I know in my heart that he's still there.

D. E.: So look at him and look at the B. you were with at first. What do you see?

J. T.: They are two different people.

D. E.: How is the first B. different from the second?

J. T.: The first one's much more together.

D. E.: And what are your feelings about the first one?

J. T.: The second kind of pushed him away . . . erased him.

D. E.: So in your image the first B. you were with has gone.

J. T.: Faded . . . [inaudible].

D. E.: Did he really exist?

J. T.: In my fantasy [crying].

D. E.: Can you run the movie backwards to where you're with the first B. at the beginning? . . . Speak to the first B.

J. T.: It's really hard to get rid of the other.

D. E.: Try saying, "You only exist in my fantasy."

J. T.: You only exist in my fantasy.

D. E.: "You're not real."

J. T.: You're not real.

D. E.: "And I'm really sad about that."

J. T.: [Lively, but sad] I am really sad [crying].

D. E.: "I've got to try to let you go."

J. T.: [Pause] I'll try to let you go . . .

D. E.: . . . What's happening now?

J. T.: I'm thinking that if I can look at him as the second one . . . maybe [inaudible due to street noise].

D. E.: Can you do that in the image? Leave the fantasy one behind?

J. T.: [With energy] He knocked the first one out. He erased it. He was so overpowering. The first one just melted away. And I think that's what happened. When we first got married, I had these illusions of what he was and who he was, and that I couldn't live without him, and he was just the strength and intelligence and the capable one of the two of us . . It took me a long time to realise that he wasn't.

D. E.: And could never be.

J. T.: I don't know about could never be, but certainly can't ever be . . . and he certainly wasn't. . . . [inaudible]. Sometimes I feel like . . . I guess I wanted to . . . that's the way I survived all this . . .

In this session, J. T. was able to directly portray her fantasy of her ex-husband as an ideal lover who could perfectly meet her needs for love, support, and sharing. When she imagined walking with the idealized B. to meet the real B., the image of the idealized B. faded. This was a vivid presentation to her of the incompatibility of the two images. The next step was to discover whether she could let go of the unrealistic, idealized version. That is why I had her say goodbye so directly. She recognized that keeping the idealized image had served as a coping mechanism ("That's the way I survived all this"). If she still needed this as a coping mechanism, saying goodbye would have evoked fear of loneliness or thoughts about herself as weak and inadequate. As it is, the giving up of the fantasy evoked a normal sadness, but nothing more, showing that with her present level of maturity she could appropriately mourn her idealized lover and no longer needed the fantasy to help her cope.

## INTEGRATING IMAGERY WORK INTO COGNITIVE THERAPY

Like any technique in cognitive therapy, imagery restructuring must be used in the context of an understanding of the patient's underlying problem. Beck and Emery (1985) emphasize the importance of working from a thorough conceptualization, out of which a specific strategy can be chosen, and within that strategy a specific tactic. C. D.'s problem was conceptualized cognitively as a failure to develop a separate self-schema. Strategies used included rehearsing assertive responses to her mother and learning that she actively created and maintained a fantasy of her mother, a process over which she could gain control. Tactics included specific applications of techniques such as directed dialogue or prompted transformation. J. T.'s problem was conceptualized as a failure to reality-test and give up an idealised version of her ex-husband. The strategy was to invite her to do this. Specific tactics included directed transformation in which the real and idealized lover appeared together, and directed dialogue giving up and saying goodbye to the idealized one.

The more well-developed and accurate is the conceptualization, the more powerful the imagery tool becomes. The conceptualization itself can be tested and enriched through the assessment component of the imagery work. The therapist can discover the nature of the client's feelings and the structure of her or his beliefs, test his or her understanding of how different assumptions interlock with each other, and assess the client's readiness to challenge particular aspects of the entire cognitive structure.

The client who understands the theory of verbal restructuring can easily grasp how the imagery work functions as a restructuring tool, because, like the purely verbal methods, it makes it possible to contact and make explicit certain beliefs and assumptions, to see their relationship to disturbing emotions, and to challenge and alter them where they are dysfunctional. The work can be integrated with the verbal work of previous and subsequent sessions by showing the client how certain beliefs and assumptions that were emerging previously have been represented in the imagery. Afterwards, it may be useful to review the imagery and have the client notice specific assumptions that were identified and the manner in which they were challenged. Sometimes this is so clear that little time needs to be spent on it.

In other cases, it is important to help the client make the connections explicitly. It may be useful to show clearly how the assumptions presented in the imagery affect specific life situations the client finds problematic, if this is not obvious from the imagery content. In some cases, where the issues revealed by imagery are complex, it may be useful to ask the client to write out the guided imagery sequence as a preamble to further work on identifying and restructuring assumptions. As with verbal work, it is important to check that the client continues to challenge the dysfunctional assumptions in everyday life. This can be done through homework tasks and, later, by questioning about behavioral changes that occur spontaneously subsequent to the session. This often reveals that the new assumptions are guiding current behavior and that the old ones have been discarded.

Sometimes developments in spontaneous imagery or dreams serve as indicators of progress. One client obtained an image of a small coffin-shaped box tightly closed with flies teeming round it. It had the numbers "16–17" written on it, which were ages at which he had many painful and avoided memories. Several weeks later, he obtained an image of the box with the lid open, and the flies were swarming less densely. This was an indication that some progress had been made in reprocessing the avoided material. Later in therapy, C. D. (see Case Example 1) reported a dream that showed that she was integrating new beliefs about herself as able to be independent. In the dream she saw herself in church getting married. Her father was there and disapproved of her choice. She was angry with him and told him that she would now make her own choices. This indicated that she was developing confidence in making and sticking to her own decisions when they conflicted with the views of her family.

Although the components of the work with imagery all have their analogies in the standard verbal techniques, there are two advantages of the imagery method. The first is that it is more effectively able to achieve restructuring outside the conceptual reasoning system in the developmentally more primitive structures. Affectively charged material cannot always be reached adequately through verbal questioning. This is even more the case where the client has a strongly intellectualizing style that serves to perpetuate cognitive avoidance when affectively charged issues are being dealt with. Greenberg and Safran (1984) emphasize that the abstract conceptual system functions in an integrated way with a facial/motor system responsible for the feeling quality of emotion and its facial and other physical expression, and a schematic emotional memory mechanism. Beck (1985) and Guidano and Liotti (1983) stress the need to achieve restructuring in these more primitive structures. Edwards (in press) shows how imagery restructuring can be used to achieve change in the schematic memory mechanism.

The second advantage of imagery over purely verbal work is that some clients have a particular aptitude for working in this modality. Bandler and Grinder's theory of neurolinguistic programming proposes that the visual, auditory, and kinesthetic are three major cognitive systems for representing the world, and that each person has a preferred modality (King, Novik, & Citrenbaum, 1983). If this is true, then those whose preferred representational system is visual will be able to achieve a more meaningful and effective cognitive restructuring through imagery than through verbal techniques.

DAVID J. A.
EDWARDS

SUMMARY

In this chapter, a guided imagery method used in gestalt therapy was described in detail and analyzed into its specific components. The basic principles underlying the imagery work were shown to be analogous to those upon which standard cognitive therapy is founded, and this was illustrated by means of case examples, first from one of Perls' dreamwork seminars and then from the author's case files.

It was shown how the method could be used to elicit the idiosyncratic meanings of the client in relation to a specific theme and to identify core dysfunctional assumptions. Illustrations were given of specific techniques that could be employed to challenge and restructure these cognitions. The benefits of the imagery modality are that it provides: (1) access to cognitions underlying emotional responses that may be difficult to identify through questioning, (2) a holistic presentation of networks of beliefs, and (3) a means of keeping the client in contact with avoided painful affect.

Once a good conceptualization of the client's problem has been achieved, guided imagery provides a modality within which specific strategies for cognitive restructuring can be facilitated through guided discovery. Therapists who are willing to explore this modality and find an aptitude for it will be gaining access to something that will greatly enrich their potential for helping and can provide exciting avenues for developing their own creativity in the challenging work of enabling clients to identify and free themselves from dysfunctional personal meaning systems.

ACKNOWLEDGMENTS. The author wishes to thank Arthur Freeman for his helpful advice, and those who participated in seminars and commented on the early drafts.

REFERENCES

Assagioli, R. (1965). *Psychosynthesis*. New York: Hobbs Dorman.

Arnkoff, D. B. (1981). Flexibility in practicing cognitive therapy. In G. Emery, S. Hollon, & R. C. Bedrosian (Eds.), *New directions in cognitive therapy: A casebook* (pp. 203–223). New York: Guilford.

Beck, A. T. (1970). The role of fantasies in psychotherapy and psychopathology. *Journal of Nervous and Mental Disease, 150*, 3–17.

Beck, A. T. (1976). *Cognitive therapy and the emotional disorders*. New York: International Universities Press.

Beck, A. T. (1985). Cognitive therapy, behavior therapy, psychoanalysis and pharmacotherapy: A cognitive continuum. In M. J. Mahoney & A. Freeman (Eds.), *Cognition and psychotherapy* (pp. 325–347). New York: Plenum Press.

Beck, A. T., & Emery, G. (1985). *Anxiety disorders and phobias: A cognitive perspective*. New York: Basic Books.

Beck, A. T., Rush, A. J., Shaw, B. F., & Emery, G. (1979). *Cognitive therapy of depression*. New York: Wiley.

Bresler, B. (1984). Mind-controlled analgesia: The inner way to pain control. In A. A. Sheikh (Ed.), *Imagination and healing* (pp. 211–230). Farmingdale, NY: Baywood.

Edwards, D. J. A. (in press). Cognitive therapy and the restructuring of early memories through guided imagery. *Journal of Cognitive Psychotherapy: An International Quarterly*.

Freeman, A. (1981). Dreams and images in cognitive therapy. In G. Emery, S. D. Hollon & R. C. Bedrosian (Eds.), *New directions in cognitive therapy: A casebook* (pp. 224–238). New York: Guilford.

Gendlin, E. T. (1978). *Focusing*. New York: Everest House.

Gendlin, E. T., Grindler, D., & McGuire, M. (1984). Imagery, body and space in focussing. In A. A. Sheikh (Ed.), *Imagination and healing* (pp. 259–286). Farmingdale, NY: Baywood.

Greenberg, L. S., & Safran, J. D. (1984). Integrating affect and cognition: A perspective on the process of therapeutic change. *Cognitive therapy and research, 8*, 559–578.

Guidano, V. F., & Liotti, G. (1983). *Cognitive processes and emotional disorders*. New York: Guilford.

Habeck, B. K., & Sheikh, A. A. (1984). Imagery and the treatment of phobic disorders. In A. A. Sheikh (Ed.), *Imagination and healing.* Farmingdale, NY: Baywood (pp. 171–196).

Hall, H. (1984). Imagery and cancer. In A. A. Sheikh (Ed.), *Imagination and healing* (pp. 159–169). Farmingdale, NY: Baywood.

King, M., Novik, L., & Citrenbaum, C. (1983). *Irresistible communication.* Philadelphia: W. B. Saunders.

Leuner, H. (1984). *Guided affective imagery: Mental imagery in short term psychotherapy.* New York: Thieme-Stratton.

McMahon, C. E., & Sheikh, A. A. (1984). Imagination in disease and healing processes: A historical perspective. In A. A. Sheikh (Ed.), *Imagination and healing* (pp. 7–34). Farmingdale, NY: Baywood.

Perls, F. S. (1971). *Gestalt therapy verbatim.* New York: Bantam.

Polster, E., & Polster, M. (1974). *Gestalt therapy integrated.* New York: Vintage.

Samuels, M., & Samuels, N. (1975). *Seeing with the mind's eye: The history, techniques and uses of visualization.* New York: Random House.

Schultz, K. D. (1984). The use of imagery in alleviating depression. In A. A. Sheikh (Ed.), *Imagination and healing* (pp. 129–158). Farmingdale, NY: Baywood.

Sheikh, A. A. (Ed.). (1984). *Imagination and healing.* Farmingdale, NY: Baywood.

Singer, J. L. (1974). *Imagery and daydream methods in psychotherapy and behavior modification.* New York: Academic.

Stevens, J. O. (1971). *Awareness: exploring, experimenting, experiencing.* Moab, UT: Real People Press.

Watkins, M. (1976). *Waking dreams.* Harper: New York.

# 16

# Cognitive Therapy with the Adult Depressed Patient

Carlo Perris

Cognitive therapy, as originally conceived and developed during the last few decades by Beck and his associates (Beck, 1967, 1970, 1976, 1982, 1986; Beck et al., 1979a; Bedrosian & Beck, 1980; Emery, 1981; Freeman, 1983; Freeman & Greenwood, 1987; Kovacs & Beck, 1978; Young & Beck, 1982), has rapidly become an established psychotherapeutic method of treatment for depressive disorders. It has been demonstrated to be as effective in treating moderate to severe depressive syndromes as are the most frequently used antidepressant drugs. Its popularity as a therapeutic tool rests on substantial experimental documentation gathered in several controlled trials (see Blackburn, 1988, for a recent review).

This chapter will present a brief description of the theory and practice of cognitive therapy, and it will review some of the evidence that lends support both to the theoretical foundations and to the claims for therapeutic effectiveness of the model.

Depression is one of the most ubiquitous of emotions. The widespread nature of the disorder has led some authors to argue that we have left behind the "age of anxiety" and the "age of anger" that dominated the periods around World War II and that we are now entering the "age of melancholy" (Hagnell, Lanky, Rorsman, & Öjesjö, 1982; Klerman, 1978). The accuracy of such a generalization aside, recent epidemiological investigations from the United States and Europe (Helgasson, 1964; Hagnell et al., 1982; Weissman & Myers, 1978) suggest that the frequency of depressive disorders is apparently increasing, contributing to a sizable proportion of the total psychiatric morbidity in the general population.

If it is accepted that feelings of sadness, despondency, and helplessness may accompany any experience of significant loss, then it is not difficult to accept that everyone is at risk of experiencing at least transient depressive feelings during his or her lifetime and that the experience of such feelings is an important part of our human heritage.

As clinicians, however, we conceive of depression in a more restricted way. We think of it as a disorder marked by the occurrence of certain well-defined symptoms and by the distinct

Carlo Perris • Department of Psychiatry, University of Umea, S-901-85 Umea, Sweden.

absence of others. The response in the patient is often subjective discomfort and an objective impairment of his or her social, vocational, and interpersonal life for a period of time.

Given the frequency of occurrence in clinical practice, there is still surprising disagreement as to whether depressive disorders should be viewed as developing along a continuum or if a division into subgroups is justified and meaningful. The list of proposed subtypes of depression could be endless because almost all of its aspects (for instance, course, severity, reactivity to external events, age at onset, biological variables, and response to treatment) have been used to claim the specificity of some subtype. On the other hand, such a long list may tell us simply that we are still uncertain as to the correct use of one of the most fundamental terms in the psychopathological lexicon and would, in turn, support the view that psychiatry, as a science, is still in a preparadigmatic stage (Pera, 1982; Perris, 1985a).

Undoubtedly, the introduction of operationalized diagnostic criteria by the St. Louis group (Feighner *et al.,* 1972) and the successive elaboration and final endorsement of these criteria in the *Diagnostic and Statistical Manual of Mental Disorders* (American Psychiatric Association, 1980, 1987) have represented important steps toward increased consistency in the use of diagnostic labels. The achievement of operational definitions should be regarded, however, as a means to enable more precise studies of better defined patient populations, rather than as an end in itself. In fact, agreement on a diagnostic construct based on symptomatology, severity, and course (as in the DSM-III or III-R), says little about the true nature of a disorder thus defined. On the other hand, reference to well-defined syndromes does allow for improved communication. In this discussion, for example, it is an advantage to be able to describe the depressive syndromes referred to as comprising the morbid conditions classified in DSM-III-R under the headings "major affective disorders," and "dysthymic disorders." The focus here will be on episodic or recurrent depressive types, rather than on the depressive episodes that are part of a bipolar disorder (Perris, 1966).

At this point, a frequently voiced misconception should be corrected. Cognitive psychotherapy, it is erroneously believed, suits only those patients suffering from milder depressive syndromes. In practice, just the opposite is true: In fact, because of its flexibility, cognitive psychotherapy can be adapted to suit most kinds of depressed patients.

Cognitive therapy is a structured, active, directive, flexible, time-limited, insight-promoting psychotherapy viable for a broad category of patients of different ages. Usually used with individuals, it is also usable in groups, or with couples and pairs. Cognitive therapy can be used with inpatients and with outpatients in a clinical practice.

The therapist–patient relationship, therapy sessions, and the overall therapeutic process are organized according to a well-defined format, a *structure,* to which both therapist and patient have agreed. Among the elements that characterize the structure are the stipulation of a contract of therapeutic goals; the development of a collaborative relationship between therapist and patient; and the establishment and maintenance of a general framework for each session (including agreement on an agenda, an assignment, the review of homework, etc.).

Both therapist and patient are expected to engage actively in the treatment process. Activity may refer both to the use of different cognitive and behavioral techniques and to the setting up of reality-testing experiments, and so forth. The therapist may use self-disclosure, where appropriate, to demonstrate a particular point to the patient. The therapist shares the responsibility to ensure that an appropriate pace is maintained during each session, so that the most effective use can be made of time, energy, and emotional resources.

Part of the therapist's activity must be *directed*—aimed toward keeping the topic of each session within the framework that has been agreed upon and coaching the patient in the performance of activities (behavioral experiments) expected to be of therapeutic value.

Another characteristic, as pointed out by Beck (1970) and others (Arnkoff, 1981; Perris, 1986) is therapeutic *flexibility*. In practice, the choice of different techniques, the pace of the treatment, and the planning of appropriate homework assignments can be specifically tailored to suit the needs and the resources of each patient. These choices are obviously not made haphazardly but in keeping with the conceptual system and constructs of cognitive therapy (Beck, 1976).

A common understanding is that cognitive therapy must be, by definition, *time-limited*. Recent reviews, in fact, include cognitive therapy among the "brief" individual psychotherapies (for example, Ursano & Hales, 1986). The phrase *time-limited,* however, needs clarification. Although the treatment of uncomplicated depressive disorders might not require more than 15 to 20 sessions (Beck *et al.,* 1979a), cognitive therapy with patients suffering from other disorders, for example, schizophrenic syndromes (Perris, 1988a,b) or personality disorders (Freeman, 1986a,b; Padesky, 1986b; Simon, 1986) usually requires a much longer time. Its use in such situations places cognitive therapy among the long-term psychotherapies. Generally, the research model of 15 to 20 sessions (Blackburn, Bishop, Glen, Whalley, & Christie, 1981; Murphy *et al.,* 1984; Rush *et al.,* 1977) has been found to be effective. The goal of cognitive therapy is not merely to effect the removal of symptoms but also to *promote insight.* Successful treatment brings to the patient's awareness the dysfunctional way of looking upon the self and relating to the environment, and it hopes to effect a change in outlook that will last beyond the recovery from a current episode. Cognitive therapy also stresses the importance of such qualities as empathy, genuineness, rapport, and concern for the patient's human value (Young & Beck, 1982). Its *humanistic* content should not be overlooked.

There are no age limitations for the use of cognitive therapy with depressed patients. Children (Padesky, 1986a), adolescents (Bedrosian, 1981; Wilkes, 1987), and aged depressives (Emery, 1981; Gallagher & Thompson, 1982; Perris, 1985) all seem amenable to this type of treatment. Although cognitive therapy is most frequently used in an individual setting, it has been used in groups (Covi et al., 1982; Hollon & Shaw, 1979; Rush & Watkins, 1981) and with couples (Epstein, 1983; Rush et al., 1980). As a rule, cognitive therapy is carried out in an outpatient basis; it is also used with inpatients (Perris, H., 1985; Shaw, 1981) when the risk of suicide is pronounced.

Beck's (1963, 1964, 1967) cognitive theory of depression is based on the assumption that depressed people interpret a wide variety of events in a distorted way, independent of objectively based disconfirmatory information. Kovacs (1980) states it well:

> since man is a thinking, evaluating, judging, and inquiring being, a patient's suffering and functional impairment is best understood and ameliorated by an exposition and correction of his or her psychological-cognitive systems. (p. 129)

So although traditional approaches to depression focus on its affective component, cognitive therapy holds that dysfunctional cognitions are responsible, in large part, for the alterations in mood, behavior, and vegetative functioning that characterize depression (Beck, 1976). The negative impact of dysfunctional cognitions on mood and behavior should not be understood to occur only in a unidirectional way, however. A cognitive-emotive-behavioral loop works to self-perpetuate the depressive response.

In focusing on the primacy of dysfunctional cognitions, Beck reestablishes a connection with a tradition of thought that can be traced back to classical times. Cicero, in fact, is credited with one of the earliest detailed descriptions of emotional disorders (Perris, 1988c) to focus on disordered thinking. He emphasized, in his *Tusculanarum Disputationum* (45 B.C.), that *"aegritudo* [his term for depression] did not depend upon the objective reality of the things, but on a subjective judgment" ("Ex quo intelligitur non in natura, sed in opinion esse aegritudinem"–*Tusc. Disp.* III, XXVIII:71). Even Plater, in his *Pratix Medica,* first published in Switzerland in 1602, stressed that melancholia rests upon a foundation of false conceptions.

The cognitive theory of depression takes into account four key cognitive elements: (1) the negative triad, comprising a negative view of self, of the world and experience, and of the future; (2) the automatic occurrence of negative thoughts; (3) the occurrence of systematic errors in the perception and processing of information; and (4) the occurrence of basic, mostly tacit, dysfunctional assumptions (also called dysfunctional schemata, or dysfunctional cognitive meaning structures). Although these concepts are discussed in several publications (Beck, 1976; Beck et al., 1979a; Bedrosian & Beck, 1980; Rush & Giles, 1982), a brief review will lay a foundation for the treatment model.

The first element of the "negative triad" refers to the depressed patient's view of self as unworthy, inadequate, or morally or physically defective. There is a well-documented tendency of depressed patients to blame themselves for past negative outcomes (Krantz & Hammer, 1979; Kuiper, 1978; Rizley, 1978) and to rate themselves as socially undesirable (Beck, 1967). The patient's relation to his or her environment, the second component of the triad, is also perceived negatively. Interactions with the environment are experienced as demanding; the world is full of obstacles and unsolvable problems. Finally, a pessimistic outlook constitutes the third element of the triad. The future is viewed as bleak, unpromising, with only continued failure anticipated.

According to the theory (Beck, 1967), these negative cognitive constructs will account for most of the symptoms that characterize the depressive syndrome. Increased dependency, indecision, apathy, hopelessness, and fatigue become easily understandable when considered against a cognitive set predisposed to underestimate personal competency and to view all activity as leading to failure.

The automatic occurrence of negative thoughts is another important component of the cognitive theory of depression. These dysfunctional cognitions, always very close to the patient's innermost problems, are automatic in the sense that they occur without previous reflection or reasoning. Because they are related to the patient's most basic dysfunctional assumptions, they are uncritically accepted by the patient without examination. One additional particular characteristic of this type of dysfunctional thinking is that it may occur so rapidly as to make it difficult for the patient even to be aware of it. One of the initial goals of cognitive therapy is to instruct the patient on how to focus on the automatic thoughts and to become aware of the extent to which such thoughts negatively influence mood and behavior.

Closely related to the patient's dysfunctional opinions of him- or herself are several errors in the perception or processing of information that Beck (1967, 1976) has identified in depressed patients. Examples of these faulty cognitions include:

- *Selective perception* of details of a situation whereas more salient aspects are neglected
- *Magnification* of the importance of negative events; and/or:
- *Minimization* of the significance of positive incidents
- *Arbitrary* inferences that imply conclusions drawn in the absence of, or contrary to, factual evidence
- *Dichotomous thinking*—the labeling of situations or events as black or white, good or bad
- *Personalization,* including consistent self-blame for the misfortunes of others and for everyday mishaps
- *Overgeneralization,* or the tendency to draw general rules from isolated events and to apply them across unrelated situations

It should be noted, however, that cognitive errors of this sort are neither specific nor exclusive to depressed patients. Healthy people may frequently commit some of the them, and similar faulty cognitions can be found in other types of patients. What is characteristic of the depressed patient is both the frequency of such thoughts and their pervasiveness, and the fact that they seem to be outside the patient's ability to correct them. Further, all those cognitive distortions act to continuously confirm the dysfunctional self-opinions in an individual's self-schemata (see Figure 1). The identification and the correction of the cognitive errors discussed here is one major focus of the therapeutic work.

The fourth and most important concept associated with the cognitive theory of depression is that of *basic dysfunctional assumptions* (or dysfunctional schema). These assumptions or beliefs represent ingrained, relatively enduring characteristics of the individual that have become established throughout life (though most frequently in early childhood). Examples of such dysfunctional opinions about the self and the relational world might include the conviction that one's worth depends exclusively on the complete success of whatever one attempts to do, or the belief that one has to have complete control over every aspect of life. Opinions of this kind are continuously confirmed by the cognitive distortions discussed before and represent a kind of guiding rule by which the individual evaluates whatever occurs. Figure 2 shows a schematic illustration of this process.

To allow for a fuller understanding of this very important process, it might be convenient to consider the concepts of cognitive-emotional structure or schema currently used by developmental psychologists to conceptualize an individual's characteristic way of construing himself or herself and his or her world.

Cognitive structures or schemata (Bartlett, 1932; Piaget, 1952) are organized representations of prior experience that facilitate recall. They also have the negative effect, however, of introducing bias and distortion into both the initial construction and the later reconstruction (Neisser, 1967). Within the framework of a structuralistic developmental theory, it is commonly assumed that the human infant enters the world with a set of rudimentary structures, genetically determined, for organizing the world. As a result of interaction with the environment, these structures unfold and are constantly being reconstructed through the dual processes of assimilation and accommodation. A frequently voiced misunderstanding is that the concept of cognitive structure does not take into account an affective component. A thorough analysis of this problem has been presented by Lundh (1983, 1987). Lundh emphasized the affective component of the schemata by suggesting the use of the term *meaning structure*. According to Lundh, ''a person's meaning structures include his knowledge and beliefs, but also his emotional and motivational disposition'' (1983, p. 16). Bowlby (1969–1980), who prefers the

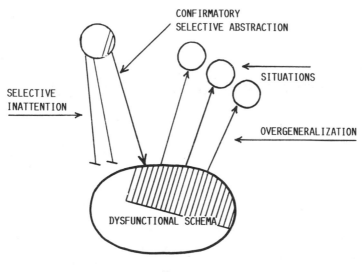

FIGURE 1

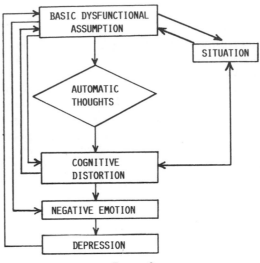

FIGURE 2

term *working models* rather than *cognitive structures* to underline even more their constructivist characteristic also emphasized their emotional component.

Although it is important for cognitive therapists to be aware of the concept of self-schemata (Markus, 1977), short-term cognitive therapy is not primarily concerned with a reconstructive analysis of what might have caused the development of dysfunctional self-schemata. It is generally acknowledged, however, that disturbances in early object relations represent one major source of the development of dysfunctional self-representations that may predispose to a depressive breakdown (Arieti & Bemporad, 1978; Beck, 1987; Bowlby, 1980). Research work carried out in our department suggests that depressed individuals have experienced their parents as lacking emotional warmth and that such experience is significantly correlated to the occurrence of dysfunctional self-opinions (Perris, 1988). The development of dysfunctional self-schemata should be regarded as the very core of an integrative concept of vulnerability common to all psychopathology (Perris, 1988, 1988a,b). The sources of these

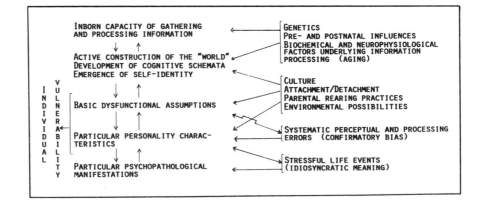

FIGURE 3

dysfunctional schemata are of different relevance for different individuals. The heuristic theoretical framework on which this hypothesis is based is shown in Figure 3. It should be kept in mind, however, that though most of the arrows in the figure point in only one direction, a continuous dialectic transaction (Magnusson, 1983; Sameroff & Chandler, 1975) between the individual and his or her environment is postulated.

The proposed framework allows for considering life events in a proper idiosyncratic context. Although no single life event, however traumatic, has proved to be consistently depressogenic, evidence is now emerging that events that may be pathogenic are related to the particular characteristics of the individual experiencing them (H. Perris, 1982) and to the individual's dysfunctional self-opinions (Hammen, Marks, Mayol, & deMayo, 1985; Olinger, Kuiper, & Shaw, 1986).

## ASSESSMENT

As with all other psychotherapies, a thorough evaluation of the patient's present state must be carried out before starting the therapeutic work. Along with past history and present living conditions, the following main points should always be covered in the initial evaluation:

1. *A thorough assessment of the risk of suicide.* A decision must be made as to as to whether the patient can be safely treated on an outpatient basis, or if treatment in a hospital setting is more appropriate. Though the accuracy of such an assessment depends, in large part, on the diagnostic skills and empathic sensitivity of the therapist, appropriate ratings scales can also be helpful. One such scale aimed at evaluating suicidal ideation (Scale for Suicidal Ideation) has been developed by Beck, Kovacs, and Weissman (1979). Some indirect indication of suicide risk can also be obtained by using the Hopelessness Scale developed by Beck, Resnik, & Lettieri (1974). It is reasonable to assume that the deeper the feeling of hopelessness, the greater the risk of suicide. Research by Minkoff, Bergman, Beck, and Beck (1973) and by Beck and his co-workers (1974b) support this assumption.

2. *An assessment of the nature and severity of the depressive syndrome.* It is important to establish whether the patient's depressive syndrome is one part of a bipolar affective disorder. Although such evidence would not, in principle, represent a contraindication to cognitive psychotherapy, it would make the addition of appropriate medication a consideration. Documentation of the effectiveness of cognitive psychotherapy in the treatment of a depressive phase of a manic-depressive disorder is still lacking. It is very difficult to distinguish a bipolar from a unipolar affective disorder if the patient is suffering from a first episode (Perris, 1982), and it is possible that bipolar depressed patients have already been included in trials of depressives successfully treated with cognitive therapy. (A recent report of hypomania in a patient treated with cognitive therapy for depression [Kingdon et al., 1986] supports this hypothesis.)

In terms of severity, a distinction should be made between psychotic and nonpsychotic patients. For the former group, both the necessity of hospitalization and the need for additional medication should be evaluated.

3. *An appraisal of the patient's home environment.* Although a large majority of patients suffering from a major depressive disorder can be best treated at home, situations exist that might require hospitalization: for example, if the home environment is too conflictual for the patient or if the patient lives alone without any assistance between sessions. The assessment must then be based on the balance between the advantages of outpatient treatment and the risks that the apparent lack of support might imply.

4. *An evaluation of general health.* It is particularly important to exclude the possibility of concurrent complicating factors that might negatively influence the course of the therapy: for

instance, severe somatic illness, organic brain damage, alcohol or drug abuse, or mental retardation.

Motivation for treatment is an important prerequisite for psychotherapy. Most proponents of short-term psychodynamic psychotherapies (Flegenheimer, 1982) consider the patient's readiness to actively participate in the treatment situation to be a key selection criterion. It would be impossible to carry out any kind of psychotherapy without some degree of voluntary participation from the patient. On the other hand, the depressed patient, because of his or her negative view of self and of the future, may be more reluctant than other patients to engage in a treatment that may require some effort from his or her side. The development of a good therapeutic relationship from the very first encounter can encourage the patient's involvement in treatment. If difficulties occur, the therapist can work with the patient to evaluate the negative beliefs held by the patient about the possibility of being cured. In the case of a lack of motivation based on negative beliefs, the following proposal for a short trial of therapy might be used:

> P.: I don't think I want to try this kind of therapy.
>
> T.: Is there any particular reason?
>
> P.: I don't believe that anything can really help me.
>
> T.: I understand that you may think so because you see everything in shades of black right now. Nevertheless, I would suggest that we meet for several sessions to test together whether I can be of some help to you.
>
> P.: It would be meaningless. I know that nothing will help.
>
> T.: OK. You think that nothing will help you, but what would you lose if we met for a few sessions?
>
> P.: Nothing. I have nothing left to lose anymore.
>
> T.: Then if you won't be losing anything, let's make an agreement. I will schedule an appointment for you for tomorrow, and you can decide whether you will continue or not.
>
> P.: OK. I'll come tomorrow, but I know that it won't be any use. I'll just be wasting your time.
>
> T.: It's kind of you to be concerned with my time. But, you see, I feel confident that we will be able to work together and that our joint efforts will have an impact on your depression.

Though the therapist must show confidence in the possibility of helping the patient and give the patient assurance, expressions of exaggerated optimism should be avoided. It is preferable to simply tell the patient that the proposed treatment has been used in hundreds of similar cases and has proved effective.

The pace of the patient's introduction and socialization to the principles of cognitive therapy must be dictated by his or her condition at the time of the evaluation interviews. With very severely depressed or poorly motivated patients, the boundary between the end of evaluation and the beginning of therapy is, as a rule, very fluid. The therapist may have to explain the principles of cognitive therapy several times over the course of the therapy. Long lectures should be avoided. With a large proportion of patients, however, it is both possible and necessary to give substantial information on the rationale of cognitive therapy, and on its conduct, at the end of the evaluation procedure. Explanations should be in simple terms and, whenever possible, should be illustrated by examples or metaphors. Appropriate readings can be suggested to the patient as a first homework assignment. One most suitable initial reading is the booklet *Coping with Depression* (Beck & Greenberg, 1974).

To emphasize the importance of the reading of this booklet, the patient should be asked to underline in one color everything that the patient believes applies to him or her and to underline in another color everything he or she thinks is not relevant for his or her condition. Compliance with such an assignment will provide the therapist with relevant material for the coming therapeutic sessions and begin the patient's socialization to the important notion of doing homework.

As a data-based model of therapy, cognitive therapy makes use of a number of different rating scales to standardize the collection of data. Some are used at the beginning and at the end of treatment, others at almost every session. At the beginning of treatment, both the therapist's ratings and a self-rating are usually made. The therapist's ought to use at least some scale for the evaluation of severity: for example, Hamilton's Depression Scale (Hamilton, 1967) or the subscale for Depression (Perris, Eisemann, von Knorring, & Perris, 1984) of the Comprehensive Psychopathology Rating Scale (Asberg, Perris, Schalling, & Sedvall, 1978). For patients' self-ratings, the most commonly used instruments are the Beck Depression Inventory (BDI; Beck, Ward, Mendelson, Mock, & Erbaugh, 1961), the Automatic Thoughts Questionnaire (ATQ; Hollon & Kendall, 1980), and either the A or B form of the Dysfunctional Attitudes Scale (DAS; Weissman & Beck, 1978). The therapist's rating, the ATQ, and the DAS (whichever has not already been used at the beginning) should be repeated at the end of the treatment. The BDI is used during therapy for a continuous monitoring of the progress of the treatment. Of course, the therapist can add those instruments that he or she feels familiar with or those that are of research interest. Care must always be taken, however, not to burden the patient with too many ratings.

Optimally, the patient should not receive any medication other than an occasional hypnotic if sleep disturbances are a great concern. There is a body of evidence suggesting that the efficacy of cognitive therapy is quite comparable to that of the most commonly used antidepressants. But there are neither ideological nor practical indications against concurrent use of antidepressive drugs should they be judged appropriate. The final decision on this issue completely depends on the condition of the patient. With patients who show a marked retardation and pronounced concentration difficulties, drugs might contribute to facilitate the therapeutic process. If a patient has to be treated with drugs, cognitive therapy is particularly useful in assessing the patient's possible negative attitudes toward medication and in correcting misconceptions by using the same principles and techniques applicable to other kinds of cognitive distortions.

It is good practice to meet the patient's closest relatives. In particular, the patient's husband or wife should be routinely invited to an early appointment. One reason for such a meeting is to get supplementary information about the circumstances related to the onset of depression in the patient. Because it is assumed that the depressed patient has a negative view of self and of the environment, it is necessary to be able to disentangle which problems reported by the patient are viewed distortedly because of the depressive illness and which are real ones. Given the nature of the depressive syndrome, real problems may be magnified by the patient. A second reason for seeing the family is to evaluate whether the relatives will be allies in the treatment process or if changes in the patient's mental state through treatment may become the source of new problems within the patient's family. Beck *et al.* (1979a) recommend that contact with the patient's relatives should be made directly by the therapist and not through the patient. There is a risk, in fact, that the patient, either because of inhibition, or because of a pessimistic outlook, would simply not carry the message. Further, the relatives of patients in psychotherapy might have a distorted view of what the treatment is about and possibly suspect they are discussed during the therapy sessions as being responsible for the patient's condition. Finally, an overprotective relative might counteract the efforts of the therapist to keep the patient active from the very start of the treatment.

At the end of the evaluative process, the experienced therapist should be in the position to make a preliminary assessment of the patient's basic dysfunctional assumptions about himself or herself and of which fundamental dysfunctional beliefs/rules contribute to the dysfunctional thoughts and behaviors.

Beck (1982) has been elaborating upon two personality characteristics that may powerfully reflect the patient's dysfunctional beliefs. According to Beck, the two main personality types can be identified as the *sociotropic* and the *autonomous*. (It should be pointed out, however, that a blend of sociotropy and autonomy is regarded as the most common situation and that one can safely speak only of a preeminence of either characteristic.) The "autonomous" person is assumed to be ruled by a striving for independence, a dislike for asking for help, and an orientation toward action. This person has a set of internalized high standards and criteria for achievement, is less reflective, and focuses on getting positive results. In contrast, the sociotropic person is socially dependent, needing to be near to people to feel safe and experience gratification. The sociotropic individual has difficulty taking risks, needs continual reassurance, and needs/demands the stability of a relationship. For the socially dependent person, rejection is worse than aloneness. Beck has suggested, on the basis of his clinical experience, that the patterning and the meaning of symptoms might be different in the two types. Further investigations on additional subjects are still required to verify this hypothesis. On the other hand, an assessment of the dominating personality type might be relevant for the therapeutic strategy to be adopted. In fact, the autonomous patient is more interested in finding a solution to his or her problems than in a warm therapeutic relationship. Thus the therapeutic effort should be focused on activities that can lead to mastery experiences rather than on introspection. In contrast, a warm relationship and a focus on the patient's definition of his or her lovableness represent a more appropriate approach to the sociotropic patient.

Beck's classic treatment manual of cognitive psychotherapy with depressed patients (Beck, Rush, Shaw, & Emery, 1979) has been followed by several volumes further detailing and delineating the treatment (Freeman, Simon, Perris, 1986; Pretzer & Fleming, 1988). The following description will outline the general characteristics of a typical therapy session and then will describe some of the most common techniques used in treating depressed patients.

## THERAPEUTIC STRUCTURE

It is good practice to meet more than once a week in the early phase of treatment of a depressed patient. In our experience, depressively retarded patients, prone to withdrawal and passivity, should be met daily during the first week of treatment. The rationale of such a high frequency is to counteract the risk of increasing passivity and to distract the patient, as far as possible, from self-defeating ruminations. Two or three sessions during the first week work well with most patients suffering from a moderate depression. Later in treatment, the frequency of the sessions can be limited to once weekly, and the last few sessions can be spaced out on a bimonthly or even monthly basis, if appropriate. A duration of 45 to 50 minutes for each session is the rule, but some flexibility should be allowed, especially in the early phase of treatment. Both shorter and longer sessions can occur, mostly depending on the mental state of the patient.

In principle, each session should include an inquiry about the experiences that the patient might have had since the last session, the review of homework assignments, an agreement on the topics to be dealt with in the present session, the assignment of homework, and a short summing up of what has been discussed during the session. It may also be helpful to actually write down the agenda for each session. Beyond the review of experiences since the previous session and the homework, further content of the agenda is a collaborative venture between therapist and patient. If the patient proves unable to make any fruitful suggestion, the therapist may pinpoint some problematic areas that have emerged during previous interviews and suggest topics to start with. When the therapy has been ongoing, there is generally little difficulty in getting a good start for the session by appropriate questioning related to relevant issues already known by the therapist.

The rationale of agreeing on an agenda is to avoid a haphazard drifting in the session. It is the task of the therapist to keep the patient on focus if the dialogue tends to get sidetracked. On the other hand, the agreement on an agenda does not imply that the therapist stops being empathic about what is going on within the patient during the session. On the contrary, the therapist must always be attentive to any verbal and nonverbal communication that requires attention, independent of any previous agreement. The agenda is a guide for the session work, rather than a program engraved in granite.

Because a depressed patient might show pronounced difficulty concentrating and a marked response latency, the pace of the session must be in tune with the state of the patient. Long, unproductive pauses, however, should be actively broken. On the other hand, a large proportion of patients accepted for psychotherapy do not show extreme retardation and are able to interact in a quite ordinary way with the therapist.

## THERAPEUTIC TECHNIQUE

The main task of the therapist is to help the patient in identifying, challenging, and eventually correcting the dysfunctional assumptions that rule his or her view of self, of the relational world, and of the future, and in recognizing the distorted cognitive mechanisms that contribute to sustaining and reenforcing those basic dysfunctional beliefs. Accordingly, both behavioral and cognitive (semantic) techniques are routinely used. The style of therapeutic interaction is to use direct questioning to facilitate this task. Although comprehensive textbooks provide exhaustive coverage of the different techniques that can be used (Beck *et al.*, 1979a; Guidano & Liotti, 1983; Jansson, 1986; Perris, 1986), some of the most common will be briefly reviewed here.

It is necessary for the therapist to help the patient in *distancing* him- or herself from basic dysfunctional beliefs and to become aware of the cognitive distortions that help perpetuate those beliefs. Also, the focus should be not on ''symptoms'' but on ''problems''—problems

| SITUATION | EMOTION(S) | AUTOMATIC THOUGHT(S) | RATIONAL RESPONSE |
|---|---|---|---|
|  |  |  |  |

FIGURE 4

on whose solution the patient can work in collaboration with the therapist. Thus, at the beginning of the therapy, the patient should become acquainted with the concepts of *automatic thoughts* and *cognitive distortions* and learn how to recognize and monitor them.

The most routinely used technique to help make the patient aware of his or her cognitive distortions is to ask the patient to pinpoint a situation that was felt to be distressing and to indicate on a four-column form the emotion felt and the thoughts that had occurred in the circumstance (Figure 4). The patient is also asked to grade on a hypothetical scale the intensity of the emotion and the degree to which he or she believes in the accompanying thoughts. The therapeutic task is to help the patient to analyze and challenge the validity of the dysfunctional thoughts and to reach a more appropriate interpretation of the stimulus situation that had contributed to the negative emotion. Afterwards, the patient is asked to introduce in the fourth column of the form the alternative interpretation of the situation that he or she has been able to reach and to reevaluate both the intensity of the emotion and the belief in the original thoughts.

Let us look at the example illustrated in Figure 4 to follow this process. The situation pinpointed by the patient was an unexpected telephone call from a boyfriend to ask if it were all right to defer a date she had looked forward to as a possible beginning of a more enduring relationship. Rather than happiness or pleasure at his call or pleasure at the expectation of the date, at whatever time, the immediate feeling had been of sadness and rejection, and the automatic thoughts: "He doesn't want to see me any more because he has discovered that I'm not worth his attention. I know that nobody will ever become fond of me."

A preliminary analysis of the patient's immediate thoughts quickly reveals several cognitive distortions: for example, the unsupported conclusion that the boyfriend did not want to meet her anymore (an *arbitrary inference*); an unwarranted opinion of unworthiness (*misattribution*); and an unjustified negative generalization to future events (*overgeneralization*). The patient could be guided to reappraise the stimulus situation more appropriately, and, accordingly, to experience a marked reduction in the intensity of her negative emotion and in the degree to which she believed in her original thoughts.

What is important in this corrective process is that the therapist and the patient must work together as two research workers who have put forward a hypothesis and want to verify its validity. Put in other words, the therapist's task is not to furnish alternative interpretations of the alleged situation on which the patient may or may not agree, nor to argue or debate the patient's dysfunctional thinking, but to guide the patient, by using Socratic questioning, to reach a more appropriate conclusion (Beck *et al.*, 1979a). Let us see how a therapeutic dialogue between our hypothetical patient and her therapist might have been:

T.: I see you felt sad and rejected when X phoned you to change your date.

P.: Well, yes. I felt I had been naïve in expecting that he would keep his promise to take me out to dinner.

T.: And when he phoned you realized that, and you concluded he didn't want to meet you anymore.

P.: Yes.

T.: Did he actually tell you he didn't want to meet you anymore?

P.: Well, no. He only said he had gotten some unexpected extra work at the office.

T.: Do you have any particular reason to believe it was just an excuse?

P.: I really don't know . . .

T.: Well, let's see. Do you know anything at all about his work?

P.: A little. He once told me his boss was unpredictable and assigned things unexpectedly.

T.: I see. Let's go back for a while to what he actually said to you on the phone. Can you remember?

P.: Well . . . I'm not sure if I can . . . I was so upset . . . I think he said he had some unexpected work out of town and he would call me back in two days.

T.: Did he sound happy about the prospect of canceling the date if you couldn't make the new day?

P.: Well . . . no . . . . Actually, he said he was very disappointed.

T.: Then let's sum up what we know so far. As I understand it, your boyfriend has a job that can involve extra work at short notice. He sounded very disappointed when he told you the unexpected had happened, and he still wanted to see you. Is that correct?

P.: Well . . . yes.

T.: If our reconstruction of what really happened is correct, could there be any other conclusion besides the one you have written down?

P.: I see the point. I guess my immediate reaction was mostly unjustified. But you see, I'm never sure about myself.

T.: Well, we will work a lot on just this uncertainty of yours. But for the moment, let me ask whether you feel as intensely sad and rejected now as you felt when you wrote down the events.

P.: Well, actually not. Now I can see things from a new angle.

T.: Do you still believe that your previous interpretation is the only correct one?

P.: You are right, I don't think that it is . . .

Were this hypothetical example to occur in a therapy session, the therapist would have enough material to work on to help the patient to become aware of her basic assumption of being unworthy and of some of her self-confirming cognitive distortions. In fact, it would reasonably be expected that similar cognitive errors would occur if any situation that could be misinterpreted as a direct blow to her already low self-esteem. A suitable approach in this case would be to assign to the patient, as homework, to write down on a similar form other possible occasions when she felt sad or rejected, to make a note of her automatic thoughts, to identify possible cognitive distortions and to search for less distressing alternative interpretations of the stimulus situation. Before embarking on this task, however, the patient must clearly understand its rationale and must have had an opportunity to learn the most common cognitive distortions. A few examples practiced during a session might be appropriate to accomplish this.

Depressed patients often complain of an incapacity to do things that should be done and feel guilty for the inability to do them. One frequent reason for the patient's incapacity relates to what amounts to "slavery" to the imperative of several *must, should,* and *ought-to* statements, coupled with difficulty in sorting things out and establishing priorities. The patient feels overwhelmed by the different and contrasting tasks he or she should accomplish and is unable to carry any of them to its proper end. When such a situation occurs, the therapist should help the patient in preparing a list of what has to be done in order to investigate together what the patient is able to do and in what order. This might then represent the basis for coming homework assignments. It is essential for the therapist to correctly evaluate the patient's capacity to succeed in the assigned task. If appropriate, a *cognitive or behavioral rehearsal* of the task to be performed can be done during the session. This technique allows for the identification of interfering thoughts that may occur to the patient as he or she visualizes the sequences of the projected task.

EXAMPLE

Mrs M., a 46-year-old, divorced cleaning woman who lived alone, complained she was unable to do anything on her return home from work. She mentioned that she could spend the whole evening pacing around in her small apartment, thinking of what she ought to do. She reported that her only daughter lived in another town and frequently wrote to her, but she did not write back for some months and then felt it was now too late to write. She felt guilty for not writing to her only daughter and maintained that her present behavior was just a confirmation that she had been an altogether bad mother. She had a lot of unsorted bills to go through and some other mail to answer. Her TV set had to be repaired, but this was impossible because she could not carry it to a shop and she was not at home during working hours to have a serviceman come to her apartment. Apparently, the list of what should be done seemed never to end. She felt overwhelmed, and the result was that she went from one task to another without carrying out any of them. She would get food without any particular interest in how it was cooked and then went to bed very early in the evening to lie sleepless for a long time ruminating about the "fact" that she was a total failure. When her problem list was reviewed in order to establish priorities, it became evident that not having answered her daughter's letters was a major cause of her guilt feelings coupled with a negative global opinion of being a "bad mother." She maintained she was absolutely unable to concentrate on writing a meaningful letter. Because the patient rated the writing of such a letter higher than her other problems, we agreed that she should tell me what she would have liked to write *if* she were to write a letter. Very soon, the patient proved able to make several sensible suggestions and the previously "impossible" letter began to unfold. She accepted the suggestion to take notes of what she was telling me, and, before the end of the session, she had been able to write a whole letter. On the strength of this success, it was later possible to reach an agreement on a further schedule for other tasks she could perform at home, some before the next session.

A frequent objection from patients (when asked to do what appear to be elementary tasks at home) is that, even if they succeeded, it would only confirm that they needed guidance for activities that others would regard as trivial. In such cases, the use of a metaphorical reference to a somatic illness may be appropriate for comparison. For example, it is not difficult to have the patient admit that even the accomplishment of an easy task would be regarded as "masterful" if the person performing it had a broken leg. Accordingly, even the carrying out of elementary routine work can be regarded as masterful when suffering from a depressive illness that impairs motivation and reduces initiative.

Besides assistance in the structuring of particular problems, a depressed patient might need assistance in structuring the whole day. In this context, the therapist should try to identify which activities have given pleasure to the patient in the past and to assess how often the patient engages in such activities at the present time. For that purpose, a special form can be used with a line for every hour of the day, on which the patient has to write down what he has done at each time and whether the reported activity has given him a sense of mastery and/or pleasure. In reviewing this mastery/pleasure schedule, the therapist has a basis to promote an increase in those activities the patient himself or herself finds most pleasant and rewarding.

Systematic behavioral assignments as home-practice activities have been traditionally used in behavior therapy (for example, Dunlap, 1932), and several therapeutic approaches make of it their major focus (Kelly's fixed role therapy; Kanfer's direct learning, 1970; Haley's directive therapy, 1976; Shelton & Ackerman's systematic homework, 1974). Occasionally, behavioral assignments have been used in psychoanalytically oriented psychotherapy, for instance, by Arieti (1974) in the treatment of patients suffering from schizophrenic syndromes. In the cognitive therapies (Beck, 1976; Ellis, 1970), homework assignments have been systematically incorporated from the very beginning of the therapeutic procedure. There are several reasons for using homework assignments. First, the use of homework provides a structure for extending the therapeutic work between sessions. Second, the assignments contribute toward making therapy more specific. Third, they facilitate the transfer of insights gained in the sessions to real-life situations. Fourth, the results of homework assignments represent an important source of feedback to the therapist about the patient's progress. Finally, and perhaps most importantly, the carrying out of homework assignments contributes to the patient's being an active participant in the therapeutic work.

For homework assignments to be purposeful, the following rules should be followed:

1. The assignment of homework must be a systematic and consistent part of the treatment on which therapist and patient agree from the very beginning.
2. Homework assignments must be based on individual planning so that the patient is able to understand them as pertinent to his or her real problems.
3. As far as possible, homework should be based on the patient's own proposals.
4. Assignments must be constructed that correspond to the patient's present resources.
5. The results of homework must always be reviewed in the following session.

The issue of "graded" assignments is of particular importance with patients suffering from depressive syndromes. In fact, because one major goal of the therapeutic work is to promote an increased level of self-esteem and a sense of mastery, assigned homework must never be far beyond the fringes of the patient's present resources.

There is a frequent misconception that cognitive therapists are purposefully unaware of and unconcerned with transference and countertransference reactions. Such misunderstanding is more surprising if one takes into account that both the major proponents of cognitive therapy, Aaron Beck and Albert Ellis, were trained analysts and thus were well familiar with this type of reaction.

Issues of transference and countertransference in the treatment of depressed patients are dealt with at some length by Beck *et al.* (1979a) and, as concerns schizophrenic patients, by Perris (1988a,b). Still, the development of transference is obviously not a major focus of cognitive therapy. If anything, the aim of cognitive therapy is to promote the development of an empathic collaborative relationship. This type of relationship should be clearly distinguished from an antitherapeutic positive transference that would foster dependency and make termination more difficult. Whenever they occur, transference reactions that could counteract the therapeutic work (including exaggerated positive reactions) are treated as additional instances of cognitive distortion and are dealt with straightforwardly, following the same principles used to analyze and to correct other distortions. Examples of negative therapeutic reactions are oppositionalism, attempts at manipulating the therapist, infatuation with the therapist, or feelings of being rejected. Instances of countertransference may include the therapist's becoming frustrated by the patient's indecision and lack of initiative (which are viewed to be willful) or the therapist's buying into the patient's negative view of reality.

Because of its active characteristic and because a time limit is agreed upon at the beginning of therapy, termination does not pose complex problems of the type that can occur in other longer therapies. Most depressed patients do not present with difficulties in terminating treatment when they feel relieved from their depressive symptomatology. It is good practice to touch on the issue of termination on different occasions throughout therapy and to emphasize that one aim of the treatment is to equip the patient with a set of new skills so that he or she will be able to continue to develop in the future, after therapy has come to an end. If an exaggerated concern about termination becomes evident, the dysfunctional thoughts behind the patient's concern must be brought to the fore and worked through accordingly. The consistent planning of one or more *booster session(s)* a few months after termination can reduce the anxiety related to separation from the therapist and facilitate termination.

Cognitive therapists, from the very beginning, have shared with behavior therapists a concern for documenting their therapeutic results. Because the treatment of patients with depressive syndromes might be regarded as the paradigm for the use of cognitive therapy, it is understandable that a large number of published studies have been concerned with the treatment of this type of mental disorder. These studies have made controlled comparisons of cognitive therapy with the other psychological treatments and with the most commonly used tricyclic antidepressants (TAD). Because critical, comprehensive reviews of the major studies published so far are available (Beck *et al.,* 1979a; Blackburn, 1988; Jansson & Öst, 1985; Rush & Giles, 1982), only a few of the most important results need be discussed here. The studies cited are those that maintained a strict adherence to the therapeutic manual developed by Beck and his co-workers (Beck *et al.,* 1979a). (The previously mentioned reviews, on the other hand, include studies in which a different cognitive-behavioral approach has been used.)

Patients in these studies were carefully chosen outpatients meeting the Research Diagnostic Criteria (Spitzer, Endicott, & Robins, 1978) or the St. Louis criteria (Feighner *et al.,* 1972) for major unipolar, nonpsychotic depression. So far, at least seven carefully designed studies have been published (Beck *et al.,* 1979; Beck, Hollon, Young, Bedrosian, & Budens, 1985; Blackburn, Bishop, Glen, Whalley, & Christie, 1981; Murphy *et al.,* 1984; Rush, Beck, Kovacs, & Hollon, 1977; Rush & Watkins, 1981; Teasdale, Fennell, Hibbert, & Amies, 1984) comprising in all 316 patients. In these studies, cognitive therapy has proved to be equally effective (Murphy, Simons, Wetzel, & Lustman, 1984) or more so than treatment with TAD (Blackburn *et al.,* 1981; Rush *et al.,* 1977, general practice patients). Comparisons concerning combined treatment have yielded similar results. In fact, the combination of cognitive therapy and TAD has been found either as effective as cognitive therapy alone (Beck *et al.,* 1979a, 1985) or superior to either cognitive therapy or TAD alone (Teasdale *et al.,* 1984).

A few of the studies mentioned so far have included follow-ups of various lengths—12 to 24 months (Beck *et al.,* 1985; Blackburn, Eunson, & Bishop, 1986; Kovacs, Rush, Beck, & Hollon, 1981; Simons, Murphy, Levine, & Wetzel, 1986). On the whole, all follow-up studies show some preliminary evidence in support of the hypothesis that cognitive therapy might have a long-term morbidity-suppressive effect on depression.

Unfortunately, the final results of the most comprehensive multicenter study of cognitive psychotherapy and interpersonal psychotherapy (Klerman, Rounsaville, Chevron, Neu, &

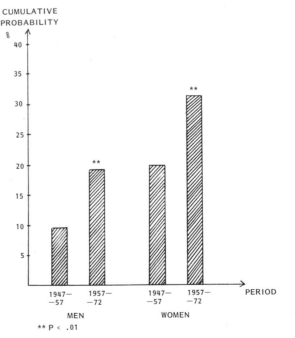

FIGURE 5

Weissman, 1979) in the treatment of depression, carried out under the aegis of the National Institutes of Mental Health (Elkin, Parloff, Hadley, & Autry, 1985), are not yet available. There are, however, studies in which cognitive therapy has been compared with other psychological treatments (Gallagher & Thompson, 1982; Shaw, 1977; Taylor & Marshall, 1977; Wilson, Goldin, & Chasbonneau-Powis, 1983). With the exception of the study by Gallagher and Thompson, which used severely depressed older patients, the others have probably included only patients suffering from a mild or moderately severe depressive illness. In all but the Shaw study (in which cognitive therapy appeared to be superior to behavior therapy), cognitive therapy and the other treatments (behavior therapy, social skills training, psychodynamic psychotherapy) showed similar efficacy in the resolution of the acute episode. At the follow-up, there was a slight tendency toward a better result with cognitive therapy than with psychodynamic psychotherapy in the study by Gallagher and Thompson. This study, however, had a very small number of patients in each group.

As mentioned in the introduction, a sizable proportion of the general population is at risk for developing a depressive disorder. According to calculations made in Sweden by Hagnell and his co-workers (Hagnell *et al.*, 1982), the cumulative probability of developing a moderate to severe depressive illness has significantly increased during the last decades (Figure 5). In the United States, the President's Commission on Mental Health (1978) estimated that about 20% of American citizens will have an affective disorder in their lifetime. Besides the suffering that depression always implies for the individual, depressive patients represent the group at highest risk to commit suicide.

During the last two to three decades effective drugs have been developed which allow the treatment of most depressive conditions. Not all patients, however, want or can be treated with drugs. Pregnant women, patients with concomitant severe somatic disorders, and most older patients often cannot be treated with the available antidepressants at adequate dosages. Also, a consistent number of depressed patients (between 20%–40%) respond poorly to drug treatment, or drop out prematurely because of side effects. Thus there is a need for an effective therapeutic alternative.

Cognitive therapy, as proposed by Beck (1976), has all the characteristics of being such an alternative. It is based on a comprehensive and plausible theory of psychopathology, and it comprises a set of strategies and techniques that can be consistently applied by different therapists. It is relatively easy to teach and is economical in terms of both time and money. In addition, several carefully conducted, controlled studies support the claim that cognitive therapy is at least as effective as the most commonly used tricyclic antidepressants in the treatment of moderate to severe major depressive disorders and suggest that it might also have a morbidity–suppressive effect in the long run.

ACKNOWLEDGMENT. This research was supported (in part) by a grant from the Swedish Medical Research Council (Grant no. 5244).

## REFERENCES

American Psychiatric Association. (1980). *Diagnostic and Statistical Manual of Mental Disorders* (3rd ed.). Washington, DC: Author.

American Psychiatric Association. (1987). *Diagnostic and Statistical Manual of Mental Disorders* (3rd ed., rev.). Washington, DC: Author.

Arieti, S. (1974). Individual psychotherapy of schizophrenia. In S. Arieti (Ed), *American Handbook of Psychiatry* (2nd ed, Vol. 3) New York: Basic Books.

Arieti, S., & Bemporad, J. (1978). *Severe and mild depression*. New York: Basic Books.

Arnkoff, D. (1981). Flexibility in practicing cognitive therapy. In G. Emery, S. D. Hollon, & R. C. Bedrosian (Eds.), *New directions in cognitive therapy* (pp. 203–223). New York: Guilford Press.

Asberg, M., Perris, C., Schalling, D., & Sedvall, G. (1978). The CPRS. Development and applications of a psychiatric rating scale. *Acta Psychiatrica Scandinavia* (Suppl. 271).

Bartlett, F. C. (1932). *Remembering.* Cambridge, England: Cambridge University Press.

Beck, A. T. (1963). Thinking and depression. Part I. Archives of General Psychiatry 9, 324–333.

Beck, A. T. (1964). Thinking and depression. Part II. *Archives General of Psychiatry, 10,* 561–571.

Beck, A. T. (1967). Depression: Clinical, experimental, and theoretical aspects. New York: Hoeber.

Beck, A. T. (1970). Cognitive therapy: Nature and relation to behavior therapy. *Behavior Therapy, 1,* 184–200.

Beck, A. T. (1976). Cognitive therapy and the emotional disorders. New York: International Universities Press.

Beck, A. T. (1982). Cognitive therapy of depression: New perspectives. In P. Clayton (Ed.), *Depression.* New York: Raven Press.

Beck, A. T. (1986). *Cognitive therapy: A 20 years retrospective.* Paper read at the 2nd International Congress of Cognitive Psychotherapy, Umeà, Sweden, September 18–20.

Beck, A. T., & Greenberg, R. L. (1974). Coping with depression. Institute for Rational Living, Inc., 45 East 65th Street, New York, N.Y. 10021.

Beck, A. T., Ward, C. M., Mendelson, M., Mock, J., & Erbaugh, J. (1961). An inventory for measuring depression. *Archives of General Psychiatry, 4,* 561–571.

Beck, A. T., Weissman, A., Lester, D., & Trexler, R. (1974a). The measurement of pessimism. The Hopelesness Scale. *Journal of Consulting and Clinical Psychology, 42,* 861–865.

Beck, A. T., Resnik, H. L. P., & Lettieri, D. (1974b). *The prediction of suicide.* Bowie: Charles Press.

Beck, A. T., Rush, A. J., Shaw, B. F., & Emery, G. (1979a). *Cognitive therapy of depression.* New York: Guilford Press.

Beck, A. T., Kovacs, M., & Weissman, A. (1979b). Assessment of suicidal intention. The scale for suicidal ideation. *Journal of Consulting and Clinical Psychology, 47,* 343–352.

Beck, A. T., Hollon, S. D., Young, J., Bedrosian, R. C., & Budens, D. (1985). Treatment of depression with cognitive therapy and amitriptyline. *Archives of General Psychiatry, 42,* 142–148.

Bedrosian, R. C. (1981). The application of cognitive therapy with adolescents. In G. Emery, S. D. Hollon, & R. C. Bedrosian (Eds.), *New directions in cognitive therapy* (pp. 68–83). New York: Guilford Press.

Bedrosian, R. C., & Beck, A. T. (1980). Principles of cognitive therapy. In M. J. Mahoney (Ed.), *Psychotherapy process* (pp. 127–152). New York: Plenum Press.

Bibring, E. (1953). The mechanism of depression. In P. Greenacre (Ed.), *Affective disorders* (pp. 13–48). New York: International Universities Press.

Blackburn, I. M. (1988). An appraisal of cognitive trials of cognitive therapy for depression. In C. Perris, I. M. Blackburn, & H. Perris (Eds.) *Cognitive psychotherapy* (pp. 329–364). Heidelberg: Springer.

Blackburn, I. M., Bishop, S., Glen, A. I. M., Whalley, L. J., & Christie, J. E. (1981). The efficacy of cognitive therapy in depression: A treatment trial using cognitive therapy and pharmacotherapy, each alone and in combination. *British Journal of Psychiatry, 139,* 181–189.

Blackburn, I. M., Eunson, K. M., & Bishop, S. (1986). A two-year naturalistic follow-up of depressed patients treated with cognitive therapy, pharmacotherapy and a combination of both. *Journal of Affective Disorders, 10,* 67–75.

Bowlby, J. (1969–1980). *Attachment and Loss* (Vol. 1–3). New York: Basic Books.

Covi, L., Roth, D., & Lipman, R. S. (1982). Cognitive group psychotherapy of depression. The close-ended group. *American Journal of Psychotherapy, 36,* 459–469.

Dunlap, K. (1932). *Habits. Their making and unmaking.* New York: Liveright.

Elkin, I., Parloff, M. B., Hadley, S. W., & Autry, J. H. (1985). NIMH treatment of depression collaborative research program. *Archives of General Psychiatry, 42,* 305–316.

Ellis, A. (1970). *The essence of rational psychotherapy: A comprehensive approach* to treatment. New York: Institute for Rational Living.

Emery, G. (1981). Cognitive therapy with the elderly. In G. Emery, S. D. Hollon, & R. C. Bedrosian (Eds.), *New directions in cognitive therapy* (pp. 84–98). New York: Guilford Press.

Feighner, J. P., Robins, E., Guze, S. B., Woodruff, R. A., Winokur, G., & Munoz, R. (1972). Diagnostic criteria for use in psychiatric research. *Archives of General Psychiatry, 26,* 57–63.

Flegenheimer, W. V. (1982). Techniques of brief psychotherapy. New York: Aronson.

Freeman, A. (1983). *Cognitive therapy with couples and groups.* New York: Plenum Press.

Freeman, A. (1986a). *General treatment considerations with personality disorders.* Paper read at the 2nd International Congress of Cognitive Psychotherapy, Umeà, Sweden, September 18–20, 1986.

Freeman, A. (1986b). *Treatment of narcissistic personality.* Paper read at the 2nd International Congress of Cognitive Therapy.

Freeman, A., & Greenwood, V. C. (1987). *Cognitive therapy. Applications in psychiatric and medical settings.* London: Human Sciences Press.

Gallagher, D. E., & Thompson, L. W. (1982). Treatment of major depressive disorder in older adult outpatients with brief psychotherapies. *Psychotherapy Theory of Research Practice, 19,* 482–490.

Guidano, V. F., & Liotti, G. (1983). Cognitive processes and emotional disorders. New York: Guilford Press.

Hagnell, O., Lanke, J., Rorsman, B., & Öjesjö, L. (1982). Are we entering an age of melancholy? Depressive illnesses in a prospective epidemiological study over 25 years. *Psychological Medicine, 12,* 279–289.

Haley, J. (1976). *Problem solving therapy.* San Francisco: Jossey Bass.

Hammen, C., Marks, T., Mayol, A., & de Mayo, R. (1985). Depressive self-schemas, life stress, and vulnerability to depression. *Journal of Abnormal Psychology, 94,* 308–319.

Helgason, T. (1964). Epidemiology of mental disorders in Iceland. *Acta Psychiatry Scandinavica,* (Suppl. 173).

Hollon, S. D., & Kendall, P. C. (1980). Cognitive self-statements in depression: Development of an automatic thoughts questionnaire. *Cognitive Therapy and Research, 4,* 383–395.

Hollon, S. D., & Shaw, B. F. (1979). Group cognitive therapy for depressed patients. In A. T. Beck, A. J. Rush, B. F. Shaw, & G. Emery, (Eds.), *Cognitive therapy of depression* (pp. 328–353). New York: Guilford Press.

Jansson, L. (1986). *Handbok i kognitiv terapi vid depression. Natur och Kultur,* Stockholm.

Jansson, L., & Öst, L.-G. (1985). *Kognitiv terapi för depression.* En översikt av 17 kontrollerade studier. Läkartidningen *82,* 1764–1767.

Kanfer, F. H. (1970). Self-monitoring: Methodlogical limitations and clinical applications. *Journal of Consulting and Clinical Psychology, 35,* 148–152.

Kelly, G. (1955). The psychology of personal constructs. (2 Vols.). New York: Norton.

Kingdon, D., Farr, P., Murphy, S., & Tyrer, P. (1986). Hypomania following cognitive therapy. *British Journal of Psychiatry, 148,* 103–104.

Klerman, G. L. (1978). Affective disorders. In A. M. Nicholi (Ed.), *The Harvard guide to modern psychiatry.* Cambridge: Belknap.

Klerman, G. L., Rounsaville, B., Chevron, E. S., Neu, C., & Weissman, M. (1979). *Manual for short-term interpersonal psychotherapy (IPT) of depression.* Mimeographed.

Kovacs, M. (1980). Cognitive therapy in depression. *Journal of the American Academy of Psychoanalysis, 8,* 127–144.

Kovacs, M., & Beck, A. T. (1978). Maladaptive cognitive structures in depression. *American Journal of Psychiatry, 135,* 525–533.

Kovacs, M., Rush, A. J., Beck, A. T., & Hollon, S. D. (1981). Depressed patients treated with cognitive therapy and pharmacotherapy: A one year follow-up. *Archives of General Psychiatry, 38,* 33–39.

Krantz, S., & Hammen, C. (1979). Assessment of cognitive bias in depression. *Journal of Abnormal Psychology, 88,* 611–619.

Kuiper, N. A. (1978). Depression and causal attribution for success and failure. Journal of Personal Social Psychology, *36,* 236–246.

Lundh, L. G. (1983). Mind and Meaning. *Acta Universitatis Upsaliensis.* Studia Psychological Upsaliensia No. 10, Uppsala, Sweden.

Lundh, L.-G. (1988). Cognitive therapy and the analysis of meaning structures. In C. Perris, I. M. Blakcburn, & H. Perris (Eds.), *Cognitive Psychotherapy* (pp. 99–131). Heidelberg: Springer.

Magnusson, D. (1983). Implications of an interactional paradigm for research in human development. Report of the Department of Psychology of University of Stockholm, Suppl. 59, Stockholm, Sweden.

Markus, H. (1977). Self-schemata and processing information about the self. *Journal of Personal Social Psychology, 35,* 63–73.

Minkoff, K., Bergman, E., Beck, A. T., & Beck, R. (1973). Hopelessness, depression, and attempted suicide. *American Journal of Psychiatry, 130,* 455–459.

Murphy, G., Simons, A. D., Wetzel, R. D., & Lustman, P. (1984). Cognitive therapy and pharmacotherapy. Singly and together in the treatment of depression. *Archives of General Psychiatry, 41,* 33–41.

Neisser, U. (1967). *Cognitive psychology.* New York: Appleton-Century-Crofts.

Olinger, L. J., Kuiper, N. A., & Shaw, B. F. (1986). Dysfunctional attitudes and stressful life events: An interactive model of depression. *Cognitive Therapy and Research, 11,* 25–40.

Padesky, C. (1986a). *Cognitive therapy approaches for treating depression and anxiety in children.* Paper read at the 2nd International Congress of Cognitive Psychotherapy, Umeå, Sweden, September 18–20, 1986.

Padesky, C. (1986b). *Cognitive therapy of avoidant personality.* Paper read at the 2nd International Congress of Cognitive Psychotherapy.

Pera, M. (1982). Metodologia della scienza e filosofia della mente. La psichiatria al bivio. In V. Andreoli (Ed.), *Controversie in Psichiatria*. Milano: Masson.

Perris, C. (1966). A study of bipolar (manic depressive) and unipolar recurrent depressive psychoses. *Acta Psychiatrica Scandinavica*, (Suppl 194).

Perris, C. (1982). The distinction between bipolar and unipolar affective disorders. In E. S. Paykel (Ed.), *Handbook of affective disorders* (pp. 45–58). Edinburgh: Churchill Livingstone.

Perris, C. (1985). *Cognitive-behavioural psychotherapy with elderly patients*. Principles, feasibility and limits. Paper read at the 2nd International Congress of Psychogeriatric Medicine, Umeå, Sweden August 1985.

Perris, C. (1985b). *Cognitive therapy*. The emergence of a new paradigm in psychotherapy and in psychiatry. Paper read at the WPA International Symposium on Affective Disorders, Athens, Greece, October 13–17, 1985.

Perris, C. (1986). *Kognitiv terapi i teori och i praktik*. Natur och Kultur, Stockholm.

Perris, C. (1988). A theoretical framework for linking the experience of dysfunctional parental rearing attitudes with manifest psychopathology. *Acta Psychiatrica Scandinavica* (Suppl. 344), 93–109.

Perris, C. (1988a). Intensive cognitive-behavioural psychotherapy with patients suffering from schizophrenic syndromes. Theoretical and practical aspects. In C. Perris, I. M. Blackburn, & H. Perris (Eds.), *Cognitive psychotherapy* (pp. 324–375). Heidelberg: Springer.

Perris, C. (1988b). Kognitiv psykoterapi med patienter med schizofrena störningar. Miljöterapi och individuell terapi. Pilgrim Förlag, Stockholm.

Perris, C. (1988c). The foundations of cognitive psychotherapy and its standing in relation to other therapies. In C. Perris, I. M. Blackburn, & H. Perris (Eds.), *Cognitive psychotherapy: Theory and practice* (pp. 1–43). Heidelberg: Springer.

Perris, C., Eisemann, M., von Knorring, L., & Perris, H. (1984). Presentation of a subscale for the rating of depression and some additional items to the Comprehensive Psychopathological Rating Scale. *Acta Psychiatrica Scandinavica, 70*, 261–274.

Perris, H. (1982). A multifactorial study of life events in depressed patients. *Umeå University Medical Dissertations*, New Series, No. 78, Umeå, Sweden.

Perris, H. (1985). *Intensive cognitive therapy with partially hospitalized depressed patients*. Paper read at the WPA International Symposium on Affective Disorders, Athens, Greece, October 13–17, 1985.

Piaget, J. (1952). The origins of intelligence in children. New York: International Universities Press.

Rizley, R. (1978). Depression and distortion in the attribution of causality. *Journal of Abnormal Psychology, 87*, 32–48.

Rush, A. J., & Giles, D. E. (1982). Cognitive therapy: Theory and research. In A. J. Rush (Ed.), *Short-term psychotherapies for depression*. New York: Wiley.

Rush, A. J., & Watkins, J. T. (1981). Group versus individual cognitive therapy: A pilot study. *Cognitive Therapy and Research, 5*, 95–103.

Rush, A. J., Shaw, B. F., & Kathami, M. (1980). Cognitive therapy of depression utilizing the couples system. *Cognitive Therapy and Research, 4*, 103–113.

Rush, A. J., Beck, A. T., Kovacs, M., & Hollon, S. D. (1977). Comparative efficacy of cognitive therapy and pharmacotherapy in the treatment of depressed outpatients. *Cognitive Therapy and Research, 1*, 17–37.

Sameroff, A. J., & Chandler, M. J. (1975). Reproductive risk and the continuum of caretaking. In F. Horowitz (Ed.), *Review of child development research*. Chicago: University of Chicago Press.

Shaw, B. F. (1977). Comparison of cognitive therapy and behaviour therapy in the treatment of depression. *Journal of Consulting & Clinical Psychology, 45*, 543–551.

Shaw, B. F. (1981). Cognitive therapy with an inpatient population. In G. Emery, S. D. Hollon, & R. C. Bedrosian (Eds.), *New directions in cognitive therapy* (pp. 29–49). New York: Guilford Press.

Shelton, J. L., & Ackerman, J. M. (1974). *Homework in counseling and psychotherapy*. Springfield: C. Thomas.

Simon, K. (1986). *Treatment of borderline disorders*. Paper read at the 2nd International Congress of Cognitive Psychotherapy, Umeå, Sweden, September 17–20, 1986.

Simons, A. D., Murphy, G. E., Levine, J. L., & Wetzel, R. D. (1986). Cognitive therapy and pharmacotherapy for depression. Sustained improvement over one year. *Archives of General Psychiatry, 43*, 43–48.

Spitzer, R. L., Endicott, J., & Robins, E. (1978). Research diagnostic criteria: Rationale and reliability. *Archives of General Psychiatry, 35*, 773–782.

Taylor, F. G., & Marshall, W. L. (1977). Experimental analysis of cognitive-behavioural therapy for depression. *Cognitive Therapy and Research, 1*, 59–72.

Teasdale, J. D., Fennell, M. J. V., Hibbert, G. A., & Amics, P. L. (1984). Cognitive therapy for major depressive disorder in primary care. *British Journal of Psychiatry, 144*, 400–406.

U.S. President's Commission on Mental Health. (1978). *Report to the President from the President's Commission on Mental Health.* Washington, DC, Superintendent of Documents, U.S. Government Printing Office.

Ursano, R. J., & Hales, R. E. (1986). A review of brief individual psychotherapies. *American Journal of Psychiatry, 143,* 1507–1517.

Weissman, A., & Beck, A. T. (1978). *Development and validation of the Dysfunctional Attitude Scale.* Paper read at the meeting of the Am. Educ. Res. Assoc. Toronto, Canada, March 1978.

Weissman, M. M., & Myers, J. K. (1978). Affective disorders in a U. S. urban community. *Archives of General Psychiatry, 35,* 1304–1311.

Wilkes, T. C. R. (1987). Cognitive therapy with depressed adolescents. In C. Perris, I. M. Blackburn, & H. Perris (Eds.), *cognitive psychotherapy* (pp. 396–408). Heidelberg: Springer.

Wilson, P. H., Goldin, J. C., & Charbonneau-Powis, M. (1983). Comparative efficacy of behavioural and cognitive treatments of depression. *Cognitive Therapy and Reserach, 7,* 111–124.

Young, J., & Beck, A. T. (1982). Cognitive therapy: Clinical applications. In A. J. Rush (Ed.), *Short-term psychotherapies for depression* (pp. 182–214). New York: Wiley.

# 17

# The Treatment of Suicidal Behavior

ARTHUR FREEMAN AND DAVID M. WHITE

> *I've thought it through very carefully. I've suffered more abuse than I should ever have to suffer. The best thing for me to do is end it all. Then I'll finally have some peace.*
>
> *The bastards! How can they be so mean? This will show them. This will fix them. I can just picture their faces when they find me. . . .*
>
> *It's a little dangerous, sure. But it feels so good. Have you ever used this stuff? It's pretty safe it you're careful; I can be careful.*
>
> *I've been called. The angel Gabriel has asked me to climb upon his wings and fly to heaven. I'm scared. What if I fall off?*

Suicide, whether an act of planned self-destruction or a passive act of allowing one's demise, has meaning not only for the patient and his or her family but for the therapist as well. Even the most experienced therapist will react with an adrenaline surge when it becomes clear that a patient has placed a time limit on his or her life. The patient might communicate the suicidal intention in any number of ways. The patient might have difficulty controlling impulses: "I can't stop myself. I sit at the table with the knife pressed to my belly and start pressing in." The patient may wish to punish someone: "I'm waiting until he graduates, and then, on the night of his party, I'll kill myself." Or the patient's anniversary date might seem an auspicious moment to die: "My husband died a year ago. I've been too long without him . . ." Given the severity of its consequence, it is essential that the therapist have an understanding of the causes, assessment, process, and treatment of suicidal behavior so that effective problem solutions can be initiated immediately.

The clinical literature on suicide has grown substantially over the last several years. Part

ARTHUR FREEMAN • Center for Cognitive Therapy, Department of Psychiatry, University of Pennsylvania, Philadelphia, Pennsylvania 19104. DAVID M. WHITE • Department of Mental Health Sciences, Hahnemann University, Philadelphia, Pennsylvania 19102.

ARTHUR FREEMAN
and DAVID M. WHITE

of the impetus for the growth of epidemiology and treatment studies has been the reported increase in suicide among children and adolescents. *The Journal of Suicide and Life-Threatening Behaviors* and the newsletter of the American Association of Suicidology have developed to offer continuing information to mental health professionals. The suicidal act has been the focus of television shows, both dramatic and documentary, and has been written about in the popular press. It is a topic of great public concern and interest.

A large body of clinical lore has developed about suicide over the years. Some of this lore is reality and research based, and some folklore, based upon untested theories and clinical concepts. Familiarity with the realities of suicide is essential for any therapist. Operating from the clinical mythology that is often shared from one generation of therapists to another may result in underassessment of lethality, underestimation of risk, difficulty in conceptualizing the problem, and, most serious of all, difficulty developing and implementing effective interventions.

Before addressing the cognitive therapy of suicidal behavior, it will be important to examine some of the common beliefs about suicidality:

1. *Talking about suicide decreases the risk.* The idea that the patient who talks about suicide is unlikely to make an attempt is unsupported by research. This notion is based on the assumption that talking about an impulse dissipates its energy and that the release of the energy eliminates the compulsion to act on the impulse. However, simply talking about an impulse will not make it disappear. Numerous early studies have shown that from 60% to 80% of persons who commit suicide have talked about it beforehand (e.g., Pokorny, 1960). More important than talking is what the person talks about. Depending on the content of the verbalizations, talking can increase, decrease, or have no effect on the intention to commit suicide. The act of discussing suicidal thoughts with a helping professional, pastor, or friend may help the patient develop solutions to the problems distressing him or her and the resolution of issues that contribute to the suicidal thinking. But simply talking about suicidal intentions cannot be relied upon to reduce the risk of suicide.

2. *"Gestures" are not serious.* The patient who makes a suicidal gesture or attempt and then immediately calls a hospital or significant other is often seen as not "serious" in his or her suicidality. It is assumed that if he or she were "really" suicidal, he or she would have resolutely followed through on the attempt. The seriousness of the attempt is judged by how close to death the individual comes. But, although the pattern of attempt/correction may reveal ambivalence about suicide or manipulative intent, it does not guarantee the situation is risk-free or that future attempts will not follow a similar pattern. The great majority of people who commit suicide have given advance notice (Robins, Gassner, Kayes, Wilkinson, & Kayes, 1959). If an individual makes a suicide gesture and expects a significant other to rescue him or her and the significant other is not available, the "half-hearted" attempt may eventuate in a full-blown death. The most frequent means of indicating suicide intent is a direct statement. Other common modes include off-hand comments about being better off dead, a desire to die, or methods of committing suicide. The patient might also leave a note, write a will, or give others expensive gifts without apparent reason (Beck, Morris, & Lester, 1974; Kovacs, Beck, & Weissman, 1976).

3. *Suicide attempts are a cry for help.* If we view the suicide attempt as a cry for help, we may fail to appreciate the gravity of the patient's problem. An attempt intended as a cry for help might always result in death. Typically, an attempt represents much more than a request or demand for help. Clinically, it is far more useful to view the suicide attempt as a statement that the individual has, in his or her own view, few alternative options left in his or her life. The patient may believe also that his or her problem-solving capacity has been exhausted and his or her problem-solving skills are unequal to the task. It does not indicate that the individual's suicide risk is low. Rather, a significant risk of additional attempts exists either until the individual's view of the situation and options changes, or, he or she dies.

4. *Holidays are a time of high suicide risk.* The so-called holiday blues, occurring between Thanksgiving and New Year's Day, are often believed to engender suicide. However, no evidence exists of higher rates of suicide, hospitalization, or depression at the holiday seasons (Christensen, 1984; Lester & Beck, 1975). In point of fact, the suicide rate and rate of attempts is higher in the spring (Rogot, Falsitz, & Feinlieb, 1976).

5. *Discussing or asking questions about suicide may suggest it to a patient.* Novice therapists often are afraid to address directly the topic of suicide because they might "put the idea in the patient's head" or make the idea of suicide more acceptable if he or she is already thinking about it. However, in our experience, discussing suicide intentions with a patient in a sensitive, direct manner tends to decrease rather than increase the risk of eventual suicide. Interventions are possible if the therapist can discuss suicide in a forthright manner. The therapist can work with the patient to establish safeguards (e.g., turning over weapons to a trusted individual), take precautions for behavior control (i.e., entering a hospital), or relieve the cognitive and emotional factors associated with the suicidality. Few interventions are possible if the therapist is unable or unwilling to discuss suicide directly.

6. *All suicide methods are equally lethal.* Some attempts involve passive behaviors; the individual does not perform activities that are needed to survive (i.e., taking proper medication, maintaining a specially needed diet, or caring for physical safety). The individual might also take more active steps to injure, maim, or kill him or herself. These might involve a range of activity from taking an overdose of pills, jumping off of a bridge, or shooting oneself. Several studies have found that men tend to utilize the more active methods, women more passive ones (Lester, Beck, & Bruno, 1976). The reasons for suicide have been found, also, to vary with gender (see, Lester, 1983; Wilson, 1981). Men consider vocational and career issues as reasons for suicide. Women tend to see relationship difficulties as the major stressor leading to suicide.

7. *Patients have a right to take their own lives.* Does the patient have the right to take his or her life? Should the therapist intervene? One can make the case that the therapist has no right to intervene and the patient's existential choice should be made freely. However, our experience has been that few patients select suicide as a free choice but feel compelled to attempt suicide by virtue of their perception that their options are very limited, that they have no other options available to them. They think that they have no freedom at all. They are governed by dysfunctional thoughts that dictate the single option of death. The goal of therapy is to enhance the patient's free will, not restrict his or her freedom of choice.

8. *Suicide runs in families.* A major predictor of suicide is the occurrence of suicide in family members. Suicide is more likely if members of the patient's family have attempted or committed suicide. However, there is little evidence that suicide intentions are genetically determined. Although the data from twin studies have been examined and concordance rates for completed suicides are higher for monozygotic than dizygotic twins (Juel-Nielsen & Videbeck, 1970; Tsuang, 1977), none of the these studies managed to investigate monozygotic twins reared apart. Although tentative evidence exists that genetics play a small role in suicide, no methodologically adequate study has shown this adequately. Environmental events, especially childhood experiences, appear to play a equally prominent role. Child abuse (Rogers & Leunes, 1979), early loss of the parents (Stein, Levy, & Glasberg, 1974), and modeling of suicidal behavior of significant others (Diekstra, 1974; Garfinkel, Froese, & Golombek, 1979) all place the patient at risk for suicide.

9. *Patients are less likely to make suicide attempts as they get less depressed.* This generally is false. Many patients are vegetatively depressed; they cannot get out of bed to care for their health and cleanliness needs. Such patients lack the energy to carry through a suicide attempt. As patients become less depressed, they have more energy, both psychic and physical, that can be focused on the suicide (Keith-Spiegel, & Spiegel, 1967). The more typical depressed individual in outpatient treatment does not become suicidal when helped from from moderate depression to mild depression, or from mild depression to no depression.

10. *Child and adolescent suicide rates have increased.* Child and adolescent suicides appear to have increased in recent years, and several "epidemics" of teen suicide have received nationwide attention. Research, however, is inconclusive as to whether there is an actual increase, or better (or different) reporting procedures. Several explanations for the apparent increase have been offered, including a greater hopelessness on the part of today's youth, the possibility of global destruction, depletion of natural resources, or widespread unemployment. Research suggests that no increase exists but that a greater awareness of suicide has led to an overdiagnosis of suicide in accident situations (Barraclough, 1973).

11. *Suicide is contagious.* The so-called cluster suicides have been reported widely. The rash of suicides that follow a death or deaths by suicide among adolescents seem to have as their core three factors. First, there is a romanticization of the act; second, disinhibition with drugs or alcohol; and third, a combination of hopelessness and a strong histrionic personality streak.

12. *Medication can stop suicidal behavior.* Many nonmedical therapists react to suicidal behavior by trying to get the patient to a psychiatrist for an immediate initiation of a course of antidepressant medication. The antidepressant medication may not have a substantial effect for a period from 1 to 3 weeks. Though potentially useful for long-term treatment, the medication may not be effective for the patient's immediate depression. In fact, tricyclic antidepressants can be quite lethal in overdose.

14. *Hospitalization is required for the suicidal patient.* Related to the medication issue is the notion that the suicidal patient must be immediately hospitalized. This presents two problems for the therapist. The operative word in most laws regarding involuntary hospitalization is "imminent"; if it cannot be demonstrated that the patient is an imminent danger to himself or others, an involuntary hospitalization is unlikely. The therapist can, of course, try to convince the patient that entering the hospital is in his or her best interest. Placing the suicidal patient in the hospital may have several effects, some positive, others negative. The positive effects are that it places the seriously suicidal patient in a safe environment (although patients can, and do, make suicide attempts in hospitals). A patient on suicide watch can be observed closely. Further, the patient in the hospital can be observed and stabilized on medication easily. Moreover, placing a patient in the hospital removes him or her from the therapist's case load and allows the therapist to share responsibility for the patient with other professionals. In the hospital setting, the patient may be taken out of a pressuring home, job, or life situation. The generally negative effects are that the hospitalized patient is isolated from family and other available support systems. The patient may be stigmatized by the psychiatric hospitalization. The therapist needs to consider carefully the qualities of the individual setting and the long-term effect of the hospitalization on the patient and his or her family.

14. *Patients with a well-developed method of suicide are more likely to make an attempt.* Patients who have well-formulated plans, leave notes, or have the means at hand to effect a suicide are far greater risks than the individual who has none of the foregoing. However, absence of a plan does not eliminate the risk of an attempt. In particular, patients with poor impulse control are at risk at any point because they lack the internal controls necessary to avoid self-destructive action.

## CLINICAL ASSESSMENT

A complete clinical assessment of the patient's suicidal ideation is essential. This assessment is part of the initial evaluation as well as the ongoing evaluation of the patient in treatment. The therapist must take any indications of suicide seriously and evaluate them with care. The clinician must be sensitive to subtle distinctions of meaning, or the subtle meanings of behaviors. The statement, "I would like to die," may mean for one patient that life has no meaning and that, at times, he or she wishes to die during sleep. This is a very different from the patient who finds his or her life situation unbearable and says, "I would like to die; how can I go about it?" Even the most sensitive clinician cannot safely assume that he or she understands fully the meaning of suicidal ideation without asking the patient directly about the ideas and thoughts.

The same care must be utilized for assessment of subtle behaviors that reflect suicidal ideation or intent. The patient who has updated his or her will, taken care of legal odds and ends, or given away possessions may be conveying a message. The assessment and understanding of the patient's view of his or her options is critical. The patient who sees few or no options is at far more serious risk than the patient who maintains that options, although limited or undesirable, exist. In making a clinical assessment of suicidality, the therapist must be aware of his or her own cognitions so that information is not lost or never sought in an attempt to gain a modicum of comfort. The therapist who is discomforted by the idea of discussing suicide may be collaborating actively with the patient's suicide attempt.

In addition to exploring the patient's cognitions and behavior, there are several additional points to consider in assessing the potentially suicidal patient: (a) Has the patient made attempts previously? (b) When was the last attempt? How frequent have the attempts been? What have been the circumstances of the attempts? Is a family history of suicide in evidence? Have either parents or grandparents made suicide attempts? Have these attempts been successful?

Several tools can be used to assist clinicians in their assessment of suicidality.

The Beck Depression Inventory, a 21-item self-report measure of depression (Beck, Ward, Mendelson, Mock, & Erbaugh, 1961) can offer the clinician a measure of the patient's general level of depression by using the total BDI score. The clinician can also assess the specific areas of depression by examining the specific items endorsed by the patient. Of particular importance are the patient responses to items 2 (Hopelessness) and 9 (Suicidality).*

The Hopelessness Scale (HS; Beck, Weissman, Lester, & Trexler, 1975) assesses directly the hopelessness component of depression. Inasmuch as the cognitive model sees hopelessness as the prime ingredient in suicide, such direct assessment is essential. By evaluating both the overall score and changes in the score over time and conducting a content analysis, the therapist can develop a conceptualization of the problems that are fueling the patient's suicidal thinking. Specific themes emerge from the scale that can be utilized in the therapy.

The Scale of Suicidal Ideation (SSI; Beck, Kovacs, & Weissman, 1980) offers the clinician a list of questions that need to be asked of the suicidal patient. They include "When you think of living, do you think that your wish to live is a strong wish to live, a moderate wish to live, a low wish to live, or no wish to live?". The SSI can be used to assess the patient's perception on the day of the interview (the right side of the form), and the patient's perceptions of how he or she might have filled out the scale at a time of greater crisis (left side of the form).

The SSI questions are imbedded in an interview format. "When you think about dying, do you find that you have a strong wish to die, a moderate wish to die, a weak wish to die, or do you have no wish to die?". "How about wishing to live. Do you have a strong wish to live, a moderate wish to live, a weak wish to live, or no wish to live at all?". Questions in each of the areas are asked in the same manner. The therapist can ask for elaboration at any time. Because suicidality is not a trait, it is best that suicidal ideation be assessed at different times and situations throughout the therapy.

The Suicide Intent Scale (SIS; Beck 1985), as with the previous Scale of Suicidal Ideation, codifies a number of issues that must be clarified immediately in assessing a patient's suicide potential. This scale is used with those patients who have made an attempt at some time

*Review the discussion of the uses of the BDI Chapter 4.

in the past. The presence of suicidal ideation does not imply necessarily that the individual intends to act. Intent indicates that actual planning has begun. Both ideation and intent must be evaluated on the day of the interview as well as for the point of greatest crisis to evaluate any possible change or variance. In addition, the clinician needs to be alert to indications of suicidal ideation throughout treatment and carefully evaluate the patient's ideation and intent whenever such ideation seems present.

## LETHALITY

The clinician should be aware of the potential lethality of any of a number of suicidal behaviors and not underestimate any of them. Although Valium has a very high margin of safety (*Physicians Desk Reference,* 1988, there are reports of patients surviving single doses of 600 mg), the ingestion of any quantity of drugs with the intention of dying must be viewed as a lethal attempt. The following clinical example illustrates the therapist's need for familiarity with the lethality levels of various drugs.

> The patient called the therapist to report that she had taken what was left in a bottle of Valium, 10 in all. On inquiry, it was discovered that the Valium was 2 mg. This total dose of approximately 20 mg of Valium would *probably* not be lethal for *most* individuals but given her size, health, and the ingestion of additional drugs and/or alcohol, the attempt was seen as having lethal intent. She took all the medication available with the full intention of dying and may well have expected to do so. Her call to the therapist did not alter her intent but suggested that she exercised her one last option with the hope that the therapist would be available and intervene (in this case, calling the police/fire emergency squad to the patient's home so that they might take her to a hospital).

# A COGNITIVE-BEHAVIORAL CONCEPTUALIZATION OF SUICIDE

The major ingredient in suicide is hopelessness (Beck, 1985). When the depressed individual believes that he or she has no more options left, death may seem to be a welcome relief. The therapist must appreciate several variations on the hopelessness theme so that he or she can best understand and treat the patient's suicidal thinking and behavior. We divide suicidal behavior into four broad types: (1) hopeless suiciders, (2) histrionic suiciders, (3) psychotic suiciders, and (4) rational suiciders. None of these types is mutually exclusive with respect to the others. The four types will be presented individually for the purposes of exposition.

In the first type, the patient maintains the belief that there is no hope of improving and therefore no longer any reason for continuing life. Four patients, all of whom are depressed, will be considered as examples.

Client A is depressed and considers suicide but feels that before exercising the suicidal option, he has 27 other options. Client B, also depressed, sees herself as having 91 other options, before suicide. Client C has 8 other possible options. Client D has 14 other options.

If all four patients were, because of world economics, personal tragedy, or cognitive distortion, to have 8 options vanish, Clients A, B, and D, although becoming more depressed, would not likely become suicidal as they have additional options to pursue. Client C, however, having exhausted all other options, would see himself as having no choice but either to commit suicide or live in unending misery. All people have their own implicit option list of the actions they might undertake in any one of a number of circumstances. For the majority of individuals, the option of suicide never is exercised. For others, it is an infrequent but annoying presence;

for still others a constant, persistent, unwanted companion. For a small group, it is an option that is not only exercised but dominates their thoughts and actions for years prior and/or subsequent to the suicide attempt.

Because suicide is at the bottom of everyone's options list, it becomes an issue only as the individual gets closer to the bottom of the list. When any individual feels that he or she has no further options, suicide becomes a viable alternative. For many patients, available options appear objectively to remain the same. However, the patient's *perception* of the available options causes him or her to feel very hopeless. Throughout history, there have been individuals who, although suicide contradicted their religious beliefs, have chosen death by their own hand as preferable to the other alternatives they have faced (e.g., the defenders of Masada). Even though their options may be limited, most individuals continually add options to their lists so that they never reach that rock-bottom point. By seeing a small victory as a reason to continue life, an additional option is generated. The following case will serve to illustrate the nature of the hopeless suicider:

> Les, a 35-year-old male, came to therapy because of severe depression. Early in the treatment, Les discussed his general hopelessness. He saw his marriage as coming to an end, his children lost to him, his job and income lost, his debts overwhelming, and his health failing. Although each of his concerns was realistic, in part (i.e., he did have marital problems, and his wife had threatened to return, with the children, to her parents in Oregon), his wife thought that he exaggerated his problems and wanted to maintain the relationship.

The second type of suicider is what we label the *histrionic suicider*. Different individuals manifest different stimulus needs. Conceptually, this type of individual has a high need for excitement. To understand the need, we might see one person as perfectly happy to spend 2 weeks of vacation on a beach doing absolutely nothing. They would not read, listen to music, walk, swim, or play. Their idea of a good time would be to do nothing except lay in the sun and tan or relax by sitting in a rowboat all day with a fishing pole. For other individuals, this type of vacation would be anathema. Their idea of an enjoyable vacation would be to travel, be active, sightsee, and play. There are, of course, many points between these two positions. Given the need for activity on the part of many individuals, the therapist may see patients for whom activity and excitement are necessary parts of their lives. When such patients feel "anxious," "nervous," "itchy," or "bored," they often will act to self-stimulate in a variety of ways such as taking drugs or alcohol in quantity, speeding in cars or motorcycles. These would all add to the excitement of life. The net result may very well be physical damage or even loss of life; however, such individuals may even utilize the suicide attempt as a source of stimulation or excitement. Three case examples serve to illustrate this type of attempter.

> Case 1 involves a 27-year-old male. He reported a number of what his previous therapist labeled serious attempts. He reported feeling itchy or nervous. His manner of coping with this nervousness was one of two things. First, he drove his car at great speeds, often exceeding 100 m.p.h. He reported a great relief after the driving episodes. His second strategy was to drive along back roads to small highway bridges over streams or creeks. He would then jump from the bridges. He would get wet and muddy but was never injured. If a tree trunk, large rock, or other debris were in the stream he might be injured or killed. This excitement was sufficient to take the edge off of his nervousness.

> Case 2 was a 35-year-old woman diagnosed with a borderline personality disorder. When she became "bored," she would sit at her kitchen table and slowly draw a knife, razor, or piece of broken glass across her forearms. She reported that the blood

welling up within the cuts would ease her boredom and anxiety. She would wrap her arms in kitchen towels after the cutting and run to the emergency room of her local hospital. Upon entering the emergency room with her arms wrapped in bloody towels, a major furor would ensue. The triage nurse and medical/surgical resident would attempt to staunch the bleeding (which had often clotted) and then contact the psychiatry resident for her admission to the psychiatry unit. After several attempts, they became accustomed to her behavior and would stop the bleeding and send her home. After the attempt, she would return home and not make another attempt for a while.

At times, the hopeless patient reports an attempt that leaves the therapist both extremely concerned yet hard pressed not to smile. The hapless attempt may appear very naive. As a result of the hapless attempt, the individual may or may not succeed at killing him- or herself.

Case 3 involves a young woman despondent over a lost love. She made all the plans to die of asphyxiation. She closed the kitchen window tightly and stuffed kitchen towels about the door to make it airtight. She then turned on the oven and put her head in the oven so that she could breathe the gas deeply. Her oven, however, was electric, and all she did was singe her hair. Her intent, however, was most serious.

Histrionic suicide attempts are flamboyant and may be repetitive. These attempts may be questioned as actual suicide attempts and classified as manipulative or motivated by a need for attention. Even so, the possibility of a histrionic attempt being lethal exists, and the suicidal ideation and attempts need to be taken seriously.

The *psychotic suicider* attempts suicide as a direct result of command hallucinations, or voices from within. It is essential to assess whether the attempt is psychotic, for, in psychotic individuals, it is not the hopelessness that must be addressed but the voices that prompt them to suicide. The primary intervention with patients who experience command hallucinations is pharmacological combined with inpatient treatment. The antipsychotic medication reduces the delusional and hallucinatory phenomena. In addition, however, individuals having command hallucinations can be helped to address two basic issues: (a) the power to respond and (b) the nature of the voices.

*The power to respond.* As a general therapeutic strategy, the patient with command hallucinations needs to be helped to gain power over the internal stimuli. This might take the form of helping the patient generate new self-statements. For example, when the voices say, "Cut your wrists, cut your wrists," the patient can refuse and say, "I don't have to. I won't, I won't, I won't." When the voices state, "You have no right to live, your life is not worth living, you need to die," it is important to help the patient respond. For example, the patient might be instructed to say repeatedly to himself or herself, "I want to live, I want to live," and to respond to the voices in an almost disputational way. The therapist may find that the use of positive self-statements and self-instructional strategies may serve to help the patient gain more control. The therapist working with psychotic patients who suffer command hallucinations to suicide needs to quickly and precisely assess the nature of the commands. Questioning the patient very directly about the content, nature, press, and power of the thought is essential. The therapist must know who and what he or she is dealing with so that interventions can be tailored directly to the individual patient.

*The nature of the voices.* The therapist needs to determine also the nature of the voices. If possible, to help the patient recognize them as not "all powerful", that is, the patient does not need to respond immediately to them. Pharmacological interventions typically are essential with the psychotic suicider. The proper medication, carefully controlled, is a vital part of the treatment plan. The danger with medication is that, unless carefully controlled and dispensed, the patient can hoard and utilize it as part of a suicide attempt.

The fourth type is the *rational suicider*. These are individuals for whom the choice to die is based on some rational consideration. These individuals rarely seek therapy to discuss their rational decision. Therapists generally see these individuals after a failed attempt. The type of situation generally offered as the model for rational suicide is that of the terminally ill cancer patient in intractable pain (Siegel, 1986). The popular media refer to the "right to die." The patient may demand that life-support systems be withdrawn and that extraordinary means of life support be terminated. The intended result is that death will shortly follow. The entire issue of an individual's right to die is a bio–medical–ethical–legal issue that is hotly debated and continues to be challenged in the courts. We have found, however, that many suicidal individuals believe their ideas are rational, reasonable, and intelligent. With therapy, the rational suicider may discover other options.

## TREATMENT OF SUICIDAL BEHAVIOR

A full understanding of the cognitive model is essential for any therapist planning to use cognitive therapy (The reader is referred to Beck, Rush, Shaw & Emery, 1979; Freeman, 1988; Freeman & Reinecke, in press; Perris, Chapter 16, this volume). Therapy cannot be a mere collection of strategies and techniques. Rather, an understanding of the cognitive underpinnings of suicidal ideation and intent is required. With that conceptual framework, the cognitive therapist can understand quickly the nature of the suicidality and develop interventions, both inter- and intrapersonally. Specifically, cognitive therapists work in a very direct manner with patients, proposing hypotheses, developing strategies for testing the hypotheses, developing a range of specific skills as needed, and teaching the patient a model for more effective coping/adaptation to the world. Probably no patient requires a direct problem-solving approach as much as the suicidal patient. The focus of the therapy is collaborative, although the collaboration may not always be 50-50. With the severely depressed and suicidal individual, the therapist's activity level must be high enough to supply the initial energy to develop the therapy work, so that the collaboration might start out 80-20, or even 90-10. In point of fact, the therapist may be far more active than he or she is with other patients. Because of the seriousness of the patient's condition, and the severity of the consequences, the therapist cannot rely simply on offering a restatement of patient problems but must use an active restructuring of thoughts, behaviors, and affect.

A problem focus that was stressed earlier (Perris, Chapter 16 this volume) is essential with the suicidal patient to help supply the direction rather than encourage a vague and aimless wandering about the broad issue of hopelessness. It is necessary that the therapist be more directive and focused in regard to the suicidal ideation, intent, and sense of hopelessness that fuels the patient's suicidal wishes. The initial goal in working with the suicidal patient is to work quickly to establish rapport. The therapist must be perceived as an individual who can be trusted, supportive, resourceful, and available, and who is allied closely with the patient. The therapist's openness, lack of self-consciousness in questioning directly the nature of the hopelessness and thoughts of suicide, utilizing the data from the psychological measures, history, and level of depression, can serve to put the patient at ease. As one patient reported after an initial crisis interview, "I really felt uncomfortable when you asked all those questions. Yet you touched on the thoughts I was having, but was afraid to say, thinking you would think me crazy for having those thoughts. When you asked those questions so directly, I knew that you must of asked them before and that maybe I wasn't so crazy, perhaps just really upset. Also, since you had heard this all before, maybe you could help me."

Having established the rapport, the therapist needs to work actively and directly on the hopelessness. The patients must be worked *with* rather than *on,* so that the patient feels part of a therapeutic team. This is especially important with suicidal patients who must see that they can, as a result of therapy, develop alternatives and options. They need to appreciate that it is not merely the therapist telling them what to do or giving them instructions. This might feed into their hopelessness with the concept, "See I can't even manage my life. I need to be told what to do." The therapist should bear this in mind when working with the suicidal patient whose energy level is low, who feels paralyzed, and whose general level of motivation may be lacking. For the individuals who have settled upon suicide as the option of choice, the therapist may need to contribute more than 50% to the collaboration until the patient makes the decision to live.

INTERVENTION TECHNIQUES

Cognitive therapy techniques are used to develop adaptive responses to dysfunctional thinking. The format for intervention is Socratic questioning (Beck *et al.,* 1979). It seems far more congruent with a collaborative model to question rather than interpret. Interpretations may be perceived by the patients as anticollaborative in that they suggest the therapist knows what is going on in the patient's mind. Although true in some cases, the patient might experience interpretations as an intrusion but questions as helpful prompts toward uncovering ideation. By questioning, the therapist offers the patient an idea, hypothesis, or prompt to his or her thinking, feeling, and experience. The cognitive techniques are all designed to challenge automatic thoughts. The therapist must master them all and use them in various combinations in the therapy work. The various techniques are essential for the patient to learn as he or she builds an armamentarium of coping skills. The techniques will be considered in the following section, with specific application to the suicidal patient.

1. *Understanding idiosyncratic meaning.* It is not safe for the therapist to assume that he or she completely understands the terms used by the patient without asking for clarification. If a group of 100 professionals were asked to indicate what they considered the prime descriptor of depression, we would not get unanimity of response. Out of 100 responses, descriptors might include sad, hopelessness, sleep difficulty, and eating problems. Given the differing meanings even among professionals, one cannot be sure of what patients mean when they use the words *depressed, suicidal, anxious,* or *upset.* Therefore it is essential to question the patients directly on the meaning of their verbalizations. This is essential to make sure that the therapist is not merely in the right ballpark in understanding but is right on target. This might be called the "Columbo technique." The TV character played by Peter Falk solved crimes not by interpreting and telling people what he thought they had done but by assuming that he did not know and being willing to ask what appeared to be obvious or even "dumb" questions. For example:

PATIENT: I'm a loser!

THERAPIST: You call yourself a loser. Just what *is* a loser? What does being a loser mean to you?

PATIENT: You know, a LOSER. You know what a loser is, don't you? I'm a LOSER, A LOSER, and I deserve to die.

THERAPIST: I know what I mean when I use the term *loser,* but I would like to know what you mean by the term *loser.*

2. *Questioning the evidence.* One effective way to challenge a dysfunctional thought is to examine the extent to which it is supported by the available evidence and whether other interpretations better fit the evidence. People use certain evidence to maintain their ideas and beliefs. It is essential to teach the patient to identify and to then question the evidence he or she uses to maintain or strengthen an idea or belief. Questioning the evidence also requires examining the source of the data. The patient who is depressed and suicidal often gives equal weight to all sources. A stranger in the street who appears to frown when the patient passes may be used as evidence for the need to kill oneself. The patient who uses selective abstraction

has the ability to ignore some data and focus on other data that support his suicidogenic view. By having the patient question the evidence, a fuller accounting of the life data and situation can be had. For example:

PATIENT: No way in the world is he interested in me. Because he's not, there's no use for me going on.

THERAPIST: You raise two issues, one that he's not interested in you, and second that if he's not there's no use continuing. Before you consider killing yourself, how do you know that he's not interested? What evidence do you have?

PATIENT: Come on. If he were interested in me he would have asked me out . . . and he hasn't.

THERAPIST: It is true he hasn't asked you out yet. Has he done anything else to let you know that he's interested? Does he spend time talking to you? How about the small gifts he bought for you?

PATIENT: That's all true, but the real test is whether or not he asked me out.

THERAPIST: So the evidence is mixed at this point?

PATIENT: Well . . . yeah.

3. *Reattribution.* A statement commonly heard among patients is, "It's all my fault." This is heard especially in situations of relationship difficulty, separation, or divorce. Although one cannot dismiss out of hand the possibility of such a statement's truth, it is unlikely that the patient is totally responsible for all that has gone wrong. Some patients take responsibility for events and situations that are only minimally attributable to them, whereas some tend to blame others and take no responsibility. The therapist can help the patient distribute responsibility reasonably among the relevant parties. If the therapist takes a position of total support (i.e., "It wasn't your fault," "She isn't worth it," "You're better off without her" or "There are other fish in the ocean"), he or she ends up sounding like friends, family, and other lay people whom the patient has already dismissed as a supportive cheering squad. In fact, the patient may thereby perceive the therapist as not understanding the patient. The therapist can, by taking a middle ground, help the patient to reattribute responsibility and not take all of the blame nor unrealistically shift all blame to other people. For example:

PATIENT: It's all my fault. I really screwed things up this time. If I could only have handled things differently, the relationship could have worked. If only I hadn't been so demanding. It could have been good, I blew it. What's left?

THERAPIST: There's much that you did both good and bad in the relationship. Is it *all* your fault that things didn't work out?

PATIENT: Yeah. Who else?

THERAPIST: What role did Alicia play in the breakup? Was she involved at all in contributing to the difficulty? I know that you feel that it was all your fault. I think it would be helpful to examine just what you contributed and what Alicia contributed to the ending of this relationship.

PATIENT: No, it's my fault.

THERAPIST: Did Alicia do anything at all to contribute to the problem?

PATIENT: You mean besides being a bitch?

THERAPIST: Let's start with that. . . .

4. *Examining options and alternatives.* The suicidal patient often sees him- or herself as having lost all options. Alternatively, he or she might see the options as so limited that among their few choices, death seems to be the easiest or simplest choice. This cognitive strategy

involves working with the patient to generate additional options. If the therapist adopts the position that suicide is "unacceptable," "wrong," "bad," or otherwise not a viable option, the therapist runs the risk of being in direct opposition to the patient. This conflict position may force the patient into a harder stance vis-à-vis suicide, distance the patient from the therapist, and undermine the therapist's neutrality and credibility. Suicide is always an option, albeit a negative one. We cannot deny that option no matter how loudly or longly we protest. The therapist's primary task is to help the patient to generate other options. For the patient with the single option of suicide, one more option increases the available options by 100%. For example:

PATIENT: What else is left for me? My life is as good as over! The only thing left for me to do is to die. I'll probably mess that up too.

THERAPIST: Dying is one option. Are there any others?

PATIENT: No. None that I can think of or want to try.

THERAPIST: Let's look at that. On the one hand, you say there are no options. On the other hand, you suggest options that you have in mind but either don't want to try or that you dismiss. I'd like to help you to look at the options, as limited as they seem to be.

PATIENT: It's not just the way I see them. That's the way it is.

THERAPIST: I know that it looks bleak right now. Dying seems the best choice. Let's see if you and I can generate another possibility.

PATIENT: I don't care. . . . about anything. That's not true, I do care.

THERAPIST: Then what can you do, in addition of course, to killing yourself?

5. *Decatastrophizing*. If the patient sees an experience as potentially catastrophic, the therapist can help the patient see whether he or she is overestimating the catastrophic nature of the situation. Questions that might be asked of the patient include, "What is the worst thing that can happen to you?" or "If it does happen, how will your life be different 3 months from now?" The therapist working against the *chicken-little* style of thinking can help the patient see the consequence of his or her or her life actions as not all or nothing and thereby less catastrophic. It is important that this technique be used with great gentleness and sensitivity so that the patient does not feel ridiculed by the therapist. For example:

PATIENT: She'll think I'm an idiot. A moron. A loser.

THERAPIST: And what if she does? What would be so horrible if she, or anyone else for that matter, thinks you're an idiot. Does that make you one? Why would this be so horrible?

PATIENT: It *would* be awful.

THERAPIST: Let's go over that again. What if she does think something about you? First, is it true, and second, how do you know what she's thinking?

PATIENT: [Smiling] Well, the world will continue to orbit, so it's not that terrible, but it would be horrible personally.

THERAPIST: Yeah . . . the world will stay in orbit.

6. *Fantasized consequences*. In this technique, the patient is asked to fantasize a situation and describe his or her images and concerns. Often the patient describes his or her concerns and by so verbalizing them can see the irrationality of the ideas. If the fantasized consequences are realistic, the therapist can work with the patient to assess realistically the danger and to develop appropriate coping strategies. This technique allows the patient to bring into the consulting room imagined events, situations, or interactions that have happened previously or that he or she believes will happen in the future. By having the patient move the fantasy to the

"reality" of being spoken, the images become grist for the therapeutic mill. The fantasy, being colored by the same dysfunctional thinking that alters many of the patient's perceptions, may be overly negative. The explication and investigation of the style, format, and content of such fantasies can yield valuable material for the therapy work. For example:

THERAPIST: I'd like you to close your eyes for a moment. Picture what you think will happen when you get your exam scores back.

PATIENT: I can picture walking into the kitchen at home. My parents are both there, and my father asks me about the exam.

THERAPIST: What does he say or do?

PATIENT: He'll get furious when I tell him that I've failed. He'll yell at me for the millionth time about my wasting his hard-earned money. He'll say that I might as well drop out of school . . . no, he wouldn't do what I was thinking.

THERAPIST: What was that?

PATIENT: My thought was that he would throw me out of the house and force me to drop out of school. He'd probably tell me that I had been doing a lousy job and then carry on for days about my work.

THERAPIST: What would he do then?

PATIENT: He'd be angry for a while, a long while, maybe days, but eventually he'd calm down.

THERAPIST: Let's stay with the image. In your image, he would throw you out of the house and have you drop out of school.

PATIENT: Nah! [Laughs.] He worries if I come home late. He's not going to throw me out. And school—he would *pass* out if I dropped out.

7. *Advantages and disadvantages.* Having the patient list the advantages and disadvantages of maintaining or changing the suicidal belief or behavior can help him or her gain balance and perspective. A scaling technique helps the patient move away from an all-or-nothing position to one that explores the possibility of experiences, feelings or behaviors that have both negative and positive qualities. The depressed patient who has dichotomized life events may see only one side. By asking that he or she examine both the advantages *and* disadvantages of both sides of an issue, a broader perspective can be achieved. Although there will, undoubtably, be some overlap between the two lists, important differences will emerge. This technique can be used to examine the advantages and disadvantages of acting a certain way (e.g., engaging in dangerous behaviors), thinking a particular way (e.g., thinking of dying), or feeling a certain way (e.g., sad). Although the patient often will claim that he or she cannot control his or her or her feelings, actions, and thoughts, it is precisely the development of such control that is the strength of cognitive therapy. For example:

PATIENT: I can't stay in this marriage. If I stay, I'll die.

THERAPIST: There are many parts to the relationship from what you've described, both good and bad. Leaving has lots of consequences.

PATIENT: I don't care anymore.

THERAPIST: Let's explore the possibilities. We can work at making two lists: The first can be the advantages and the disadvantages of staying with Steve; the second can be the advantages and disadvantages of leaving.

PATIENT: Aren't they the same?

THERAPIST: Not really. There will be some overlap, but the lists will, I think, show some very different ideas. I'm going to draw a line down the center of this page. On the left, let's put down the pros or pluses of staying with Steve. On the left the cons or negatives. We will then do that with the idea of leaving, both pro and con. We can then weight them in terms of how important each of these ideas are to you.

8. *Turning adversity to advantage.* There are times when a seeming disaster can be used to one's advantage. Losing one's job may seem a disaster but may, in some cases, be the entry point to a new job or career. An imposed deadline may be seen as oppressive and unfair but can be used as a motivator. This cognitive therapy technique requires the patient to look for the silver lining of a cloud. Given that the depressed individual has taken a view that eventuates in finding the darkened lining to every silver cloud, looking for the positive aspects in a situation initially can be very difficult. Many patients simply may not see the positive. Patients will sometimes respond to the therapist's efforts to point out positive aspects with greater negativity and opposition. They may accuse the therapist of being unrealistic and a Pollyanna (or Mary Poppins). The therapist can point out that the view being offered is no less realistic than the patient's negative view. For example:

PATIENT: Now I'm without a job. What do I do? I've got nothing. All that I've worked for is gone, there's nothing left.

THERAPIST: With the job gone, what keeps you in food service? You've considered other jobs, in fact we've spoken of some new career directions. What about those?

PATIENT: That's true. I don't have to sweat quitting. There's no job to quit. I guess in some ways that it makes me free. I hated the job. But I don't know whether I'm ready to do something new at this point.

THERAPIST: Let's explore that idea.

9. *Labeling of distortions.* One of the first steps toward self-knowledge is an identification of the errors in one's thinking. In therapy, patients may find it useful to label the particular cognitive distortions that they notice among their automatic thoughts. The list of distortions offered earlier in this book can be learned by the patient. Once learned, the patient can recognize the ''personalizing'' or ''mind-reading'' that he or she is engaging in. The labeling is helpful for some patients to begin to speak the therapist's language, ''see'' things in a cognitive therapy manner, and learn the style and format of their distorting (*Feeling Good,* Burns, 1980, is an excellent self-help book for the purpose of educating patients about cognitive therapy and the cognitive distortions). For example:

PATIENT: This always happens to me. Whenever I'm in a hurry, there's always a traffic jam.

THERAPIST: What are you doing now?

PATIENT: Yeah, I'm personalizing.

THERAPIST: Do you really believe that the traffic jam had to do with you?

PATIENT: [Laughing] Hey, I'm depressed, not crazy!

10. *Guided Association/Discovery.* Through simple questions such as ''Then what?'', ''What would that mean?'', ''What would happen then?'', the therapist can help the patient explore the personal significance of life experiences. The goal of this technique is to help the patient ''unpack'' the particular baggage that he or she is carrying around. Often, it is only the tip of the iceberg that we see. This collaborative therapist-guided technique stands in opposition to free association in psychoanalysis. The idea behind the free-association strategy is that a ''free'' wandering mind will lead to the hot areas of conflict and concern. In the chained or guided association technique, the therapist works with the patient to connect ideas, thoughts,

and images. The therapist provides conjunctions to the patient's verbalizations. The use of statements like "And then what?", "What evidence do we have that that is true?" and the like allow the therapist to guide the patient along various therapeutic paths, depending on the therapeutic conceptualization and goals. For example:

PATIENT: She'd laugh.

THERAPIST: And then what would happen?

PATIENT: I'd feel like a fool.

THERAPIST: And then what?

PATIENT: I'd be embarrassed, terribly embarrassed.

THERAPIST: Then what?

PATIENT: I don't know. That's as far as I've taken it.

11. *Paradox or exaggeration.* By taking an idea to its extreme, the therapist can help to move the patient to a more central position vis-à-vis a particular belief. Care must be taken to not insult, ridicule, or embarrass the patient. Given a hypersensitivity to criticism and ridicule, some patients may experience the therapist who uses such strategies as making light of their problems. The suicidal patient may see things in their most extreme form. When the therapist takes a *more* extreme stance (i.e., focusing on the absolutes *never, always, no one, everyone*), the patient will often be forced to move from his or her extreme view to a position closer to center. There is the risk, however, that the patient may take the therapist's statement as reinforcement of his or her position of abject hopelessness. The therapist who chooses to use paradox or exaggeration must meet three criteria: (1) a strong working relationship with the patient, (2) superb timing, and (3) the good sense to know when to back away from the technique. For example:

PATIENT: No one would help me, no one cares.

THERAPIST: No one? No one in the whole world?

PATIENT: Well, my parents care, but no one else.

THERAPIST: Let's look at that. It's not true that no one would care. Your parents would, anyone else?

12. *Scaling.* For the suicidal patient who sees things in an "all-or-nothing" fashion, the technique of scaling or seeing things as existing on a continuum can be very helpful. The scaling of a level of belief or feeling can help the patient to utilize the strategy of gaining distance and perspective. Because the patient is at a point of extreme thoughts and extreme behaviors, any movement toward a midpoint is helpful. For example:

THERAPIST: If you put your sadness on a scale of 1–100, how sad are you?

PATIENT: 90–95.

THERAPIST: That's a lot. Can you think of the saddest you have ever been in your life? When was that?

PATIENT: That's easy. When my mother died.

THERAPIST: How sad were you then?

PATIENT: 100!

THERAPIST: Can you remember a time that you were the happiest you have ever been?

PATIENT: Not really.

THERAPIST: No time at all?

PATIENT: Well if you want me to say something happy. . . .

THERAPIST: I was wondering if you have *ever* been happy?

PATIENT: Yeah. On my fifth birthday, I got a train set.

THERAPIST: If that was a happy time, label that a "1" . . . or "0" for sadness. Use those two events, your fifth birthday party as "0" sadness and your mom's death as "100" sadness. Compared to those events, how sad are you now?

PATIENT: Well, compared to that, this is a 50, maybe 45.

13. *Replacement imagery.* Not all automatic thoughts are verbal in nature. The patient's images and dreams are valuable sources of material in the therapy as well. If the patient has dysfunctional images, we can help him or her to generate more effective and functional coping images to replace the depressogenic or anxiogenic ones. Athletes have discovered that the use of coping and successful images can lead to enhanced performance. This performance might be anything from a higher high jump to lifting heavier weights.*

PATIENT: I can just picture myself standing at the bathroom sink. It scares me so. I can see myself reaching for the pills. Just thinking about the image scares me. I can't control it.

THERAPIST: Picture yourself at the sink.

PATIENT: It's hard. I can't do it. I'm scared.

THERAPIST: Try. Picture yourself at the sink. You're looking at the pill bottles in the cabinet. Picture yourself closing the cabinet and walking out of the bathroom. Let's practice that image.

14. *Externalization of voices.* By having the therapist role-play part of the dysfunctional thoughts, the patient can get practice in adaptive responding. At first, the patient can verbalize his or her dysfunctional thoughts, and the therapist can model adaptive responding. After modeling the functional and adaptive thinking, the therapist can, in a gradual manner, become an increasingly difficult dysfunctional voice for the patient to respond to. Patients normally "hear" the dysfunctional voices only in their heads. When they externalize these voices, both patient and therapist are in a better position to modify the voices/messages in a variety of ways. The patient can, hopefully, recognize the dysfunctional nature of the thoughts. The therapist can hear the tone, content, and context of the thoughts and generate strategies for intervention. For example:

THERAPIST: I'd like to be your negative voice. I'd like to help you to be a more positive and functional voice.

PATIENT: I don't think it will make much of a difference, but I'll try.

THERAPIST: Okay. Let's begin. You really don't know what you're talking about!

PATIENT: That's not true. At times I may be over my head, but overall I really do know my stuff.

15. *Cognitive rehearsal.* By visualizing an event in the mind's eye, the patient can covertly practice particular behaviors. A number of athletes use this technique to enhance performance, for example, lifting more weight, jumping higher jumps, scoring more baskets, or taking a horse over a higher jump. By first generating a reasonable scene, the patient can

---

*For a fuller discussion of the use of imagery and dreams in cognitive therapy, see Edwards, Chapter 15, this volume, and Freeman, 1981.

practice it imaginally and can investigate several possibilities. This is akin to a pilot practicing on a simulator to gain aviation skills. For example:

THERAPIST: I'd like you to close your eyes. Picture speaking with your girlfriend. Can you picture this?

PATIENT: Yeah. I don't like it.

THERAPIST: What don't you like?

PATIENT: What I'm seeing.

THERAPIST: What do you see? Describe it.

PATIENT: I see her listening to me and then turning away. I start crying and begging her to stay, and then I start feeling embarrassed and want to die.

THERAPIST: Can you picture not doing the crying and begging?

PATIENT: Not really.

THERAPIST: Let's try to construct a picture that you can live with, both literally and figuratively. What would be a scene you would like to see happen?

16. *Self instruction.* We all talk to ourselves. We give ourselves orders, directions, instructions, or information necessary to solve problems. Meichenbaum (1977) has developed an extensive model for understanding self-instruction. According to Meichenbaum's model, the child moves from overt verbalization of instructions to subvocalization to nonverbalization. This same process can be developed in the adult. For example, in learning impulse control, the patient can start with direct verbalization of self-instructions aloud. With practice, the patient can learn to say the instructions without the actual verbalizations, and the instructions eventually can come more automatically. The patient can be taught to offer direct self-instructions, or in some cases, counterinstructions. The therapist is not introducing a new technique to the patient. Rather, the patient is helped to utilize and strengthen a technique that he or she uses other times. For example:

PATIENT: What do you expect me to do? I just act this way.

THERAPIST: How might you deal more effectively with Jon [the son] when he starts to act up?

PATIENT: Well now, I just respond. I need some space. I want to throw him out of the window.

THERAPIST: What would happen if you could tell yourself the following: I need to just walk away and not respond. I need to walk away and not respond.

PATIENT: Well, if I listened to myself, I might be in better shape.

THERAPIST: That's interesting! If you could tell yourself, very directly, very forcefully to leave the situation, both you and Jon would do better. Is that so?

PATIENT: I suppose. But how can I talk rationally to myself when I'm so angry?

THERAPIST: Let's practice.

17. *Thought stopping.* Dysfunctional thoughts often have a snowball effect for the individual. What may start as a small and insignificant problem can, if left to roll along, gather weight, speed, and momentum. Once on the roll, the thoughts have a force of their own and are very hard to stop. This can be life-threatening for the suicidal patient. Thought stopping is best used when the thoughts *start,* not in the middle of the process. The patient can be taught to picture a stop sign, "hear" a bell, picture a wall, or think the word *stop.* Any of these procedures can help stop the progression and growth of the thoughts. A therapist hitting the desk sharply or ringing a small bell can serve to help the patient to stop the thoughts within a

session. The memory of that intervention can then be used by the client to assist his or her thought stopping between sessions. There is both a distractive and aversive quality to the technique. For example:

PATIENT: I keep thinking about causing plane crashes. God, I'm sweating just thinking about it. My thoughts won't stop. I'm really getting upset. . . . I should be punished.

THERAPIST: [Slapping the desk loudly] STOP!

PATIENT: . . .I . . . I . . . OK.

THERAPIST: When you start, it's really important to stop before you lose control. What just happened? What allowed you to stop?

PATIENT: The noise, I guess.

18. *Focusing.* There is a limit to how many things a person can think about at once. By occupying his or her mind with neutral thoughts, the client can block dysfunctional thoughts for a limited time period. This might involve counting, focusing on calming and pleasant images, or focusing on external stimuli. Although a short-term technique, it can be very useful to allow the patient time to learn some degree of control over his or her or her thinking. This time can then be used to utilize other cognitive techniques. For example:

THERAPIST: I would like to have you subtract the number 17 from 183, and then continue to subtract 17s successively.

PATIENT: That's hard.

THERAPIST: I know. We want to see if the counting can interfere with the rush of suicidal thinking you described.

PATIENT: Let's see. 183, 166, 159, no, 149, 132. This is silly!

THERAPIST: Keep going. 132 . . .

PATIENT: 132, 115, 98, here I go, 81, 64, 47, is that right? 30, 13; that's it.

THERAPIST: Good. How are you feeling?

PATIENT: A bit better, I guess. The thoughts did seem to go away.

19. *Direct disputation.* Although we do not advocate arguing with a patient, there are times when direct disputation may be necessary. A major guideline for its necessity is the imminence of a suicide attempt. When it seems clear to the clinician that the patient is going to make an attempt, the therapist must directly and quickly work to challenge the hopelessness. Disputation generally is not the treatment technique of choice for suicidal patients. The therapist risks becoming embroiled in a power struggle or argument with the patient. Disputation coming from outside the patient may, in fact, engender passive resistance and a passive-aggressive response that might include suicide. Disputation, argument, or debate are potentially dangerous tools. They must be used carefully, judiciously, and with skill. If the therapist becomes one more carping contact, the patient may stop listening and avoid the therapist completely. For example:

THERAPIST: I understand that you are terrified of going crazy, but obviously I'm not as concerned as you are. Would you like to know why?

PATIENT: I guess so.

THERAPIST: The reason is that this isn't the way craziness starts. You're very scared, but there are no signs of craziness. Being afraid of craziness is very different from being crazy.

PATIENT: You mean I'm not crazy? Then why do I have these thoughts?

THERAPIST: No, you're not crazy! The thoughts about killing yourself are not crazy. They are part of being depressed. That's something else.

20. *Cognitive dissonance.* When one's thinking and feeling are in conflict, anxiety can result. Although there are several explanations of this cognitive dissonance phenomenon, it is important to recognize that it exists and can be used therapeutically. The patient who is considering suicide often is dissonant for family (Pfeffer, Conte, Plutchik, & Jerret, 1979), cultural (Goss & Reed, 1971), or religious reasons (Kramer, Pollack, Redick, & Locke, 1972). Their previous learning tells them that suicide may be seen as bad, wrong, or sinful. As long as there is dissonance, suicide is less likely. When the patient resolves his or her dissonance, he or she often feels less pressure and free to make an attempt. The goal of utilizing dissonance with suicidal patients is to generate anxiety and then help them to resolve it in a more effective nonsuicidal way. They might complain that their death will be meaningless or go unnoticed. Having them examine the effect of their death on their children or family can be effective as a deterrent. By fueling the patient's dissonance and increasing the anxiety level, the therapist can help the patient resolve dissonance in an adaptive way. For example:

THERAPIST: What effect will this have on your kids?

PATIENT: They'll survive!

THERAPIST: I'm sure that they will survive, but with what effect? How will what you do influence how they think, feel, or behave in the future?

PATIENT: I don't want to think of it.

THERAPIST: I know, but it is something that's there. You might at least look at this.

PATIENT: Why? Why do I have to look at it? Once I'm gone . . .

THERAPIST: Once you're gone, the effect will linger.

## BEHAVIORAL INTERVENTIONS

There are times when the therapy approach with the suicidal patient will be *cognitive*-behavioral, where the clinical decision is to change the suicidal thoughts and ideation as the focus of the therapy. At other times, especially with the more depressed and vegetative patient, the therapeutic approach may have to be *behavioral*-cognitive, with the initial interventions (or indeed the major focus of therapy) being to change maladaptive behavior. The exact point of delineation between cognition and behavior is debatable.

The goals in using behavioral techniques are twofold. The first goal is to utilize direct behavioral strategies and techniques to alter suicidal behavior as quickly as possible. The behavioral interventions can be used to achieve the short-term but immediate impact often necessary with suicidal patients. The second goal involves the utilization of the behavioral techniques as short-term interventions that allow for the collection of data about the suicidality in the service of longer term cognitive change. In effect, the behavioral component can be the ongoing and longer term ''laboratory'' work of the therapy.

We will discuss several of the most effective behavioral strategies and techniques for working with the suicidal patient. The use of any particular behavioral technique(s) is based on the clinician's assessment of patient need, the patient's ability (either physical or emotional) to comply with a therapeutic regimen, and the therapist's skill in utilizing a particular strategy or intervention.

Working with the suicidal patient can be an uphill struggle against great inertia or an ongoing battle against keen and powerful resistance. The patient may well respond to any interventions with the typical statement, "What's the use, nothing will change." (For a discussion of noncompliance in therapy, see Freeman & Leaf, Chapter 21 this volume).

1. *Activity scheduling.* Common self-statements for many patients include "I'm overwhelmed," "There aren't enough hours in the day to do all that I need to do," "Given my inability to do what needs to be done, I might as well die," "I just sit around all day doing nothing, what's the use of living. I'm just a waste." The same individuals who feel overloaded and unable to cope with what they view as insurmountable demands rarely consider attempting to cope with their perceived load by scheduling time to do what needs to be done. It might only require planning an hour, day, week, or 2 weeks in advance. Given that the suicidal patient is feeling hopeless, the notion of a future orientation, even for an hour, may seem out of line with his or her present thinking. The goal of activity scheduling is not simply to maximize the patient's potential for productivity but to make use of the available time. For the depressed patient generally and the suicidal patient who sees him- or herself as "doing nothing of value," the activity schedule can become evidence that the patient is, or is not, doing anything of value. Three uses of the schedule are assessment, planning, and mastery/pleasure ratings.

By utilizing the activity schedule in the first session as a part of the session work or a homework assignment for the next session, the therapist can assess the patient's present use of time in order to reality-test his or her idea that he or she is doing nothing. It can be used to help him or her plan better and more productive use of time to attack the hopelessness, and finally, to begin to socialize the patient to the idea of doing homework.

If the activity schedule is used as part of the session work, the therapist can either coach the patient on the best use of the schedule or fill the schedule out based on the patient's data. What must be avoided is falling into the trap of the patient's hopelessness and labeling whole blocks of time as *sitting, in bed, watching TV,* or *doing nothing.* Even when watching TV, other behaviors, no matter how minimal, are probably being manifested. The cognitive and behavioral techniques are not mutually exclusive. The very work on the activity scheduling will probably bring out the negative cognitions that need to be responded to. If the task seems to be overwhelming to the patient, the therapist can work it a day at a time, starting with the day of the session.

The following activity schedule was completed by a 60-year-old physician recently diagnosed with metastasized bone cancer. He has been treated successfully and presently had residual pain from the treatments.

As can be seen, he is doing very little. He was feeling useless, sensing no chance to do more, and therefore concluded that he might as well succumb to the cancer and die. Any attempt on the part of his wife and son to schedule activity had been met with, "What's the use, there is nothing I can do." The goal of activity scheduling was to start with very simple and nonstressful activities. If activities could be developed that were slightly engaging, the data could be used to help refute the idea that he could do nothing and that death was his only alternative.

The activity scheduling attempted to generate activity and thereby begin to reduce his suicidality. Utilizing the activity schedule prospectively, the therapist and patient work collaboratively within the first few sessions to schedule activities for the rest of that day and the following day. Follow-up activity scheduling can be completed by phone so that there can be reinforcement of the activity engaged in, decatastrophizing the noncompliance and strengthening the therapeutic alliance. The activity schedule, once utilized, needs to be checked at each session so that the patient does not get the message that the scheduling work is not important. For suicidal patients, having a goal, meaning, and focus to their lives may serve to temporarily lessen their suicidality. Activity scheduling can then be used to help structure their lives and to serve as evidence of their ability to do more than they once thought themselves capable. A common patient belief that interferes with compliance is the notion that activities *should not* have to be scheduled. Activities should happen naturally and spontaneously. These cognitions must be dealt with immediately and directly.

A third use of the activity schedule is to have the patient rate the mastery and pleasure derived from the activities. Inasmuch as the suicidal patient rarely experiences either mastery or pleasure, it then becomes a therapeutic focus to assess and develop mastery and pleasure activities as techniques for lessening the suicidality.

2. *Mastery and Pleasure Ratings.* The patient can begin to list, examine, and reality-test mastery (M = how well they see themselves as doing something) and pleasure (P = how much they enjoyed something). The activity schedule can be utilized not only for assessing the present levels of M and P but also to begin to generate and plan more and greater mastery and pleasure experiences. The patient's significant others can be enjoined, in many cases, to help the patient be more active. By having the patient examine what he or she would like to do, we can assess the reality and likelihood that he or she will do what he or she desires. For example, a 52-year-old woman was depressed and hopeless about ever working again as a creative artist. She had worked in all media and was especially interested in sculpting. She could not, she claimed, find the time to do her artwork, given the incessant demands of others on her time and energy. She rated sculpting as a 9/10 on a 10 scale. Mastery was equally high (8/9). The therapeutic goal was to attempt to plan an hour per day that she could set aside to do her artwork. She refused, saying that it would take her that much time to get ready to work. Time would be taken away from other activities that she was loath to do. By working toward an effective schedule, time was set aside to allow her some artwork rather than none, thereby allowing her both mastery and pleasure in her life with a concomitant lessening of her hopelessness and suicidal ideation.

A second example is of a 32-year-old woman who indicated that her pleasure ratings for the hours of 7 to 10 P.M. on a Friday evening were 7, the highest they had been in weeks. She had gone to the theatre, something she did three times a year. When she was asked whether she could schedule more theatre going as part of her pleasure activities, she responded that it had never occurred to her to go more often.

3. *Graded task assignments.* The patient who feels hopeless sees him- or herself as unable to change his or her life. He or she perceives a scenario that cannot be altered wherein life tasks are perceived as overwhelming. The manner in which the patient reacts and responds to people and situations and the perceived powerlessness to change the situations in which they find themselves involved contribute to the hopelessness. The graded task work is a "shaping" strategy. Each small, sequential step approximates the eventual goal and can help the patient expand his or her activities in a gradual manner. It is important to avoid taking too large an initial step, for the patient may experience failure if he or she is not cautioned to "watch the first step, it's a beauty." For the suicidal patient, any step may appear too large. Several small steps can be reinforcing as the patient starts to experience mastery or achievement. However, for some patients, especially those who are demanding, their response to small sequential steps is often "so what," "big deal," or "it's not enough." A colleague reported the following interaction:

> The patient was severely depressed, bed-bound, hopeless, and unwilling to become active. The therapist initiated a sequence of behaviors starting with having the patient place his foot out from under the covers. This was followed by a series of steps eventuating in asking the patient to leave the bed, walk across the room, and touch the opposite wall. When the patient finally left the bed and touched the wall, the patient turned to the therapist and said, "BIG DEAL," and went back to bed.

The initial behavior in the sequence must be well within the range the patient can easily accomplish.

4. *Behavioral rehearsal.* The session can be used to practice potential behaviors or interactions, that is, dealing directly with a significant other, a boss, or a friend. The therapist can give feedback on the patient's performance, and coach the patient both on more effective

specific responses and response styles or model new behaviors. This strategy may be used for the practice of existing skills, or, if necessary, skill building.

If a patient had concern that he or she would sound too angry and aggressive, scripting the interaction (Bower & Bower, 1976) can be helpful. Role-playing specific interactions using different words or approaches allows the patient to leave the session feeling greater confidence in his or her ability to address particular life issues having had some practice.

Skill building would include both social skills and assertiveness training. When a patient describes having social difficulty, or the therapist observes social difficulties in the therapeutic interaction, the therapist cannot assume that the problem exists because the patient does not want to behave differently. There may be a skills deficit and not just a motivational deficit. Part of the work of therapy involves helping the patient gain the social skills that have been missed during normal development and that are now contributing to the hopelessness. For example:

> The patient entered therapy and early in the initial interview began to talk about his chronic loneliness. He thought that no woman would ever want to be with him and that it was of little use to continue to try to go to bars, clubs, or parties. His social skills were poor; his assessment in that regard was quite accurate. One goal of therapy was directed at building social skills.

6. *In vivo exposure.* For many problems, the most effective manner of intervention may be direct modeling in an *in-vivo* setting. Agoraphobia, social phobia, or social anxiety difficulties can be treated with the therapist working with the patient in the very situations that generate the "heat." This is far more effective than getting patient reports of the problems a week later. *In vivo* work might include traveling with the patient, making home visits, or practicing assertiveness skills at a shopping center.

7. *Relaxation, meditation, and breathing exercises.* For the anxious patient, the use of progressive relaxation, focused breathing, and meditation can help to provide distraction and thereby help the patient begin to gain a sense of control over the anxiety response. Hyperventilation and other focused breathing techniques are useful for mastering overbreathing (cf. Freeman & Simon, Chapter 18, this volume).

8. *Homework.* The patient's socialization to the cognitive therapy model must include an explanation of the importance, purpose, and potential benefits of homework. The premise of the homework is that it will help the patient feel less suicidal. The homework can begin in the first session by having the patient complete a relatively simple and straightforward assignment for discussion at the second session. A good homework assignment for this first therapy session can be the activity schedule, as discussed previously.

Basic to the practice of cognitive therapy is the recognition that the therapy is not totally accomplished in the hour or two per week that the patient is in the therapist's office. A major part of the patient's contribution to the collaboration is completing self-help work at home. Clinical experience suggests that the patients who do more self-help work make progress more quickly in therapy and are able to meet their stated therapy goals more quickly, as well. Self-help work includes any and all of the cognitive and behavioral techniques described before. The nature and number of interventions and the amount of work all need to be appropriate to the problem, within the skill range of the patient, and collaboratively developed. Homework for the suicidal patient must be developed with a graded task focus. Setting homework beyond the present energy or attentional level of the patient may, in point of fact, add to the patient's hopelessness. Conversely, accomplishing even simple tasks outside of the session can enhance the patient's sense of hopefulness. The homework review is noted early in the agenda-setting phase of the session and then included and discussed as part of the session material (see Perris, Chapter 16, this volume).

The patient who has overcome the suicidal crisis can be helped in a more traditional cognitive behavioral therapy to challenge dysfunctional thinking, question evidence, look at alternatives, reattribute responsibility, and assess consequences.

343

TREATMENT OF
SUICIDAL BEHAVIOR

## LEGAL AND ETHICAL RESPONSIBILITIES

The law in most jurisdictions states simply that if an individual is an *imminent* danger to him- or herself or others, he or she should be considered for hospitalization. Ideally, the individual can be helped to enter the hospital setting voluntarily, but, in some cases, the therapist may need to initiate or assist the patient's family to effect a nonvoluntary admission. Hospitalization is used as a way of helping a suicidal patient into a setting where he or she will be protected, and where appropriate treatment can be administered and monitored. A patient in a hospital may be on suicide watch or suicide precautions. However, hospitalization in and of itself is not sufficient to prevent an individual from committing suicide. Although it is much more difficult to effect a suicide in a hospital setting, the insistant individual can always find a way. That way may be to act in a reasonable "nonsuicidal" way for a period of time so that precautions are relaxed. Therefore it is crucial to address the hopelessness, whether the patient is treated on an inpatient or outpatient basis.

There are a number of steps in the evaluation of suicidal potential. The patient is asked whether he or she has suicidal motives, plans, and means (e.g., presence of a weapon or lethal doses of medication). The adequacy of the patient's social network (e.g., whether someone is present as a support and monitor) is examined along with any history (remote or recent) of self-destructive behavior. *The most important initial strategy in working with the suicide patient, having assessed the plan and method of suicide, is to dispose of the means of the suicide.* This might include asking the individual who collects guns and has a favorite gun waiting to be used to turn it to the police, give the gun to a significant other, or even bring it in to the therapist. One patient reported that he had three handguns loaded and available to use in a planned suicide attempt. After a rather lengthy discussion, he was convinced to turn over the guns to his brother who would keep them indefinitely. The patient was asked to call the therapist that evening to confirm that the guns had indeed been turned over to his brother. What the patient reported instead was the he had a change of heart and rather than turning the guns over to his brother, he went to the river and tossed the guns, in a paper bag, over the side and watched them sink beneath the water. How can the therapist be sure that the guns were safely on the bottom of the river? There was, of course, no sure method. The patient may have kept the guns and without the word of the brother or significant other as to the guns being in their possession for safekeeping, the patient may have kept his or her suicide option open.

Another patient who had reported amassing vast quantities of medication was asked to bring the medication into the therapist. The medication that the patient brought in literally filled a shoebox and included Thorazine, Valium, Librium, Sinequan, Ludiomil, Elavil, Dalmane, Aventyl, and Ritalin. Individuals who are potentially suicidal should be prescribed the smallest amounts possible without the ability to renew the prescription constantly. Although giving small amounts of drugs does not prevent the patient from hoarding, giving large amounts of drugs makes it too easy. Enlisting a significant other to monitor or dispense the medication may relieve both the therapist and the patient. Individuals who feel compelled to cut or slash should be encouraged to dispose of razor blades and other extremely sharp objects.

A second intervention that must be considered is one required by law, that is, informing a significant other of the patient's suicidal intent. If a patient makes it clear to the therapist that he or she plans to imminently exercise the suicide option and the therapist does not make any attempt to contact the significant other, the therapist might find him- or herself in legal jeopardy. Confidentiality does not preclude sharing of suicidal intent when the therapist feels that suicide is imminent. On this point, there might be some disagreement among therapists. Many feel that to inform a significant other of the patient's suicidal intent is a breech of confidence that destroys the therapeutic relationship. The therapist must report an imminent suicidal act. Our position is that a live patient will live to see another therapist; a dead patient's suicide terminates the possibility of further therapy.

### The Therapist as Survivor

The suicide of a patient can be an incredibly harrowing experience for the therapist (Brown, 1987; Chemtob, Hamada, Bauer, Kinney, & Torigoe, 1988; Goldstein & Buongiorno, 1984). The experience can be especially difficult because the therapist has often expended great time, energy, effort, and emotion helping the patient. The therapist also may view the suicide as a personal failure. The therapist of the suicidal patient can often carry the heaviest burden of any of the survivors of a suicide or suicide attempt (Binder, 1978; Henn, 1978; Litman, 1965). After all, the therapist is the acknowledged expert who is expected to prevent suicide. The average psychotherapist is not accustomed to coping with the death of a patient and does not have the extensive experience in dealing with death that many of our medical colleagues have. The rarity of the experience and our lack of sophistication in dealing with it make a therapist even more vulnerable to significant cognitive distortions and extreme reactions in response to a patient's suicide. Chemtob *et al.* (1988) found that psychiatrists who had had a patient suicide reported that it significantly disrupted every aspect of life.

Very few relationships have the intimacy and power of the patient–therapist relationship. On the patient's side it involves risk-taking, exposing one's faults and flaws, looking at one's dysfunctional thinking and maladaptive behavior, and verbalizing unspoken fears and thoughts that are often not shared for any of a variety of reasons with one's most significant others. From the therapist's side, it is a total focus on the patient. Few interruptions come between patient and therapist. The therapist's attention is focused on helping the patient develop strategies for coping with inter- and intrapersonal problems of life, making a therapist appear to be a very altruistic and unselfish character. The therapist does not demand payment in time (i.e., now you have unburdened yourself, let me unburden myself), rather payment and tender are of another kind—money. Although it has been said that the patient "buys" the therapist's time, attention, love, and caring, truthfully the only thing that can be "bought" is the time. Yet the therapist may experience a strong personal investment in the patient's well-being. The following quotes are from practicing therapists in response to the experience of having a patient suicide.

> Therapist No 1—I have been in practice for about 30 years. My very first experience with a patient suicide happened when I was an intern. Nobody talked about it; everyone ignored it. My supervisors and administrators just didn't talk about it. It seemed appropriate that I not talk about it. It took me over a year to put the pieces together for myself. During all that time, I was extremely depressed and upset and thought almost everyday of leaving medicine.

> Therapist No. 2.—I had only seen him three times. I had some real questions about whether there were significant organic factors with this guy, but I never did get a chance to check him out because he killed himself right after our third session. I couldn't help but feel that there was something I could have done but didn't do. Maybe I should have been more attentive to what he said. I am sure he must have given me clues as to how suicidal he was. I experienced the same stages as anyone who is faced with death. At first, there was disbelief and nonacceptance, followed by resignation, and finally an acceptance of his or her death. I am still uncomfortable with it, but the thing that helped most was to talk about it. Those people who offered themselves to talk with me about the experience were the most helpful. Some people seemed embarrassed and put off and were very ill at ease in discussing it. That situation upset me a whole lot. I really had a need to talk.

> Therapist No. 3—I don't want anyone talking about her. Talking about her won't bring her back, and I can't see what value it would serve to even mention her name. I know it is difficult, but I think I just have to forget her.

Therapist No. 4—When she died, I had the thought that I would be blamed. Her family knew she was in therapy, and her boyfriend had come to see me so he knew who I was. If she died, he would sue me. They would probably make a case that I'd done something wrong, and, God knows, I may have. It really got crazy because I exaggerated and had this image of having to be in court and being questioned about what I did and then finally having the parents give me a group of psychologists and psychiatrists to swear that I had done the wrong things. It is really strange. I was really upset because I didn't want her to die, but I think at times I was less concerned about her dying than with the effect it would have on me. She even said to me, "It is going to be your fault. You don't care about me. Nobody cares. You think you can stop me? Nobody can! Maybe I won't do it today or tonight, but one day when I can't take anymore, I'm going, and I hope that you, my mother, and my boss feel guilty because you are all shitty to me."

If we feel strongly that the theory and technique we espouse, namely the cognitive-behavioral model, is an appropriate treatment for our patients, why should it be any less so for ourselves or our colleagues? An important, if not essential, part in dealing with the suicide of a patient is to talk with a colleague, a supervisor, and/or a peer and to make explicit the concerns, thoughts, and emotions that we are having at that time. The therapist working with suicidal patients needs an opportunity to talk with peers to air specific cognitive distortions and to speak with supervisors about the particular treatment so that an assessment can be made as to whether he or she is implementing the most appropriate and efficacious interventions possible. If, after the best efforts on the part of the therapist, the patient does attempt suicide, it is incumbent upon the colleagues and co-workers to help the therapist by not treating him or her as though he or she was a leper but by offering as much support and caring as if the therapist had lost a loved relative. The loss of a relative is often easier to adjust to in that it is a personal loss, whereas the lost patient is not only a personal loss but also a blow to one's competence, self-esteem, prestige, and ability to help others.

## SUMMARY

By directly intervening at the level of hopelessness, the future-oriented negative cognition, we can make a rapid and substantial inroad into suicidal ideation. By addressing hopelessness directly, the patient perceives the therapist as being understanding and having a greater sense of what he or she is experiencing. The goal of the therapist is to then offer the patient both alternatives and options. As for the interventions for those patients who have said they have been in therapy before and have not been successful, we can ask if they have ever been in cognitive therapy before. If the answer then is no (and it probably will be), we can ask that they prolong their suicidal decision until they have given cognitive therapy a chance to work.

## REFERENCES

Barraclough, B. (1973). Differences between national suicide rates. *British Journal of Psychiatry, 122,* 247–256.

Beck, A. T. (1985). *Anxiety disorders and phobias.* New York: Basic Books (1985).

Beck, A. T., Kovacs, M., & Weissman, A. (1979). Assessment of suicidal intention: The Scale for Suicidal Ideation, *Journal of Clinical and Consulting Psychology, 47,* 343–352.

Beck, A. T., Ward, C. H., Mendelson, M., Mock, J. & Erbaugh, J. (1961). An inventory for measuring depression. *Archives of General Psychiatry, 4,* 561–571.

Beck, R., Morris, J., & Lester, D. (1974). Suicide notes and risk of future suicide. *Journal of the American Medical Association, 228,* 495–496.

Beck, A. T., Weissman, A., Lester, D., & Trexler, L. (1975). The measurement of pessimism: The Hopelessness Scale. *Journal of Consulting and Clinical Psychology, 42,* 861–865.

Beck, A. T., Rush, A. J., Shaw, B. F., & Emery, G. (1979). *Cognitive therapy of depression*. New York: Guilford Press.

Binder, R. (1978). Dealing with patients suicide. *American Journal of Psychiatry, 135,* 1113.

Bower, S. A., & Bower, G. H. (1976). *Asserting yourself*. Reading, MA: Addison-Wesley.

Brown, H. N. (1987). The impact of suicide on psychiatrists in training. *Comprehensive Psychitry, 28,* 101–112.

Burns, (1980). *Feeling good*. New York: Morrow.

Chemtob, C. M., Hamada, R. S., Bauer, G., Kinney, B., & Torigoe, R. Y. (1988). Patients' suicides: Frequency and impact on psychiatrists. *American Journal of Psychiatry, 145,* 224–228.

Christensen, R. (1984). The misdiagnosis of holiday and winter complaints: An unconscious shift in criteria? *Psychotherapy, 21,* 401.

Diekstra, R. (1974). A social learning theory approach to the prevention of suicidal behavior. *Proceedings of the 7th International Congress for Suicide Prevention* (pp. 55–66). Amsterdam: Swets & Zeitlinger, BV.

Freeman, A. (1981). The use of dreams and imagery in cognitive therapy. In G. Emery, S. D. Hollon, & R. C. Bedrosian (Eds.), *New directions in cognitive therapy* (pp. 224–238). New York: Guilford Press.

Freeman, A. (1988). Cognitive therapy of personality disorders. In C. Perris, H. Perris & I. Blackburn. *The theory and practice of cognitive therapy*. Heidelberg: Springer Verlag.

Freeman, A, & Reinecke, M. (1989). *Cognitive therapy of suicidal behavior*. New York: Springer Publishers.

Garfinkel, B., Froese, A., & Golombek, H. (1979). Suicidal behavior in a pediatric population. *Proceedings of the 10th International Congress for Suicide Prevention* (pp. 302–312). Ottawa: IASP.

Goldstein, L. S., & Buongiorno, P. A. (1984). Psychotherapists as suicide survivors. *American Journal of Psychotherapy, 38,* 392–398.

Goss, M., & Reed, J. (1971). Suicide and religion. *Life Threatening Behavior, 1,* 163–177.

Henn, R. F. (1978). Patient suicide as part of psychiatric residency. *American Journal of Psychiatry, 135,* 745–746.

Juel-Nielsen, N., & Videbeck, T. (1970). A twin study of suicide. *Acta Genetica. Med. Gemmellol., 19,* 307–310.

Kramer, M., Pollack, E., Redick, R., & Locke, B. (1972). *Mental Disorders/Suicide*. Cambridge: Harvard University Press.

Keith-Spiegel, P., & Spiegel, D. E. Affective states of patients immediately preceding suicide. *Journal of Psychiatric Research, 5,* 89–93.

Kovacs, M., Beck, A. T., & Weissman, A. (1976). The communication of suicidal intent. *Archives of General Psychiatry, 33,* 198–201.

Lester, D. (1983). *Why people kill themselves*. Springfield, IL: Thomas.

Lester, D., & Beck, A. (1975). Suicide in the spring. *Psychological Reports, 35,* 893–894.

Lester, D., Beck, A., & Bruno, S. (1976). Correlates of choice of method for suicide. *Psychological Reports, 13,* 70–73.

Litman, R. E. (1965). When patients commit suicide. *American Journal of Psychotherapy, 19,* 570–576.

Meichenbaum. (1977). *Cognitive behavior modification*. New York: Plenum Press.

Pfeffer, C., Conte, H., Plutchik, R., & Jerret, I. (1979). Suicidal behavior in latency age children. *Journal of the American Academy of Child Psychiatry, 18,* 679–692.

*Physicians Desk Reference*. (1988). Ordell, NJ: Medical Economics.

Pokorny, A. (1960). Characteristics of forty-four patients who subsequently committed suicide. *Archives of General Psychiatry, 2,* 314.

Robins, E., Gassner, S., Kayes, J., Wilkinson, R. H., & Kayes, J. (1959). Some clinical considerations in the prevention of suicide based on a study of 134 successful suicides. *American Journal of Public Health, 49,* 888.

Rogers, S., & Luenes, A. (1979). A psychometric and behavioral comparison of delinquents who were abused as children with their nonabused peers. *Journal of Clinical Psychology, 35,* 470–472.

Rogot, E., Fabsitz, R., & Feinleib, M. (1976). Daily variations in USA mortality. *American Journal of Epidemiology, 103,* 198–211.

Stein, M., Levy, M., & Glasberg, M. (1974). Separations in black and white suicide attempters. *Archives of General Psychiatry, 31,* 815–821.

Tsuang, M. (1977). Genetic factors in suicide. *Disorders of the Nervous System, 38,* 498–501.

Wilson, M. (1981). Suicidal behavior: Toward an explanation of differences in female and male rates. *Suicide and Life Threatening Behavior, 11,* 131–140.

# 18

# Cognitive Therapy of Anxiety

ARTHUR FREEMAN AND KAREN M. SIMON

Anxiety is among the most common of human responses. When experienced in moderate quantity, it can serve to motivate, energize, and mobilize the individual (Izard & Blumberg, 1985; Lindsley, 1952, 1957, 1960). Many people maintain that they "work best under pressure," that is, when their anxiety level is high enough, they are motivated to do their best, or only, work. On the other hand, the anxiety level may be so high that it can debilitate the individual and cause both emotional and physical discomfort and pain (Lindsley, 1952, 1957, 1960). Although the particular permutations of cognitive and behavioral anxiety symptoms differ from person to person, the basic physiological concomittants of the experience are common to all people. We *experience* the emotion of anxiety because of the physiological correlates (Gray, 1985; Schacter, 1964, 1967; Spielberger 1966, 1972; Stokes, 1985; Weiner, 1985). These physiological sequalae can affect every system of the body causing dermal, respiratory, circulatory, gastrointestinal, or muscular systems. In some cases, the problems can be severe enough to cause health problems, that is, ulcers, hypertension (Agras, 1985; Dimsdale, 1985). Given the potentially life-threatening impact of anxiety, it has persisted as a human response throughout human existence. Some authors have speculated that anxiety as a response mechanism has had survival value for the race (Plutchik, 1980), or a "significant evolutionary advantage" that "must have contributed in significant ways to adaptation to a dangerous environment" (Beck, 1985, p. 185).

According to DSM-II (APA, 1968), *anxiety* was defined as "the chief characteristic of the neuroses" (p. 39). Consistent with psychoanalytic theory, DSM-II held that the different neurotic states were simply different manifestations of the same problem. In anxiety neurosis, the anxiety was directly expressed, whereas in the other neurotic states (phobic neurosis, hysterical neurosis, obsessive compulsive neurosis, depressive neurosis, neurasthenic neurosis, depersonalization neurosis, or hypochondriacal neurosis), the anxiety was somehow masked and converted so as to cause depression or some other problematic symptom. Freud (1933) considered anxiety manifestations to be a deflection or conversion of sexual energy, with the particular symptoms seen to be substitutes for the sexual activity. Whether the anxiety

ARTHUR FREEMAN AND KAREN M. SIMON • Center for Cognitive Therapy, Department of Psychiatry, University of Pennsylvania, Philadelphia, Pennsylvania 10104.

was free-floating and thereby generating a general apprehensiveness or anticipatory state, whether the anxiety was firmly attached though exaggerated, as in phobia, or as an attack or persistant state, as in severe neuroses, the core of the. problem was the repression of basic libidinal impulses. Depression and anxiety were consequently seen to be a part of a continuum, that is, people get so anxious that they become depressed, or people are so depressed that they become anxious. Clinically, we often see anxiety and depression as coexisting in the same patient, thereby yielding two diagnoses. The rationale for this view is offered by psycho-analytic theory, which conceptualizes anxiety as caused by the intrapsychic battle to maintain good "objects," both internalized and externalized (Klein, 1948). Horney (1937) utilized the term *basic anxiety* to describe the person's general feelings of loneliness and helplessness in a potentially hostile world.

The anxiety response may manifest itself directly as anxiety, where the individual experiences the increased respiration, blood pressure changes, increased heart rate, or changes to the galvanic skin response at various times with various levels of severity. The anxiety may be focused on a particular situation or object and trouble the individual as a phobic response. Or the individual may depend on a primitive magical and repetitive thought or action to protect himself or herself and ward off the anxiety as in the obsessive-compulsive reactions and hypochondria. The severity of the anxiety response runs the gamut from a minor irritant to a panic response that is severely debilitating. Despite the range of responses to various internal and external stimuli that constitute the anxiety syndrome, effective treatment strategies and techniques can be utilized to control and cope with runaway anxiety.

The basic themes of anxiety are the threat or actuality of danger (Beck & Emery, 1985). Whether the threat is to person or domain, psychological or physical, real or imagined, threat is the common thread through the anxiety states. Campbell (1981) differentiates between fear and anxiety. He states that "fear is a reaction to a real or threatened danger, while anxiety is more typically a reaction to an unreal or imagined danger" (p. 42). Anxiety can be viewed in three different ways, that is, as "real" anxiety, "neurotic" anxiety, and "moral" anxiety. Real anxiety involves real danger, as objectively viewed: For example, a person with a gun approaches you and asks for your money or else he threatens to kill you. A general consensus of people would show anxiety to be the normative experience in that situation. Anxiety can also be viewed as as "neurotic" anxiety, which is a dysfunctional, idiosyncratic response: For example, 10 people may see a small dog confined in a fenced yard, and perhaps one will experience fear. Finally, there is moral anxiety or guilt that is the response to having violated personal, societal, or religious rules or schema: For example, a child lies to her parents and experiences guilt for being "bad."

## A COGNITIVE MODEL OF ANXIETY

Anxiety involves the individual's perception of danger or threat. This threat is seen to be directed at self or domain (focus of threat), from the world (locus of theat), and involving present and future consequences (direction of threat) (Beek, 1970).

The basic Cognitive Therapy model of anxiety (Freeman, Pretzer, Fleming, & Simon, 1989), involves several elements. The individual starts with an actual situation and then has a perception of that situation based on beliefs and assumptions (basic schema). The individual must make an assessment of perceived threat or perceived self-efficacy. If a situation is perceived as a threat, the person will feel endangered. If the perception is not threat but challenge, the person will feel excitement and enthusiasm. We might use the example of two skiers at the top of a high slope. Skier 1 is an experienced and well-practiced skier and sees the slope as a challenge that will be exhilarating and great fun. Skier 2 has skied only once before and sees the slope as just slightly higher than the Matterhorn and a great threat. Thus, the perception of threat and self-efficacy importantly determine our emotional reactions to life situations.

If we see a situation as involving no danger at all, we remain calm. When we are already feeling anxious, we become even more vigilant to perceived threats and begin to see threat where none existed. If we perceive a situation as dangerous and we enter that situation and are able to cope successfully, we may increase our sense of self-efficacy depending upon our attributions for our success. If, however, we avoid situations as phobics do, we will experience a decreased sense of self-efficacy.

Our perceptions are organized around basic schema (Beck *et al.*, 1979; Freeman, 1986), which are the assumptions underlying our perceptions of reality and the rules by which we live. Schema are learned from the major socializing agents (home, school, and religion) and may be in place as early as middle childhood (age 8). These schema can be personal, religious, cultural, gender, or family based. In general, schema can be viewed along two continua for purposes of predicting emotional and behavioral reactions—active/dormant and compelling/noncompelling. The active/dormant continuum implies that certain schemata are active and govern our day-to-day behavior, whereas other schema are dormant, that is, they exist but do not govern day-to-day functioning. The dormant schema emerge when the individual is under stress. The newly active schema will serve to direct behavior for as long as needed and then return to the previous dormant state. For example, most people would abide by the rule, "Thou shalt not kill." Some people would not only refrain from killing but would not eat the flesh of a butchered animal. The active schema/rule vis-à-vis killing is that "killing is wrong/bad/unacceptable." However, if a person were put into a situation wherein his or her children were being threatened with bodily harm or death by an attacker, this individual might be capable of killing the attacker to protect his or her children. The dormant rule, "protect your children," may be stimulated into an active state and will then direct behavior. When the threat or stressor is past, the dormant schema returns to its previous state of dormancy. The person who kills to protect his or her family will not likely acquire a blood lust.

As noted, schema may also be compelling or noncompelling. An individual can rather easily abandon a noncompelling schema but would find it virtually impossible to abandon a more compelling schema. The compelling schema is seen as "self," rather than as simply some part of self. For example, many people have a reluctance to eat snails but with some prodding might be willing to take a small taste. If they liked what they tasted, they might abandon the idea that snails are disgusting crawly things, and are, instead, tasty. On the other hand, the history of religion has many examples of martyrs giving their lives to avoid abandoning their religion. Thus certain schema will be more important and basic for conceptualizing a particular person than will others. To the extent that therapy is challenging compelling schema, the course will understandably be slower and more difficult than when therapy is challenging noncompelling schema.

The schema are important on a day-to-day basis even if the patient has never actually articulated them because it is the schema that generate the patient's automatic thoughts. The automatic thoughts appear to arise spontaneously and automatically in response to life events and give meaning to those events. These thoughts tend to be dysfunctional among patient populations because they include many cognitive distortions (Beck *et al.*, 1979). This distorted thinking is a key component in many of psychological problems. The therapist can, by carefully tracking the dysfunctional thoughts, gain a sense of the direction, content, and style of the schema. For example, the patient who has thoughts such as, "A 98 on a test is like a failing grade," may have many other perfectionistic and demanding thoughts that may all relate to a schema like, "To be loved/thought well of/approved of, I must be perfect." The rule regarding one's personal value being judged by performance has its roots in cultural, familial, gender, or personal schema (Freeman, 1986; Good & Kleinman, 1985).

The principles of Cognitive Therapy have been capsuled by Beck and Emery (1985) as follows:

*Principle 1: Cognitive therapy is based on the cognitive model of emotional disorders.* Cognitive Therapy involves more than merely applying a list of intervention techniques to a particular problem. The Cognitive Therapist works within the dynamic framework of the relationship between thought-feelings-behavior and underlying schema, which is based on the cognitive model of emotion (Beck, 1976; Beck *et al.,* 1979). This requires a conceptualization of the case that takes into account the patient's idiosyncratic assumptions and rules of life and requires an understanding of how this individual's automatic thoughts give rise to problematic emotional and behavioral reactions. Only when a working conceptualization has been developed can appropriate interventions be chosen that can be expected to be helpful.

*Principle 2: Cognitive therapy is brief, time-limited, and focused.* Keeping therapy brief helps both the therapist and patient to maintain a problem focus and to get to the business of therapy without undue delay. It also helps to avoid the dependency upon therapy and therapist that is a pitfall for patients participating in long-term models of treatment.

*Principle 3: A sound therapeutic relationship is a necessary condition for effective cognitive therapy.* The requirements of good therapy remain the same, regardless of the therapeutic model. The ability of the therapist to develop a working alliance with the patient is essential. Empathy, effective listening skills, and a concern for the well-being of the patient are essential aspects of therapy.

*Principle 4: Therapy is a collaborative effort between therapist and patient.* The therapeutic collaboration involved in cognitive therapy means that the patient and therapist work together as partners, collaborators, or "co-scientists" (Beck *et al.,* 1979). This means that both have input into decisions regarding therapeutic goals, the pacing of therapy, homework assignments, and so on. The collaboration is not necessarily 50/50. The more depressed or passive the patient, the greater the role of the therapist in the collaboration; once the time for termination is approaching, the patient would be expected to take the greater role. This collaboration has great value in helping to foster independence, a sense of responsibility for solving one's own problems, and for reducing the likelihood of noncompliance. However, patients who have come to therapy to be "therapized," that is, to have therapy "done" to them, will have difficulty being an active collaborator and may not be as involved in the process of the therapy.

*Principle 5: Cognitive therapy uses primarily the Socratic method.* The Socratic method involves the use of strategic questions to help the patient arrive at his or her own revelations and answers, rather than being told the answers. The use of a questioning model as a therapy tool as opposed to direct disputation, restatement, or direct sharing of information is generally preferred in cognitive therapy for a variety of reasons. Questions can serve to help the patient: (1) become aware of the content of his or her thoughts, (2) begin to identify his or her style of thinking, (3) examine his or her thoughts for particular cognitive distortions, (4) substitute more adaptive thoughts (content or style), (5) plan future strategies for dealing with his or her thoughts or actions.

Most clinicians have been taught the cardinal rule in questioning, which is to *always* use open-ended questions. However, our recommendation is to use *closed-ended* questioning with anxious patients. Although this may seem heretical, intrusive, and noncollaborative, it is, in fact, more collaborative, less intrusive, but still heretical. The anxious patient, when faced with open-ended questions may become even more anxious. By asking relatvely simple, direct questions, his or her anxiety level will be lowered. The therapist can then insert an open-ended question, to be followed by a series of closed-ended questions. For example, rather than, "tell me why you have come," the therapist can ask, "can you tell me three reasons that bring you in here." (This technique works especially well with adolescents who come into therapy anxious by virtue of being forced to come and speak to an adult).

*Principle 6: Cognitive therapy is structured and directive.* One of the most important contributions of brief therapy has been the notion of maintaining a high degree of structure. The therapist can, by keeping the therapy structured and focused, work on the discrete parts of a problem rather than attempting to work on the entire problem at once. The latter model is akin to trying to eat an entire meal in a mouthful. The meal will be better digested a mouthful at a time.

Furthermore, for the many patients who come to therapy to try to organize their lives, a free-floating, loosely organized, and unstructured psychotherapy is contraindicated. To help the anxious patient deal with the uncertainty inherent in his or her anxiety, a strong focus for the therapy and a directive stance for the therapist are important.

*Principle 7: Cognitive therapy is problem oriented.* The basic cognitive therapy model involves setting out an explicit problem list, prioritizing the list, and then actively working on the problems. This enables a greater amount of therapeutic work to be done in a shorter time than in the nonproblem-oriented treatment model. It also ensures that the patient's needs and goals will be addressed, rather than using a model wherein the therapist has a vague, unstated agenda.

*Principle 8: Cognitive therapy is based on an educational model.* The psychoeducational nature of cognitive therapy involves a sharing of information through bibliotherapy, direct information from the therapist, and the therapist being available as a resource for the patient. Limited self-disclosure may be appropriate, depending on the patient.

*Principle 9: The theory and techniques of cognitive therapy rely on the inductive method.* Just as the cognitive therapist generates private and public hypotheses to be tested in the therapy through questioning and data collection, the patient in cognitive therapy is trained to be more of a "scientist," that is, not accepting unconfirmed automatic thoughts but rather testing ideas by data collection.

*Principle 10: Homework is a central feature of cognitive therapy.* It may be unrealistic to expect that the work of therapy can take place in one or two sessions per week in the therapist's office. The more that patients can be encouraged to do for and by themselves, the faster the therapy work will progress. It is far less effective to have a patient come to the therapy office to discuss the fear that he or she has about doing something than it is for him or her to try to do the feared behavior and assess the results. The homework of therapy can be cognitive homework (examining automatic thoughts and images) or behavioral homework (*in vivo* exposure).

COURSE OF THERAPY

The course of therapy will involve the following steps:

1. Initiating and building rapport and a working alliance
2. Assessment of the problem
3. Introduction of the CT model
4. Explanation and decatastrophizing of the anxiety symptoms
5. Cognitive and behavioral techniques to ameliorate the distress
6. Practice adaptive skills both within and without therapy sessions
7. Relapse prevention
8. Termination
9. Follow-up and practice

## ASSESSMENT

In treating any psychological problem, an in-depth assessment is the key to developing a conceptualization of the problem. The preliminary, and ongoing, conceptualization is essential for developing an effective treatment plan. The following model for the assessment of anxiety is designed to gather information, develop a conceptualization of the problems(s), generate treatment strategies, and suggest possible intervention techniques.

## THRESHOLD

The first area to be assessed is the patient's threshold. Each person has a general anxiety threshold and/or thresholds for specific situations and experiences. These thresholds may shift. In times of stress, thresholds may lower, and the individual becomes sensitive to experiences that in ordinary circumstances had little or no effect. At other times, there may be an adaptation or habituation to the stressor so that it may no longer have the same effect. We can understand the concept of threshold by utilizing a scale from 0 to 100. As noted earlier, we have, over eons, evolved a safety system that allows our nervous systems to shift from voluntary to automatic (autonomic) when danger threatens. When we are below threshold, we are in general control of our responses. However, when stress builds so that we move above threshold, we shift into an automatic mode. For example, the individual who has a threshold of 10 may get up in the morning, look out of the window, and see that the sun is out and immediately become anxious. On the other hand, that same individual may see that it is raining out and immediately become anxious about that. He or she may be anxious most of the time because of his or her extremely low threshold for anxiety. This individual may be labeled as having *low frustration tolerence, generalized anxiety,* or *pansituational anxiety.* Another person may have a threshold of 90 and never seem to get anxious. This individual is often perceived as the strong pillar of the family or the community and may be seen as someone who will be able to successfully cope in any stressful situation. When such ''Rocks of Gibralter'' suddenly get anxious, people often do not understand. After all, he or she has always been so strong. They wonder what happened? What has happened is that this person has just gone over threshold to 91. It is important for the therapist to understand the threshold so that he or she can point out to the patients the threshold problem. They can then be aware of it so that we can try to alter the threshold. If that is not always possible, the patient can be given skills to help them him or her to keep below threshold. He or she is thereby better able to assume voluntary control of his or her behavior.

## COGNITIVE CONTENT

A second specific assessment issue is the cognitive content of the anxiety. In general, different psychiatric problems are associated with automatic thoughts whose content differs. For example, in depression there is the negative view of self, world, and the future; in hypomania there is an inflated view of self, world, and the future; in generalized anxiety there is a fear or threat of physical or psychological danger; in panic disorders there is not simply a fear or threat but a catastrophic misinterpretation of external or proprioceptive cues. It is more than ''I'm really worried about that'' but rather ''I'm going to die.'' In phobia the cognitive content involves danger or threat in a specific situation or circumstance or fear of an object. In hysteria, there is an overresponse to sensory abnormality, whereas in obsessive thinking there is an ongoing threat that becomes a cause for constant attention or continued worry. In compulsive behavior, repetitive acts are believed to ward off the threat. Finally, in hypochondriasis, the attribution of danger involves the belief that there is something seriously medically wrong.

Thus accurate diagnosis can help the therapist have some indication of the content of the automatic thoughts likely to be generating anxiety in a particular type of patient. However, this is only a starting place for hypothesis testing and cannot be considered as a substitute for more specific cognitive assessment. In order to fully understand the content of a particular individual's cognitions, one must sample those cognitions either verbally or in writing. Without such an assessment, therapy is not likely to be fully productive.

When we enter a novel or potentially threatening situation, we tend to make two evaluations. The first is, "What risk do I perceive for myself in that situation." The second is, "What personal or environmental resources do I perceive that I have available in this particular situation." For example, an individual may enter a situation that he or she perceives to be one of great risk but also perceives that he or she has the resources necessary to deal with it. If the risk is perceived to be higher than the available resources, we experience anxiety. If we perceive our resources as adequate to cope with the risk, we do not experience anxiety. This is not a single evaluation but an ongoing series of evaluations. For example, an individual may go into a situation that is initially seen as being one that involves great risk but is also seen as one in which he or she has the available resources to effectively cope. As the individual stays in that situation, he or she starts to perceive the risk to increase. When the risk exceeds the perceived resources, the person will begin to experience growing levels of anxiety. Conversely, an individual may go into a situation in which he or she experiences anxiety but once involved in the situation may perceive lowered risk or increased resources and thereby experiences a diminution of the anxiety.

An essential differentiation for the therapist to make is whether there is a *perception* of skill deficit or an actual skill deficit, a *perception* of high or low resources, or the reality of high or low resources. For example, a 24-year-old man was self-referred for therapy because of social anxiety. He was concerned about meeting people. His goal was to be able to be able to walk up to anyone and start a conversation, but he was too anxious and upset to do so. He said, "I just can't do it," "I'm just no good at it." As part of his session, he and his therapist walked onto the main campus. It was a nice sunny day, and there were many people out. He was asked if there was anyone he would like to meet. He pointed to a woman who was sitting at a table asking people to sign petitions for some cause. He walked up to her and started talking to her. It seemed clear from his body language and posture and by her response (they were both smiling and nodding) that he was doing quite well. When he broke off the conversation and said goodbye, she waved goodbye and smiled. He then approached his therapist and said, "See, I screwed up again." In this case the individual had the resources but perceived himself as being unskilled. Through such assessment, the therapist can begin to determine whether the need is to work on the cognitive/perceptual issues or behavioral/skill training. These are, of course, not mutually exclusive.

## PERSONALITY FACTORS

The fourth area to be evaluated is the personality factors of autonomy and dependence. These two factors have been found to be found relevant to the anxiety response (Beck, Epstein, & Harrison, 1983). Autonomy and dependence are usually thought of as anchor points on a linear continuum. At one end is the person who is very dependent, and at the other end is a person who is autonomous. Beck *et al.* (1983) found that autonomy and dependence are not part of a linear continuum but are orthogonally related. The particular combination of behavioral patterns may differ markedly from person to person. An individual may be both low dependent/low autonomous, that is, generally dependent across most life situations or, high dependent/high autonomous, that is, very dependent in some situations and very autonomous in others. For example, a very successful, 49-year-old divorced business man was referred because of high anxiety, depression, and suicidal thinking. His "reason" for his depression was that his girlfriend of about 1 year had walked out. She was, he said, making demands on him, that is, "I want to spend more time together." His response to her request was to buy her a Mercedes Benz. When she asked again, he bought her a diamond ring. She told him that she did not want diamond rings or a car but to spend more time with him. When he did not make

ARTHUR FREEMAN
and KAREN M. SIMON

more time available she left. His thoughts were, "Now I must die," "I can't live without her." What was interesting about this man was that in business he was known as a "shark," that is, someone who obtains the balance sheet for a company and sees that the business is in trouble. He would then approach the company president and offer 41 cents on the dollar for the entire business. His typical form of approach was to tell the president that "if you take my offer, I'll give you the money in cash. By 5:00 today the offer will go down to 37 cents on the dollar. By tomorrow I'll give you 28 cents. Why don't you call your accountant I'll be back in an hour." An hour later he would come back and buy the business for 49 cents on the dollar. He would then merge the business with another business he owned or sell off the stock. He did not care about firing people because he is in business to make money. The therapist asked him what would happen if a business deal fell through. What would you do? He said, "I would just pack my bag and go somewhere else." When he was asked why he did not pack his bag and find another woman, he responded, "Oh no, you don't understand, I can't live without her."

Most of us live somewhere in the middle. In certain situations, one may be high anxious and in certain situations one may be high dependent. When people are predominantly dependent or autonomous, their responses to stress are quite different one from the other. Conceptually, in occupational areas, he was high autonomous and in personal areas, he was high dependent.

The usual responses to stress are fight, flight, or freeze. The autonomous individual, when stressed, will rarely seek help and does not come into therapy willingly. He or she comes into therapy because a significant other says, "If you don't get into therapy I'll kill you." The autonomous individual will say to the therapist in the first session, "I don't think you can help me! I know me better than anybody else, and if I can't help me how can you?" When the therapist tells the autonomous person that he or she would like to see him or her once a week, the autonomous patient will often say that he or she is too busy to come in once a week, but can come in every other week. If the therapist insists on the every week schedule, the patient may cancel alternate sessions so as to come in once a month. The autonomous individual wants to keep everything at arms length. He or she will often report his or her anxiety in terms of vague physiological symptoms, "I kinda just feel this lump in my chest . . . ," " . . . "or in my throat," " . . . a little bit of neausea." The autonomous individual tends to feel trapped and encroached upon (in an almost claustropobic like manner). The therapist who tries to engender a warm, close rapport with the autonomous patient may find the patient becoming more anxious and possibly leaving therapy. An individual who finds herself involved in a relationship with an autonomous individual may find that things are getting cozier and cozier. The person may feel very good in the relationship and then the partner come up to her and talk about needing "space," "room," or distance. "Why don't we both date others for a while?" As the relationship gets closer and closer, the autonomous person feels more and more trapped.

The dependent individual enters therapy willingly, again and again. Rather than avoid therapy, this patient says, "Oh! God yes I need help, please help me". The dependent individual asks how often he or she can come for therapy. This person is concerned about the time that the therapist will be away on vacation and may ask where the therapist is going. He or she may ask to have the therapist's home phone number? How late can one call? Does the therapist take calls on weekends? The dependent patient offers the therapist very specific information about his or her symptoms, often more than the therapist would ever want to know. Dependent patients are concerned that if they do not tell the therapist *everything,* the therapist's ability to help will be impaired. When stressed, the dependent patient becomes very vulnerable to being isolated or abandoned. Thus, if the therapist is late for an appointment with a dependent patient, the patient may experience anxiety as he or she becomes afraid of being left all alone.

Anxiety is not a unitary phenomonon so that it must be broken up into its component symptoms and to look at the weight of each symptom for the patient. By assessing the particular symptoms that the patient is expecting, or has experienced, the therapist can begin to structure the therapy to deal with the symptoms. Not all anxieties are the same in terms of the symptom picture. One person may have predominantly physical symptoms, that is, difficulty breathing, indigestion, wobbliness, hot flashes, necessitating the structuring of one sort of intervention. If, however, the patient experiences fear of the worst happening and being terrified and fearful of losing control, the therapist is dealing with a very different set of symptoms. Of course, if the patient has all of the symptoms, therapy needs to be structured for all the different symptoms. The therapy would involve setting up the symptom list so therapy would start with the symptoms that are most dysfunctional and that the person perceives as severely limiting (''I can barely stand them'').

## ENVIRONMENTAL STRESSORS

The environmental stressors that the individual lives with are identified on Axis IV of the DSM-III-R (APA, 1987) multiaxial diagnostic system. What realistic environmental stress is there in this individual's life? How severe is it? The scale utilized in DSM-III-R (1987, p. 11) can be used as a gross screening tool to assess environmental stress from data gathered in the interview. It is important to keep in mind that what may be a very severe stresser for one person may be a relief for someone else.

## VULNERABILITY FACTORS

There are certain situations and circumstances that often render the individual more vulnerable to stressors. The acronym S.H.A.L.T. is a simple way of helping the patient to identify these factors. The construct is used in Acoholics Anonymous and stands for *h*ungry, *a*ngry, *l*onely, and *t*ired. To these we would add *s*ick. When people find themselves in one of those five conditions, they are more vulnerable to stress. The S.H.A.L.T. times are when the individual is more likely to drink, overeat or to use/abuse drugs, or to respond poorly to stress situations. In assessing anxiety, the therapist should determine when the anxiety experience is most likely to occur, that is, ''When I'm sitting alone at home at night'' or ''When I come home after a day's work.'' The therapist can work with the patient very directly by developing specific homework assignments for each of the vulnerability conditions: For example, to avoid hunger, the patient can plan to eating on a regular basis or, if that is difficult to arrange, to keep snack foods available as ''emergency rations.'' For the individual that becomes especially anxious when alone, a system of calling a friend or being involved in a group activity might serve to limit the vulnerability. Obviously, if one is tired, he or she needs to rest.

## PERSONAL AND FAMILY HISTORY

A patient reported that ''basically, everybody in my family is anxious. We've all always been anxious.'' DSM III-R (APA, 1987) states that

> ''Panic disorder, Phobic disorders, and Obsessive Compulsive disorder are all apparently more common among the first degree biologic relatives of people with each of these disorders than among the general population. (p. 235)

It is important to note when a patient reports a long personal or family history of anxiety, panic, phobia, or avoidant behavior, the argument over whether the anxiety is biological or psychological becomes academic. The patient has habituated to an anxiety response. Has the patient experienced a single episode of anxiety or chronic anxiety? A full anxiety response history needs to be elicited. If data can be collected from a family member, they can be used to verify or contradict the patient's perception.

## Personal Schema

It is essential to the therapy to understand the patient's personal rules or schema. As discussed earlier, these rules will often dictate the anxiety experience and responses. These rules will then dictate much of the manner, style, frequency, and content of the anxiety response. The patient who comes from a family where *hypervigilence* was the watchword, will be careful or avoidant in many different life situations.

> In trying to use exaggeration to make a point, the therapist painted the following image for an anxious patient, "You often behave in the following way: You want to cross a street. You look to the left and then to the right and then run one mile to the left to make sure that no cars are coming. You then return to your starting point and run one mile to your right to make sure no cars are coming. After returning to your starting point, you are still too frightened to chance crossing the street." The patient responded by saying, "That's just what my mother does. When she drives she stops at every corner, regardless of the color of the light or the existence of a stop sign. She looks both ways at every corner to avoid getting hit broadside by another car. However, she has been rear-ended several times." An understanding of the patient's schema is essential for the development of the treatment strategies and choice of the specific techniques.

## Physiological/Medical Problems

DSM III-R has introduced the diagnosis of organic anxiety syndrome that involves either generalized anxiety or recurrent, prominent panic attacks. These anxiety manifestations are caused by a specific organic factor. The etiological factors might include hyper- and hypothyroidism, pheochromocytoma, fasting hypoglycemia, hypercortisolism, pulmonary embolus, chronic obstructive pulmonary disease, aspirin intolerence, collagen-vascular disease, and brucellosis. An assessment of medical history, both individual and family, and clearance by a physician are important prior to making a diagnosis of anxiety.

## Drugs/Chemicals

The use of caffeine, cocaine, and amphetamines has also been related to the organic anxiety syndrome. Further, withdrawal from CNS depressants, such as alcohol or sedatives, may cause anxiety syndrome response (APA, 1987, p. 113). A patient reported that he was aware of the possible connection between the intake of caffeine and his anxiety symptoms. "I've cut out all coffee, tea, and colas. I only drink clear sodas like 7-Up or Mountain Dew." (It should be noted that Mountain Dew *does* contain rather significant amounts of caffeine). "My anxiety persists, so I don't think it relates to the caffeine." When asked the quantity of soda consumed, he reported, "about 12 cans a day."

## Imaginal Facility

One difference between depressed patients and anxiety patients is the ability to image (Beck, 1985). The anxiety patient does not simply discuss what he or she is afraid of but rather paints a vivid and powerful image of the imminent danger. The power of the patient's imaginal facility must be evaluated by the therapist. The imaging of the successful competition of an event can increase the likelihood of success in that event. These images may be brief and transitory or pervasive and long lasting. A 34 year old woman described the following. "I just know I'm going to get cancer. I'll be covered with large, oozing sores all over my body. I can smell the putrid ooze coming out of them." As she described the scene in great and disgusting detail, her anxiety level visibly increased.

A second patient entered therapy anxious, depressed, and suicidal. Her boyfriend of 3 months (an autonomous individual) announced his need for more space. Even though the patient had ended an engagement a year earlier with no sequelae, this broken relationship rendered her hopeless.

> Don't you understand? This was special. We had so much in common. We would be walking down the street and see an Irish Setter, and we both agreed that a Setter was the most wonderful dog in the world. We had driven past homes and liked the same kind of house [colonial], the same cars [sports], the same type of furniture [Chippendale and Queen Anne], and the same number of children [two, a girl then a boy]."

When the therapist questioned her about the boyfriend leaving, the patient could not understand why he left or why she was so upset. The patient had, over the 3 months of the relationship begun to build images and fantasies. These images were rehearsed again and again until they became sharply etched in her mind. These well-practiced images can be termed *memories of the future*. The image had been so well rehearsed that the image was not one of what might have been but one that seemed to have been.

## TREATMENT INTERVENTIONS—COGNITIVE

Once the therapist has developed a conceptualization of the problem, a problem list, and has prioritized the list, he or she can begin to develop a treatment strategy. The treatment strategy is the overall focus or goal of treatment. Examples of such strategies include reducing anxiety, encouraging greater mobility from home, or speaking in front of a group. The treatment strategy is implemented through the use of both cognitive and behavioral techniques. The cognitive techniques include:

1. *Understanding idiosyncratic meaning.* This involves helping the patient to explicate his or her specific definitions for the terms he or she uses. When a patient says, "I'm anxious," the therapist must understand exactly what that particular patient uses the word *anxious* to mean.

2. *Questioning the evidence.* This technique, especially valuable in the treatment of depression, is less powerful when used with anxiety patients. By asking the patient to identify the evidence that he or she is using to maintain a particular idea or behavior, the therapist can structure experiences to test the evidence. The depressed patient, who believes that "nothing will change" can see that some things can, and do, change. Anxiety patients who say "I *may* fail" cannot be as easily challenged. After all, they *may* fail, they *may* succeed, or they *may* have a neutral experience. Nonetheless, this technique can be profitably used with such patients. For example, if the patient uses as evidence of an impending heart attack certain symptoms that she has experienced many times before (without experiencing any heart attacks), the therapist may question the evidence that familiar symptoms now predict a totally new result. The patient may learn to respond, instead, that she is experiencing her anxiety symptoms again and that there is no evidence that anything more significant or dangerous is happening to her.

3. *Reattribution.* When the patient places sole responsibility for his or her difficulty on

ARTHUR FREEMAN
and KAREN M. SIMON

self or on others, the therapist can help to effect a more reasonable distribution of responsibility. When the patient says, "My anxiety is all because of my biology," the therapist can help to develop a reattribution, for example, "It may be partially biology. Let us work on the psychological portions of the anxiety and utilize medication to help with the biology."

4. *Developing alternatives.* When the patient has options and alternatives for thinking and behaving, he or she has greater freedom of choice. The anxious/panicky style of responding is only one choice among many. When the anxious patient can see other options, he or she begins to assume greater control over thoughts and actions.

5. *Decatastrophizing.* The anxiety-prone patient, especially the panic-prone patient, tends to catastrophize. The smallest bodily sensation becomes a major illness or disease. The smallest error becomes monumental in size and consequence. The therapist can work toward lessening the catastrophic thinking by helping the patient to generate noncatastrophic possibilities and coping strategies for dealing with catastrophies.

6. *Examining the fantasized consequences.* Given the strong propensity toward the use of imagery in the anxious patient, having the patient verbalize the feared event, situation, or object helps the therapist to tune in and understand what the patient's fears involve.

7. *Advantages versus disadvantages.* The patient needs to assess the utility or advantages gained from maintaining a particular format of thought and behavior. By listing the advantages in one column and the disadvantages in a second column, and then weighting each of the items, the patient can be helped to effect more reasonable problem solving.

8. *Turning adversity to advantage.* Does any particular situation have a "silver lining"? Is it possible to turn an adverse situation to one's advantage, gain or profit, that is, the loss of a relationship allows one to be free to pursue new relationships.

9. *Labeling of distortions.* The fear of the unknown is a frequent issue for anxiety patients. The more that the therapist can do to identify the nature of anxiety and to help label the types of distortions that the patient utilizes, the less frightening the entire process becomes.

10. *Guided association.* The common cognitive style for the anxiety patient is a "free-associative" style. That is, the anxious individual allows his or her mind to run freely through the morass of fearsome situations. By helping the patient to structure the associations, the patient can be helped to control and organize the runaway thoughts.

11. *Exaggeration/paradox.* Both exaggeration and paradox must be used with the utmost care. To effectively use either of these techniques, the therapist must have: (1) an excellent working relationship with the patient, (2) superb timing, and (3) an excellent sense of humor. Without these three requirements, a paradoxical intervention may be seen by the patient as sarcastic or demeaning. The use of exaggeration can be used to help the patient put his or her already exaggerated thoughts into greater relief.

12. *Scaling.* Rather than seeing all experiences at their extremes, scaling allows the patient to put experiences into a life-referenced framework. The patient is asked to first rate an anxiety experience from 0–100. The patient is then asked for anchor points to put the present situation into a life context, for example, "Think of the most anxious you have ever been in your life and label that experience as 100. Now please think of the most relaxed and calm you have ever been and label that 0. Now on that scale, where does your present anxiety fit." Patients can often (though not always) experience a rather rapid reduction in their perception of the severity of their anxiety once it is in a life context.

13. *Developing replacement imagery.* Inasmuch as anxiety is constantly being generated by the patient's imagery, the patient can be helped to develop coping images, rather than imaging failure, defeat, or embarassment. Once well practiced, the patient can do image substitution on his or her own.

14. *Externalization of voices.* The therapist can ask the patient to verbalize his or her internal dialogue. Once made manifest, the therapist can begin to develop challenges and disputation to the anxiogenic thoughts. By changing roles, the therapist and patient can

practice more adaptive responding. The therapist can be the dysfunctional voice, and the patient can practice responding.

15. *Thought stopping.* Once the anxious thoughts "take over," it is very difficult for the patient to regain control. By picturing a stop sign, a red light, or simply saying "stop!", the patient can try to reassert control. The use of a rubber band placed on the wrist and snapped when a repetitive thought occurs can be used to shock the patient into attending to his or her thoughts, rather than allowing the thoughts free reign. This technique must be used in conjunction with subsequent refocusing of attention to compelling, nonanxiety-provoking activities in order to be effective in reducing the rate and frequency of anxious thoughts. The patient must also be prepared to use these techniques many times before significant gains are realized.

16. *Distraction.* It is almost impossible to maintain two thoughts at the same strength simultaneously. If the patient is having anxiogenic thoughts, it generally precludes more adaptive thinking. Conversely, a focused thought distracts from the anxiogenic thoughts. By having the patient focus on complex counting, addition, or subtraction, he or she is rather easily distracted from other thoughts. (N.B. Take care that the person is not math/number phobic, in which case the counting will work to increase the anxiety). Having the patient count to 200 by 13s is very effective. When out of doors, counting cars, people wearing the color red, or any cognitively engaging task will work.

## TREATMENT INTERVENTIONS—BEHAVIORAL

The goals in utilizing the behavioral techniques are twofold. First, behavioral techniques can be used to effect direct behavior change. Second, the behavioral techniques can be used as experiments to collect data to be used in the service of the longer term, cognitive changes.

1. *Activity scheduling.* The activity schedule is an ubiquitous form in the therapist's armamentarium. For the patient who is feeling overwhelmed, the activity schedule can be used to plan more effective time usage. The schedule is both a retrospective tool to assess past time utilization and a prospective tool to then plan better time use.

2. *Mastery and pleasure ratings.* The activity schedule can also be used to assess and plan activities that offer the patient both a sense of personal efficacy (mastery, 1–10) (see figure 8). The greater the mastery and pleasure, the lower the rates of anxiety and depression. By discovering the low- or high-anxiety activities, plans can be made to increase the former and decrease the latter.

3. *Social skills training.* If the patient's reality testing is good and he or she does lack specific skills, it is incumbent upon the therapist to either help the patient to gain the skills or to make a referral for skills training. The skill acquisition may involve anything from teaching the patient how to shake hands to practicing conversational skills (Glass, Gottman, & Shrunk, 1976; Goldfried, Linden, & Smith, 1978; Holroyd, 1976).

4. *Assertiveness training.* As with the social skills training, assertiveness training may be an essential part of the therapy. The patient who is socially anxious can be helped to develop the skills to be responsibly assertive (Jakubowski & Lange, 1978).

5. *Bibliotherapy.* Several excellent books can be assigned as readings for homework. These books can be used to socialize or educate the patient to the basic CT model, emphasize specific points made in the session, or to introduce new ideas for discussion at future sessions.

6. *Graded tasks assignments.* This technique involves using a shaping procedure of small sequential steps that lead to the desired goal. By setting out a task and then arranging the necessary steps in a hierarchy, the patient can be helped to make reasonable progress with a minimum of stress. As the patient attempts each step, the therapist can be available for support and guidance.

7. *Behavioral rehearsal/role playing*. The therapy session is an ideal place to practice many behaviors. The therapist can serve as teacher and guide offering direct feedback on performance. The therapist can monitor the patient's performance, offer suggestions for improvement, and model new behaviors.

8. *In vivo exposure*. There are times when the consulting room needs to be abandoned if therapy is to progress. For example, in treating a phobic patient, the therapist can go with him or her into the feared bridge, go to the feared shopping mall, or travel on the feared bus. The *in vivo* exposure can bring together the office-based practice and the patient-generated homework into a laboratory experience.

9. *Relaxation training*. The anxious patient can profit from relaxation training inasmuch as the anxiety response and the quieting relaxation response are mutually exclusive. The relaxation training can be taught in the office and then practiced by the patient for homework. Ready-made relaxation tapes can be purchased, or the therapist can easily make a tape for a patient. The therapist-made tape can include the patient's name and can focus on the patient's particular symptoms. The tape can be modified, as needed.

## RELAPSE PREVENTION

The goal of the therapy is to help the patient to be successful at coping with his or her anxiety. Through the use of the various skill building techniques, the patient's personal efficacy can be increased. Prior to termination, the patient needs to inoculated against future relapse. Toward the end of therapy, as the patient is able to practice the necessary techniques, the therapist can begin to use the session time for intensive practice. By working at generating anxiety images and dealing with the images, the patient can see how successful he or she can be at effective coping. We have found it to be important to emphasize for the patient that he or she will not be anxiety-free forever. As the anxiety condition is part of the human condition, it will be part of life. The anxiety would not have to be viewed as the same catastrophic experience it was in the past. In point of fact, the return of the anxiety will be an opportunity to demonstrate the success of the therapy. Often, the patient can be helped to prepare a "crisis list." This list, generated by the patient, with the help of the therapist, can anticipate crisis situations and have, for each, a list of techniques that will help to effectively cope. By having this list of crisis, the unexpected nature of anxiety is modified. By having a list of coping techniques, the patient has an armamentarium of adaptive cognitive and behavioral responses.

## TERMINATION

Termination in cognitive therapy begins in the first session. Because the goal of CT is not cure, but rather more effective coping, the Cognitive Therapist does not plan for therapy to continue indefinitely. As a skill-building model of psychotherapy, the therapist's goal is to assist the patient in acquiring the skills to deal with the internal and external stressors. When the patient's self-report, therapist observation, and the report of significant others confirm better adaptive ability, the therapy can move toward final termination. The termination is accomplished slowly so as to allow time for ongoing modifications and corrections. Rather than the termination being an abrupt cessation of sessions, it is accomplished more gradually. Sessions are tapered off from once weekly to biweekly. From that point on, sessions can be set on a monthly basis, with follow-up sessions at 3 and 6 months. After that point, the therapy contact can be ended. Patients can, of course, call and set an appointment in the event of an emergency. Sometimes, patients will call simply to get some information, a reinforcement of a particular behavior, or to report a success. With the Cognitive Therapist in the role of a consultant/collaborator, this continued contact is appropriate and important.

## CASE STUDIES

The following cases will serve to illustrate the applications of the techniques discussed in this chapter.

### Case No. 1—Dave P.

Dave, a 45-year-old businessman, was referred for Cognitive Therapy by a neighbor. The neighbor, a successful businessman had been in therapy and was extolling the virtues of Cognitive Therapy and the therapist. Dave was extremely successful. He owned several flower shops in local shopping malls. His presenting complaint was that his wife and son, both of whom were active in the running of the business, had "pressured" him into opening another store in a new mall. Although protesting his inability to deal with the pressure of the additional store, he had moved ahead with completing the details of acquiring a lease, fixtures, and merchandise, all under protest. This pattern of high anxiety prior to opening a store had been repeated prior to the opening of every one of his stores. At intake, Dave's Beck Anxiety Inventory score was 48 (Figure 8).

His family, developmental, school, and occupational history were unremarkable. When asked whether his anxiety began with the pressure of the new store, Dave reported that he had always been "nervous," "worried," "excitable," "jumpy," or "anxious." He had sought therapy over the years, beginning at age 20 and had seen various therapists for periods of time ranging from two sessions to 3 years on a weekly basis. No therapist was able to ease his worry for more than a few weeks. Pharmacotherapy had been tried with minimal effect. At the time of his starting CT, he was taking ½ mg of Xanax, PRN. He generally took 1 mg daily. The summary of his presenting symptoms can be seen on the anxiety summary (Figure 9).

The initial goals of therapy were to reduce Dave's worrying in terms of both frequency and amplitude, decatastrophize his present life situation, and to begin to teach him specific coping techniques. The initial technique that was utilized was distraction. Inasmuch as he reported that the constant rumination about the potential "disaster" about to befall him took up much of his waking time, distraction and thought stopping were helpful. The distraction involved counting cars with out-of-state license plates while driving, stopping his rumination by counting to 300 by 13s, or counting people wearing red clothing in a mall. The thought stopping involved picturing a large stop sign and saying "STOP" to himself. Both of these techniques were initially helpful but lost their effectiveness within 10 days. By this time, however, he had been introduced to relaxation techniques, counterimagery, and the dysfunctional thought record.

In the course of therapy, it became apparent that Dave was also extremely dependent on his wife. He requested that she be included in the therapy to "help in doing the exercises." This was arranged, and his wife became a willing partner in the therapy. After 4 weeks of twice-weekly therapy sessions, Dave's anxiety was reduced by half. Sessions were then arranged on a weekly basis for 12 weeks. At that point Dave was able to contemplate the store opening with minimal anxiety that was easily accepted. His use of Xanax was reduced, though not eliminated. Sessions were continued for the next 6 months on an alternate week basis. In that time, there were several anxiety attacks. Phone calls to the therapist helped Dave to weather the attacks, see them as limited in duration, and not, in any way, life-threatening.

ARTHUR FREEMAN
and KAREN M. SIMON

Carla was a 33-year-old, married, white Catholic woman who complained of severe anxiety and moderate depression and hopelessness. She began therapy in order to be able to stop taking antidepressant and antianxiety medication so that she and her husband could begin a family. She worked part-time as a typist in a doctor's office; her husband of 3 years was an engineer. Although Carla had suffered from anxiety for years, her symptoms had increased markedly upon the death of her one remaining parent—her mother. This loss was exacerbated by the loss of friends who married and moved away or who had children and therefore had little time to maintain their friendship.

Carla's developmental, school, and occupational history were unremarkable. Her family history was significant in that several close relatives, including her mother, had experienced episodes of anxiety and depression. Carla's father died when when was six years old, and she and her mother became exceptionally close after that.

Carla entered therapy complaining of a wide variety of physiological symptoms, including colitis, high blood pressure, palpitations, tachycardia, sweating, hot and cold flashes, trembling, restlessness, impaired concentration, difficulty falling asleep, startling easily, muscular aches and pains, stiffness, flatulence, sighing, dry mouth, flushing, frequent urination, feeling faint, and twitching. Recurrent automatic thoughts included "What's wrong with me?" "It isn't normal to feel this much anxiety." "I'll never be happy or confident." "I've lost everyone." "I'll never have a family." "I'm going crazy." Her test scores were as follows: Beck Depression Inventory—26; Beck Anxiety Inventory—27; Hopelessness Scale—13.

When Carla began therapy, she was taking subclinical levels of Sinequon and Xanax on a regular basis. We first arranged with her physician that her Sinequon dosage be increased to 150 mg and that she be withdrawn from the Xanax. The Sinequon helped to control her anxiety at a manageable level while we began our treatment program

Based upon our initial interview and the Weekly Activity Schedule the patient filled out after the first session, several goals were agreed upon: (1) increase pleasurable activities, (2) increase social interactions with other women, (3) apply for other job positions that required more self-direction, (4) increase assertiveness with her husband, (5) learn relaxation techniques, and (6) reduce depressive affect through rational responding.

Carla's homework included Weekly Activity Schedules, on which we monitored pleasant and depression and anxiety-provoking events to discover the relationship between events and emotions as well as to monitor Carla's compliance with the therapeutic regimen. The patient was told that it was highly unlikely that she would overcome her depression without becoming more actively involved in pleasurable activities. Because her husband was not inclined to make such plans for them, it was Carla's responsibility to do so. She was told to plan activities for the two of them for weekends and for herself during the week. As she began to carry through on this homework, her depression began to lift.

She was also introduced to the Daily Record of Dysfunctional Thoughts (DTR) in order to teach her to respond more adaptively to her negative thoughts and to elucidate her underlying schemata. It turned out that the most prominent depressogenic and anxiogenic cognitive themes were of personal loss and of self-criticism for being anxious. Carla was helped to see that, because her losses were real, it was understandable that she would periodically be sad when she thought of them. However, it was her choice as to how often and how much time she would spend thinking about them. She was also helped to realize that criticizing herself for an understandable reaction did not make sense and only made her feel worse and more out of control.

The anxiety was dealt with directly through the use of relaxation tapes. She was given a variety to try and liked the Jacobson progressive relaxation technique best. She used this tape three evenings each week. Carla was also helped to recognize life situations that had a greater anxiety stimulation potential and to try to avoid them. This was done by teaching Carla to schedule pleasure and relaxation breaks throughout her day and to avoid overly ambitious schedules. Finally, Carla was taught to respond adaptively to her "pressuring" thoughts.

As Carla's anxiety and depression scores came down to the midteens, her Sinequon was reduced by 25 mg per week until she was drug-free and coping effectively.

## SUMMARY

Anxiety is one of the most common problems encountered in clinical practice. It can affect virtually all response systems either individually or in combination. The symptoms of anxiety may be experienced as affective/emotional, behavioral, physiological, or cognitive and are often disabling in personal, social, or occupational functioning.

The cognitive model of anxiety stresses the role played by the individual's perceptions, thoughts, images, beliefs, and other cognitive phenomena in the origins and maintenance of anxiety. Specifically, the central themes in the cognitions of anxious persons are danger, threat, and vulnerability. Further, the automatic thoughts and images that involve such themes are generated by underlying schema or assumptions of a dysfunctional nature. These schema, often in place since early or middle childhood, may be culturally, religiously, gender, or family based.

Cognitive Therapy involves: (a) the establishment of a working alliance with the patient; (b) assessment and conceptualization of the problem(s); (c) socialization of the client to the therapy model; (d) explanation of the nature of anxiety; (e) decatastrophizing the anxiety symptoms; (f) the use of cognitive and behavioral techniques aimed at the relief of symptoms; and (g) the practicing of adaptive behaviors, both within and without the therapy session.

Careful assessment facilitates the effective use of appropriate strategies and techniques. Assessment within CT includes the assessment of the patient's threshold for anxiety, the cognitive content of the anxiety, the risk versus resource ratio, personality factors of sociotropy/autonomy, the symptom constellation, the patient's environmental stressors, the patient's personal schema, and specific vulnerability factors. The therapy utilizes the broad range of cognitive and behavioral techniques to help the patient to cope more effectively with anxiety-producing situations and to reduce the frequency and amplitude of the anxiety response.

The common problems encountered in the treatment of the anxious patient may be averted or reduced by virtue of the therapy being maintained as structured, problem-solving, and educative. In addition, the emphasis on skill building serves to facilitate generalization and maintenance of gain. CT works to provide the anxious patient with the tools to effectively cope with the present anxiety and with future anxiety episodes.

## REFERENCES

Agras, S. (1985). Stress, panic and the cardiovascular system. In A. Hussain Tuma & Jack D. Maser (Eds.), *Anxiety and the anxiety disorders* (pp. 363–368). Hillsdale, NJ: Lawrence Erlbaum.

American Psychiatric Association. (1968). *Diagnostic and statistical manual* (2nd ed.). Washington, DC.: American Psychiatric Press.

American Psychiatric Association. (1987). *Diagnostic and statistical manual* (3rd ed. rev.). Washington, DC.: American Psychiatric Press.

Beck, A. T. (1970a). Roles of fantasies in psychotherapy and psychopathology. *Journal of Nervous and Mental Diseases, 150*(1), 3–17.

Beck, A. T. (1970b). The core problem in depression: The cognitive triad. In J. H. Masserman (Ed.), *Depression: Theories and therapies* (pp. 47–55). New York: Grune & Stratton.

Beck, A. T. (1976). *Cognitive therapy and the emotional disorders.* New York: International Universities Press.

Beck, A. T. (1985). Theoretical perspectives on anxiety. In A. Hussain Tuma & Jack D. Maser (Eds.), *Anxiety and the anxiety disorders* (pp. 183–196). Hillsdale, NJ: Lawrence Erlbaum.

Beck, A. T., Rush, A. J., Shaw, B. F., & Emery, G. (1979). Cognitive therapy of depression. New York: Guilford.

Beck, A. T., & Emery, G. (1985). *Anxiety disorders and phobias: A cognitive perspective.* New York: Basic Books.

Beck, A. T., Epstein, N., & Harrison, R. (1983). Cognitions, attitudes and personality dimensions in depression. *British Journal of Cognitive Psychotherapy, 1*(1), 1–16.

Campbell, R. J. (1981). *Psychiatric dictionary.* New York: Oxford University Press.

Dimsdale, J. E. (1985). A psychosomatic perspective on anxiety disorders. In A. Hussain Tuma & Jack D. Maser (Eds.), *Anxiety and the anxiety disorders* (pp. 355–362). Hillsdale, NJ: Lawrence Erlbaum.

Freeman, A. (1986). Understanding personal, cultural, and family schema in psychotherapy. In A. Freeman, N. Epstein, & K. M. Simon (Eds.), *Depression in the family* (pp. 79–99). New York: Haworth Press.

Freeman, A., Pretzer, J., Fleming, B., & Simon, K. M. (1989). *Clinical applications of cognitive therapy.* New York: Plenum Press.

Freud, S. (1933). *New Introductory lectures in psychoanalysis.* New York: Norton.

Glass, C. R., Gottman, J. M., & Shmurak, S. H. (1976). Response acquisation and cognitive self-statement modification approaches to dating skills training. *Journal of Counselling Psychology, 23,* 520–526.

Goldfried, M. R., Linehan, M. M., & Smith, J. L. (1978). Reduction of test anxiety through cognitive restructuring. *Journal of Consulting and Clinical Psychology, 46,* 32–39.

Good, B., & Kleinman, A. (1985). Culture and anxiety: Cross cultural evidence for the patterning of anxiety disorders. In A. Hussain Tuma & Jack D. Maser (Eds.), *Anxiety and the anxiety disorders* (pp. 297–324). Hillsdale, NJ: Lawrence Erlbaum.

Gray, J. A. (1985). Issues in the neuropsychology of anxiety. In A. Hussain Tuma & Jack D. Maser (Eds.), *Anxiety and the anxiety disorders* (pp. 5–25). Hillsdale, NJ: Lawrence Erlbaum.

Holroyd, K. (1976). Cognition and desensitization in the group treatment of test anxiety. *Journal of Consulting and Clinical Psychology, 44,* 991–1001.

Horney, K. (1937). *The neurotic personality of our time.* New York: Norton.

Izard, C. E., & Blumberg, S. H. (1985). Emotion theory and the role of emotions in anxiety in children and adults. In A. Hussain Tuma & Jack D. Maser (Eds.), *Anxiety and the anxiety disorders* (pp. 109–129). Hillsdale, NJ: Lawrence Erlbaum.

Jakubowski, P., & Lange, A. J. (1978). *The assertive option: Your rights and responsibilities.* Champaign, IL: Research Press.

Klein M. (1948). *Contributions to psychoanalysis 1921–45.* London: Hogarth Press.

Lindsay, W. R., Gamsu, C. V., McLaughlin, E., Hood, E. M., & Espie, C. A. (1987). A controlled trial of treatments for generalized anxiety. *British Journal of Clinical Psychology, 26,* 3–15.

Lindsley, D. B. (1952). Psychological phenomena and the electroencephalogram. *Electroencephalography and Clinical Neurophysiology, 4,* 443–456.

Lindsley, D. B. (1957). Psychophysiology and motivation. In M. R. Jones (Ed.), *Nebraska symposium on motivation* (pp. 45–105). Lincoln: University of Nebraska Press.

Lindsley, D. B. (1960). Attention, consciousness, sleep, and wakefulness. In J. Field & H. W. Magoun (Eds.), *Handbook of physiology* (Vol. 3; pp. 1553–1593). Washington, DC: American Physiology Society.

Plutchik, R. (1980). *Emotion: A psychoevolutionary synthesis.* New York: Harper & Row.

Schacter, S. (1964). The interaction of cognitive and physiological determinants of emotional state. In L. Berkowitz (Ed.), *Advances in experimental social psychology* (Vol. 1; pp. 49–80). New York: Academic Press.

Schacter, S. (1967). Cognitive effects on bodily functioning: Studies of obesity and eating. In D. C. Glass (Ed.), *Neurophysiology and emotion* (pp. 117–144). New York: Rockefeller University Press.

Shepherd, M., Cooper, B., Brown, A. C., & Kalton, G. W. (1966). *Psychiatric illness in general practice.* London: Oxford University Press.

Spielberger, C. D. (1966). The effects of anxiety on complex learning and academic achievement. In C. D. Spielberger (Ed.), *Anxiety and behavior* (pp. 361–398). New York: Academic Press.

Spielberger, C. D. (1972). Anxiety as an emotional state. In C. D. Spielberger (Ed.), *Anxiety: Current trends in theory and research* (Vol. 1; pp. 23–49). New York: Academic Press.

Stokes, P. (1985). The neuroendocrinology of anxiety. In A. Hussain Tuma & Jack D. Maser (Eds.), *Anxiety and the anxiety disorders* (pp. 53–76). Hillsdale, NJ: Lawrence Erlbaum.

Weiner, H. (1985). The psychobiology and pthophysiology of anxiety and fear. In A. Hussain Tuma & Jack D. Maser (Eds.), *Anxiety and the anxiety disorders* (pp. 333–354). Hillsdale, NJ: Lawrence Erlbaum.

Woodward, R., & Jones, R. B. (1980). Cognitive restructuring treatment; A controlled trial with anxious patients. *Behavior Research and Therapy, 18,* 401–407.

# 19

# Cognitive and Behavioral Approaches to the Treatment of Anorexia Nervosa

JANET SASSON EDGETTE AND MAURICE F. PROUT

Anorexia nervosa can be a devastating illness resulting in physical impoverishment and grossly impaired psychosocial functioning. It is characterized primarily by a refusal to eat a sufficient amount of food to sustain an adequate level of nourishment (Slade, 1982). One diagnostic criterion is the maintenance of weight at least 25% below the norm for one's age (American Psychiatric Association, 1980). Such extensive weight loss plays havoc with a body that is often already under the physiological stress of puberty. Disturbed attitudes toward eating, manifested in preoccupations with food and peculiar patterns of handling food, is another noted feature of the disorder (Cooper & Fairburn, 1984; Garner, 1986; Garner & Bemis, 1982; Halmi, 1982; McFarlane, Bellissimo, & Upton, 1982; Muuss, 1985). Other features include intense fears of weight gain, behaviors directed toward weight loss, excessive physical activity, disturbances in body image, and, in females, amenorrhea (Halmi, 1982; Kissel & Arkins, 1973; Minuchin, Rosman, & Baker, 1978; Muuss, 1985; Slade, 1982).

Anorexia nervosa occurs primarily in adolescent females, with the percentage of males ranging an estimated 5% to 15% (Bemis, 1978; Kissel & Arkins, 1973; Muuss, 1985; Ziesat & Ferguson, 1984). Once believed to be a rare disorder, its incidence has increased dramatically over the past two decades (Bemis, 1978). Reported incidences include 1 in 250 females in the United States between the ages of 12 and 18 (American Psychiatric Association, 1980) and 1 severe case for every 200 adolescent females (Garner & Garfinkel, 1985). Higher incidences of 1 severe case per 100 English girls 16 years of age or older (Crisp, Palmer & Kalucy, 1976) and of 1 severe case per 150 Swedish adolescent girls (Nylander, 1971) have also been noted. College-age females manifesting less severe symptomatology have been reported with even higher incidence (Clarke & Palmer, 1983; Muuss, 1985).

JANET SASSON EDGETTE • Department of Mental Health Sciences, Hahnemann University, Philadelphia, Pennsylvania 19102.    MAURICE F. PROUT • Institute for Graduate Clinical Psychology, Widener University, Chester, Pennsylvania 19013.

JANET SASSON
EDGETTE and
MAURICE F. PROUT

Anorexia nervosa is generally considered to be a multidetermined disorder (Fundudis, 1986; Garner & Bemis, 1985; Vandereycken & Meerman, 1984). The complex interplay of different predisposing factors calls for a multidimensional approach to treatment utilizing a broad range of interventions. Garner and Garfinkel (1980) and Garfinkel and Garner (1982) have developed an elaborate schema of predisposing psychological and sociocultural factors that play important roles in the etiology and maintenance of this disorder.

Despite the multidetermined nature of anorexia nervosa, its onset is typically marked by an elective restriction of food intake based on the belief that one is overweight (Fundudis, 1986). Bruch (1962) characterizes anorexics as having profound disturbances in perception and conception that are manifested in delusional distortions of body image. Thus, despite extreme slenderness or even apparent emaciation, anorexics view themselves as not being thin enough. Furthermore, these perceptual and conceptual disturbances result in the inaccurate perception or cognitive interpretation of stimuli arising from within one's own body. The individual is therefore frequently unable to recognize hunger or fatigue. Such a misassessment of internal stimuli, as well as the anorexic's pronounced hyperactivity, contrasts strikingly with the physiological state of malnutrition with which anorexics present.

In part, Bruch views the symptomatology of anorexia nervosa as an outgrowth of the paralyzing sense of ineffectiveness characterizing the psychological functioning of anorexics. She describes the anorexic's life experience as one of acting only in response to the demands of others. Self-starvation is understood as a struggle for autonomy, competence, control, and self-respect. Whipple and Manning (1978) note deficiencies in such areas of ego development as self-identity and the sense of autonomy and state that the self-regulation of food may provide the anorexic with the one area in which she feels she can maintain some sense of control over her life.

Anorexia nervosa is regarded as being quite refractory to therapeutic intervention (Cooper & Fairburn, 1984; Garner & Bemis, 1982; Halmi, 1982; Muuss, 1985; Powers & Powers, 1984). Denial of the illness and disinterest in ameliorative efforts are common. Even when patients have been considered successfully treated, abnormal body weights and psychosocial and psychosexual disturbances persist (Whipple & Manning, 1978). Anorexia can also be life-threatening: Between 5% and 20% of the treated population die due to starvation, suicide, or organ failure secondary to the illness (Powers & Powers, 1984; Whipple & Manning, 1978). The mortality rate of the many cases that go unrecognized and untreated remains unknown.

Disagreement about the management and treatment of choice for anorexia nervosa continues to exist (Dickstein, 1985; Fundudis, 1986; Muuss, 1985). Fundudis (1986) reports major areas of controversy as including the use of inpatient versus outpatient settings and the relative effectiveness of different therapeutic approaches. Several authors, however, have emphasized the need for a multifaceted treatment approach in view of the multiplicity of causative factors and the heterogeneity of personality features (Bemis, 1978; Halmi, 1982; Peake & Borduin, 1977). A two-phase approach to intervention is frequently instituted with the initial aim of treatment being the medical management of the disorder and the normalization of weight and eating. The second, longer term phase typically addresses the different areas of psychological maladjustment, weight maintenance, and the consolidation of new adaptive eating habits.

## BEHAVIORAL APPROACHES

Traditional behavioral approaches to the etiology of anorexia nervosa focus on social learning theories and the principles of operant conditioning. Peake and Borduin (1977) point out that within this model, anorexic symptomatology is generally considered to be a manifestation of a maladaptive learning pattern. They state that the behavioral approach addresses the eating and interpersonal conflict issues as symptoms whose reinforcements need to be discovered and altered.

Slade's (1982) behavioral functional analysis of the etiology of anorexia describes antecedent events and consequences thought to be significant variables in the development and maintenance of the disorder. Psychological, biological, and social factors are all taken into account. Antecedent events are predisposing conditions that may include a general dissatisfaction with life and oneself and precipitating psychosocial stimuli such as comments about body shape and weight gain. Consequences of successful dieting behavior include both positive and negative reinforcers. One very important positive reinforcer is the powerful feeling of self-satisfaction and control derived from dieting and weight loss. Slade comments that its strong influence on otherwise maladaptive behaviors is a function of "successful behavior in the context of perceived failure in all other areas of functioning" (1982, p. 173). Negative reinforcement occurs through the avoidance of aversive stimuli such as weight gain. Other stimuli include those developmental and psychological conflicts that may have initially given rise to the onset of the illness. The anorexic's obsessional preoccupation with food, eating, weight, and body size allows her to avoid a direct confrontation with these anxiety-provoking issues.

Behavior therapy with anorexic patients predominantly involves the application of learning principles to extinguish the maladaptive eating and weight control patterns of behavior. Interventions generally aim at the alleviation of symptoms through altering the contingencies by which they are supported. Behavioral analyses are conducted in order to identify the specific response chains for each individual that may have resulted in the inhibition of eating. A treatment paradigm is then engineered whereby desirable behaviors are rewarded and undesirable ones discouraged.

With respect to anorexia nervosa, behavior therapy has been recognized as being most effective in the acute phase of the illness where the stabilization and normalization of weight and eating may be urgent (Cinciripini, Kornblith, Turner, & Hersen, 1983; Halmi, 1982, 1985; McFarlane et al., 1982). Indeed, the majority of clinicians using a behavioral approach employ operant conditioning programs within inpatient hospitalization settings. Positive reinforcers such as increased social privileges, access to visitors, and allowances for physical activity are made contingent upon the demonstration of increasingly adaptive eating behaviors or, more typically, of weight gain. Negative reinforcers for limited food intake, weight loss, or vomiting after meals include isolation, enforced bed rest and in extreme cases, tube feeding (Cinciripini et al., 1983; Eckert, Goldberg, Halmi, Casper & Davis, 1979; Halmi, 1983). Halmi (1985) notes that, for some patients, the hospitalization and separation from family are alone sufficient negative reinforcers to induce weight gain.

Halmi (1985) recommends that the behavioral program be modified once the patient has reached her target weight. She suggests that the escalating anxiety surrounding the ability to maintain the new weight become the principal focus, best addressed by expanding the range of activities and privileges for as long as the weight remains within a reasonable range and restricting the patient to the ward whenever it does not. The patient should be given increasing control over her diet and allowed to practice eating at home with family members and in restaurants. An aftercare program, supplementing behavioral management with individual psychotherapy and family counseling in order to address identified problems in the transition to the home environment is advised. Other clinicians (Bemis, 1978; Garner & Bemis, 1982, 1985; McFarlane et al., 1982; Peake & Borduin, 1977) have also emphasized a need for treatment strategies in addition to behavioral ones to effect long-term eradication of symptoms. Halmi (1985) notes that few anorexics are treated with behavior therapy alone.

Bachrach, Erwin, and Mohr (1965) are credited with the first explicit use of operant conditioning with specifically selected reinforcers in the treatment of anorexia nervosa. Their treatment of a 37-year-old female focused on the identification and subsequent manipulation of those variables that would most effectively restore the desired behaviors. Using social attention and social access as positive reinforcers, eating behaviors were modified by shaping the patient's approaches to food intake. Gradually, reinforcement became contingent upon the amount of food eaten, and eventually, upon weight gain itself in order to circumvent the problem of the patient vomiting after meals.

Other early studies of the behavioral management of anorexia nervosa include that of Leitenberg, Agras, and Thompson (1968), which was one of few to use experimental control procedures. Blinder, Freeman, and Stunkard (1970) were the first to use the anorexic's compulsive hyperactivity in constructing an operant paradigm, wherein access to physical activity was used as a positive reinforcer. Scrignar (1971) and Neumann and Gaoni (1975) evaluated the effects of using favored foods as positive reinforcements, with no emphasis on weight gain.

Agras, Barlow, Chapin, Abel, and Leitenberg (1974) ran a series of single-case experiments designed to separate the effectiveness of several therapeutic variables. Their study was prompted by the results of an earlier study (Leitenberg *et al.,* 1968) in which caloric intake and weight gain continued despite the removal of the hypothesized positive reinforcer. This had raised the possibility that other environmental variables were playing a role in conditioning the desired behaviors.

The variables studied for differential effectiveness were positive reinforcement, informational feedback, and meal size. The authors' first experiment resulted in the discovery of a fourth variable responsible for weight gain: the negative reinforcement of remaining in the hospital. The patients maintained their increased food intake and weight gain despite a return to a nonreinforcing baseline phase in an effort to secure a prompt discharge.

Agras *et al.* (1974) subsequently designed a second experiment that controlled for the effects of this negative reinforcement by contracting with the patient for a 12-week hospital stay regardless of weight gain. Examining the respective roles of positive reinforcement, informational feedback, and meal size in promoting the desired behaviors led the authors to conclude that the feedback on the number of calories consumed, mouthfuls eaten, and weight gained was the most influential. Positive reinforcement was followed in effectiveness by the serving of large meals. The authors added, however, that maximum therapeutic success would be best achieved by using a combination of all three variables.

Eckert *et al.* (1979) reported the only controlled treatment study with random assignment of patients to behavior therapy or its absence. Designed to compare the effectiveness of behavior therapy and milieu therapy, and of cyproheptadine and placebo, patients were randomly assigned to one of four treatment cells: (1) behavior therapy and cyproheptadine, (2) behavior therapy and placebo, (3) no behavior therapy and cyproheptadine, and (4) no behavior therapy and placebo. The behavior therapy followed an operant conditioning paradigm. The results, assessed after 35 days, revealed no significant difference in weight gain between those patients receiving behavior therapy (9 lb) and those receiving milieu therapy (8 lb). Explanations for this outcome suggested by the authors include the use of constant rather than individualized reinforcers, the schedule of delayed rather than immediate daily reinforcers, and the possibility that various milieu programs and isolation may have, in themselves, produced a maximal possible weight gain (Halmi, 1985). The authors did note, however, a significant difference in weight gain between the subsets of patients in each of the therapeutic groups that had not received any prior outpatient treatment of any kind. Within this context, behavioral therapy was more effective than milieu. This may have implications for the selection of patients more likely than others to benefit from behavioral interventions.

Another approach to the treatment of anorexia nervosa has been to conceptualize it as a phobic disorder. Hallsten (1965) had outlined an etiological model of an intense fear of weight gain in a 12-year-old female anorexic. Maladaptive eating patterns were understood to have erupted as a result of the rejection the patient had received for her obesity. Although weight loss during the early phases of the illness was positively reinforced, the dropping of her weight below normal levels was responded to by family and friends with rejection and punishment. Unable to make the distinction between the different contingencies that gave rise to the same subjective experience, the patient generalized the rejection from the former situation of obesity to the current one of exaggerated weight loss. The girl responded to this new situation with the same means of anxiety reduction that had been effective with her earlier fear of weight gain: food avoidance and the need to become thinner.

Mavissakalian (1982) attempted to directly treat phobic compulsive behavior in anorexics through response prevention and prolonged exposure within an operant paradigm. Two teenage anorexic females were positively reinforced with social privileges and hospital day passes only when meals were completed within a 30-minute time limit, and, in addition the patient remained seated for an hour after each meal. This program therefore systematically incorporated response prevention of the compulsive exercising after meals characteristic of many anorexics and insured that exposure to phobic stimuli related to food and weight gain was maintained for a full 90 minutes at each meal. Both patients gained ½ lb per day during their 35 and 48 respective days of hospitalization. Follow-up 3½ months later revealed continued weight gains for each.

Mavissakalian reserved judgment on the attribution of these results to the direct effectiveness of treating anorexia nervosa as a phobic disorder until more studies were done comparing, psychophysiologically, the fears of anorexics with those of clinically tested phobics. Salkind, Fincham, and Silverstone (1980) designed skin conductance studies to explore the issue of whether or not anorexia nervosa can appropriately be called, and treated as, a phobic disorder. Because it had previously been demonstrated that patients suffering from specific phobic disorders have an increase in skin conductance when exposed to the feared object, the authors sought to assess changes in the skin conductance of anorexics presented with food- and weight-related stimuli.

The most consistent finding was that the skin conductance responses to stimuli in anorexics were low compared with those from subjects with classic phobic disorders. This was subsequently determined not to be due to impairments of the sweat gland mechanisms secondary to the illness. The experimenters concluded that avoidance behaviors in anorexics is associated with a different psychopathological mechanism than that ordinarily found in phobic individuals.

Garner and Bemis (1985) also distinguish anorexia nervosa from simple phobic disorders for the reason that the anorexic symptoms are maintained by positive as well as negative reinforcement. Weight loss is not only a solution for avoiding the anxiety-provoking situation of fatness but provides a considerable degree of gratification in its own right. The sense of mastery, self-control and competence derived from successful dieting constitute potent cognitive self-reinforcements that maintain the behavior. The authors state that hunger acquires new meaning as it becomes associated with higher order accomplishments. Weight control or loss thus become a barometer of achievement and a referent for self-evaluation.

It has behooved many clinicians to address the need for adjunctive therapies to behavioral interventions in the treatment of anorexia nervosa. Behavioral approaches have generally been viewed as appropriate and effective for the purposes of immediate weight gain, restoration of adaptive eating habits, and the amelioration of reinforcing variables within the patient's environment. However, a number of researchers and therapists have expressed the view that the use of a therapeutic program that does not directly speak to such issues as dysfunctional family relationships, feelings of ineffectiveness, autonomy, one's sense of control, and the resolution of developmental conflicts risks losing, in the long run, any initial gains made with behavior therapy (Bemis, 1978; Minuchin *et al.*, 1978; Slade, 1982; Whipple & Manning,

JANET SASSON
EDGETTE and
MAURICE F. PROUT

1978). These clinicians, including those deeply embedded in the behavioral tradition, have encouraged the development of interventive programs that address other psychological conflicts in the anorexic patient that play a role in the maintenance of the illness.

Minuchin (Minuchin *et al.,* 1978) reported a high degree of success with anorexics using a comprehensive systems model of approach and intervention that combines principles and strategies from behavior and family schools of therapies. He conceptualizes anorexia nervosa as an interpersonal, rather than individual problem, and focuses on a restructuring of the dysfunctional family system that uses the symptoms of the illness as a mechanism to avoid interpersonal conflicts among its members. The importance of addressing such family patterns as rigidity, poor conflict resolution, and overinvolvement is well stated in Minuchin's own words: "To expect the anorexic to maintain autonomous changes in the face of an unchanged family system is unrealistic" (p. 90).

The initial part of Minuchin's treatment program is strictly behavioral. Operant paradigms are designed for patients, who may or may not be hospitalized. Rewards are contingent upon weight gain, and it is understood by the patient that it is her responsibility to decide whether or not she will eat. Minuchin stated that it is imperative that the behavioral component not be recognized as the focal point of treatment but rather for its ability to diffuse the power struggle over eating and teach the anorexic patient that her domain of power rests in the ability to influence her situation and control her own activities.

Minuchin reported that most patients begin to gain weight within 5 to 7 days of the program's initiation. Once this occurs, the focus of attention shifts away from the anorexic patient onto dysfunctional family patterns. A "family lunch session" is scheduled during which the patient, therapist, and family all dine together. The therapist takes advantage of this situation, typically quite emotionally charged, in order to cue-in on the dynamics of the family interactional patterns. Suggestions and solutions are offered as conflicts arise within the mealtime setting. Prior to discharge, both the patient and family are involved in the development of an appropriate outpatient management program that will continue the therapeutic process set into motion during these first 2 weeks.

A follow-up survey by Minuchin (average period of 2 years) on those individuals treated with his systems model revealed a success rate greater than 85%. This is significantly higher than those rates cited by other experimenters of all therapeutic orientations, including behavioral (Bemis, 1978; Bhanji & Thompson, 1974; Schwartz & Thompson, 1981). Pertschuk (1977) remarked that Minuchin's results are not generalizable due to the fact that the population treated (average age 13) was younger than those usually reported in treatment studies and therefore had a briefer duration of the illness.

Nevertheless, one can postulate that the success of Minuchin's program reflects not so much the advantages of working with subjects whose maladaptive patterns of behavior might be less highly entrenched as it does the particular theoretical underpinnings and techniques of the therapy itself. Notions of shared responsibility and increased autonomy, family involvement from the outset, minimal behavioral manipulation on the part of staff, and removal of the patient from the locus of pathology may prove to be elements of great impact in designing behaviorally oriented treatment programs. Minuchin does not, however, operationalize his definition of the successfully treated anorexic, and one remains unsure whether this emphasizes the maintenance of weight gain and appropriate eating behaviors or includes a wider spectrum of corrected psychosocial and family interactional functioning.

Although inpatient operant conditioning programs have generally been effective in abating life-threatening weight loss in anorexics, they have often not resulted in long-term maintenance of these weight gains (Ollendick, 1979). Clinicians have emphasized the need to institute outpatient management programs to ensure the transfer and maintenance of therapeutic gains to the home environment.

Erwin (1977) outlined an outpatient contingency management plan for a 37-year-old female anorexic who had been treated behaviorally in a rigidly controlled hospital environment. Family assistance was an integral part of the plan. Family members were given specific instructions that essentially duplicated the rigid environment from which the patient had just been released. They were asked specifically to avoid reinforcement of maladaptive behaviors, verbally reward the maintenance of weight, follow a rigid schedule for meals, discuss only pleasant topics at mealtime, and not make an issue of eating nor prepare special diets. Following this patient's release from the hospital, she endured a course of widely fluctuating weights. Although she reported improvements in the areas of social activity and familial independence, 16 years later she had lost all but 8 pounds of the initial in-hospital weight gain. In retrospect, Erwin felt that the addition of intermittent behavior treatments during these years would have been of great value in assisting the patient with her struggle for recovery.

The results of Erwin's study suggest that outpatient programs that are primarily an extension of the externally controlled operant paradigm used during hospitalization are not as effective in preventing relapses as might be a program designed to emphasize the anorexic's self-monitoring and sense of mastery over her illness. Bachrach *et al.* (1965) found that the social reinforcements from co-workers and peers, personal reinforcements such as the reappearance of healthy skin and hair, increased energy levels, and the renewed ability to work and socialize were of great value in maintaining one former anorexic's adaptive eating patterns.

Hauserman and Lavin (1977) devised an outpatient plan that was successful in maintaining the weight a 20-year-old female anorexic had gained during a 1-month inpatient operant contingency program. The components of the plan were twofold: an extended behavioral contract that allowed the patient to remain at home, contingent upon a specified amount of continued weight gain, and cognitive restructuring of irrational belief systems coupled with training in the recognition and expression of emotions. A follow-up study 2 years later showed the patient stabilized at 125 lb, 30 lb above her discharge weight. She reported that she was attending school full-time, was more assertive in family interactions, and was quite satisfied with life as a whole.

The increased attention and interest in the use of behavior therapy has been complemented by a barrage of criticism from both those clinicians who believe in its efficacy and hope to improve various aspects of its application and those who maintain that other modes of interventions are more appropriate and effective. Bemis (1978) outlined several areas for improvement that can foster the acceptance and validity of behavior therapy as used with anorexics. A strong criticism of his is the small sample size of reported studies and the lack of discriminating diagnostic criteria. Furthermore, the supplemental use of pharmacologic agents, family therapy, and psychotherapy during the course of an operant conditioning program make it difficult to attribute successful results to behavioral interventions.

Bemis also faults the emphasis on rapid weight gain in many of the inpatient behavior therapy programs. An eagerness to demonstrate the effectiveness of behavioral techniques may cause some clinicians to subordinate caution for expediency. Recent studies, however, have established more moderated contingency standards for weight gain and have begun to emphasize a more global approach to the treatment of anorexia nervosa that focuses on other dysfunctional aspects of the individual's personality and behavior that are symptomatic of the illness.

Bruch (1974) has been the most outspoken critic of the use of behavior therapy with anorexics. She feels that inpatient contingency programs emphasizing rapid weight gain are coercive and humiliating and that such an experience is counterproductive to the development of a sense of inner control, competence, and autonomy that she sees as critical for complete recovery. She suggests, instead, a therapeutic approach combining the reinstitution of normal weight through cognitive restructuring of perceptual and conceptual disturbances and a psychodynamic treatment of the underlying issues of control and autonomy. The essential therapeutic task is not the analytic interpretation of the patient's behaviors but encouraging the patient's awareness of those feelings and impulses that originate within herself. The therapist helps the patient to recognize these feelings and act accordingly.

Garner and Bemis (1982) shed a different light on inpatient behavior therapy programs. They suggest that hospitalization should be presented to the patient not as a means of enforcing weight gain but as a way of gaining control over distressing patterns of behavior. They describe behavioral paradigms within hospital settings as an opportunity for change rather than as a coercive program of last resort. Patients should be well prepared for the contingency plans and for the psychological and physical concomitants of weight gain. Pertschuk (1977) stated that hospitalization is not intended to be curative but should serve as the first step toward recovery.

Many clinicians employing behaviorally oriented therapy with patients suffering from anorexia nervosa are well aware of the multiple dimensions of this illness and the complexity of its origins and manifestations. Blinder *et al.* has, for many years, contributed to the study of behavioral intervention with these individuals and wisely acknowledges that "the power of the operant treatment method requires caution in its application" (1970, pp. 1096–1097). Such is the case with any form of psychotherapy.

The advantage of behavior therapy with anorexics warrants its continued use and refinement. Few other therapies have been able to approach its success in inducing rapid weight gains, thus eliminating the need for drastic somatic therapies such as tube feeding and tranquilization in cases of imminent starvation. Operant paradigms where the positive contingencies are clearly outlined allow the patient a sense of responsibility for changes in her eating behaviors and minimize the possibility of confrontations with staff over the eating itself (Garfinkel, Moldofsky, & Garner, 1977).

## COGNITIVE-BEHAVIORAL APPROACHES

The important role of cognitive factors in the development and maintenance of anorexia nervosa has received much attention (Bruch, 1962; Garner, 1986; Garner & Bemis, 1982, 1985) as clinicians have recognized limitations in conceptualizing the disorder strictly in behavioral terms. The underlying premise of a cognitive approach is that the central feature of anorexia is the persistence of underlying faulty beliefs and values regarding body shape and weight (Cooper & Fairburn, 1984; Garner & Bemis, 1982, 1985).

Garner & Bemis (1982, 1985) describe the cognitive model of anorexia nervosa as a paradigm of causal and maintaining variables in which the former converge in the anorexic's belief that it is of paramount importance that she be thin. The seemingly irrational behaviors are seen as a direct result of a set of distorted beliefs, attitudes, and assumptions about the meaning of body weight. The developmental distresses of adolescence are allayed through a pursuit of thinness, and feelings of self-doubt and deficiency are overridden by maintaining a figure believed to be the envy of all others. Citing Bandura's (1978) and Beck's (1970) comments that entrenched cognitive sets may be so powerfully controlling as to be impervious to external contingencies, Garner and Bemis (1982) point out that anorexics may effectively be insulated from information or experiences that could modify their belief systems. They add that the sequelae to starvation, which includes concrete thinking, rigidity, social withdrawal, and emotional liability, among other features, may further isolate the anorexic and leave her more vulnerable to the influence of her distorted perceptions.

Cognitive labeling factors and the misperception of bodily cues have been the focus of Bruch's (1962) investigations into the etiology of anorexia nervosa. Faulty hunger awareness is believed to result from early interactional patterns that were unresponsive to the child's needs. Because these needs were determined more by parental influence than by internal physical states, such children never learn to appropriately identify and respond to signals coming from within their own bodies (cited in Ross, 1980).

Garner (1986) writes that cognitive therapy for anorexics offers powerful strategies for modifying the distorted beliefs associated with eating and body shape and for addressing the developmental, interpersonal, and self-attributional themes underpinning the disorder. He states that a particular advantage of this therapeutic modality is its compatibility with other approaches, including the more traditional ones where developmental deficits may be seen as central pathognomonic factors. He does point out, however, that conventional cognitive therapy approaches need to be adapted to the specific therapeutic needs of anorexic patients. These needs include the following:

1. Idiosyncratic beliefs related to food and weight,
2. The interaction between physical and psychological components of the disorder,
3. The patient's desire to retain certain focal symptoms,
4. The development of motivation for treatment with an emphasis on the gradual evolution of a trusting therapeutic relationship,
5. A prominence of fundamental self-concept deficits related to self-esteem and trust in internal state, and
6. The longer duration of therapy than is typical for depression or anxiety disorders because of the time required to reverse the patient's deteriorated physical state and because of the nature of her focal symptoms. (1986, pp. 303–304)

Garner and Bemis (1982, 1985) developed a comprehensive cognitive-behavioral treatment approach for anorexia nervosa modeled after the cognitive therapy program for depressed and neurotic patients designed by Beck and his colleagues (Beck, 1970, 1976; Beck, Rush, Shaw, & Emery, 1979). Some of their methods were adapted from other cognitive approaches as well (Ellis, 1962; Goldfried, 1971; Mahoney, 1974; Meichenbaum, 1974). Citing Hollon and Beck (1979), the authors state that the essence of cognitive-behavioral therapy involves teaching patients to examine the validity of their beliefs on a moment-to-moment basis. The thrust of this approach with anorexia nervosa, then, is the identification and modification of the underlying assumptions and reasonings of the anorexic around which the system of irrational beliefs and expectations organize. The authors add, however, that the faulty cognitions are not considered to be the sole etiological factor nor the sole focus of intervention.

The following premises are identified by Garner and Bemis as characteristic of the anorexic's cognitive structure:

1. The assumption that body weight or shape can serve as the sole criterion for self-worth
2. The assumption that complete self-control and regimentation are desirable
3. The conviction that there is a perfect balance between hunger and satiation that would eliminate the need for constant readjustment

The most critical injunction offered by the authors is that the therapy must not degenerate into arguments over the validity of these premises lest such challenges on the part of the therapist be construed as a personal attack. Frequently, a great part of the anorexic's identity is tied in with these belief systems, and the sole use of logic to undercut them is usually counterproductive. A more effective approach has been found to be the use of behavioral exercises in conjunction with various cognitive techniques where the patient is encouraged to recognize and verbalize previously unspoken premises. Such frank acknowledgment of one's underlying belief system may work to mitigate its power over the patient.

Garner and Bemis discourage the use of traditional *in vivo* behavioral techniques for approaching the object of avoidance because the feared stimulus may be more the self at undesirable weight levels than the food. The behavioral techniques used in their model include rehearsal of the patient's reaction to weight gain, the scheduling of pleasant reinforcing events unassociated with weight loss or self-control in order to expand the set of active reinforcers, and exercises designed to modify maladaptive eating patterns. The supplementary use of operant conditioning, desensitization, and social skills training is also encouraged.

The authors believe that cognitive interventions are important adjuncts to the standard behavioral techniques used in treating anorexia nervosa because of the disorder's tendency to elicit strong positive reinforcements outside of the treatment setting. Once the therapist has helped the anorexic patient become motivated to gain weight and discontinue the dangerous weight control practices, the following interventions are used to modify the dysfunctional belief systems:

*Operationalizing* distorted beliefs is a form of cognitive restructuring that teaches the patient to examine the validity of her beliefs on a moment-to-moment basis. For example, a patient who equates competence with thinness can be helped to develop a working definition of competence that permits a determination of whether or not it is affected by changes in weight.

*Articulating beliefs* may, in itself, lead to belief change. The following are some types of cognitive distortions that manifest from the anorexic's belief system and can be modified with this intervention: all-or-none reasoning whereby the anorexic thinks in absolute terms ("If I gain one pound I'll go on to gain a hundred"); overgeneralizing on the basis of one event ("I used to be of normal weight and wasn't happy, so gaining weight won't make me feel any better"); magnifying the significance of undesirable consequent events ("If others comment on my weight gain I won't be able to stand it"); egocentric interpretations of impersonal events ("Two people laughed when I walked by—they were probably saying that I was fat"). By having the patient articulate precisely what her fears are and define her terms, therapy can begin the task of evaluating their validity.

*Decentering* the egocentric perspective helps the patient to evaluate beliefs from different perspectives, allowing for the development of more realistic attitudes. For example, she may be instructed to establish a set of criteria for evaluating when her appearance or behavior are eliciting responses from the environment.

*Decatastrophizing* is used to combat the anxiety generated from magnifying the negative consequences of a particular event. Vague predictions of calamity are modified by asking such questions as "What if the feared situation occurred?" "Would it really be as devastating as imagined?" "Could coping strategies be generated?"

*Challenging the "shoulds"* explores the moralistic and arbitrary nature of self-commands such as "I should always diet" or "I should exercise daily" that evoke subsequent feelings of inadequacy due to their unattainability.

*Projective hypothesis testing* involves the translation of specific predictions and conclusions into formal hypotheses. These can then be evaluated by collecting data on planned experiments.

*Reattribution techniques* are used to assist anorexics in altering the interpretation of their self-perceptions. Garner and Bemis choose to conceptualize disturbances in the assessment of body shape as a cognitive, rather than perceptual, phenomenon. Hence, the therapeutic strategy is to change how the anorexic interprets what she sees instead of modifying her "misperception." The patient is encouraged to view her perception of herself as obese not as an accurate response to the stimulus but as a manifestation of the disease process. This serves to avoid confrontations that might erupt from direct attempts to contradict the patient's self-perception.

Garner and Bemis suggest that the application of cognitive-behavior therapy should not be restricted to the symptoms of anorexia nervosa alone but used to address other issues of concern for the individual. They note that anorexics often do not feel that they have the right to voice other complaints once their weight gain has been stabilized. The withdrawal of attention by both the therapist and family as soon as the maladaptive symptoms have abated may lead to a relapse by reinforcing the use of the illness for secondary gain or by leaving significant psychological problems unresolved.

The treatment approach proposed by Garner and Bemis is a multifaceted one, and the reader is directed to their writings for an elaboration of the techniques employed and of the therapeutic rationale. In sum, the authors consider this cognitive-behavioral model a promising one for treating anorexia nervosa, although still describing their hypothesis regarding its appropriate application as somewhat tentative. They report that to date, the techniques discussed have not been applied systematically in clinical settings. Thus, although the authors' impressions of their efficacy are favorable, they note that no rigorous testing has yet been conducted in the service of either supporting or refuting them. The specificity with which Garner and Bemis have presented this model is in part meant to encourage its replication and evaluation by other investigators.

Cognitive-behavioral interventions have also been an important therapeutic vehicle in an inpatient milieu treatment strategy that has been shown to be effective with chronic anorexics. Levendusky, Berglas, Dooley, and Landau (1983) designed The Therapeutic Contract Program (TCP) as an alternative to the inpatient operant paradigms and token economies where the generalization of behavior change beyond the sphere of structured contingency programs is limited. The goal of TCP is the fostering of self-control repertoires and a sense of personal responsibility (Berglas & Levendusky, 1985). This is approached through a core program augmented with a series of supplemental therapeutic interventions tailored to each patient's needs. Underpinning this strategy is the belief that the view of oneself as responsible for behavioral change is instrumental in the generalization and maintenance of therapeutic gains after discharge.

The core program is referred to as self-defined behavior contracting and serves to promote patient involvement in treatment goals and postdischarge plans. (Berglas & Levendusky, 1985). The treatment contract is a series of "intentional" statements conveying an expectation that certain behaviors will be effected or initiated in the upcoming week. Long-term goals, addressed by a series of short-term objectives, are developed with staff assistance through functional analyses of each patient's treatment needs. The essence of these contracts is that the goals and objectives developed are composed of self-imposed and self-generated standards that, when achieved, are attributed to internal rather than external factors. The staff's ongoing use of social reinforcements for the completion of contract items does, however, provide some degree of extrinsic inducement and reward in order to support the added behavior-changing influence of operant paradigms. Structured meetings for all members of the TCP community are held weekly. Each patient's contract is publically reviewed, and patient and staff feedback are offered on the degree of goal achievement. Interferences with contract compliance or with the harmonious functioning of the community result in open-door seclusion, which was found to be a very effective reinforcer. The incentive to leave is more than just the termination of a noxious stimulus but the wish to return to a desired and rewarding, but inaccessible, social environment. Levendusky and Dooley (1985) state that the support through a public contract process is particularly important in the treatment of anorexia where the issues of control and secrecy are often critical.

Another component of The Therapeutic Contract Program is Self-Control Training which takes place in a group format (Berglas & Levendusky, 1985). Training procedures based on an analysis of the patient's symptomatology and personal style are designed to modify cognitions and foster the internal attribution of change. Rational restructuring and systematic desensitization are among the techniques used.

Group Social Skill Training is a third component of the program and is composed of a three-tiered group sequence. Participation in a social interaction group is followed by involvement in a communications group, teaching assertiveness skills and adaptive social functioning

JANET SASSON
EDGETTE and
MAURICE F. PROUT

through role play and homework. In the cognitive restructuring group, the most advanced of the three, patients learn the basic principles of cognitive-behavior therapy. Negative self-statements, tendencies toward catastrophic thinking, and irrational assumptions are identified and challenged in the context of a process-oriented group experience. This experience provides group members with an interactive format, with situations from outside the group and therapeutic community serving as foci for discussion. Levendusky and Dooley (1985) write that the group component of the TCP is of paramount importance when treating anorexics. Viewing anorexia as a social as well as an eating disorder in which significant social interaction deficits are in evidence, they suggest the need for rudimentary didactic training with a heavy emphasis on role playing, video training, and facilitation of group interaction.

In addition to the components already described, anorexic inpatients participate in the integrated treatment protocol. Composed of three phases, this component is a rigorous operant approach designed to manage the maladaptive eating behaviors (Levendusky & Dooley, 1985). An introduction phase both exposes the newly admitted patient to the orientation procedures available to all incoming patients and allows the staff an opportunity to observe the patient. For the majority of patients who do not modify their eating patterns solely by virtue of being in a therapeutic environment, a self-control phase is initiated wherein a set of expectations regarding caloric intake, weight gain, number of meals and snacks per day, and the limitation of exercise are established for each individual. Extremely symptomatic or emaciated patients requiring a more restrictive environment move into the staff-control phase of the integrated treatment protocol. Criteria for discharge from the program include graduation through the self-control phase, achievement of an ideal weight, and the setting up of an aftercare program.

Levendusky and Dooley (1985) cite an outcome comparison study by Dooley, Landau, and Levendusky (in press) in which the treatment of anorexics using the TCP was compared to the more traditionally oriented approach of a private psychiatric hospital. Although both groups of eight patients were similar on measures related to the severity of their illness, the length of hospitalization for the TCP group was 50% shorter and the treatment outcome better in terms of weight gain. The authors conclude that the data demonstrate the effectiveness of the TCP in the treatment of severely symptomatic low-weight anorexics both in terms of weight gain and weight maintenance following discharge.

## FOLLOW-UP STUDIES

The short-term success of any treatment program designed to treat anorexics does not imply long-term cure. Bemis (1978) cited that, although the initial response to all forms of treatment is generally favorable, follow-up studies have shown that fewer than half of all patients treated for anorexia nervosa achieve long-term satisfactory adjustment. Physical and psychological symptoms reappear in 25% to 50% of these patients, and as many as one third may require rehospitalization within 2 years of treatment.

Schwartz and Thompson (1981) reviewed data from 12 major outcome studies of anorexia nervosa published between 1965 and 1977 and found that only half of the patients reported full recovery. Another 31% reported improvements in weight gains. Out of the 602 patients followed, 18% claimed no significant change at all. Social-marital adjustment was poor for 45% of the 478 patients on whom these data were available, and 46% of 407 reported signs of psychiatric impairment.

Citing studies done by Crisp (1983) and Agras and Werne (1978), Agras and Kraemer (1983) report that nearly two thirds of a previously hospitalized anorexic population will return to normal weight, with a majority experiencing regular menses. However, approximately half the population will continue to manifest eating disturbances and psychosocial impairments (Agras & Werne, 1978; Hsu, 1980).

There appears a dearth of long-term follow-up information on patients treated exclusively with behaviorally oriented therapies. Even fewer studies on the long-term effectiveness of cognitive therapy are available. Furthermore, little has been done to assess the differential effectiveness of various treatment modalities. Agras and Kraemer (1983) evaluated the results of 21 studies in order to compare the effectiveness of medical treatment, behavior therapy, and drug therapy on weight gain in anorexic patients. They found no difference between medical treatment and behavior therapy, although they temper this conclusion with the fact that entry weights for those treated medically were higher. Another finding was that, although mean weight gains in the three categories were similar, those in the behavior therapy group gained at a faster rate, sustaining the weight gain over the relatively short period of follow-up.

Hsu (1980) conducted an overview of outcome studies that were published between 1954 and 1978. He reported many of these studies as having shown that weight restoration immediately after treatment is not directly correlated with long-term maintenance. The short duration of follow-up done on many single-case studies does not accurately assess long-term outcome for either weight, eating behaviors, or psychological functioning. Small sample sizes and the lack of uniform definitions for "recovery," "satisfactory adjustment," and "cured" are other methodological flaws common to follow-up studies of anorexics.

Pertschuk (1977) completed an in-depth follow-up evaluation of 27 patients treated for anorexia nervosa at the University of Pennsylvania Psychiatric Service since March 1972. Almost every one of these patients had been placed on a behavioral contract that was supplemented by family therapy. Antidepressant medication was given to those suffering from severe depression. Treatment for weight gain had been successful for 25 of these patients. As a group, they had continued to gain weight after discharge, but Pertschuk noted that correlations between the percentage of weight gained during hospitalization and at follow-up were not significant. Only 2 of the 27 patients were reported as having completely recovered, with no residual adjustment or eating problems. Rehospitalization was required for 4 patients who had attempted suicide and 2 who were clinically depressed. Another 4 needed to return for another inpatient weight-gain program.

Pertschuk also discovered in his study that the normalization of weight was not paralleled by a normalization of eating patterns; most patients at follow-up continued to express an inordinate concern with food. The treatment program at the University of Pennsylvania had emphasized weight gain and not the extinction of maladaptive eating habits. The author advised clinicians of behavior therapy to assess the importance of resolving pathologic eating behaviors in the treatment of anorexia nervosa.

## CONCLUSION

An important consideration for those clinicians treating anorexics with behaviorally oriented and cognitive-behavioral therapies is the delineation of the goals of treatment. Although many programs emphasize the return to near normal weights as their immediate goal, long-range goals often remain ambiguous. Nevertheless, there appears to be an increasing awareness that ultimate goals in the treatment of these patients include not only the maintenance of healthy weight and eating habits but concommitant improvements in their psychological, sexual, and social adjustments, as well as a return to satisfactory functioning in their daily lives. Slade (1982) emphasizes the need for clinicians to work with the anorexic patient in the development of successful behaviors and alternative interests that can provide other sources of positive reinforcement to replace those received by the individual through her anorexic symptoms. Once this occurs, the anorexic can begin to break the vicious cycle of dieting and weight control and the powerful satisfaction that it provides. What follows is a case study of a young woman treated for anorexia nervosa over the course of 10 months, using primarily a cognitive-behavioral approach. The development of new, more adaptive behaviors and of alternative interests was an integral part of the psychotherapy.

## CASE STUDY

### Introduction

Carol was referred for therapy after taking a medical leave of absence from her college. She was 18 years of age at the time of the initial evaluation. Her parents were physicians (surgeon, internist) who prided themselves on offering a family environment marked by both intellectual and social achievements. Carol was noted to be quite popular in high school, belonging to a number of organizations. She was intellectually gifted, graduating in the upper 2% of her high-school class and attaining mid-1400s on her SATs.

Much to the delight of her parents, Carol was accepted to an Ivy League university on full academic scholarship. Unfortunately, she soon found herself in competition with other gifted and socially adept students. Four months into her freshman year, a long-standing boyfriend from high-school days announced that he was interested in someone else and terminated the relationship. At the end of her first semester, she evaluated her life as follows:

1. "My grades weren't what they should have been, I was getting B's and C's."
2. "I was really miserable without Craig—crying, feeling lost."
3. "I found other students were voted officers of clubs instead of me; I became just another member."

Carol's parents became concerned with her academic performance and urged her to commit more effort to her studies. Indeed, her father called the university and, after some negotiation, was able to arrange individual tutoring for three of her subjects. Upon entering her second semester, Carol was spending considerably more time with academics and less with social activities. She did not date and began to eat more. Concomitant with increased studying and eating was a modicum of improvement in her grades and an increase of approximately 25 lb in a 7-week period.

Because her grades were now improved, Carol felt some freedom to begin dating. A date was arranged via a roommate and, as luck would have it, she became quite infatuated with the young man. Unfortunately, his interest soon dwindled, with the relationship ending quite suddenly. She later stated that she had felt "tossed away, like I couldn't do anything right." She continued to eat, gain weight, and remain socially isolated. Upon a weekend visit, both parents were surprised by her weight gain but did not comment except to praise her for the grade improvement. During the same visit, her brother stated, "You sure have gotten fat." Carol remembers that approximately 2 weeks after that visit she decided it was time to take charge of her life.

Carol began a diligent regimen of starvation. She religiously avoided most food and commenced upon a strenuous 7-days-per-week aerobics program. Over a 4-week period her weight dropped considerably. Initially, others were complimentary; they soon, however, became concerned. Hospitalization was precipitated by Carol's fainting on her way to class.

A complete medical work-up was instituted at the university hospital, and no organic etiology was discovered to account for the profound weight loss. The diagnosis was anorexia nervosa. Therapists should be aware that in treating eating-disordered patients, ongoing consultation with an internist familiar with the condition is essential. These patients are vulnerable to a variety of medical disturbances—some life threatening—and the appropriate medical backup must be maintained from the beginning of treatment.

Psychotherapy consisted of instituting an operant model, similar to those discussed in the earlier part of this chapter. Although weight gain was gradually achieved, Carol remained unhappy. She was discharged from the hospital, a medical leave from school was arranged, and she returned home. Soon thereafter Carol began to lose weight and was referred again for treatment.

## Rationale for Treatment

Although there are numerous research and case studies attesting to the various efficacies of operant approaches to eating disorders, we advocate an individual approach driven by a cognitive and behavioral analysis. By this we mean not only an assessment of eating behaviors but, in addition, an appreciation of the patient's cognitive map, that is, way of understanding or making sense of the world and events. In the case of Carol, the initial operant program resulted in a good outcome with poor follow-up results. Although this approach may have been successful for some patients, it did not hold in this case. The ultimate failure, from the therapists' perspective, was due to a lack of completeness in comprehending the case. Issues related to perception of self, schemata, cognitive distortions, problem-solving ability, and interpersonal assertiveness were never addressed.

## Brief Review of Interventions

Upon her return home, Carol's initial Beck Depressive Inventory score was 32. Although she was not suicidal, a review of the BDI revealed themes of demoralization and helplessness. An initial review of the Daily Record of Dysfunctional Thoughts indicated a high degree of sensitivity to potential interpersonal rejection. Her weekly activity schedule was entirely focused upon the kitchen (counting calories), her room (reading, watching TV), and her local Y (exercising). In short order, it became clear that the only activity of significance through which Carol experienced a sense of control and mastery was in obsessively managing her weight.

The therapeutic process targeted a number of areas in need of attention. Assertiveness training was instituted, along with videotaped replay. The rationale for this stemmed from Carol's own statement that her popularity seemed dependent upon always doing for others. Various scenarios were developed to offer her exposure to other ways of responding to interpersonal situations. When she experienced difficulty with a particular scene, playback allowed her to determine whether it was due to a lack of skill or to anxiety. More often than not, the latter was identified, and this then provided access to underlying assumptions, cognitive distortions, and the like. One silent rule governing Carol's behavior was, "If I don't always do for others, they won't like me." Not only was this worked within the standard cognitive therapy manner but, in appreciation of her worst case fantasy, alternative responses other than falling apart were explored and developed. This was done through a problem-solving mode wherein she would state the problem, outline her typical response, list possible alternatives, view the consequences, and evaluate the results.

Partly responsible for Carol's decrease in social activity was her assumption that if she couldn't be a "star" in the activity or organization, it was not worth pursuing. As therapy proceeded, she was willing to attempt a variety of activities to test-out this hypothesis. To her surprise, she discovered that she could actually enjoy certain activities without having to be the center of attention. Indeed, she admitted to a certain relief at not having to be "on" all the time.

Interaction with the opposite sex turned out to be the proverbial albatross for Carol. Her silent assumptions were mainly personalized. If a relationship did not continue, she automatically assumed that she was the causative factor, that she was unlikable, too fat, not attractive, and the like. Although not dismissing outright her potential contribution to the demise of a relationship, systematic questioning and investigation led to her acknowledgment that the other party might, for a variety of reasons, wish to discontinue a relationship and that these alternative possibilities might have nothing to do with her worthiness.

Finally, the silent as well as spoken demands of academic excellence needed to be addressed. Carol gradually came to rate her level of happiness as nil under her current academic regimen. Although receiving an A was gratifying, the cost was severe restrictions in other areas of her life. Despite a family meeting, both parents remained adamant that she maintain her GPA. Carol was able to hold her own with her parents, agreeing to return to college only if B's and C's were acceptable to them. After much haggling, the parents reluctantly agreed.

This patient has to date a 7-year follow-up. She completed her undergraduate degree and as well as an MBA. Her weight is maintained at appropriate levels, and there is no bulimia or addictions. Although her work is stressful, she builds in "buffers" for relaxation. She still continues to experience urges to excel at all costs and in all activities (work, social) but is able to identify the underlying rules, assess the costs, and develop reasonable alternatives. She states that she continues to feel in control of her life and remains asymptomatic.

## SUMMARY

In presenting this case, the authors are advocating that a thorough assessment of patients be undertaken. Appreciation of only a behavioral or cognitive dimension can be clinically disastrous for the anorexic patient. Although operant approaches clearly work for some, they are not effective for all; this is so for cognitive approaches as well.

Clinicians are urged to conceptualize the anorexic's operant environment as existing well beyond eating behavior. Certainly, family and social consequences need to be appreciated within the context of treatment. Also, the patient's perceptions of the world, her guiding assumptions, and level of transactional skill serve as potentially fertile ground for intervention. The probability of successful outcome is heightened when both cognitive and behavioral domains are clinically assessed.

## REFERENCES

Agras, S., Barlow, D. H., Chapin, H. N., Abel, G. G., & Leitenberg, H. (1974). Behavior modification of anorexia nervosa. *Archives of General Psychiatry, 30,* 279–286.

Agras, W. S., & Kraemer, H. C. (1983). The treatment of anorexia nervosa: Do different treatments have different outcomes? *Psychiatric Annals, 13,* 928–935.

Agras, W. S., & Werne, J. (1978). Behavior therapy in anorexia nervosa: A data-based approach to the question. In J. P. Brady & H. K. H. Brodie (Eds.), *Controversy in psychiatry* (pp. 655–675). Philadelphia: W. B. Saunders.

American Psychiatric Association. (1980). *Diagnostic and Statistical Manual of Mental Disorders* (3rd ed.). Washington, DC: Author.

Bachrach, A. J., Erwin, W. J., & Mohr, J. P. (1965). The control of eating behavior in an anorexic by operant conditioning techniques. In L. P. Ullman & L. Krasner (Eds.), *Case studies in behavior modification* (pp. 153–163). New York: Holt, Rinehart & Winston.

Bandura, A. (1978). The self-system in reciprocal determinism. *American Psychologist, 33,* 344–358.

Beck, A. T. (1970). Role of fantasies in psychotherapy and psychopathology. *Journal of Nervous and Mental Disease, 150,* 3–17.

Beck, A. T. (1976). *Cognitive therapy and the emotional disorders.* New York: International Universities Press.

Beck, A. T., Rush, A. J., Shaw, B. F., & Emery, G. (1979). *Cognitive therapy of depression: A treatment manual.* New York: Guilford.

Bemis, K. M. (1978). Current approaches to the etiology and treatment of anorexia nervosa. *Psychological Bulletin, 85,* 593–613.

Berglas, S., & Levendusky, P. G. (1985). The Therapeutic Contract Program: An individual-oriented psychological treatment community. *Psychotherapy, 22,* 36–45.

Bhanji, S., & Thompson, J. (1974). Operant conditioning in the treatment of anorexia nervosa: A review and retrospective study of 11 cases. *British Journal of Psychiatry, 124,* 166–172.

Blinder, B. J., Freeman, D. M. A., & Stunkard, A. J. (1970). Behavior therapy of anorexia nervosa: Effectiveness of activity as a reinforcer of weight gain. *American Journal of Psychiatry, 128,* 77–82.

Bruch, H. (1962). Perceptual and conceptual disturbances in anorexia nervosa. *Psychosomatic Medicine, 24,* 187–194.

Bruch, H. (1974). Perils of behavior modification in the treatment of anorexia nervosa. *Journal of the American Medical Association, 230,* 1419–1422.

Cinciripini, P. M., Kornblith, S. J., Turner, S. M., & Hersen, M. (1983). A behavioral program for the management of anorexia and bulimia. *Journal of Nervous and Mental Disease, 171,* 186–189.

Clarke, M. G., & Palmer, R. L. (1983). Eating attitudes and neurotic symptoms in university students. *British Journal of Psychiatry, 142,* 299–304.

Cooper, P. J., & Fairburn, C. G. (1984). Cognitive behaviour therapy for anorexia nervosa: Some preliminary findings. *Journal of Psychosomatic Research, 28,* 493–499.

Crisp, A. H. (1983). Treatment and outcome in anorexia nervosa. In R. K. Goodstein (Ed.), *Eating and weight disorders* (pp. 91–104). New York: Springer.

Crisp, A. H., Palmer, R. L., & Kalucy, R. S. (1976). How common is anorexia nervosa? A prevalence study. *British Journal of Psychiatry, 128,* 549–554.

Dickstein, L. J. (1985). Anorexia nervosa and bulimia: A review of clinical issues. *Hospital and Community Psychiatry, 36,* 1086–1092.

Dooley, C. P., Landau, R. J., & Levenduskly, P. G. (In press). *Integrated treatment protocol: A comprehensive approach to the treatment of anorexia nervosa.* Manuscript submitted for publication.

Eckert, E. D., Goldberg, S. C., Halmi, K. A., Casper, R. C., & Davis, J. M. (1979). Behavior therapy in anorexia nervosa. *British Journal of Psychiatry, 134,* 55–59.

Ellis, A. (1962). *Reason and emotion in psychotherapy.* (Secaucus, NJ: Lyle Stuart.

Erwin, W. J. (1977). A 16-year follow-up of a case of severe anorexia nervosa. *Journal of Behavior Therapy and Experimental Psychiatry, 8,* 157–160.

Fundudis, T. (1986). Anorexia nervosa in a pre-adolescent girl: Multimodal behaviour therapy approach. *Journal of Child Psychology and Psychiatry, 27,* 261–273.

Garfinkel, P. E., & Garner, D. M. (1982). *Anorexia nervosa: A multidimensional perspective.* New York: Brunner/Mazel.

Garfinkel, P. E., Moldofsky, H., & Garner, D. M. (1977). The outcome of anorexia nervosa: Significance of clinical features, body image, and behavior modification. In R. A. Vigersky (Ed.), *Anorexia nervosa* (pp. 315–329). New York: Raven.

Garner, D. M. (1986). Cognitive therapy for anorexia nervosa. In K. D. Brownell & J. P. Foreyt (Eds.), *Handbook of eating disorders* (pp. 301–327). New York: Basic Books.

Garner, D. M., & Bemis, K. M. (1982). A cognitive-behavioral approach to anorexia nervosa. *Cognitive Therapy and Research, 6,* 123–150.

Garner, D. M., & Bemis, K. M. (1985). Cognitive therapy for anorexia nervosa. In D. M. Garner & P. E. Garfinkel (Eds.), *Handbook of psychotherapy for anorexia nervosa and bulimia* (pp. 107–146). New York: The Guilford Press.

Garner, D. M., & Garfinkel, P. E. (1980). Socio-cultural factors in the development of anorexia nervosa. *Psychological Medicine, 10,* 647–656.

Garner, D. M., & Garfinkel, P. E. (1985). Introduction. In D. M. Garner & P. E. Garfinkel (Eds.). *Handbook of psychotherapy for anorexia nervosa and bulimia* (pp. 3–6). New York: Guilford.

Goldfried, M. R. (1971). Systematic desensitization as training in self-control. *Journal of Consulting and Clinical Psychology, 37,* 228–234.

Hallsten, Jr., E. A. (1965). Adolescent anorexia nervosa treated by desensitization. *Behavior Research and Therapy, 3,* 87–91.

Halmi, K. A. (1982). Pragmatic information on the eating disorders. *Psychiatric Clinics of North America, 5,* 371–377.

Halmi, K. A. (1983). Anorexia nervosa and bulimia. *Psychosomatics, 24,* 111–129.

Halmi, K. A. (1985). Behavioral management for anorexia nervosa. In D. M. Garner & P. E. Garfinkel (Eds.), *Handbook of psychotherapy for anorexia nervosa and bulimia* (pp. 147–159). New York: Guilford.

Hauserman, N., & Lavin, P. (1977). Post-hospitalization continuation treatment of anorexia nervosa. *Journal of Behavior Therapy and Experimental Psychiatry, 8,* 309–313.

Hollon, S. D., & Beck, A. T. (1979). Cognitive therapy of depression. In P. C. Kendall & S. D. Hollon (Eds.), *Cognitive-behavioral interventions: Theory, research and procedures* (pp. 153–203). New York: Academic Press.

Hsu, L. K. G. (1980). Outcome of anorexia nervosa: A review of the literature (1954 to 1978). *Archives of General Psychiatry, 37,* 1041–1043.

Kissel, S., & Arkins, V. (1973). Anorexia nervosa reexamined. *Child Psychiatry and Human Development, 3,* 255–263.

Leitenberg, H. Agras, W. S., & Thompson, L. (1968). A sequential analysis of the effect of selective positive reinforcement in modifying anorexia nervosa. *Behavior Research and Therapy, 6,* 211–218.

Levendusky, P. G., & Dooley, C. P. (1985). An inpatient model for the treatment of anorexia nervosa. In S. Emmett (Ed.), *Theory and treatment of anorexia nervosa and bulimia—Biomedical, sociocultural and psychological perspectives* (pp. 211–233). New York: Brunner/Mazel.

Levendusky, P. G., Berglas, S., Dooley, C. P., & Landau, R. J. (1983). Therapeutic contract program: Preliminary report on a behavioral alternative to the token economy. *Behavior Research and Therapy, 21,* 137–142.

Mahoney, M. J., (1974). *Cognition and behavior modification.* Cambridge: Ballinger.

Mavissakalian, M. (1982). Anorexia nervosa treated with response prevention and prolonged exposure. *Behavior Research and Therapy, 20,* 27–31.

McFarlane, A. H., Bellissimo, A., & Upton, E. (1982). "Atypical" anorexia nervosa: Treatment and management on a behavioral medicine unit. *The Psychiatric Journal of the University of Ottawa, 7,* 158–162.

Meichenbaum, D. (1974). *Therapist manual for cognitive behavior modification.* Ontario: University of Waterloo Press.

Minuchin, S., Rosman, B., & Baker, L. (1978). *Psychosomatic families: Anorexia nervosa in context.* Cambridge: Harvard University Press.

Muuss, R. E. (1985). Adolescent eating disorder: Anorexia nervosa. *Adolescence, 20,* 525–536.

Neuman, M., & Gaoni, B. (1975). Preferred food as the reinforcing agent in a case of anorexia nervosa. *Journal of Behavior Therapy and Experimental Psychiatry, 6,* 331–333.

Nylander, I. (1971). The feeling of being fat and dieting in a school population. *Acta Socio-Medica Scandinavica, 3,* 17–26.

Ollendick, T. H. (1979). Behavioral treatment of anorexia nervosa. *Behavior Modification, 3,* 124–135.

Peake, T., & Borduin, C., (1977). Behavioral and analytical approaches to the treatment of anorexia nervosa: A case study. *Family Therapy, 4,* 49–56.

Pertschuk, M. J. (1977). Behavior therapy: Extended follow-up. In R. A. Vigersky (Ed.), *Anorexia nervosa* (pp. 305–314). New York: Raven.

Powers, P. S., & Powers, H. P. (1984). Inpatient treatment of anorexia nervosa. *Psychosomatics, 25,* 512–527.

Ross, A. O. (1980). *Psychological disorders of children: A Behavioral approach to theory, research and therapy* (2nd ed.). New York: McGraw-Hill.

Salkind, M. R., Fincham, J., & Silverstone, T. (1980). Is anorexia a phobic disorder? A psychophysiological enquiry. *Biological Psychiatry, 15,* 803–808.

Schwartz, D. M., & Thompson, M. G. (1981). Do anorexics get well? Current research and future needs. *American Journal of Psychiatry, 138,* 319–323.

Scrignar, C. B. (1971). Food as the reinforcer in the outpatient treatment of anorexia nervosa. *Journal of Behavior Therapy and Experimental Psychiatry, 2,* 31–36.

Slade, P. (1982). Towards a functional analysis of anorexia nervosa and bulimia nervosa. *British Journal of Clinical Psychology, 21,* 167–179.

Vandereycken, W., & Meermann, R. (1984). *Anorexia nervosa: A clinician's guide to treatment.* Berlin: Walter de Gruyter.

Whipple, S. B., & Manning, D. E. (1978). Anorexia nervosa: Commitment to a multifaceted treatment program. *Psychotherapy and Psychosomatics, 30,* 161–169.

Ziesat, H. A., & Ferguson, J. M. (1984). Outpatient treatment of primary anorexia nervosa in adult males. *Journal of Clinical Psychology, 40,* 680–690.

# 20

# Treatment of Obesity

F. MATTHEW KRAMER AND LAURIE A. STALKER

## INTRODUCTION

Obesity is one of the major health problems in modern society. A recent National Institutes of Health Consensus Development Conference (1985) concluded that being overweight by 20% or more of ideal body weight represents a significant risk for increased mortality and morbidity. Among the health risks associated with obesity are cardiovascular disease, hypertension, diabetes, and some types of cancers (Bray, 1985). In the United States, approximately 30% of women and 25% of men are 20% or more overweight. Obesity is also becoming increasingly common in children and adolescents (Gortmaker, Dietz, Sobal, & Wehler, 1987). From the mid-1960s to the late 1970s, the prevalence of obesity increased from 17.6% to 27.1% in 6- to 11-year-old children and from 15.8% to 21.9% in 12- to 17-year-olds.

In addition to increased health risks, there are also significant psychosocial consequences of obesity. Negative stereotypes about obesity are endemic to Western society. Obese people are commonly seen as being responsible for their obesity and generally less attractive, likable, intelligent, and capable than normal-weight individuals (Wooley, 1987). This stigmatization of obesity has important practical effects as well. Obese persons, for example, are less likely to be admitted to college than normal-weight people with similar qualifications (Canning & Mayer, 1966). Obese people are also more likely to face discrimination in the work environment (Allon, 1982) and have more difficulty obtaining employment (Roe & Eickwort, 1976). The extreme prejudice against fatness is apparent even in young children (Staffieri, 1967). Young children are more likely to rate obese silhouettes as ''stupid'', ''ugly'' and ''lazy'' than average-weight or thin silhouettes. Obese persons often internalize or passively accept these negative attitudes and thereby are apt to expect failure of themselves and criticism from others (Wooley, 1987).

The treatment of obesity would appear to be a fairly straightforward task: consume fewer calories and expend more calories. However, successful weight loss is deterred by complex biological, psychological, and social factors. For example, research indicates that there are

F. MATTHEW KRAMER • Behavioral Sciences Division, U.S. Army Natick Research, Development, and Engineering Center, Natick, Massachusetts 01760–5020.    LAURIE A. STALKER • Department of Psychiatry, University of Pennsylvania, Philadelphia, Pennsylvania 19104.

F. MATTHEW
KRAMER and LAURIE
A. STALKER

strong physiological pressures (e.g., a high number of fat cells) that help maintain obesity (Sjostrom, 1980). Furthermore, keeping excess weight off requires permanent changes in life-style. In recent years, cognitive-behavioral approaches have provided effective methods of obtaining significant weight loss. Comprehensive treatment of obesity involves the decision to seek or provide treatment, choosing the initial form(s) of intervention with appropriate revision over time (e.g., working for weight loss), and maximizing the likelihood of weight loss maintenance.

## ASSESSMENT

### THE DECISION TO LOSE WEIGHT

The client's actual weight, desired weight loss, and ideal weight (based on the Metropolitan tables—Table 1) can be examined to determine how realistic and appropriate the goal weight is. A client 20 pounds overweight who wishes to lose 30 pounds clearly presents a different situation than a person who is presently 50 pounds overweight who has never been within the ideal weight range of the Metropolitan table. Similarly, someone who hopes to lose 40 pounds in 4 weeks may pose different concerns for the clinician. A balance is necessary between what the client wishes to lose, how much on average they are above the ideal weight range, and their willingness to commit time and energy to the process of weight loss.

People seek help to lose weight for a wide range of motivations and with varying levels of readiness. The final choice of what, if any, treatment to pursue is ultimately up to the client. However, thorough assessment of a person's reasons for seeking treatment and factors related to outcome will best set the groundwork for making and following through on the decision to lose weight.

The main goal of the initial contact with the potential weight loss client is to put her or his weight goals and present weight status in an appropriate context. This includes not only components directly relevant to weight loss but also the many other aspects of the person's life (e.g., physical, social, psychological, financial). For example, if a client has severe arthritis, then vigorous walking or running will not be advisable, and physical activities such as swimming may be explored as a means to increase caloric expenditure. Likewise, a lack of assertiveness with other people may hinder efforts to control intake in social settings, and therefore assertiveness training could be incorporated into the treatment plan. Not only must the need for or importance of weight loss be addressed but also the individual's readiness. Appropriate postponement of a weight loss program may be a positive step in some situations. If the client cannot commit the time or energy needed to achieve weight loss for whatever reasons, then the clinician will probably best serve the client by deferring weight loss treatment. Alternatively, time may be spent on dealing with why such a committment cannot be made, whether it is a matter of some more pressing problem or more of a motivational issue.

The initial step is to assess the client's problems and issues. Why is she or he seeking to lose weight at the present time? Some persons, may be more motivated by external forces (e.g., physician's recommendations, pressure from family members), whereas others have personal reasons (e.g., improving one's appearance). Following Brownell (1988), the client can list reasons for and against beginning a weight loss program (Table 2).

For example, Bob would seem to have more reasons for not beginning a program at this time. Becky, on the other hand, has more reasons to lose weight then not. The therapist can be particularly helpful in assisting the client to see the potential benefits and costs of weight loss in a balanced manner. In some situations, a client may be seeking weight loss as a means to deal with other problems (e.g., marital disharmony) or have concurrent difficulties (e.g., depression). A joint decision between the therapist and client then needs to be made regarding

TABLE 1. 1983 Metropolitan Height and Weight Tables[a]

| Men | | | | |
|---|---|---|---|---|
| Height: | | | | |
| Feet | Inches | Small frame | Medium frame | Large frame |
| 5 | 2 | 128–134 | 131–141 | 138–150 |
| 5 | 3 | 130–136 | 133–143 | 140–153 |
| 5 | 4 | 132–138 | 135–145 | 142–156 |
| 5 | 5 | 134–140 | 137–148 | 144–160 |
| 5 | 6 | 136–142 | 139–151 | 149–168 |
| 5 | 7 | 138–145 | 142–154 | 149–168 |
| 5 | 8 | 140–148 | 145–157 | 152–172 |
| 5 | 9 | 142–151 | 148–160 | 155–176 |
| 5 | 10 | 144–154 | 151–163 | 158–180 |
| 5 | 11 | 146–157 | 154–166 | 161–184 |
| 6 | 0 | 149–160 | 157–170 | 164–188 |
| 6 | 1 | 152–164 | 160–174 | 168–192 |
| 6 | 2 | 155–168 | 167–182 | 172–192 |
| 6 | 3 | 158–172 | 167–182 | 176–202 |
| 6 | 4 | 162–176 | 171–187 | 181–207 |

| Women | | | | |
|---|---|---|---|---|
| Height: | | | | |
| Feet | Inches | Small frame | Medium frame | Large frame |
| 4 | 10 | 102–111 | 109–121 | 118–131 |
| 4 | 11 | 103–113 | 111–123 | 120–134 |
| 5 | 0 | 104–115 | 113–126 | 122–137 |
| 5 | 1 | 106–118 | 115–129 | 125–140 |
| 5 | 2 | 108–121 | 118–132 | 128–143 |
| 5 | 3 | 111–124 | 121–135 | 131–147 |
| 5 | 4 | 114–127 | 124–138 | 134–151 |
| 5 | 5 | 117–130 | 127–141 | 137–155 |
| 5 | 6 | 120–133 | 130–144 | 140–159 |
| 5 | 7 | 123–136 | 133–147 | 143–163 |
| 5 | 8 | 126–139 | 136–150 | 146–167 |
| 5 | 9 | 129–142 | 139–153 | 149–170 |
| 5 | 10 | 132–145 | 142–156 | 152–173 |
| 5 | 11 | 135–148 | 145–159 | 155–176 |
| 6 | 0 | 138–151 | 148–162 | 158–179 |

[a]Reprinted with permission from *Statistical Bulletin*, 1983, *64*, 2.

which concerns, if any, need to be addressed, and how these effect the decision to begin a weight loss program. For example, Bob listed reducing his wife's nagging as a potential benefits of going on a diet. If he were to go ahead with a diet, his chances of success are limited, nor has he made any positive steps in dealing with the pressure he feels from his spouse.

Examining the person's attitudes about being overweight and his or her expectations about weight loss are also important in the decision-making process. That is, in what ways does the person experience distress related to weight (e.g., lack of fitness as experienced by shortness of breath and/or a sense of being a weak-willed individual because obesity has been allowed to develop)? Clients may also hold realistic beliefs about how weight loss will improve

TABLE 2. Perceived Benefits and Sacrifices of Starting a Diet for
Two Overweight Persons[a]

|  | Bob's list |
| --- | --- |
| Benefits | Sacrifices |
| Stops wife nagging | Give up favorite food |
| Look better | Go to clinic meetings |
|  | Feel deprived |
|  | Embarrassed about diet around friends |
|  | Fatigue |
|  | Becky's list |
| Benefits | Sacrifices |
| More energy | Hard work and sacrifice |
| Better chance for job | Constant effort |
| Look better for dating | Must drink less with friends |
| Wider choice of clothes |  |
| Improve health |  |

[a]Reprinted with permission from Brownell, K. D. (1988). *The LEARN Program for
Weight Control.*

their lives, but some individuals may expect weight loss to result in immediate and dramatic improvements in satisfaction with their lives. Unrealistic attitudes or expectations need to be identified and resolved, or the efficacy of treatment is likely to suffer. One client, for example, felt that her life was a mess financially and emotionally and that her relationship with her husband was steadily deteriorating. Although the initial interview confirmed that many sources of distress were present, some open to change and others not, she repeatedly emphasized her belief that weight loss would somehow result in marked improvement in all aspects of her life. Because she was not open to dealing with problems other than her weight and unwilling to give up her belief about the effects of weight loss, a useful treatment plan was not possible.

In addition to the relatively open-ended assessment already described, the more structured evaluation of information that follows is crucial for weight loss treatment.

## WEIGHT STATUS AND WEIGHT HISTORY

The client's current degree of overweight can be most simply determined using a standard height and weight table (Metropolitan Life Insurance Company, 1983). Although such tables do not provide an exact measure of body composition they do provide a practical estimate of the desirable weight range for a given individual (see Table 2). Individuals between 20% and 40% overweight are considered to be mildly obese, 41% to 100% moderately obese, and over 100% morbidly obese. If more exact measures are desired, the most precise method is by underwater weighing (Garrow, 1978). Formulas based on skinfold measurements at several sites on the body (Durnin & Womersley, 1974) also give a good estimate of body fat.

Obesity may be manifested in either hypertrophic or hyperplastic forms. Hypertrophic obesity refers to an increase in fat cell size but not fat cell number. Hyperplastic obesity refers to an increase in fat cell number; obesity, particularly if severe, is often accompanied with increase in fat cell size and number. Individuals who become obese in childhood are more likely to have an increased number of fat cells especially if they are morbidly obese. Fat cells do not appear to be lost even with large weight losses and shrink only to a limited degree. As a result, the heavier childhood-onset person may not realistically be able to reach an ideal weight (Sjostrom, 1980). People who have repeatedly lost and regained significant amounts of weight may also have greater difficulty with weight loss due to findings that suggest that repeated dieting increases the body's metabolic efficiency (Brownell, Greenwood, Stellar, & Shrager, 1986).

Given the potential impact that type of obesity and repeated dieting have, a detailed weight history is important. Typically, the clinician starts by asking the client his or her weight at 5-year intervals since birth. Significant losses or gains as well as the perceived causes are also reported. The client may talk with parents or teachers or use photographs and so on as a means to gain more information about childhood weights. Deliberate weight loss efforts should be explored in detail. Weight loss method, duration, weight loss, time the loss was kept off, and the client's reactions are all useful information. Family history of overweight and weight-related attitudes should also obtained. Extent of previous dieting, family history, and years since onset of the obesity are all likely to be associated with a more difficult course of weight loss and especially weight loss maintenance (Dubbert & Wilson, 1983). The Stanford Eating Disorders Questionnaire (Agras *et al.*, 1976) is useful for obtaining the basic weight history information that may then be supplemented by discussion with the client. The goal here is to obtain as detailed as possible description of the client's weight history and the background characteristics and events that have influenced that history. An example of such an assessment is given in Figure 1.

PSYCHOLOGICAL ASSESSMENT

In clinical practice with obese persons, standard psychological evaluation including measures of depression (e.g., the Beck Depression Inventory), anxiety (e.g., Spielberger State-Trait Anxiety Inventory), marital and social adjustment (e.g., Locke-Wallace Marital Adjustment Test), work satisfaction, self-concept (e.g., Tennessee Self-Concept Scale), and overall psychopathology (e.g., MMPI) is appropriate. Although obesity is not necessarily linked to any particular type or level of pathology (McReynolds, 1982; Wadden & Stunkard, 1987), the evaluation may reveal factors that will effect the usefulness of weight loss treatment or influence the therapist's recommendations. In addition, psychological assessment provides a second source along with a medical evaluation for placing a person's obesity in an overall context. Thus, a client with marital problems or a significant depression may be suitable for combined weight loss and other therapy. Alternatively, problems may be dealt with on a one-at-a-time basis with, for example, treatment for weight loss being postponed while depression is treated. The crucial point here is that, whereas psychological factors may not predict treatment outcome, interventions for obesity must be conducted with an awareness of the

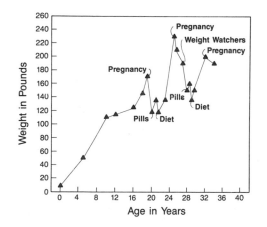

FIGURE 1. Example of a weight history graph.

person's overall functioning. Similarly, the clinician needs to be sensitive to changes during therapy as some clients do experience negative emotional (Stunkard & Rush, 1974) or social responses (Wadden & Stunkard, 1987).

The potential sources and types of social support in the client's environment should also be evaluated. Are there people in the workplace or at home who could provide support and how have these people helped or hindered past efforts at change. Clients can also describe past efforts to obtain support and their success or failure in doing so.

MEDICAL EVALUATION

Although many clients seek weight loss for reasons of appearance a significant proportion are motivated by health reasons. In either case, a pretreatment physical is appropriate. A medical evaluation will provide information about past and present physical status. The client should inform his or her physician of the plan for weight loss and seek the physician recommendations regarding any dietary or exercise restrictions. Periodic monitoring by the physician can provide useful information to the client and therapist about improvements and complications in health parameters during the course of treatment (e.g., blood pressure, cholesterol). For some individuals changes in health risks may be the primary reason for seeking weight loss and thus changes in medical status will be an important measure of treatment outcome. In this sense weight loss may serve as a valuable adjunct or alternative to medical intervention.

# TREATMENT

The treatment of choice for mild obesity (20% to 40% overweight) is a predominantly behavioral program. The safety and efficacy of behavioral interventions have been documented in nearly 200 controlled studies (Brownell & Wadden, 1986; Wilson & Brownell, 1980). In recent years, more explicit and in-depth emphasis has also been placed on the physical activity and nutritional aspects of weight loss and maintenance.

In research protocols, treatment typically lasts from 3 to 6 months. However, subjects in such programs often do not reach their goal weights and, therefore, in clinical settings, treatment sessions will usually extend over a period of many months or in some cases 1 or more years. Subjects may be seen individually or in small groups (5 or less) so that individualization of treatment methods is possible. A basic core program is provided in weekly 60- to 90-minute sessions over a 12- to 24-week period. Subsequent meetings may be scheduled less frequently (i.e., twice a month) with a focus on problem solving, and, as goal weight is approached, increasingly on long-term maintenance strategies. The chronic nature of obesity and its treatment indicate that continued treatment may be necessary. Thus, clients should be seen at 6- or 12-month intervals even after successful weight loss. Clients should also be encouraged to make appointments or phone contact as desired. The goal is to prevent or at least allow for recovery from relapse. Follow-up contact with the client is apt to be of most benefit if the focus of these sessions is on problem solving and the development of strategies and less on supportive measures alone (Perri, 1987). The specific problem or problems are identified, coping strategies or possible solutions are developed, and strategies are applied and evaluated until an effective approach is found. For example, the client might report continued problems with eating when visiting friends or relatives. Possible solutions would include increasing the client's assertive refusal of food offers, explaining the situation to other people, and planning ahead so that food consumed while visiting will not result in excessive intake. Subsequently, the client might find that food refusal works well with friends but less well with relatives. However, adjusting food intake before and after the visit to the relatives results in a satisfactory overall intake.

Substantial variety exists from one program to another, but a basic core of techniques is typically applied. There techniques can be categorized into several broad components: self-monitoring, stimulus control, changing eating behavior, and cognitive restructuring. Although early programs used these methods primarily to control and reduce food intake, more recent efforts fruitfully employ behavioral methods to incorporate nutritional and physical activity components into treatment. Programs are also increasingly incorporating a focus on long-term change as opposed to the acute emphasis of many early interventions. One of the major additions to obesity treatment has been the inclusion of a relapse prevention component. Relapse prevention is a way of conceptualizing behavior change that is particularly applicable to the maintenance of change. As will be discussed later, relapse prevention integrates behavioral and cognitive methods as a means for long-term life-style change.

At the start of treatment, the emphasis is on monitoring the client's behavior. The information gained by this method provides a setting in which to learn and apply the techniques and information described later. Each session has as an agenda, a particular topic or method as its focus, as well as reviewing particular problems clients have, and previously taught material. Thus, as treatment progresses, clients enlarge their knowledge base and the number of methods that may be employed. Moreover, through their own review of their efforts as well as in collaboration with the therapist, clients refine their thinking and behavior and develop specific ways in which to optimize change. The need for continued evaluation and modification of the weight loss program cannot be overemphasized. With the assistance of the therapist, the client is conducting a single-subject experiment with the goal of achieving long-term control of his or her energy balance.

SELF-MONITORING

Increased awareness and evaluation of one's behavior is an essential element of the behavioral program (Kirschenbaum, 1987). At the start of treatment, the client's records of her or his food intake and the circumstances surrounding that eating provide valuable information about potential areas for changes to both the client and therapist. For example, the records might indicate that specific times (e.g., late evening) or types of foods (e.g., sweets) or moods (e.g., sadness) are associated with higher calorie consumption. Beyond this use as a diagnostic tool at the start of treatment, food records serve to increase the client's awareness throughout treatment and thereby assist client and therapist in noting progress or problems as they occur. In addition, a 2- or 3-week period of self-monitoring at the start of treatment is useful in evaluating the client's readiness and motivation for treatment. Clients who are able to successfully complete the self-monitoring forms are more likely to successfully lose weight than clients who do not complete the forms. A typical self-monitoring form is shown in Table 3. The importance of these records should be stressed to the client.

Reinforcement for changes in behavior or weight may be a useful component of self-monitoring. Both the client and therapist can use the monitoring to assess the client's progress, and, as previously agreed upon goals are met, a reinforcer is given either by the client, the therapist, or significant other. Either small amounts of money or other types of symbolic rewards (e.g., a movie) are suitable. Rewards involving positive alternatives to eating or food-oriented activities are especially valuable. For example, spending time with a friend without eating (e.g., walking in the park, visiting a museum) is a good reinforcer for behavioral change and also enhances a source of pleasure that is not linked with eating.

Reinforcement by an external person (e.g., the therapist or a family member) or self-reinforcement has varying effectiveness for individual clients (Israel & Saccone, 1979). External reinforcement is often helpful in the initial weight loss efforts and, for a subset of people, may be useful in longer term efforts. Individuals able to effectively employ self-reinforcement procedures are less likely to respond well to external direction (Carroll, Yates, & Gray, 1980).

The client and therapist can then modify the source of direction to be more or less internal as is most effective. Over the course of the program, sources and methods of reinforcement may be designed so that the client can continue to apply reinforcement techniques once formal treatment is terminated.

Goal setting may also be usefully employed in the context of self-monitoring. Previous research examining both longer term goals (e.g., weekly) and shorter term goal setting (e.g., daily or more frequently) suggests that setting goals for shorter time periods is of greater benefit (Bandura & Simon, 1977; Dubbert & Wilson, 1984). At each session, the therapist and client can select goals for the following week. These goals are then broken down into daily or even morning, afternoon, and evening subgoals. For example, a calorie reduction goal of 60 calories per day could be set to achieve an endpoint of 420 fewer calories consumed per week. For many clients, making changes in gradual increments results in greater success than making large, abrupt changes. Daily goals are entered at the beginning of the day on the self-monitoring form. As the day progresses, achievement of the goals is evaluated and later goals adjusted to compensate as necessary to reach the overall goal for the day and week. Through setting and monitoring goals or behavior change, the client is better able to evaluate his or her progress and determine particularly problematic situations.

STIMULUS CONTROL

Techniques in the realm of stimulus control are intended to decrease environmental cues for problem eating and increase cues for helpful behaviors. A simple example might be the dishes of snacks (e.g., nuts, candies) that some people keep out in easily available sites. Under such conditions, many people would be apt to snack when otherwise they might not. These

TABLE 3. Record of Food Intake and Related Behavior

| Diet Diary | | | Name | | | Date | |
|---|---|---|---|---|---|---|---|
| Food | Time | Place | People | Feelings | Activity | | Calories |
| Breakfast | | | | | | | |
| ___ | ___ | ___ | ___ | ___ | ___ | | ___ |
| ___ | ___ | ___ | ___ | ___ | ___ | | ___ |
| ___ | ___ | ___ | ___ | ___ | | | ___ |
| | | | | | Total calories | | ___ |
| Lunch | | | | | | | |
| ___ | ___ | ___ | ___ | ___ | ___ | | ___ |
| ___ | ___ | ___ | ___ | ___ | ___ | | ___ |
| ___ | ___ | ___ | ___ | ___ | ___ | | ___ |
| | | | | | Total calories | | ___ |
| Dinner | | | | | | | |
| ___ | ___ | ___ | ___ | ___ | ___ | | ___ |
| ___ | ___ | ___ | ___ | ___ | ___ | | ___ |
| ___ | ___ | ___ | ___ | ___ | ___ | | ___ |
| | | | | | Total calories | | ___ |
| Snacks | | | | | | | |
| ___ | ___ | ___ | ___ | ___ | ___ | | ___ |
| ___ | ___ | ___ | ___ | ___ | ___ | | ___ |
| ___ | ___ | ___ | ___ | ___ | ___ | | ___ |
| | | | | | Total calories | | ___ |
| | | | | | Total calories for day | | ___ |

techniques were originally based on the work of Schachter and his colleagues (Schachter & Rodin, 1974) that suggested that obese persons are particularly responsive to external cues for eating such as time and place or other stimuli. Subsequent research indicates that a high level of responsiveness to external cues is by no means unique to nor characteristic of obese individuals (Rodin, 1981). As a result, stimulus control techniques may not help obese persons to behave in a "lean" manner but remain useful as a means for controlling food intake by reducing stimuli-enhancing food intake.

Particular techniques include the following. Clients eliminate or reduce visual or other sensory cues by not purchasing problem foods if possible. More important, at home, foods are put away rather than stored in the open. Leftover or extra foods that are problematic should be discarded. Clients can reduce the range the cues associated with eating by eating in only one place (e.g., the dining room table) and not engaging in other activities such as watching television. In order to reduce impulse buying, clients may make grocery lists and plan their trip for a time (or with other people) that will be least likely to be problematic. Similarly, "automatic" eating may be reduced by interrupting the chain of behavior as well as increasing the cost involved. For example, when making toast, the client would take out a slice of bread, toast it, put the bread, jam, etc., away, and finally eat the prepared toast. Not only must the person then consciously decide that he or she wants another piece of toast, but the whole routine must be repeated.

## Changing Eating Behavior

As with sensitivity to external stimuli, early evidence suggesting that obese persons eat differently than lean persons has not been born out in further study. Certain persons may eat in an "obesifying" manner during the development of obesity, but, on the whole, the available information does not indicate that certain eating styles cause obesity nor that lean and obese persons eat in a distinct manner (Spitzer & Rodin, 1981). Nonetheless, the methods originally created with the idea of teaching obese persons to eat like normal-weight individuals remain useful for the process of weight loss.

A major area in this area concerns controlling the pace of eating. Literally, this means eating fewer calories per minute during the course of the meal. Clients eat more slowly by extending pauses between bites and putting silverware down after each bite. Foods higher in bulk such as complex carbohydrates (e.g., breads or potatoes with little or no added fat) or salad vegetables are also useful in slowing the pace of intake and reducing total intake (Duncan, Bacon, & Weinsier, 1983). Clients are also asked to pause periodically while eating to assess their level of hunger and to leave at least a small amount of food on their plate at the end of the meal. This helps the person to stop eating when comfortably satisfied rather than eating until the available food is entirely eaten.

Clients may also substitute other activities in place of eating. The earlier in the chain of behavior the greater the likelihood of success. For example, Mary typically eats fairly modestly during the day and early evening when she is working and then spending time with her husband and their two young children. However, later in the evening, the children are in bed, her husband is watching television, and Mary often reports feeling restless and bored, which, in turn, frequently leads to snacking. Eating low-calorie snacks or having smaller snacks might prove effective in controlling intake. A more powerful and likely-to-succeed approach would focus on the earlier component of the behavioral chain that ends with snacking. Activities that are incompatible with eating or enjoyable alternatives to eating could be planned for the problematic time of day. If carefully chosen, those activities will be particularly effective because they will serve not only the goal of controlling eating but will be a source of pleasure in of themselves.

F. MATTHEW
KRAMER and LAURIE
A. STALKER

Beck and his colleagues (Beck, Rush, Shaw, & Emery, 1979) originally defined a cognitive triad in terms of how a person views oneself, one's experiences, and one's future. Concurrent with these three aspects of a person's beliefs and attitudes are the general as well as specific ways in which the person understands, reacts to, organizes, and otherwise interacts with both internal and external stimuli. An overweight person often may not only feel negatively about being heavy but also believe that other people feel similarly. Thus, criticism by others is not only to be expected but also deserved. Likewise, an episode of overeating may be viewed as evidence that weight loss efforts are doomed to failure. Beck's methods are useful at all points in the treatment process.

Clients may show a variety of cognitive distortions such as overgeneralizations or arbitrary inferences. In addition, clients may think in a self-defeating manner about a variety of areas such as the standards they set for themselves, how they evaluate perceived failures, or how they explain or make excuses for their behavior. At the start of treatment, the need to assess the client's expectations and attitudes about his or her obesity and weight loss has been mentioned earlier. It is at this point that the clinician may first encounter distorted thinking. If the client, for example, expresses his or her belief that she or he must lose all of her or his excess weight to feel that she or he has been successful, the therapist cannot only note this client's tendency to think in an either/or manner and to set potentially unrealistic goals but also endeavor to explore the beliefs that underly this thinking.

In a similar manner, self-defeating thoughts and beliefs should be evaluated throughout treatment. Some of these will be broader in nature (e.g., "I'm fat so it is no wonder no one respects me"), whereas others will be more specific (e.g., "Well, I've cheated again; I might as well give up for today" or "I just can't bear to not have those cookies. It's not fair that I can't ever treat myself"). Through discussion, the client can be helped to realize that, logically, one episode of overeating does not ruin the diet and that accepting such a belief is demoralizing and self-defeating. The client can gradually learn to counter such thoughts (e.g., "O.K. I did overeat this morning but that doesn't mean things are hopeless. I can plan my next two meals to balance out the extra I've had").

People's thoughts typically become automatic over time, and the underlying beliefs are difficult to articulate. Thus, expanding self-monitoring to include cognitions is often a fruitful strategy. Clients may be instructed to work on identifying and writing down their thoughts over the course of the day when events occur that are likely to provoke a self-defeating thought. For example, a client might weigh herself and find that she has not lost any weight in the last 3 days and immediately think something like "It just goes to show that I'm no good and won't ever get this fat off." The client then writes down this thought. As her ability to monitor her thought improves, she can then begin to write down more rational alternatives. Many individuals also find it useful to rate on a 0 to 100 scale their degree of belief in the original and alternative thoughts. This monitoring provides material for therapist–client interaction and a means for the client to see her progress.

Cognitive methods can be applied to help the client achieve and maintain behavioral changes in addition to countering negative thoughts. Clients may cognitively instruct themselves on various behaviors (e.g., "It is almost time to start dinner. First, I'll lay the table settings and then start cooking. I need to remember to make a little less than I usually have and to put everything away before we start eating so that I won't nibble on my son's leftovers or the extra food on the counter"). It is also of value for clients to note and reinforce themselves for their behavior (e.g., "Great. I had toast instead of a Danish for breakfast again. I've been doing a good job of that").

Combining cognitive and behavioral methods gives the therapist and client an increased number of options and optimizes the likelihood of finding a strategy that is most effective.

Cognitive intervention is especially helpful in modifying long-held beliefs that may undermine the effectiveness and continued use of behavioral methods.

## NUTRITION

The main goal of the nutritional component of a weight loss program to ensure a balanced intake of essential nutrients in the context of calorie restriction. For the majority of clients, the daily diet should be approximately 1,500 calories for men and 1,200 for women that will result in a calorie deficit of roughly 500 calories per day. These calorie levels are suggested along with modest, increases in physical activity to achieve a 1- to 2-pound-a-week rate of weight loss. The client's previous experiences and particularly the self-monitoring forms are extremely useful in altering total intake or specific types of foods as necessary. A focus on the components of the diet is probably as important as the total numbers of calories eaten (Flatt, 1987). Evidence from animal as well as human studies suggest that the high fat diet typical of Western countries (i.e., 40% of total calories) is not only associated with disease but also with increased rates of obesity. Recommendations, then, are to reduce the percentage of calories from fat to no more than 30% of the diet, those from protein to between 12% and 15%, and from carbohydrates at least 55%. The latter should be predominantly derived from complex

TABLE 4. Sample Food Exchange Plan

Specific examples of food items within each of the food exchange list

| Food exchange list | Food group | Specific food example (= means the two items are interchangeable) |
|---|---|---|
| 1 | Milk | 1 cup skim milk = 1 cup yogurt made from whole milk |
| 2 | Vegetable | ½ cup celery = ¼ cup grape juice |
| 3 | Fruit | ½ small mango = ½ cup grape juice |
| 4 | Bread | 1 slice whole wheat bread = ½ cup bran flakes |
| | | = 6 saltine crackers |
| | | = ¼ baked beans |
| | | = 1 small white potato |
| 5 | Meat (Lean) | 1 oz sirloin beef = 3 sardines |
| 6 | Meat (Medium Fat) | 1 oz boiled ham = 1 egg |
| 7 | Fat | 1 teaspoon margarine = 2 teaspoon mayonnaise |

Total food exchanges in an 1,800-KCAL diet

| Food list | No. of exchanges | Protein (g) | Carbohydrate (g) | Fat (g) | Kcal |
|---|---|---|---|---|---|
| Nonfat milk | 2 | 16 | 24 | 0 | 160 |
| Vegetables | 4 | 4 | 10 | 0 | 50 |
| Fruits | 5 | 0 | 50 | 0 | 200 |
| Bread | 9 | 18 | 135 | 0 | 630 |
| Meaty, lean | 8 | 56 | 0 | 24 | 440 |
| Fat | 7 | 0 | 0 | 35 | 315 |
| Total | | 94 | 219 | 59 | 1,795 |

F. MATTHEW
KRAMER and LAURIE
A. STALKER

carbohydrates (e.g., bread, fruits) rather than sources such as sugar or alcohol. High-calorie foods that contain substantial amounts of fat and sugar are especially risky because they are not only calorically dense but also, by their very palatability, promote overeating. Having a variety of foods is important for assuring proper nutrition as well as an enjoyable food selection. However, the variety of foods chosen as well as the preparation and display of foods can be done to enhance satisfaction and weight control. Similarly, because many people and especially dieters frequently neglect nutrition, attention must be spent—perhaps using a system such as the four food groups—to ensure adequate nutrition while reducing calories, cholesterol, sodium and so forth in the efforts to improve health.

Although some clients will be well informed about the nutritional and caloric characteristics of foods, most people will benefit from structured guidance in choosing their diets. An exchange system is a good method for assisting clients to select a variety of acceptable foods that will meet calorie and nutrition needs. Exchange lists break foods down into food groups and provide calorically equivalent portions for a large number of foods in each group. An example of a food-exchange plan and specific foods is shown in Table 4. Further information about the development and use of food exchange lists can be obtained from a registered dietician or through a detailed booklet jointly produced by the American Diabetes Association and the American Dietetic Association (booklets can be ordered from the American Dietetic Association, P.O. Box 909705, Chicago, IL 60690. Enclose $1.25 per copy plus $2.50 for shipping and handling). Depending on the individual, menus may be useful at the start of treatment. However, the goal is to instill in the client the ability to develop dietary habits that promote weight loss and maintenance. Preplanning meals is a useful way to enhance adherence and reduce impulsive eating and food purchasing.

## EXERCISE

Weight is maintained by a balance between caloric intake and caloric expenditure. In the past, weight loss programs have promoted weight loss primarily by reducing caloric intake and have given less attention to losing weight by increasing energy expenditure. In part, this bias toward food restriction stemmed from the popular conception that it takes an inordinate amount of exercise to produce a small weight loss. Because few people on weight loss diets were interested in becoming Olympic champions, it appeared easier and more efficient to shave off a few calories by forgoing a piece of apple pie. Indeed, most people appear more able or at least more willing to create a negative energy balance by eating less rather than exercising more. On the whole, studies comparing behavioral programs with and without an exercise component found that programs with an exercise component produced only slightly greater losses (Pi-Sunyer, 1987; Wirth, 1987). However, some of these same studies as well as others have shown that people exercising regularly after the completion of treatment kept off a larger percentage of weight losses. Thus, exercise appears to enhance the maintenance of weight initially lost through food restriction.

On the basis of evidence such as the foregoing, greater attention has been focused on the benefits of an exercise component in comprehensive treatment programs for the obese. Exercise is clearly an important component of the maintenance phase of any weight loss program, as indicated before. However, it can also make a number of useful contributions to the initial stages of weight loss. First, moderate levels of exercise may reduce appetite, and good evidence exists indicating that moderate increase in exercise does not increase food intake (Pi-Sunyer, 1987; Wirth, 1987). Thus moderate amounts of exercise actually help an individual make her or his calorie goals. Exercise only increases appetite and consequently food intake when there are large increases in exercise. Second, exercise may increase an individual's metabolism for short periods after exercise as well as the thermic effects of food intake. Thus, if an individual exercises shortly before eating, a somewhat smaller percentage of the calories consumed will be available for storage in adipose tissue. Third, exercise helps increase the loss of body fat and preserves lean body mass. As a result, a larger quantity of the weight lost is fat. Fourth, exercise is a constructive alternative to snacking. Going for a walk around the block not only helps to controlling intake but also uses up a small number of calories. On a regular basis, substituting modest forms of physical activities can have a marked benefit on energy balance.

Regular physical activity has a variety of positive effects on physiological and psychological functioning. Exercise can improve many of the physical consequences of obesity such as hypertension, diabetes, coronary heart disease, and arthritis. Exercise, for example, helps reduce blood pressure, changes serum lipids, and increases insulin sensitivity (Wirth, 1987). Exercise can also have a positive effect on psychological functioning (Folkins, 1976). Dieting is often associated with anxiety, depression, and other negative moods. Similarly, as described earlier, obese individuals frequently have a negative and derogatory view of their physical self and a poor self-image. Dieting may also cause considerable stress (Polivy & Herman, 1983) because food intake must be constantly monitored and because of the severe deprivation of an important ingredient of the social fabric and sustenance. Exercise has been found to be effective way to reduce depression and stress (Freemont & Craighead, 1987; Sachs & Buffone, 1984) as well as an effective way to improve self-image. Positive changes in mood appear to occur within a period of weeks and do not seem to be dependent on level of aerobic fitness. Thus, exercise may help in the management of the often transient but potentially troublesome emotional correlates of dieting. In addition, a regular program of physical activity is one way overweight persons can act to improve how they feel about themselves.

Exercise programs for the obese are typically broken down into two types: life-style and programmed exercise. Life-style exercise refers to ways of increasing energy expenditure by

TABLE 5. Calories Expended for 10 Minutes of Physical Activity

| Activity | Body weight | | | | |
|---|---|---|---|---|---|
| | 56.8[a] 125[b] | 68.2 150 | 79.5 175 | 90.9 200 | 113.6 250 |
| Sitting quietly | 10 | 12 | 14 | 16 | 20 |
| Domestic housework | 34 | 41 | 47 | 53 | 68 |
| Walking downstairs | 56 | 67 | 78 | 88 | 111 |
| Walking upstairs | 146 | 175 | 202 | 229 | 288 |
| Walking (2 mph) | 29 | 35 | 40 | 46 | 58 |
| Walking (4 mph) | 52 | 62 | 72 | 81 | 102 |
| Jogging (5.5 mph) | 90 | 108 | 125 | 142 | 178 |
| Running (7 mph) | 118 | 141 | 164 | 187 | 232 |
| Cycling (5.5 mph) | 42 | 50 | 58 | 67 | 83 |
| Cycling (13 mph) | 89 | 107 | 124 | 142 | 178 |
| Mowing grass (power) | 34 | 41 | 47 | 53 | 67 |
| Mowing grass (manual) | 38 | 45 | 52 | 58 | 74 |
| Chopping wood | 60 | 73 | 84 | 96 | 121 |
| Bowling (nonstop) | 56 | 67 | 78 | 90 | 111 |
| Dancing | 35 | 42 | 48 | 55 | 69 |
| Dancing (vigorous) | 48 | 57 | 66 | 75 | 94 |
| Golfing (walk) | 33 | 40 | 48 | 55 | 68 |
| Skiing (cross-country) | 98 | 117 | 138 | 158 | 194 |

[a]Expressed in kilograms.
[b]Expressed in pounds.

increasing the amount activity in everyday life. Examples of increased life-style activity include parking the car farther from one's destination and walking the extra distance, getting off the elevator one or two floors beneath one's destination, and walking up a couple flights of stairs, cleaning the house more vigorously by stretching while dusting, planning the sequence of household chores so that one needs to walk up and down the stairs more, and answering the phone on a different floor.

Programmed exercise refers to structured exercise programs such as aerobic and dance classes. A walking program is frequently used as an initial starting point. Subjects are instructed to start a moderate program of walking every day. They can start with any amount of walking (e.g., walking around the block) and then, over time, they increase the distance and pace of their walking. It can be pointed out that vigorous walking expends approximately the same amount of calories as jogging and is safer for bones, joints, and muscles than running.

In choosing the type of programmed exercise that will work for an individual, consideration of his or her interests should be given. If they have always wanted to swim, then joining a swimming club would be a good idea. Likewise, if possible, exercise programs should be developed around individual interests: tennis, skiing, softball, bicycling, swimming. However, vigorous sports are usually too strenuous for the obese when they are just beginning to lose weight. Therefore, a plan for gradually increasing activity is needed. For example, it may be most reasonable to start with a walking program during the initial part of a weight loss program. As fitness improves, the individual may be more ready to start with other more vigorous activities such as tennis, jogging, and bicycling. As always, it is important to get medical clearance before starting any exercise program. The exercise component of the program should aim for a 2- to 3-hundred calorie increase in daily activity. This may sound like a lot until one considers that for a 175-pound person, a slow walk will expend 200 calories in about 50 minutes. Table 5 shows the average number of calories a variety of leisure household and work activities used in a 10-minute span. Thus relatively modest changes in daily activities and a small but regular program of programmed exercise will add up to a significant increase in energy expenditure. How quickly a particular client should plan to reach the 2- to 3-hundred-calorie level will depend on initial weight, level of activity, as well as other individual characteristics.

The major problem related to physical activity programs is that over 50% of the people who begin a program either on their own or in a group format stop exercising within 6 months (Martin & Dubbert, 1982). Overweight individuals are especially likely to stop exercising. Both the client and therapist need to be aware of the fact that exercise programs will have few salient reinforcing consequences in the initial weeks of increased activity. A number of steps may help to enhance long-term involvement in an exercise program by maximizing the positive and minimizing the negative aspects of physical activity. Clients should choose activities of interest if possible and build up slowly in order to avoid injury or soreness. If possible, a variety of activities should be done to reduce boredom or mental fatigue. Exercising with others or in a setting such as a YMCA will provide a helpful support structure for many people. As with eating behavior and dietary intake, physical activity should be monitored. Similarly, self-reinforcement and goal-setting techniques may be used as a means for increasing the likelihood of sticking to a regular schedule of physical activity.

## RELAPSE PREVENTION

The relapse prevention model was developed by Marlatt and his associates (Marlatt & Gordon, 1985) as an approach to understanding and treating addictive behaviors. Clinical evidence has long suggested that individuals with problems of overdrinking, eating, and so on often are able to control intake for large periods of time. However, at some point, a situation or event inevitably arises (e.g., a party or an unpleasant day at work) resulting in a slip or lapse.

One or more lapses then frequently result in a relapse into the problem behavior for the rest of the day, week, or so on. Relapse then is likely to culminate in giving up all efforts to control the behavior.

A figure of the model (see Figure 2) shows the various components, as well as possible points and methods for intervention. The initial step in preventing relapse is identifying situations that are likely to create problems. These high-risk situations may be either interpersonal (e.g., being at a party) or intrapersonal (e.g., feeling bored). Self-monitoring plays a critical role in identifying these situations. Imaginal or role-played situations may also be useful forms of assessment.

Once the client is better able to identify problematic situations, he or she can begin to develop coping responses. In some cases, helping the person to identify alternative behaviors is useful as is planning ways to reduce or eliminate the risk; obviously, some problematic situations are unavoidable or at least are not avoidable on a long-term basis (dining out, stress). In this situation, clients also need assistance in developing appropriate skills as well as in applying skills they already possess. In some cases, a person may readily be able to use a relevant skill but fail to do so due to anxiety or other cognitive or emotional factors. Stress-reducing interventions or relaxation training may, for example, help a person be more assertive in refusing food offers. On the other hand, practice in and out of sessions combined with modeling and feedback from the therapist can aid clients to learn and apply alternatives to eating inappropriately. For example, rather than avoiding having lunch with friends in order to eliminate a high-calorie meal, the person can plan alternate activities with friends that do not revolve around eating or plan ahead where to go and what to order in order to maintain the control of intake. An important additional component is examining the client's expectations about the expected benefits of problem behavior. The person may explain how much he or she enjoys his or her meals with friends but can be helped in putting the situation into a context so that the focus is on decreasing intake while maintaining or even enhancing the source of the

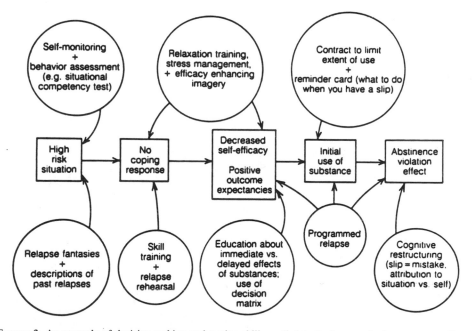

FIGURE 2. An example of decision-making and coping skills applied to the lapse and relapse process. Boxes represent the stages in the process and circles represent examples of interventions targeted at each stage. Reprinted by permission from G. A. Marlatt & Gordon, J. R. (1985). Relapse prevention: Maintenance strategies in addictive behavior change (p. 54). New York: Guilford Press.

positive feelings (i.e., spending time with a friend). Lapses or slips will naturally occur from time to time. Clients should be told that such lapses are inevitable and can be used as a way for improving their abilities to control their eating rather than as a sign of failure. Clients frequently react to a lapse by attributing it to their own weakness and feel guilty about not upholding their plan to be a "successful dieter"—"I've blown it again. If I weren't so much of a slob I could control myself. I might as well give up." Marlatt and Gordon (1985) term this reaction the abstinence violation effect (AVE). Cognitive techniques such as those described by Beck are useful in relabeling the lapse as a single mistake that does not indicate that the person is a failure and that success in the future is impossible. The therapist and client also analyze the situation in order to determine what led to the lapse and what needs to be done to handle it on other occasions. An important overall concern in working with the client is to emphasize the development of self-fulfilling (i.e., *wants* in Marlatt's approach) activities and the reduction of expected behaviors (*shoulds*). Long-term behavior change is extremely difficult if the individual continually feels that he or she is depriving him- or herself or restricting his or her life for the sole positive outcome of weight control. In sum, creating a life-style that balances the client's goals and expectations enhances the chances of continued success.

# SUMMARY

Obesity is a complex disorder requiring complex intervention and permanent changes in life-style. Although the failure of most persons to achieve permanent weight loss in relatively short-term treatment programs is often taken as evidence of the intractible nature of obesity, an equally valid conclusion is that an acute disease treatment model is inappropriate. Certainly, obesity demands serious treatment by the clinician. However, successful intervention also demands a long-term committment by both the therapist and the client. Too often, a short course of intervention is expected to produce clear-cut success. In reality, obesity is quite similar to psychiatric disorders such as depression or medical disorders such as diabetes. Initial treatment may result in large benefits for the client but continued effort and, frequently, renewed intervention is necessary.

# REFERENCES

Agras, W. S., Ferguson, J. M., Greaves, C., Qualls, B., Rand, C. S. W., Ruby, J., Stunkard, A. J., Taylor, C. B., Werne, J., & Wright, C. (1976). A clinical and research questionnaire for obese patients. In B. J. Williams, S. Martin, & J. P. Foreyt (Eds.), *Obesity: Behavioral approaches to dietary management* (pp. 168–176). New York: Brunner/Mazel.

Allon, N. (1982). The stigma of overweight in everyday life. In B. Wolman (Ed.), *Psychological aspects of obesity: A handbook* (pp. 130–174). New York: Van Nostrand Reinhold.

Bandura, A., & Simon, K. M. (1977). The role of proximal intentions in self-regulation of refractory behavior. *Cognitive Therapy and Research, 1,* 177–193.

Beck, A. T., Rush, A. J., Shaw, B. F., & Emery, G. (1979). *Cognitive therapy of depression: A treatment manual.* New York: Guilford.

Bray, G. A. (1985). Complications of obesity. *Annals of Internal Medicine, 103,* 1042–1062.

Brownell, K. D. (1988). *The LEARN program for weight control.*

Brownell, K. D., & Wadden, T. A. (1986). Behavior therapy for obesity: Modern approaches and better results. In K. D. Brownell & J. P. Foreyt (Eds.), *Handbook of eating disorders* (pp. 180–197). New York: Basic Books.

Brownell, K. D., Greenwood, M. R. C., Stellar, E., & Shrager, E. E. (1986). The effects of repeated cycles of weight loss and regain in rats. *Physiology and Behavior, 38,* 459–464.

Canning, H., & Mayer, J. (1966). Obesity—its possible effect on college acceptance. *New England Journal of Medicine, 275,* 1171–1174.

Carroll, L. J., Yates, B. T., & Gray, J. J. (1980). Predicting obesity reduction in behavioral and nonbehavioral therapy from client characteristics: The self-evaluation measure. *Behavior Therapy, 11,* 189–197.

Dubbert, P. M., & Wilson, G. T. (1983). Treatment failures in behavior therapy for obesity: Causes, correlates, and consequences. In E. Foa & P. M. G. Emmelkamp (Eds.), *Treatment failures in behavior therapy* (pp. 263–288). New York: Wiley.

Dubbert, P. M. & Wilson, G. T. (1984). Goal setting and spouse involvement in the treatment of obesity. *Behaviour Therapy and Research, 22,* 227–242.

Durnin, J. V. G. A., & Womersley, J. (1974). Body fat assessed from total body density and its estimation from skinfold thickness: Measurements on 481 men and women aged 16 to 71 years. *British Journal of Nutrition, 32,* 77–97.

Flatt, J. P. (1987). The difference in the storage capacities for carbohydrate and for fat, and its implication in the regulation of body weight. *Annals of the New York Academy of Sciences, 499,* 104–123.

Folkins, C. H. (1976). Effects of physical training on mood. *Journal of Clinical Psychology, 32,* 385–388.

Freemont, J., & Craighead, L. W. (1987). Aerobic exercise and cognitive therapy in the treatment of dysphoric moods. *Cognitive Therapy and Research, 11,* 241–251.

Garrow, T. S. (1978). *Energy balance and obesity.* Amsterdam: Elsevier/North Holland Biomedical Press.

Gortmaker, S. L., Dietz, W. H., Sobal, A. M., & Wehler, C. A. (1978). Increasing pediatric obesity in the United States. *American Journal of Diseases in Children, 141,* 535–540.

Israel, A. C., & Saccone, A. J. (1979). Follow-up effects of choice mediator and target of reinforcement on weight loss. *Behavior Therapy, 10,* 260–265.

Kirschenbaum, D. S. (1987). Self-regulatory failure: A review with clinical implications. *Clinical Psychology Review, 7,* 77–104.

Marlatt, G. A., & Gordon, J. R. (Eds.). (1985). *Relapse prevention: Maintenance strategies in addictive behavior change.* New York: Guilford.

Martin, J. E., & Dubbert, P. M. (1982). Exercise applications and promotion in behavioral medicine: Current status and future direction. *Journal of Consulting and Clinical Psychology, 50,* 1004–1017.

McReynolds, W. T. (1982). Toward a psychology of obesity: Review of research on the role of personality and level of adjustment. *International Journal of Eating Disorders, 2,* 37–57.

Metropolitan Life Insurance Company (1983). Metropolitan height and weight tables for men and woman. *Statistical Bulletin, 1,* 2–9.

NIH Health Consensus Development Conference. (1985). Health implications of obesity. *Annals of Internal Medicine, 103,* 977–1077.

Perri, M. G. (1987). Maintenance strategies for the management of obesity. In W. G. Johnson (Ed.), *Advances in eating disorders: Vol. 1. Treating and preventing obesity* (pp. 177–194). Greenwich, CT: JAI Press.

Pi-Sunyer, F. X. (1987). Exercise effects on calorie intake. *Annals of the New York Academy of Sciences, 499,* 94–103.

Polivy, J., & Herman, C. P. (1983). *Breaking the diet habit.* New York: Basic Books.

Rodin, J. (1981). The current status of the internal-external obesity hypothesis: What went wrong. *American Psychologist, 36,* 361–372.

Roe, D. A., & Eickwort, D. R. (1986). Relationships between obesity and associated health factors with unemployment among low income women. *Journal of the American Medical Women's Association, 31,* 193–194, 198–199, 203–204.

Sacks, M. L., & Buffone, G. W. (Eds.). (1984). *Running as therapy: An integrated approach.* Lincoln: University of Nebraska Press.

Schachter, S., & Rodin, J. (1974). *Obese humans and rats.* Washington, DC: Erlbaum/Wiley.

Sjostrom, L. (1980). Fat cells and body weight. In A. J. Stunkard (Ed.), *Obesity* (pp. 72–100). Philadelphia: Saunders.

Spitzer, L., & Rodin, J. (1981). Human eating behavior: A critical review of studies in normal weight and overweight individuals. *Appetite, 2,* 293–329.

Staffieri, J. R. (1967). A study of social stereotype of body image in children. *Journal of Personality and Social Psychology, 7,* 101–104.

Stunkard, A. J., & Rush, J. (1974). Dieting and depression reexamined: A critical review of reports of untoward responses during weight reduction for obesity. *Annals of Internal Medicine, 81,* 526–533.

Wadden, T. A., & Stunkard, A. J. (1987). Psychopathology and obesity. *Annals of the New York Academy of Sciences, 499,* 55–65.

Wilson, G. T., & Brownell, K. D. (1980). Behavior therapy for obesity: An evaluation of treatment outcome. *Advances in Behaviour Research and Therapy, 3,* 49–86.

Wirth, A. (1987). The role of exercise in weight control. In A. E. Bender & L. J. Brookes (Eds.), *Body weight control* (pp. 188–200). New York: Churchill Livingstone.

Wooley, S. C. (1987). Psychological and social aspects of obesity. In A. E. Bender & L. J. Binder (Eds.), *Body weight control* (pp. 81–89). New York: Churchill Livingstone.

# 21

# Cognitive Therapy Applied to Personality Disorders

ARTHUR FREEMAN AND RUSSELL C. LEAF

In the last several years, there has been a growing interest in the study and understanding of personality disorders. Patients with personality disorders have been part of the clinician's case load since the beginning of the recorded history of psychotherapy; the general psychotherapeutic literature on the treatment of personality disorders, however, has emerged more recently and is growing quickly. The main theoretical orientation in the present literature is psychoanalytic (Abend, Porder, & Willick, 1983; Chatham, 1985; Goldstein, 1985; Gunderson, 1984; Horowitz, 1977; Kernberg, 1975, 1984; Lion, 1981; Masterson, 1978, 1980, 1985; Reid, 1981; Saul & Warner, 1982). Millon (1981) is one of the few volumes in the area of personality disorders that offers a behavioral focus, and the volume by Beck, Freeman and associates (1989) will be the first to offer a specific cognitive-behavioral focus. This is of interest, in that leading cognitive therapists have been, and remain, interested in "personality disorder" and "personality change" (Hartman & Blankenstein, 1986). When Beck (1963a,b) and Ellis (1957a, 1958) first introduced cognitive approaches, they drew upon the ideas of "ego analysts," derived from Adler's critiques of early Freudian psychoanalysis. Though their therapeutic innovations were seen as radical, their earliest cognitive therapies were, in many ways, "insight therapies" in that the therapy was assumed to change a patient's overt "personality," whether or not the therapy changed some hypothesized underlying personality. Although Beck and Ellis were among the first to use a wide array of behavioral treatment techniques, including structured *in vivo* homework, they have consistently emphasized the therapeutic impact of these techniques on cognitive schemata and have argued in favor of the integration of behavioral techniques into therapy within a broad framework that has some roots in prior analytic practice (Beck, 1976; Ellis & Bernard, 1985); they and their associates have emphasized the impact of treatment for particular types, or styles, of cognitive errors on

ARTHUR FREEMAN • Center for Cognitive Therapy, Department of Psychiatry, University of Pennsylvania, Philadelphia, Pennsylvania 19104    RUSSELL C. LEAF • Department of Psychology, Rutgers University, New Brunswick, New Jersey 08903; and Institute for Rational-Emotive Therapy, New York, New York 10021.

dysfunctional self-concepts, as well as on presenting focal problems (Beck & Freeman, 1989; Ellis, 1985; Freeman, 1987).

Reviews of principles and techniques for cognitive therapy typically focus on treatment of specific clinical symptoms and syndromes. That emphasis highlights the common concerns, both theoretical and empirical, that have reshaped both cognitive and behavioral therapies during the last two decades. Psychotherapeutic assessment is now increasingly objective, symptom-oriented, and behavioral, and treatment typically integrates directive cognitive and behavioral approaches (Salkovsis, 1986).

Although some theorists still argue that global self-referential measures are inherently less useful and important for assessment and treatment evaluation than symptom-specific, focal, ones (Latimer & Sweet, 1984; Rachman & Wilson, 1980; Scharnberg, 1984), most analyses of psychotherapeutic practice have found that patients usually present with "core" problems, for example, problems that are central both for particular symptoms and for problematic self-referential cognitions (Frank, 1973). The idea that cognitive therapy is more efficacious and efficient when it focuses on "core" problems stems from the notion that important cognitive structures are categorically and hierarchically organized so that, for example, many exemplars of a patient's difficulties can be subsumed under one class and influenced by changes in single or few schemata. It is consistent with the principal contemporary theories of cognitive structure and cognitive development, all of which stress the function of schemata as determinants of rule-guided behavior (Neisser, 1976; Piaget, 1971, 1974, 1976, 1978; Schank & Abelson, 1977).

Cognitive theorists share with psychoanalysts the notion that it is usually more productive to identify and treat "core" problems but differ from them in the view of the nature of core structure, which we see as a group of schema that work to structure categorical judgment, or classification, and diverse schemata are, according to this, the tools used to guide the directions and qualities of one's daily life. Most of this process is clearly conscious. Of that which is not immediately so, much is readily accessible to consciousness. Dysfunctional feelings and conduct, according to cognitive therapeutic theory, are mainly due to features of our schemata that tend to produce consistently biased judgments and a concomitant consistent tendency to make errors in certain types of situations. Schematic errors, not unconsciousness or defensiveness *per se,* are the source of difficulties. The basic premise of the CT model is that attributional bias, rather than motivational or response bias, is the main source of dysfunctional affect and conduct (Hollon, Kendall, & Lumry, 1986; Matthews & MacLeod, 1986; MacLeod, Matthews, & Tata, 1986). Finally, other work has shown both that clinically relevant cognitive patterns are related to psychopathology in children in a way that parallels the cognitive and affective relationship patterns typically found among adults (Beardslee, Bemporad, Keller, & Klerman, 1983; Leitenberg, Yost, & Carroll-Wilson, 1986; Quay, Routh, & Shapiro, 1987) and that effective cognitive therapy can follow similar lines in children and adults (DiGiuseppe, 1983, chapter 27 this volume).

Given the long-term nature of patients' characterological problems, their general avoidance of psycotherapy, their frequent referral through family pressure of legal remand and their seeming reluctance or inability to change, these patients are often the most difficult patients in a clinician's caseload. They can, and often do, require more work within the session, a longer time for therapy, and more therapist energy than other patients. All of this without the same rate of change and satisfaction as is gained with other patients.

## REFERRAL

These patients typically come for therapy with presenting issues other than Axis II problems, most often with complaints of depression and anxiety. The reported problems of depression and anxiety may be separate and apart from the Axis II patterns, or superimposed upon and fueled by, the Axis II personality. Given the latter combination, the course of treatment is far more complicated than the typical non–Axis II patient with the same presenting complaints. The duration of treatment, frequency of treatment sessions, goals and expectations for both therapist and patient, and the techniques and available strategies need to be altered in the CT treatment of personality disorders. Given the difficulties inherent in working with the personality disorders, they are not untreatable.

The personality-disordered patient will often see the problems that he or she encounters in the world as not related to him or her but rather as outside of him or her; these patients often have no ideas about how they got to be the way they are or how to change. Their style of behaving and responding to the world is self-consonant. These patients are often referred by family members or significant others who recognize a dysfunctional pattern or who have reached their personal limit in attempting to cope with this individual. Still other patients are remanded by the judicial system. This latter group are often given a choice, that is, go to prison or go to therapy (Henn, Herjanic, & VanderPearl, 1976; Moore, Zusman, & Root, 1984).

## DIAGNOSIS

Although some personality disorders are diagnosed rather early in treatment, a clinician may not be aware of the characterological nature, chronicity, and severity of the patient's personality problems. (Fabrega, Mezzzich, Mezzich & Coffman, 1986; Karno, Hough, Burnam, Escobar, Timbers, Santana, & Boyd, 1986; Koenigsberg, Kaplan, Gilmore, & Cooper, 1985). At the Institute for Rational-Emotive Therapy, for example, 61.8% of 380 recent patients who completed Millon Clinical Multiaxial Inventories (MCMI) at intake, all of whom sought short-term cognitive therapy for Axis I problems, had scores of 85 or above that indicate pathology on the scales that assess Axis II problems (DiGiuseppe, Ellis, Leaf, Mass, Backz, Alington, & Wolfe, 1987, unpublished data). The very high rate of apparent personality disorders in this sample may, of course, reflect various inadequacies of the use of MCMI cutpoints as diagnostic criteria, but these seem to be the best available objective indicators of Axis II disorders (Gibertini, Brandenburg, & Retzlaff, 1986; Green, 1982; McMahon & Davidson, 1985; Millon, 1982; 1985; Moreland & Onstad, 1987; Widiger, Williams, Spitzer, & Frances, 1985). The high rate may also reflect the fact that negative life events are frequent in the lives of New York Metropolitan Area patients, when they are compared with those from more placid settings. Whatever the cause, the high rate highlights a central issue. Some patients come only for symptomatic treatment for acute problems. When schema-focused treatment for a personality disorder may also be indicated, the patient and therapist cannot automatically agree on an agenda of treatment goals. When Axis II problems are a focus at intake, the patient may not be willing, at treatment onset, to work on the personality disorders but rather may choose to work on the problems for which he or she was referred. It is important to remember that the patient's goals and not those of others (including the therapist) are the focus of treatment. The patient's schemata are the agent, as well as target of therapeutic change. If an externally referred patient is not willing to work on "core" issues, the therapist may work to convince the patient to be trusting and to follow the therapist's agenda. This can be set up as an experiment and as one of life's challenges. Ideational confrontation, *per se,* is not necessarily harmful to therapeutic trust but, rather, patient perception of whether or not the therapist is sincerely concerned about the patient's interests is the principal critical factor (Conoley & Beard, 1984).

Mary, a 23-year-old computer programmer came to therapy because of "tremendous work pressure, inability to enjoy life, a perfectionistic approach to virtually all tasks, and a general isolation from others." She was working very hard at her job and getting very little satisfaction from the work. She was constantly late in getting her work completed. Her boss was constantly asking her for the finished programs. "He doesn't understand that I work very slowly and carefully. He just wants the work done quickly, and I have my standards of what I consider good enough to submit". She would have to take work home on weekends and stay in the office until 7 or 8 P.M. during the week to get the work done according to her "standards."

Mary did very well throughout her schooling, getting honors at graduation. Throughout her school experience, she had little time for friends, leisure activities, or fun. "I was determined to do well. When I finished school I figured that I could then relax and have fun." Her compulsive personality traits were rewarded in school and at home. Teachers always remarked on her neat, perfect work that resulted in her receiving many awards at graduation. Without the school focus, work took all of her time, and she was no longer rewarded for her perfectionism

In point of fact, a personality disorder can help some individuals to be very successful, for example, in the military. The dependent personality may be ideal for service in the military because he or she is compliant to orders. A 66-year-old man, diagnosed as both compulsive and avoidant personality stated, "The best time in my life was in the army. I didn't have to worry about what to wear, what to do, where to go, or what to eat."

Achieving a mastery of DSM-III-R is essential in diagnosing personality disorders on Axis II. By familiarizing oneself with the diagnostic criteria, the clinician is able to further question symptom patterns or constellations. If a patient reports that he or she has several of the diagnostic criteria, the clinician can question as to whether the other criteria in that symptom picture are present. If the patient meets the Axis II criteria, it would suggest an exploration of how Axis II issues affect the patient's presenting problems. Axis II problems are not always diagnosed at treatment intake, though early diagnosis and treatment planning are likely to be more effective (Morrison & Shapiro, 1987). Many Axis II patients are silent about their problems, or deny them, as a reflection of the disorders themselves; this differs from silence or denial of medical problems only in that both the cause and the disorder are identical (Douglas & Druss, 1987; Prince, 1985; Silverman, 1987). Whether or not they are diagnosed as having personality disorders, patients sometimes believe that their personalities are an appropriate focus of treatment and sometimes fear such a focus. The effectiveness of cognitive treatment at any given point in time depends on the degree to which their expectations about therapeutic goals are congruent with those of their therapist (Martin, Martin, & Slemon, 1987). Mutual trust and request fulfillment by the therapist are important, as they are in any medical setting (Like & Zyzanski, 1987). The collaborative nature of goal setting is one of the most important features of cognitive therapy. Power struggles over conflicting goals do not usually facilitate progress (Foon, 1985).

A summary of diagnostic signs that may point to the possibility of Axis II problems include: (1) the patient or significant other may report, "Oh, he/she has always done that, since he's a little boy/girl," or the patient may report, "I've always been this way". (2) The patient is not compliant with the therapeutic regimen. Although this noncompliance (or resistance) is common in many problems and for many reasons, ongoing noncompliance should be used as a signal for further exploration of Axis II issues. (3) Therapy seems to have come to a sudden stop, with no apparent reason. The clinician working with these patients can often help the patient to reduce the referral problems of anxiety or depression only to be stopped short in the therapeutic endeavor by the personality disorder. (4) patients seem entirely unaware of the effect of their behavior on others. They report the responses of others but fail to address any stimulus behavior that they might exhibit. (5) There is a question of the motivation of the patient to change. This is especially true for those patients who have "been sent" to therapy by family members or the courts. (6) The patient may give lip service to the therapy and to the importance of change but seems to manage to avoid changing. (7) The patient's problems appear to be self-consonant. The problems that these patients report seem to be an inimical part of them as opposed to some problem outside of them, that is, a depressed patient without an Axis II diagnosis may say, ''I just want to get rid of this depression. I know what it is like to feel good, and I want to feel that way again. Axis II patients see the problems as them. ''This is how I am,'' ''This is who I am'' (8) The Axis II patient sees the problems as, ''out there.'' In terms of Beck's cognitive triad (Beck *et al.*, 1979), they see their problems in terms of the world's ''doing to'' them.

## COGNITIVE THERAPY CONCEPTUALIZATION OF PERSONALITY DISORDERS

If we visualize the personality, we may liken it to a large wheel of Swiss cheese. Different cheeses may be of differing sizes, and the wheel would probably be solid enough to support a person's weight. However, when cut through the center, the cheese will be seen to have many holes. These holes may be many or few; they many be large or small. In terms of personality disorder, the larger the holes in what are basic areas, the greater the disorder. If the ''hole'' or area of deficit is affiliation, the avoidant or schizoid personality disorders will result—autonomy (dependent personality disorder), acceptance of social norms and strictures (antisocial), impulse control (borderline, histrionic), altruism (narcissistic), or flexibility (compulsive). If there are many areas of deficit, there will, of course, be several areas of disorder. Smaller ''holes'' may cause behavior labeled eccentric or may cause some minor psychic discomfort and life difficulty. Eccentric behavior may, in fact, cause no difficulty at all. An involvement in a particular environment, occupation, or group may allow for the acceptance of behaviors that in other quarters would be seen as unacceptable.

The personality disorder is probably one of the most striking examples of Beck's notion of schema (Beck *et al.*, 1979; Freeman, 1987). One might begin to understand the personality disorders, for example, by organizing a discussion around clinically relevant schemata. The cognitive schemata that determine ''personality,'' according to this view, are those that Adler originally called ''life schema'' and later called ''lifestyles'' (Ansbacher & Ansbacher, 1963), the rules that an individual uses to organize the process of adaptation to life's challenges and changes. Lifestyle rules can be classified into a variety of useful categories, such as personal, familial, cultural, religious, gender, or occupational schemas. Further, it can be assessed through interview and history the degree to which particular schema are active or dormant, as well as the degree to which they are compelling or changeable (Freeman, 1987; Freeman, Simon, Fleming, & Pretzer, 1989; Freeman & Simon, Chapter 18, this volume). The *active schema* govern our everyday behavior. These schemas have to do with where one chooses to sit after entering a room, how one chooses to dress, and how one generally related to people and tasks. *Dormant schemas* are essentially out of awareness. They become active and available when the individual is stressed, and at that point become active and serve to govern behavior. When the stressor is no longer present, the dormant schemas recede to their previous state of dormancy. For example, if someone were asked his or her thoughts about killing, he or she might respond with the biblical maxim, ''Thou shalt not kill.'' Their beliefs about killing may or may not extend to eating meat, hunting, and the like. If, however, that person were asked about his or her behavior if the life of his or her children were threatened, he or she might now speak of the *need* to kill to protect his or her children. Stress invokes the schema, ''It is essential to protect one's children''.

Some schemata are noncompelling whereas others are very compelling. The compelling/noncompelling nature of a particular schema is part of a continuim. A noncompelling schema is one that the individual believes in but can relatively easily challenge and/or surrender. Compelling schemata are not easily challenged and are surrendered only with great difficulty, or not at all. An example would be the religious or political martyrs who chose to die rather than surrender their compelling views. Axis II patients are generally governed by very compelling schemata, so that these very powerfully held rules are not easily surrendered. The chronicity of the personality disorder comes from the schemata being in place since middle childhood or earlier. In general, however, dormant schemata are not usually most compelling (Persons & Burns, 1986).

> A man who was proud that his active lifestyle schema, which consciously guided many aspects of his daily activities, was "nonsexist" found himself highly disturbed by his mate's infidelity, even though he thought his own similar conduct was not a threat to their relationship. He sought treatment for his anger and depression and quickly discovered that he had a dormant, stress-activated, schema whose content was something like "women have sexual relations because they love someone, but men do it for thrills." Fortunately, his dormant schema was not very compelling. He was quickly able to reinterpet both his and his mate's infidelity as a threat, but not an awesome one, to their relationship, and the more appropriate feelings that resulted from this reinterpretation helped him to give up his initially maladaptive rages and find more satisfying approaches to solving his marital problems.

These schema are evolutionary and develop as the individual moves through life. They are the basic rules that people live by. From birth through middle childhood, these rules are, ideally, in a constant stage of change. Utilizing a Piagetian model, there is a constant need for adaptation to the requirements of life. Through the interactive processes of assimilation and accomodation, these schema that allow us to organize and understand our world, change. If one were to ask a 2-month-old infant for a conceptualization of what food seeking is like to the, he or she would probably tell us that, "to gain food, you have to cry until the woman with the food comes. Then you open your mouth, and the food is presented, and you are allowed to take as much as you want, sometimes out of one container, and sometimes out of the matching container." As children mature, these schema change. For many reasons, some of the schema do not mature and are maintained at an earlier level of development. This is the beginning of an Axis II problem. The schema that are basically functional in this earlier part of life are being applied during later, more demanding times. These schemata become fixed when they are reinforced and/or modeled by parents.

Although most of these early schema were at one time functional, they have long since lost their functional value by dint of never having been modified by the individual to meet changing life/world experiences. For example, if a 1-year-old child would like to be picked up, he or she conveys that message to a caretaker by lifting his or her arms and grunting or crying. The caretaker responds by picking the child up. As the child matures, the schema are altered. The schema, "I can do for myself," develops, and the child no longer has the schematic world view that "I need others to take care of me and meet my basic needs." When a child at age 1 is demanding of attention and help, it is often thought of as cute. When the same schema is manifested at age 31 it is not cute but quite dysfunctional. A second example would be the 2-year-old who acts in an impulsive manner and who tells the parent, "No one should stop me from doing what I want to do." In dealing with a 2-year-old, this behavior is expected, though not enjoyed. If, at age 42, there is a passive-aggressive view of the world or an antisocial view, the lack of impulse control is not welcome. With certain personality disorders, the individual acquires schema that direct—"I don't have to accept controls. I don't have to build controls, and I can do whatever I want to do."

Given the chronic nature of the problems, one must question as to why these behaviors are maintained. They may cause difficulty at work, school, or in personal life. In some cases, they are reinforced by the society, that is, the teachers who encourage a child who is "a real worker," "a kid that doesn't fool around," "a kid who hasn't messed around while other kids are messing around,'' ''a kid who really works hard and gets A's.'' Often compelling schemata that a patient will often ''know'' are erroneous are hard to change. Two factors seem most important: First, as DiGiuseppe (1986) has pointed out, the problem may be partly due to the difficulty people (including scientifically oriented therapists) have in making a ''paradigm shift'' from a sometimes accurate hypothesis to a less familiar one; second, as Freeman and Freeman *et al.* (1988) (1987) has noted, people often find ways to adjust to and extract short-term benefits from fundamentally biased schemata that restrict or burden their long-term capacity to deal with the challenges of life. With respect to the first problem, DiGiuseppe recommends therapeutic use of a variety of examples of the error that a particular schema produces, so that its biasing effect can be seen as having an impact on broad areas of a patient's life, and repeated explication of the consequences of an unbiased alternative. Although one would expect that therapy following these recommendations would often be prolonged, the recommended strategies for dealing with this problem are largely under the control of the therapist and can usually be implemented when indicated. The second problem is not so tractable. When patients adjust their lives to compensate for their anxieties, for example, they would have to change their lives and face their anxieties, in order to change. If a patient with both compulsive and avoidant personality disorders describes the period of his military service as ''the best time in my life'' because ''I didn't have to worry about what to wear, what to do, where to go, or what to eat,'' we would not expect the patient, at intake, to seek or embrace a therapeutic strategy that requires he practice homework exercises that expose him to a constant array of new risks (Turner, Beidel, Dancu, & Keys, 1986). Before a patient would adopt an appropriate therapeutic strategy, the therapist would probably have to try to reshape the patient's initial expectations about the goals, time course, and procedures of therapy, help the patient achieve some relatively immediate and practical gains, and develop a trusting and supportive collaborative relationship.

Freeman (1987) and Freeman *et al.* (1989) has labeled the process by which patient's learn to restrict their lives to adjust to their weaknesses as the *briar patch syndrome,* after Joel Chandler Harris's stories about Br'er Rabbit and his antagonists, Br'er Fox and Br'er Bear, as told by Chandler's archetypic storyteller Uncle Remus. The classic story of Br'er Rabbit and the Tar Baby exemplifies the avoidance of becoming vulnerable. After Br'er Rabbit has been lured out into the open and tricked into striking the tar baby, and becoming covered with the tar, he was easily caught. Cunningly, he implored Br'er Fox and Br'er Bear to do anything they wished with him but to *not* throw him into the briar patch. The briars and thorns clearly made it a painful place for anyone who entered. Although he screamed in pain when they did throw him in, he was soon shouting with laughter, in a place he did not again soon leave. ''You fools, I was born and bred in this here briar patch. This is my home.'' Though vulnerable to the occasional thorn, he was not vulnerable to foxes and bears. Unfortunately, of course, an overly timid occupant of a briar patch may pay a heavy price in reduced opportunities and reduced capacities, for his or her safety. In leaving the briar patch to search for food, the rabbit risks becoming vulnerable. The threat of capture and death evoke a high level of anxiety. So, too, the Axis II patient has difficulty leaving the restrictive briar patch of his or her personality disorder because of the high level of anxiety that would be evoked. The individual tries to find the safe walkways within that briar patch. Periodically, he or she may back up and get stuck by a briar. Although the individual does not like getting stuck, he or she fears the idea of being vulnerable.

One of the most important treatment considerations in working with personality disordered patients is to be aware of the ''briar patch syndrome.'' Therapy will evoke anxiety because the individual is being asked to give up who he or she is and to step out of the briar patch. It may be uncomfortable, limiting, and lonely in there but to go out means, ''I may get hurt and feel anxious''. Beck and Emery (1985), in discussing the treatment of agoraphobia, states:

It is crucial that the patient experience anxiety in order to ensure that the primitive cognitive levels have been activated (since these levels are directly connected to the affects). The repeated, direct, on-the-spot recognition that the danger signals do not lead to catastrophe . . . enhance(s) the responsivity of the primitive level to more realistic inputs from above. (p. 129)

Given the importance of the schematic changes, they are difficult to alter. The schemas are held firmly in place by behavioral, cognitive, and affective elements. Changing only one factor will probably not be effective at changing the schema. The therapeutic approach must take a tripartite approach. To take a cognitive approach and try to argue that patient out of his or her distortions will not work. Having the patient abreact within the session to fantasies or recollections will not be successful by itself. A therapeutic program that addresses all three areas is essential.

The patient's cognitive distortions serve as signposts that point to the schemas. The goal of the therapy is to help the patient to identify the different rules that they live by. The therapist has several options of what might be done to work with the schemas. The first options is schematic restructuring. This may be likened to urban renewal. Having decided that a structure is unsound, the decision is made to tear down the old structure and build a new structure in its place. (This has been a goal of therapy for many years, particularly psychoanalysis.) Whether this restructuring is reasonable is very questionable. An example of schematic restructuring is to have a paranoid personality become a fully trusting individual.

A second possibility is schematic modification. This involves smaller changes to the basic manner of responding to the world. An example would be to have the paranoid personality trust some people, in some situations. A second possibility is to have the paranoid personality self-instruct not to respond as the response that he or she typically gives is undesirable.

The third possibility is schematic reinterpretation. This involves helping the patient to understand and reinterpret his or her life-style and his or her schemata in more functional ways. Patients can also work on restructuring schemata—rebuilding—if that is possible. The most reasonable goals when working with an Axis II patient is to either modify or reinterpret the schema. By schematic reinterpretation, the therapist can find ways of patients dealing with their schema/rules in a more adaptive and functional manner. Given that the rules are not necessarily good or bad, it would depend on how they are interpreted. For example, if someone had a great need to be loved or admired, he or she might choose to teach preschool children, who kiss and hug the teacher. If one wants to be looked up to and respected, earning or buying a title, that is professor, doctor, or colonel, can meet the need for status. Many vocational choices are made because the career or occupation offers and opportunity to meet the schematic press. For example:

A 35-year-old patient who had never had a "straight" job entered therapy because he wanted to give up his life as an illicit drug dealer. He supported himself by selling every illegal drug that his clients, mainly middle-class employed or independently wealthy individuals in an affluent suburban community, wanted to buy. He had been convicted on drug charges only once, on a reduced misdemeanor charge when he was 20 years old, and had served only a few months in jail. He had been in a methadone maintenance program for a short time, at one point in his late 20s when he became heavily dependent on opiates. He had had a variety of sexual adventures, both heterosexual and homosexual. Despite these background factors, which together with his slightly above average intelligence make a diagnosis of antisocial personality disorder almost inevitable, his life was somewhat stable at the time when he entered treatment. He had only one sexual partner, a highly compliant woman with whom he lived. He smoked tobacco and marijuana cigarettes daily and drank alcoholic beverages and snorted cocaine daily. He smoked opium occasionally and used heroin intravenously a few times a month. His business was fairly steady and provided a moderate middle-class income from a stable customer base. He rarely took on new customers and rarely lost old ones. He was, nevertheless, tired of the daily ordeal of a dealer, with the waiting, lies, obligatory drug sampling, and risk of arrest that it entailed. The question he faced, obviously was "what could I change to?" The answer, according to his therapist, was "something straight where your experience is an asset. How about selling real estate? It's a lot like selling dope. You'll still have the waiting, the lies, and the obligatory look-sees, but it's perfectly legal. It pays about the same, and the customers are pretty much the same as the ones you have now." After some inquiry among his customers, he took this suggestion seriously. The problem, of course, was getting him through the necessary training and launched on his new career. He had no idea what people talked about when they were being straight, or how legal businesses were conducted. He had to develop and practice ordinary social skills and to invent a prior career, as a self-employed artist, and to learn to present a cover story about his life history that precluded the possibility of new acquaintances or a potential employer checking references and searching for his employment history. It took 2 years of weekly behavioral assignments, during which he took business courses at a local junior college and trained in a real estate broker's office, before he passed his licensing exam and made his first commission. At that point, he terminated the formal process of therapy, but it took 2 more years of patient effort before his income was high enough to give up dealing entirely. He still uses alcohol, cigarettes, and most of the drugs he previously sold but much less frequently, and he is largely out of his briar patch. He now usually avoids former criminal associates and former clients, has straight friends, invests in real estate instead of German cars, and has married his former girl friend. Throughout the process, a sequence was followed in which an effort to develop effective new behaviors was first planned, then the risky plans were tried out, and both positive and negative effects of these trials were discussed and dealt with. It was made clear from the beginning that a long step-by-step process was involved. The fact that each step opened up new horizons, that each was small enough so that problems could be worked through, and that acceptance and support was consistent contributed to success.

In discussing plans for therapy with a patient diagnosed at intake as borderline personality disorder, she asked, "why are you trying to teach me to control my anxiety. I'm depressed, I'm not anxious at all." At that point the therapist told her the story about the briar patch, and the need to master anxiety-reduction skills. These skills, it was pointed out, would be an essential factor in successful therapy. One patient responded that "it's good to have that safety and I don't understand why I should ever give it up." As the therapist starts to help patients be able to step outside the briar patch, patients must have ways to cope with the increased anxiety. Unless they are able to cope with the anxiety, they may leave therapy and jump right back in the briar patch again. (Space limitations preclude a detailed discussion of anxiety treatment, cf. Beck, A. T. & Emery, G. (1985). *Anxiety disorders and phobia: A cognitive perspective.* New York: Basic Books; Freeman, A., and Simons, K. M., *Cognitive therapy of anxiety* (Chapter 18, this volume). An unfortunate life history may contribute to the compelling quality of biased schemata and the development of personality disorders. An example appears in data reported by Zimmeman, Pfohl, Stangl, and Coryell (1985). They studied a sample of women who had been hospitalized for acute depressive episodes, coded as DSM-III, Axis I disorders. When they divided their sample into three groups, distinguished by differential severity on a negative life events scale designed to assess Axis IV (severity of psychosocial stressors) status, all three groups were similar on acute symptomatic measures such as the Hamilton scale and the Beck Depression Inventory. Despite the apparent similarity in presenting symptoms among the groups differing in negative life events, the severity of the cases within each life events frequency group and the difficulty of treatment for these individuals did differ significantly. Among the 30% of all patients who attempted suicide during the course of the study, the attempt rate was 4 times as high in the high-stress than in the low-stress group. Personality disorders were evident in 84.2% of the high-stress group, 48.1% of the moderate-stress group, and only 28.6% of the low-stress group. The investigators interpreted their finding that frequent negative life events were associated with personality disorder and case severity as at least partly due to the chronicity of the events and the patient's response to this chronicity; if unusually frequent negative events have occurred in someone's life, a pessimistic bias about oneself, the world, and, the future is not unlikely. In contrast, patients who successfully use their briar-patch syndromes to live in a relatively secure personal world may have very low rates of clinically evident personality disorders. In a study of psychiatric referrals in a peace-time military hospital, for example, the only striking difference between the patient population and those similarly referred in civilian settings was a very low rate of diagnosable personality disorders (Hales, Polly, Bridenbaugh, & Orman, 1986). The clinical appearance of a personality disorder is not itself a clue to whether or not patients have biased schemata. As the large literature on self-fulfilling prophecies testifies, it is possible to make consistently biased predictions from inaccurate schema and yet live in such a way, because one restricts risk taking and does not test more accurate alternative schema, that one will consistently be correct (Jones, 1977).

## COGNITIVE THERAPY OF PERSONALITY DISORDERS

The initial goal of therapy is an assessment of the problems and the development of a conceptualization of the patient problems and an appropriate treatment plan. When therapists recognize that cases involve personality disorders, they view them as especially difficult (Merbaum & Buther, 1982; Rosenbaum, Horowitz, & Wilner, 1986). Anticipated patient "resistance" is probably the main source of such perceptions. In fact, these expectations are often accurate. Whenever the briar-patch syndrome is therapeutically relevant, and we find it almost invariably so, in treating personality disorders, it may be difficult to agree about goals and to maintain good therapeutic collaboration.

For example, a prominent wealthy businessman whose principal problem, in the view of the therapist, was a narcissistic personality disorder, entered Cognitive Therapy, in response to his wife's entreaties. His goal was to deal with problems of anger, anxiety, and guilt arising from marital conflict. Like most patients who were not self-referred, he was not interested in schema therapy but only in symptom therapy (Chamberlain, Patterson, Reid, Kavanagh, & Forgatch, 1984). His guilt provided a basis for quick therapeutic gains that were later used to foster collaborative goals that were originally desired only by the therapist. Despite the fact that a great deal of content specificity in the relationships between cognitions and affect is evident when group data are considered (Beck, Brown, Steer, Eidelson and Riskin, 1987), this patient, like many with personality disorders, had a somewhat idiosyncratic description of "guilt" and its causes. He had a schema something like "other people are unimportant" and "I am infinitely more able than they are." This implied that he had great self-worth because of exceptional ability. It seemed prudent to evaluate his opinions about his superior prowess in dealing with life's circumstances and opinions he used to confirm his incredible superiority. In the course of this evaluation, he agreed with an interpretation by the therapist, who had hypothesized that the patient's guilt might stem from negatively evaluating his self-worth because he was unable to get his wife to stop nagging him about his failure to pay some large financial obligations. The therapist helped him see that other individuals he admired because of their ability to get their way also had, in each instance, some failure to control a part of their lives. He modified his dominant schema somewhat, so that an occasional irritating lack of prowess did not detract from his wonderfulness, and his guilt became much less severe. In addition, he was able to give up some of his anxiety about his wife's prowess, because it was only limited to one area of his life, and he also gave up some of the anger toward her that had covered up much of this anxiety. The therapist pointed out to him that giving up his anger helped her be less upset, allowed her to work harder, therefore to make more money from her very successful business, and then contribute more to pay off his liabilities. Further, he was less often neurotically distracted when working, more effective, and therefore also able to contribute more effectively to meeting his financial obligations. He recognized that this sequence had increased his prowess over both himself and his world. He was able to see that modifying his schema was the key to getting what he wanted, and he generalized this lesson to other problems. He gave up much of his guilty, anxiety, and anger toward his wife resulting from having been, in his view, forced into committing several serious felonies to support their extremely expensive life-style. He also gave up similar feelings resulting from his need to engage in frequent sexual liaisons with other women because, in his view, his wife was not a completely proficient sexual partner, always able to satisfy all his desires. His relationship with his wife improved, and he also became more financially responsible and less frequently unfaithful. He was also able to agree with the therapist about the value of schema-oriented therapy over symptomatic therapy and became willing to discuss and accept collaborative therapeutic goals involving further schematic modifications and to consider more expansive reinterpretations. When a therapeutic colleague who happened to be treating the wife suggested that the best goal for this patient's personality problem would be, as in some cases of analytic therapy, to tear it down and build a new one, the therapist demurred. He argued that such restructuring may not always be possible, at least with the psychological resources likely to be available in this case. It would be much like urban renewal, that is, tearing down the old and constructing a new and "better" structure. It might, however, turn out like most cases of urban renewal, a worse result than the original. Whether one views the result in terms of social responsibility or in terms of learning ABC's of principles about dysfunctional feelings and thoughts, the therapist interpreted the course of therapy as reasonably successful. Obviously, the patient also did so because he paid a substantial amount for it, as well as for subsequent therapy for his wife and son (both of which were, however, somewhat less successful in his view, because the wife and son tended, as a consequence of their therapy, to develop more personal autonomy than he had wished). Others, in contrast, might argue that the therapy was either unsuccessful or unethical because the ultimate focus and some of the results were not what the patient initially expected (Williams, 1985).

Following the assessment, the therapist must make sure that there is socialization or education of the patient to the cognitive therapy model. The ideas of what cognitive therapy involves, the goals and plans of the therapy, and the importance of therapeutic collaboration are stressed.

The initial therapeutic focus may be on relieving the presenting symptoms, that is, anxiety or depression. In helping patients to deal with their anxiety or depression, the therapist can teach patients the basic cognitive therapy skills that are going to be necessary in working with the more difficult personality disorder. If the therapist can help the patient become less depressed or less anxious, the patient may accept that this therapy may have some value after all, and it may be worthwhile continuing to work in therapy. Some Axis II patients may, having brought the anxiety and depression under control with fairly standard techniques, choose to leave therapy. One technique that may be helpful with these patients is to differentiate between "symptom therapy" and "schema therapy." By explaining the importance of working on the schema, the patient may choose to stay in therapy.

The essential nature of the therapeutic collaboration stressed by Beck *et al.* (1979) is

ARTHUR FREEMAN
and RUSSELL C. LEAF

nowhere more important than with the Axis II patient. The relationship will be one of the key ingredients in the therapy of the personality disorder. The therapeutic relationship will be a microcosm of the patient's responses to others in his or her environment. The sensitive nature of the relationship means that the therapist must exercise great care in working with this patient group. Being even 2 minutes late for a session with the dependent personality may evoke anxiety about abandonment. The same 2 minutes will raise the specter of being taken advantage of by the paranoid personality. Building and maintaining trust, essential to good therapy generally, is imperative. Given the imperative nature of trust and a relationship, few patients test the patience and mettle of a therapist more than the Axis II group. Issues of the therapist's countertransference must be acknowledged and addressed directly by the therapist. For example, a 42-year-old man was referred by a therapist who had told the patient, "I think I have helped you all I can." In a conversation with the new therapist, the previous therapist said, "This is one of the most demanding guys I have worked with in 20 years of practice. I've really had it with him. He called me at 3 A.M. to tell me that a woman has stood him up for a date. When I asked what time the date was set for, the patient said 9 P.M. the previous evening. When I asked him why he didn't call then he replied, 'I didn't want to bother you then.' When I asked the patient if he was aware of the time, he replied, 'Of course, but that's why you're there.'"

The collaborative nature of the therapy must be constantly stressed. The therapy of the personality disorder must include a strong supportive/expressive component. Without the therapist's active support, the patient may quickly become frightened and disillusioned and leave therapy. The collaborative set involves setting mutually acceptable goals for therapy. These goals must be reasonable and proximal. The patient who expects that he or she will become a totally different person as a result of therapy will, invariably, be disappointed. By making small steps toward the desired goals, therapy can move ahead slowly but effectively. Therapists must keep in mind that collaboration is not always 50:50. With many patients, the collaboration may be 80:20, or 90:10.

The rate of treatment and frame of treatment must be discussed. The patient who has read of CT and expects that he or she will be "cured" in 12 to 20 sessions must be apprised of the greater severity and chronicity of these problems and that these problems will take a longer time for treatment. Twelve to 20 months (or more) is a far more reasonable time frame for the treatment of personality disorders.

The patient's significant others can be invaluable allies in the therapeutic endeavor by helping the patient to do homework, do reality testing, and offering support in making changes. The significant others can also be important sources of data about the patient's past behaviors. In a negative vein, meeting with the significant others may enable the therapist to piece together a family history of problems and what keeps the patient behaving in the same dysfunctional way. Finally, the significant others might be involved in marital or family therapy with the patient.

Noncompliance by the patient is often a sign of treatment failure. When Axis II disorders are present, it may be due to the impact of the patient's personality disorder on the therapeutic relationship, or to the therapist's reactions to the features of that disorder. Common patient problems include: (1) lack of motivation, because the patient does not anticipate benefits great enough to compensate for the required effort and risk; (2) lack of skill, because the patient may never have learned, for example, social skills that others take for granted; (3) secondary gain, because significant others reinforce the patient for staying in his or her own briar patch; (4) fear that the attempt will fail, because compelling schemata lead the patient to think "I can't do it" or other cognitions that emphasize vulnerability or hopelessness; (5) fear that others will not accept the change, because "I must not let them down," "they will leave me," or other cognitions that emphasize abandonment or rejection; (6) fear that the client will not really prefer the changed self, because "I'll feel like a phony," "I'll never be comfortable like that," or other cognitions that emphasize authenticity or consistency; and (7) characterological rigidity or low frustration tolerance.

Similarly, common therapist problems include: (1) lack of motivation, because the therapist sees the client as such a difficult case, given the rewards, that the therapist's effort lacks diligence and effortfulness; (2) lack of skill, because of poor timing of interventions, inadequate assessment, failure to appreciate the patient's desire to control or manipulate the course of therapy, and so forth; (3) secondary gain for coaxing the client into giving up, because, for example, of dogged insistence that cognitive therapy is extremely powerful and should be very short term except with unmotivated patients. If a patient needs 12 to 20 months rather than 12 to 20 sessions to show improvement, it is not a sign of therapist inadequacy or of limits of the therapeutic methods. Other therapist problems include (4) fear that the client will not change if a personality disorder, rather than, or as well as, a symptom is the target, because the goal is "too ambitious;" (5) fear that those who referred the client will not accept the change, because the patient may actually change in a way that pleases him or her even less than his or her pattern at referral; (6) fear that the patient will develop an iatrogenic disorder, because the therapist becomes embroiled in a power struggle with the patient or because increased stress from the patient's external circumstances or from the demands imposed by therapy become more than the patient can handle; and (7) characterological rigidity or low frustration tolerance. All of these problems have elements that are found in all therapy, whether or not the patients have personality disorders. They seem more frequent, however, when personality disorders are at issue.

In addition to problems due to patient, therapist, or communication deficits, there are problems that arise from poor socialization to the therapeutic model. One may skip steps when dealing with a simple symptomatic problem where therapy proceeds rapidly, but in working with personality-disordered patients, it is best to make sure they have a clear understanding of why schemata are the major focus of cognitive therapy, of the pace at which *they* can expect progress with *their* problems, and the kind of support they can and cannot expect from their therapist. If schemata were all visual, a clear picture of our schema for therapy might show a therapist pointing at maps and pictures of existing and more accurate schemata, while the patient looked at the scenes pointed to and tried to practice, with eyes closed, reconstructing eidetic images of the more accurate scenes. A more skillful or experienced therapist might have more maps and pictures than a less skillful one, but the patient's vigilance about the details of the figures and the patient's willingness and ability to recall the images when under stress are more important than the therapist's armamentarium. In addition, in order to maintain trust, it is important for these patients to understand in advance that they are on their own when they try to effect changes in their lives but can expect encouragement to proceed and moral support from their therapist whatever their performance and whatever its outcome.

## COGNITIVE AND BEHAVIORAL TECHNIQUES

The Cognitive Therapy of personality disorders progresses in the same manner as Cognitive Therapy with other disorders. The identification of the patient's distorted thinking is followed by the therapist working with the patient to test the meaning, reality, or validity of the thoughts and perceptions. The techniques can be, somewhat arbitrarily, divided into cognitive and behavioral techniques. The particular mix of cognitive and behavioral techniques is, of course, related to the needs of the patient. As discussed earlier, the more severe the pathology, the more behavioral the approach. The less severe the behavioral pathology, the more cognitive the approach (see Figure 1).

ARTHUR FREEMAN
and RUSSELL C. LEAF

Cognitive techniques that can be helpful include: (1) searches for idiosyncratic meaning because these patients often label their feelings and thoughts in unusual ways, in part because of their deviant experience patterns; (2) labeling of distortions, so that the patient can be made aware that particular automatic patterns of thought are, in fact, biased and unreasonable; (3) development of replacement imagery, to counter catastrophic or other antecedents of dysfunctional cognitions and provide a base for more accurate cognitions (Means, Wilson, & Dlugokinski, 1987); (4) guided association, through which the therapist helps the client see possible alternative and sequences that the client does not usually include in his or her schemata; (5) examining options and alternatives, so that the client comes to see beyond the briar patch; (6) examining the advantages and disadvantages of maintaining or changing a belief, so that primary and secondary gains can be clarified; (7) scaling, so that experiences can be put into life perspective, to reduce the biases due to thinking about them in isolation; (8) disputing irrational thoughts, so that evidence for and against the accuracy of compelling schemata can be explicitly evaluated; (9) reattribution, by which changes in ideas about responsibility for actions and outcomes can be assigned; and (10) coaching and self-instruction, by which clients can be prompted, encouraged, and guided to new patterns of action (Meichenbaum, 1977; Novaco, 1975).

Cognitive and behavioral techniques play complementary roles in the treatment of personality disorders. The behavioral ones serve to move the patient into a new position, and the cognitive ones serve to develop new schemata and to modify or reinterpret old ones. Ultimately, of course, the cognitive techniques probably account for most of the change that occurs (Deffenbacher, Story, Stark, Hogg, & Brandon, 1987). The cognitive work, like the behavioral, requires more care and precision than usual when clients have personality disorders. The schemata of these patients are often unusually defective, even when their behavior has been corrected, and a larger variety and longer duration of cognitive reworking is typically required. Although the first principle of treatment for personality disorders is to emphasize behavioral methods, *the final principle is to follow up with thorough cognitive ones.*

The goals of using the behavioral techniques are threefold. First, the therapist may need to work very directly to alter self-defeating behaviors. Second, patients may be skill deficient, and the therapy must include a skill-building component. Third, the behavioral assignments can be used as homework to help to test out cognitions. Behavioral techniques that can be helpful include: (1) activity monitoring and scheduling, which permits retrospective identifica-

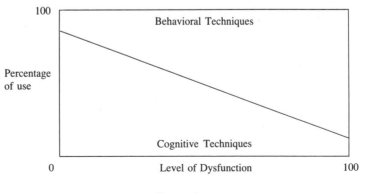

FIGURE 1

tion of briar patches and prospective planning of changes; (2) behavioral rehearsal, modeling, assertiveness training, and role playing for skill development prior to early efforts to respond more effectively, either in old problematic situations or in new ones; (3) relaxation training and behavioral distraction techniques, for use when anxiety becomes an imminent problem during efforts to change; (4) *in vivo* exposure, either by arranging conditions for a problematic situation by appointment in consultation setting or by arranging for the therapist to go with the client to a problematic setting, so that the therapist can help the client deal with dysfunctional schemata and actions that have, for whatever reason, not been tractable in the ordinary consultation setting; (5) graded task assignment, so that the patient can picture the process of changes as an incremental step-by-step process during which the difficulty of each part can be adjusted and mastery achieved in stages; and (6) mastery or pleasure ratings, so that the patient can validate the successfulness and pleasure from changed experiences, or lack thereof.

# CASE MATERIAL ILLUSTRATING THE COGNITIVE THERAPY OF PERSONALITY DISORDERS

In this final section, each of the personality disorders will be presented. Our goal in this section is to present a broad case conceptualization along with specific case material to illustrate how the typical schemata manifest themselves in the cognitive and behavioral styles of the patient. Given the range of combinations and permutations possible with schema, in content, combination, intensity of activity, the examples used are of patients where a particular disorder is clearly primary. Because many of the Axis II patients have mixed diagnoses, in DSM-III-R, more than one personality disorder can be diagnosed if the patient meets criteria (p. 336).

The personality disorders are divided into three groups or clusters. Cluster A includes the paranoid, schizoid, and schizotypal personality disorders. These disorders, by virtue of the behavioral manifestations are labeled *odd or eccentric*. Cluster B includes the antisocial, borderline, histrionic, and narcissistic personality disorders, grouped together because of the "dramatic, emotional, or erratic" manifestations. Finally, Cluster C includes avoidant, dependent, obsessive-compulsive, and passive aggressive, labeled "*anxious or fearful*" (DSM III-R, p. 337).

## Paranoid Personality Disorder

The individual with a paranoid personality disorder generally tends to interpret the actions of others as posing a specific or general threat to his or her person or property. Often, the actions of others are overinterpreted in the direction of any actions being potentially harmful. The particular bias that they bring to any situation may be used as a basis to confirm their preexisting notions of impending harm coming from others. Typical schema are:

1. People will eventually try to hurt me.
2. People cannot be trusted. They will always take advantage of me.
3. People will try to bother or annoy me.
4. Don't get mad, get even.
5. Any insult, no matter how slight, directed at me should be punished.
6. Stay on guard. Always be prepared for the worst.
7. To compromise is to surrender.

8. Avoid intimacy. If I get close to people, they can find out my weaknesses.
9. Keep alert for anyone who has power. They can hurt me.

### CASE ILLUSTRATION

John was a 29-year-old engineer. He entered therapy because of "difficulty at work." His supervisor had suggested that John "get help" and referred John to the company counseling center. Rather than go to the company counselors who John was sure would not keep confidential what he said, he sought private therapy. His condition for therapy was that his being in therapy would not be shared with his employer. In John's view, the reason for the referral was part of a personal vendetta against him by the supervisor. In point of fact, the problem at work was so severe that John was threatened with being fired if he did not change his attitude and behavior at work.

John was unmarried and did not date. He did not see his lack of a social life as either unusual or problematic. When asked about his lack of dating, he replied, "There are really few nice women out there. They're just out to get what they can from a guy, money, sex, you know what I mean?" John had never had many friends. He had two male friends since childhood, both of whom were also single. He said that he trusted both of these friends, but not totally. "You can never tell when someone will turn on you."

John worked in an office with several other men and had worked for the company for 6 years. He refused to talk with the other men in his office and insisted that they address him by his family name rather than by his given name. "We're not friends, why should I be so familiar with them?" His goal in therapy was simply to meet his employer's requirement. John intended to stay in therapy until the present crisis "blows over."

Recognizing the nature of John's difficulty as Axis II issues, the therapist chose to maintain the therapeutic relationship on a professional title basis. John was "Mr. Smith," and the therapist was "Dr. Freeman." By keeping the relationship "professional," the attempt was made to avoid exciting John's anxiety about closeness. The focus of the therapy was initially to try to help John behave differently at work so as to maintain his job. Trust needed to be built very slowly. At one point, the therapist was 5 minutes late for a session. This became "evidence" for the therapist's lack of trustworthiness. The session was spent discussing whether John would be charged for a shortened session, whether John's lateness in the future would be acceptable, and whether John could expect late behavior from the therapist in the future. When the therapist was away for a 1-week vacation, John said that he understood the therapist going on vacation, "but why at such an inconvenient time for me?"

With the focus being on changing John's work behavior, other areas of concern could be brought into the therapeutic collaboration, that is, social interaction, seeking "safe" pleasure activities.

After 18 months of therapy, on a weekly basis, John agreed to enter a group, in addition to the individual therapy. Within the group, John was willing to self-disclose on a very limited basis and experiment with the response of individuals within the group. In the individual therapy, he tried to predict the response of others and found himself to be incorrect a large percentage of the time. Given that John was so very sure of what others were thinking or planning, he experienced cognitive dissonance and anxiety. He affiliated with a woman in the group, a very dependent 32-year-old, and they began dating. John was, of course, in the position of power, but this relationship represented the first long-term relationship he had ever had. He terminated therapy shortly thereafter. His job problems had been modified, and he was now willing to talk with his co-workers. He was no longer in danger of being fired.

Schizoid individuals seem to have little or no idea about why people affiliate. They see other people involved in relationships but see relating as part of a different language, culture or universe. Typical schema are:

1. Why should I be close to people?
2. Being close to others is of little importance.
3. I am my own best friend.
4. Stay calm. Displays of emotion are unnecessary and embarrassing.
5. What others say is of little interest or importance to me.
6. Sex is okay but just for release.

## Case Illustration

Dan, a 66-year-old chemist, came for therapy because of his anxiety. He had never married but was presently dating a woman he had dated for the past 8 years. He would see her once a week on a Saturday night, go to a movie, and have sex. He would then go home. "Why stay over? I did what I came for. That's pretty funny, what I came for."

Dan had been in various therapies over the past 40 years. His first therapy experience was when he was in Europe attending medical school in Switzerland on the G.I. Bill. After a year of school he experienced panic attacks and entered a Jungian analysis. He remained in analysis for only 6 months and left when he experienced a dimunition of his anxiety. He left medical school and returned to the United States. He completed graduate school and received a PhD in chemistry.

Dan sees himself as "low keyed"; he states, "I never get angry." The therapeutic goals with Dan were first to lower his anxiety and then to explore his avoidance or lack of understanding as to why people spend time together. He came for weekly therapy sessions and seemed to enjoy the sessions. He reported that when he was 2 years old, his mother became quite ill with tuberculosis and was sent to a sanitarium for 2 years. She returned home for several months and then had to return to the sanitarium where she died. During his mother's illness, he lived with his maternal grandmother. After his mother's death, he continued to live with his grandmother until age 6. At that time, his father remarried, and he had to return to live with his father and stepmother. He did not want to leave his grandmother and barely knew his father. Dan's lack of a family feeling and his difficulty in seeing himself as connected with others probably stemmed from these early unsuccessful affiliation experiences. Through childhood, adolescence, and his young adult years relationships were avoided. A major personal schema was "Getting attached to people is not a good idea. They'll probably leave me." Therapy was focused on increasing Dan's interactions with others. He began to spend weekends with his girlfriend, attend family functions with her (weddings, Thanksgiving dinner, Christmas, and funerals) and went away on a 2-week vacation with her.

Dan was not against spending time with another person; it was never something that he ever really understood. Although it was not his first thought or choice, he did begin to spend time with his girlfriend. He needed to use self-instructional strategies to be with others. The self instruction was, "When in doubt, don't be alone." In Dan's case, the behavior was altered, though not the underlying schema. The continued interpersonal contacts served to reinforce schema about the advantages of relating that served to modify the older schema.

## Schizotypal Personality Disorder

It is very difficult to isolate specific schemata that are idiosyncratic to the schizotypal personality disorder. These patients are usually seen as strange or peculiar. These eccentricities are readily observable but not severe enough to meet criteria for schizophrenia (DSM-III-R, p. 340). The major goal in working with these patients would be similar to those in working with schizophrenics, that is, social skills training (including grooming, interpersonal skill development, and generally appearing less peculiar), anxiety reduction, and self-instructional training.

## ANTISOCIAL PERSONALITY DISORDER

The lack of a "superego" seems to be the hallmark of this disorder. These individuals tend to have little remorse subsequent to their abusive, impulse-driven, or dangerous behavior. One interesting clinical observation is that these individuals often see themselves as smarter than all others. Antisocial individuals may plan events wherein they believe that they are superior. When caught in committing a crime, their "problem" is getting caught, not committing the crime. The goal for the future may be to become a better criminal, rather than obeying the law. Typical schema are:

1. Rules are meant for others.
2. Only fools follow all of the rules.
3. Rules are meant to be broken.
4. Look out for Number 1.
5. My pleasure comes first.
6. If others are hurt, offended, or inconvenienced by my behavior, that is their problem.
7. Do it now! I will not allow myself to be frustrated.
8. I will do whatever I must to get whatever I want.
9. I'm really smarter than most everybody else.

## CASE ILLUSTRATION

Max was a 29-year-old male, currently a participant in a methadone maintenance program. He was seen in therapy, in addition to his drug counseling. He had been in trouble with both school and legal authorities since the age of 12. He was supposed to come for therapy on a twice-weekly basis but came in for therapy on the average of two to three times a month. He always had a reason for missing his sessions. His excuses were often so simple as to be naive, for example, "I had to go to New York [from Philadelphia] to get parts for a truck that I am thinking of buying, and it took 2 days to get the part." When asked from whom the truck was being purchased, Max replied, "Some guy I just met, a friend of my sister's." When asked as to why he had to buy the part for a truck he did not own, why it could not be obtained in his city, and why the part had to be gotten on days that sessions were scheduled, he would develop the story even further. Finally, the therapist asked him the make of truck, and Max replied, "a Ford." When the therapist attempted to reality-test with him, Max became offended that he was not being believed. "If you don't trust me, how can you help me," he asked of the therapist.

Treatment with Max was focused on building prosocial behaviors, in effect, building a "superego". The therapist was gentle but firm in not accepting Max's constant excuses. The focus of the therapy was on helping Max to accept responsibility. By challenging the cognitive distortions and alerting Max to the dysfunctional nature of his schemata, Max began to see how his behaviors, viewed by him as clever and complex, were in reality transparent and childlike. Max became extremely anxious when his persona was threatened. The difficulty he had in changing was that he did not see his behavior as a mask but as the only way to behave. When Max could accept that he could get even more from the world by becoming part of the system, rather than trying to always fool the system, he began to act more adaptively. His goal of getting the most for himself did not waver. He now tried to get it in ways that got him into far less trouble. He returned to school to finish his high school diploma and then continued on to a 2-year college program. On follow-up over 2 years, Max continued to stay out of legal problems.

## BORDERLINE PERSONALITY DISORDER

The common view of this disorder, prior to the publication of DSM-III, was that this patient was on the "borderline" between neurosis and psychosis. With stress, the patient might go "south of the border." When neuroses was removed from the diagnostic lexicon (DSM-III, 1980), the traditional view of the borderline collapsed. These patients are notably unstable and tend to dichotomize virtually every experience. The therapist may be seen as the greatest therapist to ever live, or within minutes, the most unfeeling, unthinking, disreputable, unethical individual to ever pretend to be a therapist. An old therapist's joke claims the heuristic differentiation between borderline and personality disorder and schizophrenia to be that schizophrenics bother almost everybody, whereas borderlines only bother their therapist. A major goal of therapy with this group is to try to teach them the need for a modulation of behavior. Their general fear of abandonment often leads to their being even more demanding, thereby causing people to retreat from them. Typical schema are:

1. I am not sure who I am.
2. I will eventually be abandoned.
3. My pain [psychic] is so intense that I cannot bear it.
4. My anger controls me; I cannot modulate my behavior.
5. My feelings overwhelm me; I cannot modulate my feelings.
6. He/she is so very, very good that I am so lucky [or alternately and quickly] he/she is so very, very awful that I cannot bear them.
7. When I am overwhelmed, I must escape [by flight or suicide].

## CASE ILLUSTRATION

Alice, a 34-year-old woman was referred by a psychiatrist because of her ongoing depression. Pharmacotherapy had been ineffective, as had a year of insight-oriented therapy. Alice had been married to an account for the past 15 years. She had completed a master's degree in education and worked as a teacher for 6 years. She left teaching because of her depression and some physical problems. At the point of entering therapy, she had not worked in 6 years. She stayed at home, "too depressed to do anything." When Alice was asked to make a list of her negative thoughts, she began her list with "I was bad before I was born, I was a bad fetus." She described her mother as having regaled her for years with how bad she [Alice] had been *in utero*. Her mother had a difficult first trimester with a great deal of nausea, could not sleep because of chronic lower back pain in the second trimester, and was bedridden for the last trimester of her pregnancy.

Alice had few friends throughout her childhood and adolescence. Her mother attempted to innoculate Alice against the "viciousness" of the world by slapping Alice across the face almost daily. If Alice cried, her mother kept hitting her, to teach her to resist the pain of the world. Finally Alice could accept the slaps without crying. At that point, Alice's mother would hit her so Alice would be more emotionally responsive.

When Alice was graduated from high school and discussed going to college, her mother became distraught. Her mother told Alice, "I can't stand the thought of you going away. I'll die without you here. You are all I have to live for. Can't you forget college and get a job in town. Please don't leave me." Alice chose a college close to home for the first 2 years and commuted to school. Her second 2 years were spent on a campus at a distance from her home.

Therapy proceeded for 13 months before Alice felt she could *begin* to trust the therapist. Therapy was a stormy road. When the therapist told Alice about an impending vacation 1 month hence, she withdrew from therapy. "What is the use of being in therapy when you are leaving," she said in response to the therapist's inquiries. When told that the therapist did intend to return, Alice questioned, "How do I know that?" Any separation was seen by Alice as irrevocable, and the therapist's return was seen by Alice as anticlimactic. She feared the coming year and the impending separation of next summer's vacation. Alice had few ideas as to how her mistrust and fear of separation (and abandonment) came to be. After the second year of therapy, Alice told the therapist about an incident that had occurred when she was 7 years old. Her father was in the U.S. Navy and stationed in Japan. Her mother had Alice spend a week in the beginning of the summer with Alice's paternal grandmother. Alice was told that during that time, Alice's father would return home and her mother and father would come to get her. Alice's grandmother worked as a matron at a state orphanage. For the first week, Alice lived in her grandmother's room. When her mother and father did not call or come to get her, Alice was moved into the girl's dormitory. She stayed in the dormitory for the balance of the summer. Plans were made for Alice to attend school at the orphanage. Three days before school was to begin, she was brought to her grandmother's room where she was greeted by her parents. Her mother's only comment was, "Your father was delayed." When questioned as to why she had never mentioned that experience, Alice replied, "I didn't think that it was all that important." Using the abandonment as a clue, the therapist inquired as to whether there were other incidents of being left abandoned, separated, or taken from her parents. Alice went on to describe several other instances of being emotionally abandoned (her mother would get angry at her and not speak to her for weeks at a time) or physically abandoned (being left sitting on a bench in a shopping mall or store and told not to move. Her mother returned hours later). Given these early experiences, Alice's schemata about being abandoned were powerfully in place. When asked about her relationship with her husband, she said that she did not trust that he would stay with her for very long.

The goals of the therapy were first, to carefully try to challenge the idea that she would be abandoned. Alice was unwilling, at first, to take a risk that the therapist would leave and return, or, that the therapist would leave, return, and still be willing to work with her. Her distortion in this regard was that the therapist would forget about her while he was away.

A second goal of therapy was to work with Alice and her husband to try to improve the marital relationship. Couples sessions were instituted to help her husband better understand Alice and her problems and for Alice to risk telling her husband of her dissatisfaction with many aspections of the relationship.

In the third year of weekly therapy, Alice was less depressed and less anxious than she was initially. She was not working, and it was questionable as to whether Alice would ever work again. The therapeutic relationship, being the microcosm of her relationship with the world, continued to be the arena for Alice to understand her fear of abandonment and to frame experiments to test this early schema.

## HISTRIONIC PERSONALITY DISORDER

The highly dramatic behavior of this type of patient is described by Eric Berne in his classic volume, *Games People Play* (1964). In "The Stocking Game,"

a woman comes into a strange group and after a very short time raises her leg, exposing herself in a provocative way, and remarks, "Oh my, I have a run in my stocking." This is calculated to arouse the men and make the other women angry . . . . What is significant is [the] lack of adaptation. She seldom waits to find out what kind of people she is dealing with or how to time her maneuver. Hence she stands out as inappropriate and affects her relationships with her associates. (p. 129)

The male variant of the "game" would involve comments regarding the tightness of one's underwear.

These patients are typically highly reactive or overresponsive to other people. They are often perceived by others as shallow and self-centered. Their overall demand on the environment is for rather immediate gratification of needs, be they emotional, physical, or creative. Physical attractiveness is a high priority for the histrionic individual. Typical schemas are:

1. Appearances are important.
2. People are judged on external appearances.
3. I must be noticed.
4. I must never be frustrated in life.
5. I must get everything I think that I want.
6. Emotions should be expressed quickly and directly.
7. Beauty is the most important consideration in judging someone.

CASE ILLUSTRATION

Leonard was a 40-year-old attorney. He was referred by his treating therapist. Although the ostensible reason for the referral was because of Leonard's unremitting depression, it soon became clear that Leonard's therapist no longer wanted to work with him. A graduate of an Ivy League university and an Ivy League law school where he was a member of the *Law Review,* Leonard was unemployed. He had lost his last job, a civil service position earning $35,000 per year. Others of his class were earning four to five times that amount as partners in major law firms.

When speaking with Leonard (never Len), the therapist had to listen to the footnotes of Leonard's speech, for example "I met with John, he's a senior partner in Green, Smith and White, a prestigious firm that is one of the largest in the city, and one of the oldest, second only to Flip, Flop, and Over. He is married to Marcia, a physician specializing in rare tropical diseases."

Leonard often became so distracted in the telling that his original goal was lost. His intent seemed to be to overwhelm the listener with his intelligence and fund of knowledge. His level of appropriateness was so low that he would give object lessons in manners to street toughs, for example, when asked for a light by a street tough saying "Hey man, give me a light", Leonard's response was, "I am certainly not your man." The street tough punched Leonard in the face.

Leonard lost wives, girlfriends, jobs, doctors, and therapists because of his inappropriateness, demandingness, and general poor sense. His physician called to tell him to find another primary care physician because Leonard would call him several times a week regaling him with symptoms and wanting to discuss the infrequent side effects of medications that Leonard had read about in the PDR. At times, Leonard affected an English accent to impress women. After speaking to them in his accent, he could never call the women for a date because they would then find out that he was not British.

At one point, Leonard called his therapist to say that he was feeling suicidal. "I have the point of a large, very sharp Sabatier pressed to my abdomen. You know how sharp this very excellent chef's knife is, don't you?"

The goals of therapy with Leonard were to set firm and consistent limits. Leonard's schemata were made explicit rather early in therapy, so that Leonard could understand why the therapist would not be responding to the broad histrionic behavior. Leonard generally took these limits well. On occasion, he began pressing the limits. On one occasion, he attempted to prolong the therapy session. Every attempt to end the session was met with, "I just need to tell you one more thing." Finally, the therapist ushered Leonard out of the office. At the door, Leonard turned and said, "You are aware that I'm thinking of killing myself within an hour of my leaving, aren't you?" The therapist's response was to inform Leonard that the emergency room was available, but the issue of the suicidality needed to be dealt with at the next session.

The limits were constantly being tested and needed to be maintained for the sake of the therapy, Leonard's well-being, and the therapist's mental health.

## NARCISSISTIC PERSONALITY DISORDER

In classical Greek mythology, Narcissus was so enamoured of the reflection of the beautiful youth in the water (himself), that he became rooted to the spot. Narcissistic patients are similar to the histrionic patient in their inflated view of themselves, the need to be noticed as special, and the need to only be with people as special as themselves. They are very demanding in their relationships and therefore also as patients. Typical schemas are:

1. I must have my way in every interaction.
2. I must not be, in any way, foiled in seeking pleasure or status.
3. I am more special than anyone else.
4. I should only have to relate to special people like me.
5. I must be admired.
6. No one should have more of anything than I have.

## CASE ILLUSTRATION

Sam was a 64-year-old surgeon and professor of surgery at a medical school. He came to therapy with great reluctance, as part of marital therapy. He had been married for 42 years, to Anita. She had suffered a "nervous breakdown" (major depressive episode), which required her being hospitalized. The treating resident strongly recommended marital therapy. As part of the assessment, Sam was seen for two sessions. He made it quite clear that he did not like being in the therapist's office, did not want to be part of the therapy, and did not think that anything wrong with his wife had anything to do with him. He was, at first, quite pleasant and charming, trying to convince the therapist that his (Sam's) involvement in therapy was unnecessary. Failing that, he became brusque, bordering on rudeness. "Why," he inquired, "am I seeing a therapist who is only an associate professor, when I am a full professor. If I have got to be part of this ridiculous business, I might as well have the best person."

The marital issue revolved around Sam demanding that his wife wait on him, hand and foot. She had little more than servant status and was expected to provide for his every whim. In recent years, his wife had become more and more "down" and finally ceased functioning and came into the hospital. His view of Anita's problem was that she was just "too moody, too weak, too spoiled, and too reluctant to do her job," which was, in his eyes, to do his bidding. Sam considered his position in life as one that was well deserved. He described himself as a tyrant in the operating theater because "I'm damn good." He described, with great relish, how he had his residents and nurses jump whenever he came into a room.

The goals of therapy, within the context of the agreed-upon marital work, was to have Sam respond differently to his wife. The reason was so that she could return to full functioning. It was pointed out to Sam that if he continued to create stress, his wife would continue to be depressed and would be unavailable to meet his needs. With this as a goal, he continued in therapy. Marital sessions were held weekly, and Sam was seen on a alternate-week basis. The therapy work with Sam was quite limited. Much of the therapy work consisted of direct instruction on more adaptive ways to behave with Anita. His more pervasive behavioral response was not dealt with in the therapy. He could, in fact, alter his response to Anita, not because he agreed with it, but because if he did not make that alteration, he would get even less of what he wanted. The focus of the work with Anita was to have her be more assertive and try to refuse doing things that she did not want to do. If Sam wanted certain things done, they could hire someone and pay them to do it, or do it himself. After 6 months of therapy, Sam and Anita terminated the therapy. She was less depressed and described Sam as more responsive. She also pointed out that any response on Sam's part was more response than she had gotten in the past.

## AVOIDANT PERSONALITY DISORDER

A question for the clinician is whether a patient is schizoid or avoidant, both of which share the common threads of general difficulty in interpersonal relationships, sensitivity to criticism, and an avoidance of contact with others. The debate between the proponents of similarity and difference between these diagnoses has been quite lively (Millon, 1985). The disorders are quite different both in the content of the disorder and in the schemata underlying the disorders. Millon (1981) differentiated between the asocial individual (schizoid) and the withdrawn individual (avoidant). The avoidant individual sees others in social situations and would like to join them, whereas the schizoid individuals are reclusive and do not generally seek interpersonal relationships (including therapy because of the very nature of psychotherapy as an intense interpersonal experience). Typical schemas are:

1. I must be liked.
2. I must not look foolish to myself or others, at any time.
3. The world is a dangerous place.
4. I must depend on others to take care of me.
5. Isolation is better than being put at risk of being hurt.
6. All criticism is the same. The slightest criticism is the same as massive condemnation.
7. People must offer me unconditional guarantees of acceptance before I commit myself to relating to that person.

## CASE ILLUSTRATION

Alan, a 20-year-old undergraduate was self-referred because of "social anxiety." (Although social anxiety was a major component of Alan's life, he met criteria for avoidant disorder.) He had decided that after 2 years at the university, he needed to make friends. He had no contact with others in his dormitory or with his next-door neighbors. He infrequently spoke to other students in his classes because of his anxiety. Alan's mother called the therapist after the first session and informed the therapist that, when at home, Alan was "funny and related well to all of his relatives." Alan's father had died when Alan was 6 years old. He was raised by his maternal grandmother while his mother worked. Being an only child, his grandmother was afraid to allow him to play with other children because he might get hurt. He was expected to return home directly after school so as to be safe. Clubs, Scouting or other extracurricullar activities were discouraged because of the potential danger involved. Alan reported the following example of childhood overprotection. "I must have been about 8 or 9. It was during the summer, and my mother and grandmother had rented a summer cottage. I was playing outdoors, and my grandmother was sitting on the porch watching me. I saw some kids playing two houses away and started walking towards them. My grandmother came off the porch towards me. I was almost to the kids when my grandmother grabbed me by the arm. The other kids saw that and started making fun of me. They called me "momma's boy," "sissy," and "fairy." My grandmother yelled at them and that made it even worse. I didn't want to go out of the house for fear of seeing those kids again."

Therapy was very problem focused. It lasted for 20 months, excluding the summer months when Alan returned home. A series of graded task assignments (i.e., asking a student in class for an assignment), role play in the office utilizing clinic staff as role-play assistants, and directly challenging Alan's distortions and the underlying schemata were the main tools. When the new school year began, Alan started speaking to other students in class and began relating to others in his dormitory. He started staying with a small group of students that Alan labeled as *nerds and losers, just like me*. His self-esteem was still quite low, but he had effectively begun the process of trying to be more social. The anxiety reduction techniques were essential in Alan's treatment. By the end of the second year of therapy, Alan was involved with others in his dormitory and had begun dating.

## DEPENDENT PERSONALITY DISORDER

As previously discussed, the appealing, helpless behavior of the 1-year-old child is inappropriate in the adult. The dependent personality disorder goes beyond the culturally dictated behaviors of being unassertive but represents an inability to initiate projects, plans, or ideas. It involves an abdication of autonomy far in excess of appropriate sharing of responsibility.

### CASE ILLUSTRATION

Sally was a 34-year-old unmarried teacher. She had been teaching first grade for the past 12 years. Her previous therapist referred her to her present therapist with the statement, "I believe Sally to be untreatable. Her great dependence precludes her ever changing." Sally was, indeed, dependent. She would not make a decision without consulting her mother, her therapist, her two best friends, and her father. She did not simply ask for opinions but rather asked for decisions. If the decisions were at variance, Sally would become very anxious. Her dating pattern was to become attached to a man after one date, and when he did not call her for a second date, she would become distraught. The following is an index of the severity of the dependent personality disorder. A man took her out for a date and tried to rape her. When she fought him off and forced him to leave her apartment, he called her a "tease" and told her he would never call her again. Sally became upset at the loss. She did not focus on the attempted rape but rather on her perception of his abandonment of her.

The goal of therapy with Sally was to have her attempt to make small decisions on her own. Almost any situation in her life became grist for the therapeutic mill. One example was Sally's taking a vacation. She had not taken a vacation in the past 10 years. Her rationale was that she never had someone to go with, could not decide where to go, when to go, how long to spend, and so forth. With the discrete goal of going on a vacation, small goals of gathering information and turning plans into action were the focus of the therapy. Sally's choice of vacation locale was England, the same vacation the therapist took the previous year. Inasmuch as the goal was *any* vacation, as better than none, no interpretation of the continued dependence was made. Sally planned the vacation to go on a tour with a group of teachers. The trip was planned and taken with the help of a guide. The successful experience of having gone on a vacation was then used to demonstrate that Sally could do things on her own. Sally has subsequently taken two other vacations.

One technique that proved to be very helpful was using Sally's pathology in the service of the therapy. She was willing to do homework, fill out dysfunctional thought records, attempt new behaviors, and relinquish old problematic behaviors after discussing the importance of change with the therapist. Not wanting to alienate the therapist, Sally was willing to take certain risks.

She has developed a relationship with a man, has changed her school-teaching assignment to another building and a new grade. She still experiences great anxiety in new situations but is now willing to take chances in those new situations.

## OBSESSIVE-COMPULSIVE PERSONALITY DISORDER

Few patients are as self- and other demanding as the obsessive-compulsive personality disorder. The perfectionistic demand, although being functional in some areas of life, at certain times, becomes dysfunctional as a general life-style. The obsessive-compulsive lives to work, as opposed to working so that they can live more comfortably. They are often perceived as "tight," "stiff," "serious," "humourless," or "constricted."

Typical schemas are:

1. There are strict rules in life.
2. By focusing on the details of a situation, one will reduce the chances of making errors.
3. A person is defined by what they do.
4. The better job you do the better person you are.
5. Rules must be adhered to without alteration.
6. Never discard anything that may be of some value.
7. Emotions must be controlled.

## CASE ILLUSTRATION

Phyllis was a 35-year-old executive working for a large corporation, earning a large salary. She had no social life, no friends, and did not date. Her workday started at 6:30 A.M. and lasted until 9:00 P.M. She would work on Saturday and Sunday for 5 hours. She had, at that point, never dated, and had never had sexual intercourse. Her referral was to deal with a germ phobia for which she had sought treatment from several therapists over the past 25 years. In all of her previous therapy, the germ phobia was the major focus of the therapy work. In establishing a problem list at the onset of therapy, the therapist tried to establish a hierarchy of problems to be worked on. Phyllis listed the germ phobia as being the most important. Given that it was a chronic symptom that did not incapacitate her but rather discomforted and inconvenienced her, the therapist questioned as to whether it might be of value to start working with other problems. The therapeutic goal was to attempt to gain some success at treating the other symptoms, rather than repeat the failures of the past by focusing all of the therapeutic energy on the germ phobia. The therapist recommended that the initial focus be on developing social interactions. The therapy work, over the first year was on skill building and experimenting with different types of social interactions. Phyllis' first dating situation ended after two dates. The man, a 40-year-old divorced attorney, was far more experienced than she. He wanted to immediately institute a sexual relationship. Her choice of this man was made on the basis of his status as an attorney with a successful practice. Her second dating experience, Henry, lasted for 1 year and included a sexual experience. Although this man was unsatisfactory for many reasons to Phyllis, his work status was impressive. Throughout the therapy work, Phyllis would talk about her germ phobia, which although a problem area, was placed lower down on the list of therapy issues.

After 1 year, Henry told Phyllis that he wanted to stop seeing her. Phyllis immediately focused on the catastrophe of the loss and was sure that she would never meet another man. Shortly afterward, she met Bill. He was right for her in many ways, except one. His job was essentially a lower status managerial one, with a lower salary. Phyllis and Bill became intimate rather quickly and within the next several months began to discuss living together and being married. Her parents were concerned that this relationship should not interfere with her work. "After all", her mother said, "There are many fish in the ocean." When Phyllis discussed this in therapy, that is, ending the relationship so that she would not be distracted from her work, the therapist pointed out that there were indeed many fish in the ocean but she had not caught that many. Therapy is ongoing. Phyllis and Bill are getting married and have purchased a house together. Phyllis has modified her work hours and slowly has become part of Bill's social circle. Her parents still would like to see her focus on work, but she has resisted that. The germ phobia remains as an irritant.

## PASSIVE-AGGRESSIVE PERSONALITY DISORDER

Berne's game of "Schlemiel" exemplifies the nature and texture of the passive-aggressive disorder. The schlemiel comes to your home for a party. He or she begins the evening by dropping Swedish meatballs on your white couch. The schlemiel quickly apologizes, commenting on his/her "clumsiness". The host/hostess responds by saying it was okay, that accidents happen. The schlemiel's next move is to spill wine on the carpet. The game repeats itself, that is, "I'm sorry"/"It's okay." The next move may involve the schlemiel stepping through the draperies, self-castigating him/herself for continued clumsiness. The host's response is, ideally, the same forgiving message.

The schlemiel, in fact, is expressing great anger and aggression in the clumsy behavior but is compelled to mask the anger and to not exhibit the anger openly. The test of this hypothesis is to not forgive the schlemiel, for example, "Thanks for your apology. I know that you must be sorry, so what I will do is send the bills for cleaning the carpet and sofa to you, along with the repair bill for the draperies." At this point, the schlemiel often becomes "hurt" or angry. "What do you mean by sending me bills for things that were accidents? You really make me mad by taking advantage of me this way." The passivity is only a thin veneer, which when scratched shows the anger underneath.

Typical schemas are:

1. I should only have to do what I want to do.
2. People should not make demands of me.
3. Others undervalue my work and worth.
4. People in authority are generally unfair.
5. I should not be asked to do so much work.
6. Deadlines and pressures are unfair and should be resisted.
7. Anger cannot be directly expressed.
8. Anger is dangerous and must be avoided.
9. Whatever can be put aside for tomorrow can be left for tomorrow.
10. Get away with whatever you can.

## CASE ILLUSTRATION

Kevin was a 32-year-old, third-year medical resident. Mary, Kevin's fiancée, had been seen for the treatment of depression. Her treatment had been very successful. She had met Kevin and planned to marry him. She requested couples therapy to help deal with "some tensions" that they were experiencing. Kevin was a chronic procrastinator and had gotten into significant difficulty with his residency director because Kevin was far behind in his reports and charts. Kevin voiced his dissatisfaction with his residency because "they're all out to screw me. I just want to get out." He broke promises to Mary and always apologized and blamed his lack of followthrough on his work load, his on-call assignments, his poor schedule, and his lack of motivation. Despite Mary's asking Kevin to tell her if he was not going to do what he promised so that she could do it, he did not comply. He was abjectly sorry when they lost a deposit on a house because he forgot to tell Mary that he did not obtain the proper signatures on a loan application.

Despite the difficulties, they married. Kevin kept promising to turn over a new leaf. On their honeymoon, they took a prepaid tour to the Bahamas. At their first dinner together as man and wife, Mary ordered a glass of wine to celebrate. When the waiter brought the wine, Kevin asked if the wine was included in the prepaid meal. When the waiter informed them that the wine was two dollars extra, Kevin sent it back. "After all," he told Mary, "we've got to watch our money very carefully now." He found reasons to inspect the contents of her purse ("I was just looking for a pen"). He insisted that she could only purchase pizza from a restaurant at a distance from home because it was one dollar less expensive, though both agreed that the pizza was inferior to that served at a restaurant closer to home (Mary had to do the traveling).

A crisis arose when Kevin was suspended from his residency 2 months prior to finishing his training. He had told the residency director that he and Mary would be taking 2 weeks for a vacation in 3 days' time. Though Kevin had earned the vacation time, his request was denied. He was informed that he knew the rule regarding vacation requests that was that requests were to be submitted 30 days in advance. Kevin informed the director that he (Kevin) had arranged for coverage of his patient load and that he was not needed. The director told Kevin that the issue was that Kevin had consistently broken, bent, and generally ignored the rules that other residents observed. Kevin asked if his request would have been approved if he had asked 30 days earlier. The director replied that it would have most certainly have been approved. "Well then," Kevin responded, "if it would have been approved 30 days ago, why make a fuss now?" Kevin was forbidden to absent himself. Kevin saw this as another issue of "them" being out to get him. He took the vacation and was suspended.

In therapy, Kevin would always see himself as the wounded, victimized, assaulted, and picked-upon member of the relationship. Despite the very clear exposition of Kevin's schema, he was determined to maintain what he saw as his "integrity." Mary eventually left Kevin. Kevin stayed in therapy for three sessions. In that time, his goal seemed to be to convince the therapist that his (Kevin's) position was correct. He then left therapy.

## SUMMARY

For every theory of personality, there is an accompanying theory of what may cause a disorder of personality. The interest in acquiring skills to treat personality disorders has become a prime focus of interest among therapists. This interest has come from the apparent increase in patients being treated for psychological disorders that include Axis II problems. Although these patients do not generally come for therapy for the Axis II problems, they often come for their Axis I problems. These patients require a longer time in treatment and more energy and time from the therapist without the same rate of gain as with patients whose problems are not complicated by personality disorders.

The Axis II problems exemplify Beck's idea of the schema being a central issue in the formation of these disorders. The personality disorder is basically a result of undeveloped or unevolved schema. Schematic representations that were once effectively used by the individual become a source of dysfunction. Given the chronic nature of the personality disorder, Cognitive Therapy can be used successfully. The arena for the treatment is the therapeutic relationship. The patient is first taught the necessary skills for dealing with the personality disorder by dealing with the Axis I problems. Through the processes of schematic restructuring, schematic modification, or schematic reinterpretation, the patient can be helped to deal with the long-standing life problems that are part of the personality disorder.

The present chapter is meant as a preliminary work. By setting out treatment ideas and sharing the authors' clinical experience, clinicians will, hopefully, be encouraged to develop their own applications of Cognitive Therapy to this difficult but treatable group.

# REFERENCES

Abend, S. M., Porder, M. S., & Willick, M. S. (1983). *Borderline patients: Psychoanalytic perspectives.* New York: International Universities Press.

Ansbacher, H. L. (1985). The significance for Alfred Adler of the concept of narcissis. *American Journal of psychiatry, 142*(2), 203–207.

Ansbacher, H., & Ansbacher, R. (1963). *The individual psychology of Alfred Adler.* New York: Basic Books.

Baumeister, R. F. (1987). How the self became a problem: A psychological review of the historical research. *Journal of Personality and Social Psychology, 52*(1), 163–176.

Beardslee, W. R., Bemporad, J., Keller, M. B., & Klerman, G. L. (1983). Children of parents with major affective disorder: A review. *American Journal of Psychiatry, 140*(7), 825–832.

Beck, A. T. (1963a). *Depression: Causes and treatment.* Philadelphia: University of Pennsylvania Press.

Beck, A. T. (1963b). Thinking and depression. *Archives of General Psychiatry, 9,* 324–333.

Beck, A. T. (1976). *Cognitive therapy and the emotional disorders.* New York: International Universities Press.

Beck, A. T., & Emery, G. (1985). *Anxiety disorders and phobias: A cognitive perspective.* New York: Basic Books.

Beck, A. T., & Freeman, A. (1989). *Cognitive therapy of personality disorders.* New York: Guilford.

Beck, A. T., Rush, A. J., Shaw, B. F., & Emery, G. (1979). *Cognitive therapy of depression.* New York: Guilford.

Beck, A. T., Brown, G., Steer, R. A., Riskind, J. H., & Eidelson, J. I. (1987). Differentiating anxiety and depression: A test of the cognitive content-specificity hypothesis. *Journal of Abnormal Psychology, 96*(3), 179–183.

Berne, E. (1964). *Games people play.* New York: Grove.

Byrne, D., & Kelley, K. (1981). *An introduction to personality* (3rd ed.). Englewood Cliffs, NJ: Prentice-Hall.

Casey, P. R., Tryer, P. J., & Platt, S. (1985). The relationship between social functioning and psychiatric functioning in primary care. *Social Psychiatry. 20*(1), 5–9.

Chamberlain, P., Patterson, G., Reid, J., Kavanaugh, K., & Forgatch, M. (1984). Observation of client resistance. *Behavior Therapy, 15,* 144–155.

Chatham, (1985).

Conoley, J. C., & Beard, M. (1984). The effects of a paradoxical intervention on therapeutic relationship measures. *Psychotherapy, 21*(2), 273–277.

Corsini, R., (ed.). (1979). *Current personality theories.* Ithasca, IL: F. E. Peacock.

Costall, A., & Still, A. (Eds.). (1987). *Cognitive psychology in question.* New York: St. Martin's Press.

Deffenbacher, J. L., Storey, D. A., Stark, R. S., Hogg, J. A., & Brandon, A. D. (1987). Cognitive-relaxation and social skills interventions in the treatment of general anger. *Journal of Counseling psychology, 34*(2), 171–176.

DiGiuseppe, R. (1983). Rational emotive therapy and conduct disorders. In A. Ellis & M. E. Bernard (Eds.). *Rational-emotive approaches to the problems of childhood* (pp. 111–138). New York: Plenum Press.

DiGiuseppe, R. (1986). The implication of the philosophy of science for rational-emotive theory and therapy. *Psychotherapy, 23*(4), 634–639.

DiGiuseppe, R., Ellis, A., Leaf, R. C., Mass, R., Backz, Alington, D. E., & Wolfe, J. (1987). Unpublished data. Institute for Rational Living.

Douglas, C. J., & Druss, R. G. (1987). Denial of illness: A reappraisal. *General Hospital Psychiatry, 9*(1), 53–57.

*DSM-1—Diagnostic and statistical manual* (1st ed.). (1952). Washington, DC: American Psychiatric Press.

*DSM-II—Diagnostic and statistical manual* (2nd ed.). (1968). Washington, DC: American Psychiatric Press.

*DSM-III—Diagnostic and statistical manual* (3rd ed.). (1980). Washington, DC: American Psychiatric Press.

*DSM-III-R-Diagnostic and statistical manual* (rev. 3rd ed.). (1987). Washington, DC: American Psychiatric Press.

Earls, F. (1981). Temperament characteristics and behavior patterns in three-year-old children. *The Journal of Nervous and Mental Disease, 169*(6), 367–371.

Ellis, A. (1957a). Rational psychotherapy and individual psychology. *Journal of Individual Psychology, 13*(1), 38–44.

Ellis, A. (1957b). Outcome of employing three techniques of psychotherapy. *Journal of Clinical Psychology, 13* (4), 344–350.

Ellis, A. (1958). Rational psychotherapy. *Journal of General Psychology, 59*, 35–49.

Ellis, A. (1985). *Overcoming resistance: Rational-emotive therapy with difficult clients.* New York: Springer Publishing Company.

Ellis, A., & Bernard, M. E. (1985). What is rational-emotive therapy (RET)? In A. Ellis & M. E. Bernard (Eds.), *Clinical applications of rational-emotive therapy* (pp. 1–30). New York: Plenum Press.

Fabrega, H., Mezzich, J. E., Mezzich, A. C., & Coffman, G. A. (1986). Descriptive validity of DSM-III depressions. *The Journal of Nervous and Mental Disease, 174*(10), 573–584.

Foon, A. E. (1985). The effect of social class and cognitive orientation on clinical expectations. *British Journal of Medical Psychology, 58*(4), 357–364.

Frank, J. D. (1973). *Persuasion and healing* (2nd ed.). Baltimore: Johns Hopkins University Press.

Freeman, A. (1987). *Understanding personal, cultural and religious schema in psychotherapy.* In A. Freeman, N. Epstein, & K. M. Simon, *Depression in the family* (pp. 79–99). New York: Haworth Press.

Gibertini, M., Brandenburg, N. A., & Retzlaff, P. D. (1986). The operating characteristics of the Millon Clinical Multiaxial Inventory. *Journal of Personality Assessment, 50*(4), 554–567.

Green, C. J. (1982). The diagnostic accuracy and utility of MMPI and MCMI computer interpretive reports. *Journal of Personality Assessment, 46*(4), 359–365.

Goldstein, W. (1985). *An introduction to the borderline conditions.* Northvale, NJ: Jason Aronson.

Gundeson, J. G. (1984). *Borderline personality disorders.* Washington, DC: American Psychiatric Press.

Hales, R. E., Polly, S., Bridenbaugh, H., & Orman, D. (1986). Psychiatric consultations in a military general hospital. A report on 1,065 cases. *General Hospital Psychiatry, 8*(3), 173–182.

Hall, C., & Lindzey, G. *Theories of personality.* New York: John Wiley & Sons.

Hamilton, S., Rothbart, M., & Dawes, R. M. (1987). Sex bias, diagnosis, and DSM-III. *Sex Roles, 15*(5/6), 269–274.

Hartman, L. M., & Blankenstein, K. R. (1986). *Perception of self in emotional disorder and psychotherapy.* New York: Plenum Press.

Henn, F. A., Herjanic, M., & VanderPearl, R. H. (1976). Forensic psychiatry: Diagnosis and criminal responsibility. *The Journal of Nervous and Mental Disease, 162*(6), 423–429.

Hollon, S. D., Kendall, P. C., & Lumry, A. (1986). Specificity of depressogenic cognitions in clinical depression. *Journal of Abnormal Psychology, 95*(1), 52–59.

Hjelle, L. A., & Ziegler, D. J. (1981). *Personality theories.* New York: McGraw-Hill.

Horowitz, M. (Ed.). (1977). *Hysterical personality.* New York: Jason Aronson.

Jones, R. A. (1977). *Self-fulfilling prophesies, social psychological, and physiological effects of expectancies,* Hillside, NJ: Lawrence Erlbaum Associates.

Karno, M., Hough, R. L., Burnam, M. A., Escobar, J. I., Timbers, D. M., Santana, F., & Boyd, J. H. (1986). Lifetime prevalence of specific psychiatric disorders among Mexican Americans and non-Hispanic whites in Los Angeles. *Archives of General Psychiatry, 44*(8), 695–701.

Kernberg, O. F. (1975). *Borderline conditions and pathological narcissism.* New York: Jason Aronson.

Kernberg, O. F. (1984). *Severe personality disorders: Psychotherapeutic strategies.* New Haven: Yale University Press.

Koenigsberg, H. W., Kaplan, R. D., Gilmore, M. M., & Cooper, A. M. (1985). The relationship between syndrome and personality disorder in DSM-III: Experience with 2,462 patients. *American Journal of Psychiatry, 142*(2), 207–217.

Latimer, P. R., & Sweet, A. A. (1984). Cognitive versus cognitive-behavioral procedures in cognitive-behavior therapy: A Critical review of the evidence. *Journal of Behavior Therapy and Experimental Psychiatry, 15* (1) 9–22.

Leitenberg, H., Yost, L. W., & Carroll-Wilson, M. (1986). Negative cognitive errors in children: Questionnaire development, normative data, and comparison between children with and without self-reported symptoms of depression, low self-esteem, and evaluation anxiety. *Journal of Consulting and Clinical Psychology, 54* (4), 528–536.

Like, R., & Zyzanski, S. J. (1987). Patient satisfaction with the clinical encounter: Social psychological determinants. *Social Science in Medicine, 24*(4), 351–357.

Lion, J. R. (Ed.). (1981). *Personality disorders: Diagnosis and management.* Baltimore: Williams & Wilkens.

MacLeod, C., Mathews, A., & Tata, P. (1986). Attention bias in emotional disorders. *Journal of Abnormal Psychology, 95*(1) 15–20.

Mahoney, M. J., & Freeman, A. (Eds.). (1985). *Cognition and psychotherapy.* New York: Plenum Press.

Martin, J., Martin, W., & Slemon, A. G. (1987). Cognitive mediation in person-centered and rational-emotive therapy. *Journal of Counseling Psychology, 34*(3), 251–260.

Masterson, J. F. (1978). *New perspectives on psychotherapy of the borderline adult.* New York: Brunner/Mazel.

Masterson, J. F. (1980). *From borderline adolescent to functioning adult: The test of time.* New York: Brunner/Mazel.

Masterson, J. F. (1985). *Treatment of the borderline adolescent: A developmental approach.* New York: Brunner/Mazel.

Mathews, A., & MacLeod, C. (1986). Discrimination of threat cues without awareness in anxiety states. *Journal of Abnormal Psychology, 95*(2), 131–138.

Maziade, M., Caperaa, P., Laplante, B., Boudreault, M., Thivierge, J., Cote, R., & Boutin, P. (1985). Value of difficult temperament among 7 year-olds in the general population for predicting psychiatric diagnosis at age 12. *American Journal of Psychiatry, 142*(80), 943–946.

McMahon, R. C., & Davidson, R. S. (1985). An examination of the relationship between personality patterns and symptom/mood patterns. *Journal of Personality Assessment, 49*(5) 552–556.

Means, J. R., Wilson, G. L., & Dlugokinski, L. J. (1987). *Self-initiated imaginal and cognitive components: Evaluation of differential effectiveness in altering unpleasant moods, imagination, cognition and personality, 6*(3), 219–226.

Meichenbaum, D. (1977). Cognitive behavior modification. New York: Plenum.

Merbaum, M., & Butcher, J. N. (1982). Therapists' liking of their psychotherapy patients; Some issues related to severity of disorder and treatability. *Psychotherapy: Theory, Research and Practice, 19*(1), 6–76.

Millon, T. (1981). *Disorders of personality.* New York: John Wiley & Sons.

Millon, T. (1985). The MCMI provides a good assessment of DSM-III disorders: The MCMI-II will prove even better. *Journal of Personality Assessment, 49*(4), 379–391.

Moore, H. A., Zusman, J., & Root, G. C. (1984). Noninstitutional treatment for sex offenders in Florida. *American Journal of Psychiatry, 142*(8), 964–967.

Moreland, K. L., & Onstad, J. M. (1987). *Validity of Millon's computerized interpretation system for the MCMI: A controlled study. Journal of Consulting and Clinical Psychology, 55*(1), 113–114.

Morrison, L. A., & Shapiro, D. A. (1987). Expectancy an outcome in prescriptive vs. exploratory psychotherapy. *British Journal of Clinical Psychology, 26*(1), 59–60.

Neisser, U. (1976). *Cognition and reality.* San Francisco: W. H. Freeman.

Novaco, R. (1975). *Anger control: The development and evaluation of an experimental treatment.* Lexington, MA: Heath & Co.

Perris, C. (1986). *Kognitiv terapi i teori och praktik.* Sweden: Natur och cultur.

Persons, J. B., & Burns, D. D. (1986). The process of cognitive therapy: The first dysfunctional thought changes less than the last one. *Behavior Research and Therapy, 24*(6), 619–624.

Piaget, J. (1971). *The construction of reality in the child* (M. Cook, Trans.). New York: Ballantine. (Original work published 1936).

Piaget, J. (1974). *Experiments in contradiction.* Chicago: University of Chicago Press.

Piaget, J. (1976). *The grasp of consciousness.* Cambridge: Harvard University Press.

Piaget, J. (1978). *Success and understanding.* Cambridge: Harvard University Press.

Pfohl, B., Coryell, W., Zimmerman, M., & Stangl, D. (1986). DSM-III personality disorders: Diagnostic overlap and internal consistency of individual DSM-III criteria. *Comprehensive Psychiatry, 27*(1), 21–34.

Prince, R. (1985). Denial: Is its use in heart disease a bad thing? *Integrative Psychiatry, 3* 66–67.

Quay, H. C., Routh, D. K., & Shapiro, S. K. (1987). Psychopathology of childhood: From description to validation. *Annual Review of Psychology, 38,* 491–532.

Rachman, S. J., & Wilson, G. T. (1980). *The effects of psychological therapy* (2nd ed.). New York: Pergamon Press.

Reich, J. (1987). Sex distribution of DSM-III personality disorders in psychiatric outpatients. *American Journal of Psychiatry, 144*(4), 485–488.

Reid, W. H. (ed.). (1981). *The treatment of the antisocial syndromes.* New York: Van Nostrand.

Rosenbaum, R. L., Horowitz, M. J., & Wilner, N. (1986). Clinician assessments of patient difficulty. *Psychotherapy, 23*(3), 417–422.

Salkovskis, P. M. (1986). The cognitive revolution: New way forward, backward somersault or full circle? *Behavioural Psychotherapy, 14,* 278–282.

Saul, L. J., & Warner, S. L. (1982). *The psychotic personality.* New York: Van Nostrand.

Schank, R. C., & Abelson, R. P. (1977). *Scripts, plans, goals and understanding.* Hillsdale, NJ: Lawrence Erlbaum.

Scharnberg, M. (1984). The myth of paradigm shift, or how to lie with methodology. Stockholm: Almquist & Wiksell International.

Searles, H. F. *Psychoanalytic therapy with the borderline adult.* In J. F. Masterson (1978). *New perspectives on psychotherapy of the borderline adult.* New York: Brunner/Mazel.

Sherman, M. (1979). *Personality: Inquiry and applications.* New York: Pergamon Press.

Shultz, D. (1981). *Theories of personality.* Monterey: Brooks/Cole.

Silverman, S. (1987). Silence as resistance to medical intervention. *General Hospital Psychiatry, 9,* 259–266.

Turner, S. M., Beidel, D. C., Dancu, C. V., & Keys, D. J. (1986). Psychopathology of social phobia and comparison. *Journal of Abnormal Psychology, 95*(4), 389–394.

Ward, L. G., Friedlander, M. L., & Solverman, W. K. (1987). Children's depressive symptoms, negative self-statements, and causal attributions for success and failure. *Cognitive Therapy and Research, 11*(2), 215–227.

Widiger, T. A., & Sanderson, C. (1987). The convergent and discriminant validity of the MCMI as a measure of DSM-III personality disorders. *Journal of Personality Assessment, 51*(2), 228–242.

Widiger, T. A., Willimas, J. B. W., Spitzer, R. L., & Frances, A. (1985). The MCMI as a measure of DSM-III. *Journal of Personality Assessment, 49,*(4), 366–378.

Widiger, T. A., Williams, J. B. W., Spitzer, R. L., & Frances, A. (1986). The MCMI and DSM-III: A brief rejoinder to Millon (1985). *Journal of Personality Assessment, 50*(2), 198–204.

Williams, M. H. The bait-and-switch tactic in psychotherapy. *Psychotherapy, 22*(1), 110–115.

Zwemer, W. A., & Deffenbacher, J. L. Irrational beliefs, anger, and anxiety. *Journal of Counseling Psychology, 31*(3), 391–393.

Zimmerman, M., Pfohl, B., Stangl, D., & Coryell, W. (1985). The validity of DSM-III Axis IV. *American Journal of Psychiatry, 142*(12), 1437–1441.

# A Cognitive-Behavioral Approach to Sex Therapy

Barry McCarthy

Sex therapy is a relatively new area of treatment formally established in 1970 with the publication of the Masters and Johnson book, *Treating Sexual Inadequacy*. Although Albert Ellis (1958) had written extensively in the sexual field, cognitive approaches have only recently received more emphasis. This chapter will examine a cognitive-behavioral approach to sex therapy. The three major components of the cognitive-behavioral approach are: (a) replacement of sexual anxiety with sexual comfort; (b) adopting positive sexual attitudes and learning sexual skills; and (c) a program of individually designed sexual exercises to be done between therapy sessions. The goal of this therapy is to develop a comfortable, functional, and satisfying sexual style. Sex therapists usually work with established couples, but sex therapy can be implemented with individuals who do not have regular sexual partners. This approach to sex therapy is based on the work of Masters and Johnson (1970), Annon (1974), Leiblum & Pervin (1980), LoPiccolo & LoPiccolo (1978), and McCarthy & McCarthy (1984). Sex therapy utilizes a broad range of cognitive-behavioral strategies and techniques tailored to the specific sexual problem.

Cognitive-behavioral sex therapy is best conceptualized as a form of couples psychotherapy. To do successful, competent sex therapy, the clinician must be knowledgeable and comfortable not only with the area of sexual function and dysfunction but also individual and couple therapy. There are three major aspects that differentiate it from marital psychotherapy: (1) the focus is on the sexual relationship; (2) the therapy contract is time-limited, usually 12 to 20 sessions; and (3) it emphasizes the practice of sexual exercises between sessions. The most common therapy format consists of one session a week with a single therapist.

---

Barry McCarthy • Department of Psychology, American University, and Washington Psychological Center, Washington, DC 20016.

BARRY McCARTHY

Assessment of sexual functioning and complaints is a critical first step, with the major tool for assessment being the detailed sex history. Referral to a physician (usually a gynecologist and/or urologist) is important whenever there is a possibility that organic factors may be causing or contributing to the sexual dysfunction. Such medical assessment can be as straightforward as a single office visit or as complex as 2 days of testing for hormonal, neurological, and vascular functioning.

The sex history is a semistructured individual interview that typically follows a chronological framework. In addition to gathering information, it is important for the clinician to establish rapport, increase comfort with sexual language, and counter sexual myths with accurate information. The sex therapist attempts to model a comfortable, tension-free attitude toward sexuality. The clinician can reduce guilt and provide a positive model by openly discussing topics such as masturbation, oral-genital stimulation, and fantasy. It is important that the client feel *permission* to talk about and experience these activities rather than *pressure* to engage in them. A clinician taking a sex history uses the following guidelines to obtain information for treatment planning: (1) beginning with nonanxiety-provoking material and progressing to that which is more emotional and intimate; (2) being nonjudgmental and encouraging the client to reveal socially undesirable or traumatic sexual experiences; (3) discussing strengths in the client's sexual development as well as problems; and (4) assessing the client's level of comfort and skill in a variety of sexual interactions.

The client is told at the beginning of the assessment interview that, if there is information he or she does not want shared with the partner, this information will be held in confidence. For example, if the difficulty brought to therapy is an inability to maintain an erection with his wife and the clinician learns that the male has erections with an extramarital partner, it is clear that an anxiety-reduction strategy to deal with the erection problem would not be the appropriate intervention.

The clinician utilizes open-ended questions and elicits information about sexual attitudes, anxieties, and skills. Typical areas of sexual anxiety include nudity, touching of partner's genitals, specific parts of one's own body being looked at or touched, guilt over sexual fantasies, avoidance of specific sexual behaviors, fear of loss of control, fear of physical harm, and fear of pregnancy. Because the clinician must rely on self-report (sex interaction is never observed), comfortable, clear, and detailed communication is essential. It is particularly important to understand the use of sexual language. Clients might utilize proper terms such as penis and intercourse, colloquial terms such as ''prick'' and ''make love,'' or have their own language such as ''junior'' and ''afternoon delight.'' It is necessary to clarify the meanings of terms so that the therapist and clients fully understand one another and make the details of sexual activities (affectionate touching, manual and oral stimulation, and intercourse techniques) clear. Many clients believe the myth that ''good lovers just naturally know what to do,'' so it is helpful for the clinician to preface discussion of skills by noting that sexual functioning is complex, learned behavior.

The ideal couple for cognitive-behavioral sex therapy has a specific sexual dysfunction, is committed to their marriage, do not have severe nonsexual relationship problems, and are willing to view learning a sexual interaction style as a couple task. Conversely, a more difficult couple has diffuse sexual and relationship problems, is angry and blaming, and has a tenuous commitment to the relationship.

## TECHNIQUES FOR TREATMENT OF SPECIFIC DYSFUNCTIONS

There are specific interventions for each problem, but each person, each couple, and each sexual dysfunction is complex and unique. So, far from being a mechanically oriented cookbook approach, successful sex therapy requires implementation of treatment principles by clinicians who use clinical judgment in timing, sequencing, and processing cognitive and sexual exercises with clients.

For males, the most common sexual dysfunctions are premature ejaculation (also called involuntary or rapid ejaculation), erectile difficulty (also called impotence), inhibited sexual desire (also called hypoactive sexual desire or low libido), and ejaculatory inhibition (also called ejaculatory incompetence or retarded ejaculation).

For females, the most common sexual dysfunctions are nonorgasmic response with partner, inhibited sexual desire, preorgasmic dysfunction (also called anorgasmic dysfunction), sexual aversion, and vaginismus.

The key elements in successful sex therapy are changes in sexual attitudes, developing sexual comfort, and sexual stimulation skills that occur during the sexual exercises. This is different from psychotherapy that focuses on change occurring within the therapy session itself. The couple learns to view sexuality as pleasure-oriented (as opposed to performance), as nondemanding, and as a cooperative, intimate couple activity. Sexual exercises done in the privacy of their home serve as *in vivo* desensitization experiences. The exercises provide the couple with the opportunity to build an increasingly complex, flexible, and problem-free sexual repertoire. The first set of exercises focuses on initiation, sensual touching, and developing feedback and guiding skills (McCarthy & McCarthy, 1984). The premise is that nondemand, nongenital exercises will increase comfort with nudity and touching as well as reduce performance anxiety. As the couple's sexual comfort increases, exploratory nondemanding genital pleasuring exercises are introduced. The couple is instructed to add to their sexual repertoire gradually and comfortably. The task focus is shared pleasure, exploration, and increased comfort rather than performance demands for sexual expertise and orgasm. Stress is placed on increasing sexual awareness without falling into the trap of becoming self-conscious and clinical about sexuality.

The cognition the client needs to learn is that each individual is responsible for his or her own comfort and arousal. This includes giving feedback to the partner and making clear, direct sexual requests. The emphasis on self-responsibility is followed by a focus on mutual couple responsibility for sexual satisfaction. You cannot ''give'' or ''make'' the partner have an erection or orgasm; however, you can facilitate the partner's sexual functioning by being active and emotionally involved and by being receptive to guidance and sexual requests. Cognitions about individual responsibility are consistently reinforced throughout the exercises and therapy sessions.

Typically, the first 2 weeks of the sex therapy exercises, regardless of the particular problem, focus on learning sexual communication and touching skills. The progress of the couple is carefully monitored, especially regarding anxiety reduction. Exercises can be repeated with modifications to maximize comfort as well as to minimize boredom.

The couple is usually requested to refrain from intercourse or from attempting orgasm during the initial phase of sex therapy in order to reduce performance orientation and to increase comfort with the pleasuring process. A crucial clinical judgment is when to lift those prohibitions. Some clinicians lift them simultaneously, although the recommended strategy is to lift the prohibition on orgasm after the second week and to keep the one on intercourse for at least a week longer. The rationale is that nonfunctional cognitions and behaviors revolving around intercourse are overlearned. Focusing on nondemanding pleasuring exercises can improve comfort and sexual skills (especially stroking, manual stimulation, and oral stimulation) without the performance pressure and rigid sexual scenario associated with intercourse.

Another crucial clinical judgment involves the degree to which the therapist focuses specifically on the sexually dysfunctional behavior. Zilbergeld and Ellison (1980) have persuasively argued that, rather than focusing on erections (which tends to increase self-consciousness and performance demands), the client should instead be encouraged to focus on comfort, pleasure, and erotic stimulation. The exercises prescribed for treatment of the specific dysfunction build on the nondemand and pleasuring experiences. Intercourse can be integrated into exercises as another pleasuring experience, rather than thought of as a totally separate sexual behavior. This allows intercourse to be relearned in the context of a comfortable, mutually satisfying couple activity and helps prevent regression to old dysfunctional intercourse patterns.

## MALE SEXUAL DYSFUNCTIONS

In considering specific strategies for treating each dysfunction, it is important to remember the *central principles* of cognitive-behavioral sex therapy: (a) to build sexual comfort, (b) to develop functional cognitive and sexual skills, and (c) to utilize specific sexual exercises. The best illustration of these principles can be seen in the treatment of premature ejaculation. The key element in premature ejaculation is the association of high sexual excitement and high performance anxiety. This association leads to a decrease in the male's awareness of his arousal pattern, especially the point of ejaculatory inevitability, and to a lack of appreciation of the sensations that accompany arousal. In helping the male to increase voluntary ejaculatory control, the first step is discrimination learning. The "do-it-yourself" techniques have emphasized trying to ignore or downplay arousal by such tricks as wearing two condoms or thinking of unpleasant things such as how much money you owe. In contrast, the sex therapist instructs the male to focus on increasing his awareness of sensations and identifying the point of ejaculatory inevitability. This can be accomplished by means of masturbation training (Zilbergeld, 1978) or use of the "stop–start" technique (Perelman, 1980). Initially, the couple is instructed to focus on learning control with extravaginal stimulation and then in the female-on-top, "quiet vagina" intercourse exercise. After control has been achieved in these exercises, the couple moves to slow thrusting controlled by the female, then slow thrusting controlled by the male, and finally to more rapid thrusting. This process is repeated, using other intercourse positions. Voluntary control is achieved by a gradual learning process.

In the "stop–start" technique, as the man approaches the point of ejaculatory inevitability, he signals his partner to stop movement and stimulation. When his urge to ejaculate subsides, he signals her to resume stimulation. As this procedure is repeated, the male gains confidence in his ability to monitor and voluntarily control his ejaculation. Eventually, rather than stopping completely, he maintains control by making subtle shifts in the speed and type of intercourse thrusting. The male develops cognitions relating to enjoying the entire pleasuring arousal/intercourse process, viewing sexuality as a cooperative, giving experience with the woman as his sexual friend, and valuing the woman's arousal as well as his own.

The second most frequent male sexual problem is secondary erectile dysfunction. This has traditionally been called *impotence,* but the term has fallen out of favor because of its negative connotations. Erectile dysfunction means that the man is having trouble getting and maintaining an erection sufficient for intercourse, not that he is less powerful or masculine.

A common sequence in the development of erectile difficulties starts with the male's trying to control ejaculation by reducing arousal, which results in the loss of erection during intercourse. This progresses to where the male loses erections at the point of intromission, loses erections during foreplay, has difficulty gaining erections, and eventually avoids sex. By the time the man comes for therapy, he is enmeshed in this negative anticipation, aversive experience, avoidance cycle.

Performance anxiety and the taking of a spectator role are key factors in erection problems. Treatment strategy is to reduce performance anxiety and to break the failure-negative anticipation cycle by putting a temporary prohibition on intercourse and orgasm. The male needs to learn about and experience the normal physiological process involved in the waxing and waning of erections. Most males immediately push toward intercourse as soon as they have obtained an erection. The series of nondemand exercises allows the man (and his partner) to learn that he can enjoy sexuality without an erection and that sexual pleasure is not dependent on intercourse and orgasm. If the arousal does not result in orgasm, his erection will naturally wane, and he can become erect again with continued sexual stimulation.

Nondemand pleasuring exercises help the male to: (1) reduce his performance anxiety; (2) reassert his role as an active and involved sexual participant; (3) identify the types of sexual stimulation that he finds most sensual and arousing; (4) improve his sexual communication skills; and (5) learn to approach intercourse not as a separate performance task but as a continuation of the pleasuring sequence (McCarthy, 1986).

Zilbergeld (1978) has suggested that, even when anxiety is low, the conditions for good sex have been met, and the stimulation is effective, there still may be times when the male has erectile difficulty. Thus it is important for the therapist to teach the client cognitive and behavioral strategies that will enable him to deal with an occasional erectile difficulty without overreacting. The male has to adopt the cognition that the normal penis is not a perfectly functioning machine and that, when he has erectile difficulties, he can satisfy his partner and himself by using manual and/or oral stimulation. Cognitively, he can learn that he is able to enjoy a sexual experience, see himself as masculine, and as a good lover whether or not he had a stiff penis. Too much of the male's self-esteem is invested in his penis—he can learn to feel good about himself as a person and a lover independent of the state of his erection.

Ejaculatory inhibition is a more commonly experienced sexual difficulty, especially of middle-years males, than previously thought (McCarthy, 1981; Schull & Sprenkle, 1980). Although traditionally described as the total inability of the male to ejaculate within the vagina, there are many varieties of this dysfunction. The most common is an intermittent pattern, where the male has regularly ejaculated intravaginally, but now is unable to, at least 25% of the time. One variant pattern is the male who is only able to ejaculate while using a fetish arousal pattern (a very narrow range of sexual stimulation). A common inhibition involves emotionally blocking oneself off from the partner and her sexual stimulation. This may be the result of anger or shyness in requesting additional stimulation.

The strategy used in treating ejaculatory inhibition is to identify and reduce blocks and inhibitions, to increase arousal by using multiple stimulation techniques, such as testicle stimulation and/or fantasy during intercourse, to identify and utilize "orgasm triggers," and to increase the sexual expressiveness of the couple by increasing verbalization and movement during sex (McCarthy, 1981).

Males are more likely to come for sex therapy than almost any other type of psycho-therapy. It is unfortunate and paradoxical that the male's rigid criterion for sexual success interferes with therapeutic progress and sexual satisfaction. The male believes that only "perfect" performance can be viewed as "masculine" and that a "real man" can function autonomously from his partner, that is, he can experience desire, erection, and orgasm, needing nothing from the woman. One of the most important cognitive changes in successful sex therapy is that the male comes to see sexuality as encompassing more than his penis and intercourse. He learns to value pleasure over performance, to see the woman as his sexual friend, can enjoy the pleasure-giving and receiving process, and develops a sense of emotional and sexual intimacy that replaces the rigid performance criterion.

## FEMALE SEXUAL DYSFUNCTIONS

The emphasis in defining female dysfunctions has been on the presence or absence of orgasm. Orgasm is a natural response to sexual arousal, a positive and integral aspect of female sexuality. However, the requirement of orgasmic response at each sexual opportunity is an unrealistic performance demand for women. This demand is a major cause of secondary nonorgasmic response, the most frequent female sexual dysfunction. The woman had at one time been orgasmic with a partner but now is either totally nonorgasmic or reaches orgasm on an infrequent or irregular basis. The causes of this dysfunction include performance anxiety, poor sexual communication, relationship problems, anger, and depression. Treatment strategy places a major emphasis on the woman's awareness and responsibility for her own sexual response.

Through nondemand pleasuring exercises, the woman has an opportunity to reexperience sensual and erotic stimulation without pressure for arousal, intercourse, or orgasm. In some cases, the woman quickly regains her ability to respond to nonintercourse stimulation.

Barbach (1980) states that each woman has a unique orgasmic pattern; this view is communicated to the couple and strongly reinforced. At a given sexual opportunity, the woman might be nonorgasmic, singly orgasmic, or multiply orgasmic. Orgasmic response might occur during the pleasuring/foreplay period, during intercourse, or during the afterglow/afterplay period. There is no "right" pattern of orgasmic response. The woman and her partner are encouraged to develop a sexual style with which they are comfortable and that is satisfactory for them.

A common complaint is the woman who is unable to reach orgasm during intercourse. If she is orgasmic during sexual activity and enjoys the intercourse experience, there is no need for sex therapy. The most helpful therapeutic intervention is for the therapist to label this sexual response style as normal and healthy, thus validating her sexuality. The woman having an orgasm during intercourse is not the definition of "normal female sexual functioning." If the woman desires to increase her sensations and responses during intercourse, several techniques can be utilized, such as intercourse with simultaneous clitoral stimulation, intercourse positions such as lateral-coital intercourse that involves greater pelvic contact, the woman controlling the timing and rhythm of coital thrusting, and the use of pubococcygeal muscle exercises during intercourse (McCarthy & McCarthy, 1984). The distinction between "vaginal" and "clitoral" orgasms is not scientifically or sexually meaningful. Physiologically, an orgasm is an orgasm, whether obtained through vibrator stimulation, masturbation, manual stimulation by partner, cunnilingus, or intercourse.

The woman learning to be more sexually assertive, to make requests, to guide her partner, and to assume responsibility for her sexual response is crucial to the development of a satisfying sexual relationship. Many men think it is the male's responsibility to ensure his partner an orgasm each time, so that the woman's orgasm has become a measure of the man's sexual prowess. This male-oriented performance pressure has proven immensely destructive to female sexuality and to couple satisfaction. The appropriate association is between "sexuality and pleasure," not "sexuality and performance." The woman is advised to take a more active, involved, expressive role in the sexual interaction. Cognitively, she can view herself as the ultimate expert on her body and her sexual expression. With the woman assuming responsibility for her sexuality, the male's role is to be an involved and caring partner who is open and responsive to her guidance and requests.

Exercises to improve sexual skills are introduced once the couple has established a comfortable, sensual, intimate relationship. These techniques focus on multiple stimulation to build arousal. Depending on the woman's desires, breast and vulva stimulation, manual and oral stimulation, fantasy, and/or vibrators can be helpful. The woman is encouraged to take a more active and guiding role during intercourse and to continue multiple stimulation, such as kissing, breast stroking, clitoral stimulation, the woman setting the coital rhythm, and fantasies. Orgasm is seen not as a performance goal but rather as a natural response to the giving and receiving of sexual pleasure.

A common dysfunction is where the woman has never been orgasmic with her partner but does reach orgasm through masturbation. This often involves a power/control issue, where she either fears "letting go" in front of the partner or feels angry or distrustful of him. A valuable technique in the former instance is for the woman to masturbate to orgasm in front of her partner (Heiman & LoPiccolo, 1988).

Anxiety and anger are the two emotional states most likely to inhibit sexual response. The nondemand pleasuring exercises followed by the multiple stimulation exercises are the treatment of choice with anxiety-based problems. Where the inhibiting factor is anger, the treatment of choice is not sex therapy but marital therapy focused on communication and problem solving.

*Preorgasmic* (also called *primary nonorgasmic*) is a term referring to women who have never been orgasmic by any means. Preorgasmic women often have the cognition that they do not deserve sexual pleasure and/or that sex is a disappointment and will never work for them. Two intervention strategies are available for treating this dysfunction. Short-term preorgasmic women's groups (Barbach, 1974) are particularly valuable for women without partners. If the woman is married or has an involved partner, an alternative strategy is to view the problem as a relationship one and treat the couple. In addition to couple pleasuring exercises, the woman engages in a personal program of self-exploration and masturbation. The rationale is that, if she is aware of her arousal pattern and can experience orgasm herself, then she can share that learning with her partner (Heiman & LoPiccolo, 1988). Initial orgasmic response occurs in either masturbatory activity or manual or oral stimulation; it is relatively rare during intercourse.

Attention has been focused on the problem of sexual aversion (Kaplan, Fyer, & Novick, 1982; Kolodny, Masters, & Johnson, 1979), which is often misdiagnosed as inhibited sexual desire or nonorgasmic response. Sexual aversion involves a specific element in the sexual interaction that is so negative that it reaches phobic proportions. Although sexual aversion occurs in males, it is predominantly a female syndrome. Common aversive stimuli include semen, buttocks, vaginal secretions, breast stimulation, smells, and tongue kissing. Some women are sexually functional if they can avoid the aversive stimuli, whereas others are dysfunctional.

*In vivo* desensitization is an effective intervention strategy. The woman gradually and comfortably approaches the aversive stimulus. Couples are instructed not to avoid sex nor to end a sexual interaction when the woman becomes anxious, because this would reinforce the discomfort and avoidance. They are advised to move to a more comfortable and secure pleasuring position and can either end the exercise at that point or resume the sexual interaction. The goal is to reach a level of comfort and mastery. The cognitions that are most valuable are that she deserves sexual pleasure, that she has a right to proceed at a pace that is comfortable for her, and that her partner is her intimate sexual friend.

A rarer sexual problem but one especially amenable to cognitive-behavioral techniques is vaginismus. The definitive diagnosis of vaginismus requires a gynecologist to perform a physical examination and observe the spasming of the vaginal introitus. The strategy for overcoming vaginismus is use of *in vivo* desensitization. The manner of desensitization can be dilators, the woman's finger, or innovative materials of increasing sizes such as candles. When comfort is established, additional stimuli including the male's finger(s) and eventually his penis are introduced. Use of additional modalities such as relaxation training, couple communication, and assertiveness training is helpful. The cognition that is most valuable is that sexual openness is a good part of her, along with the image of her bodily openness to him.

## TREATMENT OF MORE COMPLEX SEXUAL PROBLEMS

In this section, we will discuss three particularly complex sexual issues: inhibited sexual desire, couple sexual dissatisfactions, and patterns of fetish arousal.

Inhibited sexual desire (ISD) has received a good deal of attention (Kaplan, 1979;

LoPiccolo & Friedman, 1988; McCarthy, 1984). Lief (1977) estimates that approximately 30% of sex therapy referrals involved ISD, and it has been labeled *the sexual problem of the 80s.*

Assessment and treatment approaches to ISD emphasize cognitive, attitudinal, expectational, and behavioral factors, particularly the importance of the person taking responsibility for his or her sexuality (LoPiccolo & Friedman, 1988). In the assessment phase, it is crucial to identify anxieties, inhibitions, anger, and guilt that may be responsible for blocking sexual feelings. Careful assessment must be undertaken of the variety of thoughts, images, sensations, fantasies, and interpersonal feelings that the person labels *sexual.* For example, if the woman labels only intercourse and orgasm as being sexual and if she enjoys neither, she adopts a self-label as *frigid* or is so labeled by her partner. She then views sexual expression as not being "her" and develops a negative view of sexual interaction and of herself as a sexual being. This turns into a self-fulfilling prophecy, leading to continued unsatisfactory sexual experiences.

Therapeutic intervention in this self-defeating cycle involves a strategy for expanding the boundaries of what is thought of as sexual and increasing awareness of these cues. The individual taking responsibility for her or his sexuality is a cornerstone of this approach. Clients are encouraged to keep a daily diary of broadly defined sexual thoughts, feelings, and images. The clinician gives permission and encourages clients to develop a range of sexual fantasies, perhaps by reading sexual books and magazines or attending sexually explicit movies. The individual is encouraged to develop an ideal sexual scenario, including as many contextual and interpersonal cues as possible. Labeling oneself as *frigid* or *nonsexual* is directly confronted. A variety of cognitive restructuring techniques, including self-instructional training, rational disputation, and identification of cognitive distortions (Lazarus, 1981) are used to refocus the individual on comfort, receptivity, and responsivity, and away from the judgmental performance criteria of intercourse and orgasm. For example, the woman who finds intercourse disappointing because she has to concentrate and work so hard to be orgasmic during intercourse is encouraged to request the type of manual and oral pleasuring scenarios that she finds most arousing and to give herself permission to let go and experience orgasm during nonintercourse sex. She would focus on the positive feelings and sensations available to her rather than let herself be intimidated by the rigid, unrealistic model of the sexually liberated woman.

In working with couples who have a discrepancy in sexual desire, the concepts of Zilbergeld and Ellison (1980) are used to assess the motivations and patterns of both partners, not just the one with ISD. The concepts of naturally occurring discrepancies in sexual desires and preferences as well as the range of alternatives to meet sexual and emotional needs allows viewing sexual expression from a couple problem-solving perspective. It is particularly important to discuss the quality of the sexual experience rather than stay stuck on the frequency problem.

In sexual exercises, special attention is given to initiation patterns, level of involvement of the individual, and increasing assertiveness so that the expression of feelings and needs becomes part of the sexual experience. The person with ISD is encouraged to increase activity and involvement such as doing touching for themselves and/or requesting multiple stimulation rather than viewing sex as a passive "servicing" of the partner.

An important behavioral exercise involves establishing a "trust" position. This means if the person becomes anxious or uninvolved, she or he can request switching to a focus on a warm, close, comfortable interaction. Examples of trust positions include lying together and holding each other, one person puts his or her head on the other's lap and has his or her hair stroked, or where they lie back-to-chest in a "spoon" position and breathe together in a slow, rhythmic manner.

Couple interaction is an area requiring special attention in assessing and treating ISD. In some couples, sexuality is used as the arena to play-out control struggles or to act-out anger. Sexual interaction is a cooperative venture in giving and receiving pleasure. At its best, sexuality is an intimate, open sharing of feelings and sensations. Unfortunately, sex can also be an angry, coercive, and manipulative experience. In these cases, marital interventions focused on learning direct expression of anger and problem-solving approaches are necessary, either as a prerequisite or as a concomitant to sexually focused therapy. The sexual exercises elicit couple interactional issues so they can be dealt with therapeutically.

A second complex sexual problem involves couple sexual dissatisfactions. This refers to couples who do not have a specific sexual dysfunction but report chronic dissatisfaction with their sexual relationship. Sources of dissatisfaction include initiation patterns, arguments over frequency, variety issues, interfering aspects of anger, and dissatisfaction with the after-play/afterglow experience. These couples report that the arousal and orgasm phases are mechanically satisfactory, although emotional satisfaction is low.

When applying cognitive-behavioral strategies to the treatment of dissatisfied couples, it is important to clarify expectations about the role they want sexuality to play in their marital relationship (McCarthy & McCarthy, 1981). Clarifying expectations and suggesting guidelines to make marital sex more satisfying is a new concept for most couples and helps them break out of their self-defeating cycle. The therapeutic focus is on shared responsibility for developing a mutually satisfying and flexible sexual style. Each couple is unique; there is no ''right'' way to initiate, nor is there a ''normal'' number of times to have intercourse per week. Suggested guidelines include setting aside couple time, accepting occasional unsatisfactory sexual experiences, and increasing intimate communication. The primary functions of marital sex are shared pleasure, greater emotional intimacy, and tension reduction. An unsatisfying sexual style can serve to devitalize a marital relationship.

The therapeutic strategy for dealing with sexual dissatisfactions is to take the sexual interaction from the realm of a nonverbal power struggle cloaked in ''romantic mystique'' and to present it as a positive, cooperative experience open to discussion, negotiation, and problem solving. Emphasis is put on use of *I* communications combined with clear and assertive requests. The clinician has to challenge the couple's assumption that natural, spontaneous sex is best, and emphasize the value of open, intimate sharing about sexuality and the marriage.

A helpful technique is to structure a ''ping-pong'' pattern of initiation, where each person has a day when he or she is responsible for sexual initiation. Ideally, both partners would learn to initiate, to be able to say ''no'' in nonhostile ways, and to offer a variety of sensual or sexual alternatives.

The therapist confronts the myth that each sexual experience has to be equally involving and satisfying for both partners. Frank, Anderson, and Rubinstein (1978) found that, among couples who did not complain of sexual problems, less than half of their sexual experiences are rated as equally satisfying. Cognitive restructuring can be used to attack the ''every-sexual-encounter-should-be-dynamite'' myth. Couples are encouraged to be affectionate in and out of the bedroom and to be aware that touching has its own rewards rather than each touch being a prelude to intercourse.

Another complex sexual problem involves patterns of paraphiliac arousal. Behavioral interventions, especially aversive conditioning, masturbation monitoring, and cognitive restructuring have been effective with a range of paraphilias, including exhibitionism, voyeurism, and fetishes (Brownell & Barlow, 1980). Most of the literature consists of reports on individual treatment of the male. A systems viewpoint that emphasizes multiple determinants of the behavior and mutual couple responsibility for change is usually beneficial and often necessary. In this treatment regimen, the male is seen individually on a weekly basis, focusing on decreasing the paraphiliac arousal, and the couple is seen conjointly once a week to improve their sexual relationship.

Arousal to paraphiliac stimuli has little transferability to couple sex. The combination of high sexual excitement and guilt/obsessiveness attached to the sexual behavior has a multi-plicative effect that makes this an addictive sexual experience. In individual sessions, the male is encouraged to take responsibility for not acting out his patterns of paraphiliac sexual behavior. At the same time, he is encouraged to reduce his guilt about his ''deviant'' arousal by understanding the maladaptive learning process and by focusing his energy in the present and future rather than obsessing about past sexual transgressions. Guilt is not a motivator to promote positive change; rather it lowers self-esteem and contributes to the continuation of the maladaptive pattern. A number of therapeutic techniques, including aversive conditioning, especially covert sensitization, are used to stop the client from acting out the paraphiliac pattern. One frequently used technique is masturbation monitoring, where the male gradually and systematically alters the fantasies he uses as he approaches orgasm until the fetish fantasy is extinguished (Marquis, 1970).

The woman is relieved of the pressure to keep track of or worry about the man's paraphiliac behavior. During couple sessions, she is encouraged to assume mutual responsibil-ity for making their sexual relationship more satisfying by increasing her sexual and emotional involvement. These couples tend to have a passive, uninvolved, nonsatisfactory sexual rela-tionship where the entire experience revolved around the male's paraphiliac activity. Para-philias are best viewed as an intimacy disorder, and building a positive sexual relationship makes it more likely the male will maintain therapeutic gains (Schwartz & Masters, 1984).

## TREATMENT OF PEOPLE WITHOUT PARTNERS

The sex therapy model is primarily couple-oriented, but there are many individuals with sexual problems who do not have regular partners. Typically, singles are seen by a therapist of the same sex. At one time, sexual surrogates were utilized, but use of surrogate partners proved extremely problematic both in terms of legal issues and the ''burn-out'' effect on the surrogate.

''Preorgasmic'' women's groups have received widespread attention in the literature (Barbach, 1974) and are the treatment of choice for females without partners. Treatment most commonly involves 10 sessions on a twice-weekly basis. The group design includes education, permission giving, behavioral homework assignments, and modeling by group leaders (es-pecially on taking responsibility for one's own sexuality and being sexually assertive). The process also provides support, confrontation, and problem-solving opportunities.

Through self-exploration and masturbation, the woman learns her individual arousal pattern. This program has achieved considerable success in reducing anxiety and increasing awareness of orgasmic response, but the results in transferring these responses to partner sex are more ambiguous (Payn & Wakefield, 1982). Group approaches to male sexuality have been explored, though they have been less popular due to the reluctance of males to admit sexual problems to others of their gender.

Individual sex therapy for men without partners has focused on education, masturbation retraining, relaxation and guided imagery techniques, cognitive restructuring, and improve-ment of hetersocial skills (McCarthy, 1980). The male is encouraged to break self-defeating patterns of interacting with women, such as drinking to reduce anxiety, playing the ''macho'' role, and attempting intercourse on first dates. The client is encouraged to choose a partner with whom he is comfortable, is attracted to, and trusts.

Sex therapy with the individual female client involves a female therapist and follows the same basic format. As a result of culturally scripted sexual patterns, the single woman is often placed in the position of fending off unwanted sexual advances and being labeled ''frigid'' when she does so. The female therapist models the concept that the woman can be comfortable with her own sexuality and that she has the right to choose how and with whom she can most enjoy sexual expression. Cognitive restructuring and assertiveness training are used to allow the woman to feel more in control of her sexuality.

Bibliotherapy can be helpful as an adjunct to cognitive-behavioral sex therapy. Unlike many of the self-help sexuality books that overemphasize sexual variations and sexual performance, the most useful sex literature attempts to: (1) provide information; (2) set reasonable expectations; (3) reduce the negative emotional states of anxiety, guilt, and anger; and (4) establish guidelines for functional communication and stimulation techniques. Some of the books that are useful for females include *For Yourself* (Barbach, 1976), *Becoming Orgasmic* (Heiman & LoPiccolo, 1988), and *The New Our Bodies, Ourselves* (Boston Women's Health Collective, 1984). Books recommended for males are *Male Sexual Awareness* (McCarthy, 1988), *Male Sexuality* (Zilbergeld, 1978), and *Prime Time* (Schover, 1984).

## COMMON THERAPEUTIC DILEMMAS

There are several difficulties clinicians have in applying cognitive-behavioral sex techniques. These include: (1) not giving clear, direct instructions; (2) abandoning exercises at the first sign of resistance or avoidance; (3) not processing the exercises in detail; (4) emphasizing performance goals rather than increasing comfort and skills; (5) appearing aloof and uninterested in therapy; and (6) not ensuring generalization and maintenance of change.

Stopping the exercises to explore feelings, do in-depth interpretation, or point out secondary gains from the sexual problems has the effect of reinforcing avoidance of sexual interaction. The couple is encouraged to continue a sexual experience until they reach a sense of comfort or choose to end the sexual exercise in a positive manner. The problems elicited by the exercises can be dealt with in the therapy session by confronting the unrealistic cognitions and/or by redesigning the exercise.

Many clinicians are reluctant to do a detailed processing of sexual exercises. Therapists report a feeling of being a ''voyeur'' by being invasive in an area that is private and sensitive, or they may fear appearing to be sexually seductive or experiencing sexual arousal. Because the therapist does not observe the sexual behavior, there *is* a need for clear, detailed feedback, both to assess progress and to help design the next steps of the behavioral program. For example, sometimes the difference between a neutral and a highly arousing stimulus involves only a very slight modification in the pressure, rhythm, or area of stroking. These details need to be explicated in processing the sexual experience.

A typical ''performance pressure'' mistake made by clinicians is to say something like, ''Now you should have intercourse'' or ''Get an erection and insert half way in the vagina'' or ''Experience orgasm during clitoral stimulation.'' This puts pressure on the client to perform and to reach this goal immediately. A more useful strategy is not to tell the client he or she *should* experience anything but rather to give them permission to do so by removing a prohibition and telling him or her that he or she *can*. Arousal, erection, and orgasm are the natural response to involving, effective stimulation. The clinician focuses the couple on increasing comfort, improving sexual communication, and utilizing multiple stimulation.

One of the major reasons that cognitive-behavior therapy is not more popular among experienced clinicians is that they find the structure, information giving, and task assignments less personally involving and emotionally rewarding than other forms of therapies. Sometimes when doing a standard behavioral intervention, the clinician appears minimally attentive and only becomes more involved when problems or crises occur. Because an involved therapist is reinforcing to a client, couples may present problems with the structured program in an attempt to get the therapist's attention. Such problems can be avoided if the therapist reinforces success with the program throughout the course of treatment.

Generalization and maintenance of sexual changes is not fully addressed in the literature. There are assumptions in traditional psychotherapy that, once a person gains insight or gets in touch with feelings, these breakthroughs (a) result in behavioral change that (b) generalize to a large number of areas and (c) are easily maintained. These assumptions are erroneous (Lazarus, 1976), particularly in the sexual area.

Clients often regress after termination of therapy, so the therapist needs to deal directly with maintaining changes. The sex therapy has given them a basic sexually functional repertoire. The couple is encouraged to develop their own unique style of being intimate and sexual. Couples are encouraged to engage in do-it-yourself exercises, set aside at least two times a month to share emotional and sexual feelings, and to schedule a 6-month follow-up therapy session that will focus on maintenance and generalization of their marital and sexual gains.

# REFERENCES

Annon, J. (1974). *The behavioral treatment of sexual problems.* Honolulu: Enabling Systems.

Barbach, L. (1974). Group treatment of preorgasmic women. *Journal of Sex and Marital Therapy, 1,* 139–145.

Barbach, L. (1976). *For yourself.* New York: Doubleday.

Barbach, L. (1980). *Women discover orgasm.* New York: Free Press.

Boston Women's Health Collective. (1984). *The new our bodies, ourselves.* New York: Simon & Schuster.

Brownell, K., & Barlow, D. (1980). The behavioral treatment of sexual deviation. In A. Goldstein & E. Foa (Eds.), *Handbook of behavioral interventions* (pp. 604–672). New York: Wiley.

Ellis (1958). *Sex without guilt.* New York: Lyle, Stuart.

Frank, E., Anderson, C., & Rubinstein, D. (1978). Frequency of sexual dysfunction in "normal" couples. *New England Journal of Medicine, 299,* 111–115.

Heiman, J., & LoPiccolo, J. (1988). *Becoming orgasmic.* New York: Spectrum Books.

Kaplan, H. (1979). *Disorders of sexual desire.* New York: Brunner/Mazel.

Kaplan, H., Fyer, A., & Novick, A. (1982). The treatment of sexual phobias. *Journal of Sex and Marital Therapy, 8,* 3–28.

Kolodny, R., Masters, W., & Johnson, V. (1979). *Textbook of sexual medicine.* Boston: Little, Brown.

Lazarus, A. (1976). Multimodal behavior therapy. New York: Springer.

Lazarus, A. (1981). *The practice of multimodal therapy.* New York: McGraw-Hill.

Leiblum, S., & Pervin, L. (Eds.). (1980). *Principles and practice of sex therapy.* New York: Guilford.

Lief, H. (1977). Inhibited sexual desire. *Medical Aspects of Human Sexuality, 11,* 94–95.

LoPiccolo, J., & Friedman, J. (In press). Broad spectrum treatment of low sexual desire. In S. Leiblum & R. Rosen (Eds.). *Assessment and treatment of desire disorders.* New York: Guilford.

LoPiccolo, J., & LoPiccolo, L. (Eds.). (1978). *Handbook of sex therapy.* New York: Plenum Press.

Marquis, J. (1970). Orgasmic reconditioning: Changing sexual object choice through controlling masturbatory fantasies. *Journal of Behavior Therapy and Experimental Psychiatry, 1,* 263–271.

Masters, W., & Johnson, V. (1970). *Human sexual inadequacy.* Boston: Little, Brown.

McCarthy, B. (1980). Treatment of secondary erectile dysfunction in males without partners. *Journal of Sex Education and Therapy, 6,* 29–34.

McCarthy, B. (1981). Strategies and techniques for the treatment of ejaculatory inhibition. *Journal of Sex Education and Therapy, 7,* 20–23.

McCarthy, B. (1984). Strategies and techniques for the treatment of inhibited sexual desire. *Journal of Sex and Marital Therapy, 10,* 97–104.

McCarthy, B. (1988). *Male sexual awareness: Increasing sexual pleasure.* New York: Carroll and Graf.

McCarthy, B., & McCarthy, E. (1981). *Sex and satisfaction after 30.* Englewood Cliffs, NJ: Prentice-Hall.

McCarthy, B., & McCarthy, E. (1984). *Sexual awareness: Sharing sexual pleasure.* New York: Carroll and Graf.

Payn, H., & Wakefield, J. (1982). The effect of group treatment of primary orgasmic dysfunction on the marital relationship. *Journal of Sex and Marital Therapy, 8,* 133–150.

Perelman, M. (1980). Treatment of premature ejaculation. In S. Leiblum & L. Pervin (Eds.), *Principles and practice of sex therapy.* New York: Guilford.

Schwartz, M., & Masters, W. (1984). Treatment of paraphiliacs, pedophiles, and incest families. In A. Holstrom (Ed.), *Research handbook of rape.* New York: Guilford.

Schover, L. (1984). *Prime time: Sexual health for men over 50.* New York: Holt, Rinehart & Winston.

Schull, G., & Sprenkle, D. (1980). Retarded ejaculation: Reconceptualization and implications for treatment. *Journal of Sex and Marital Therapy, 6,* 234–246.

Zilbergeld, B. (1978). *Male sexuality.* Boston: Little, Brown.

Zilbergeld, B., & Ellison, D. (1980). Desire discrepancies and arousal problems in sex therapy. In S. Leiblum & L. Pervin (Eds.), *Principles and practice of sex therapy* (pp. 65–101). New York: Guilford.

# 23

# Psychotherapy for Chronic Pain
## A Cognitive Approach

Bruce N. Eimer

Chronic pain is a health problem of epidemic proportions. Debilitated victims of long-duration, intractable pain lead severely limited lives. For example, many low-back-pain patients, in addition to suffering from physical pain are chronically depressed and are unable to sleep at night, to eat properly, to take care of activities of daily living, and to remain gainfully employed. Traditional medical approaches often prove unsatisfactory for providing long-term relief from chronic pain. In addition, clinicians frequently encounter patients whose pain complaints have no discernible organic basis or where the degree of tissue damage is disproportionate to the reported pain severity. The search for efficacious alternatives has led clinicians to focus on psychological approaches to the problem of treating chronic pain patients (Barber & Adrian, 1982; Catalano, 1987; Holzman & Turk, 1986; Turk, Meichenbaum, & Genest, 1983).

Unfortunately, most chronic pain patients initially consulting a psychotherapist are resentful toward a medical system that has failed them, angry about having pain, and demoralized and depressed about their painful lives. Hence, the therapist needs to pay special attention to building a therapeutic relationship with a patient whose expectations are initially soured. This demands a high degree of activity and relevance on the part of the therapist (Bellissimo & Tunks, 1984; Turk *et al.*, 1983). In this chapter, a cognitive approach to psychotherapy with chronic pain patients will be presented that takes into account the special problems that are likely to emerge in working with this patient population. The approach described here dictates that the therapist assume an active role as a teacher or coach to encourage and guide the patient in learning strategies for managing pain, coping with related problems, and assuming a more rewarding life-style.

## ACUTE VERSUS CHRONIC PAIN

The International Society for the Study of Pain (1979), as quoted by Merskey (1982), has succinctly defined pain as "an unpleasant sensory and emotional experience which is associ-

Bruce N. Eimer • Departments of Psychiatry and Rehabilitation Medicine, Abington Memorial Hospital, Abington, Pennsylvania 19001.

ated with tissue damage or described in terms of tissue damage.'' (p. 10) The key word in this definition is *experience*. Pain is a complex subjective experience, and as such, is influenced by context, focus of attention, thoughts, feelings, attitudes, beliefs, images, and behaviors, in addition to sensory processes.

The degree to which a sensation following an injury will be interpreted by an injured individual as painful is dependent on a complex of factors. A particularly poignant example is offered in a much-cited study by Beecher (1946). He compared the reactions of World War II soldiers whose painful wounds occasioned their leaving the battle zone with the reactions of civilians awaiting surgery. More of the soldiers reported less pain, and fewer requested narcotics than did the civilians. According to Beecher, the soldiers viewed their painful wounds as a gift in that they had been given a ticket home. For the civilians awaiting surgery, there were other more psychologically painful implications. These observations highlight the important roles of cognition, personal meaning, and expectation in the experience of pain. If one witnesses the injured athlete doggedly giving his best despite an injury, one sees illustrated the primacy of context and focus of attention in pain perception.

The foregoing examples illustrate situations giving rise to acute pain. Acute pain serves as a signal that something is physically wrong. To return to the latter example, once the injured athlete is out of the game and has the opportunity to refocus his or her attention on the sensations of the injury, he or she is alerted to the necessity of preventing further damage and tending to the wound. Acute or short-duration pain by definition is pain that subsides with time. If the athlete's pain did not subside within a few months or in fact became worse, then it would be seen as having turned into chronic pain. Chronic pain is pain that has outlasted its utility as a signal of any ongoing, remediable threat (Sternbach, 1987). Some common sources of chronic, benign pain are musculoskeletal disorders, neuralgia, neuritis, vascular disorders, arthritis, excessive levels of muscle tension, gastrointestinal disorders, and maladjustment to the effects of surgery. Some common types of pain produced by the previously mentioned etiologies are low back pain, neck and shoulder pain, the burning, stabbing, and throbbing of neuritis and neuralgia, migraine and cluster headaches, the numbness and coldness in hands and feet of Raynaud's disease, chronic muscle stiffness and soreness, inflammatory joint pain, muscle contraction headaches, and gastrointestinal pains.

When pain does not subside or becomes worse, there are profound psychological ramifications. Hendler (1984) has described four stages in the progression of the pain experience. During the first, or acute, stage that lasts up to 2 months, there are no apparent psychological changes, probably because patients at this stage generally expect to get well. During the next 4 months or subacute stage, patients become concerned and frightened if their pain has not diminished or disappeared. If pain persists after 6 months, life-limiting depression and anxiety are likely to ensue as the patient enters the chronic stage. If patients have pain for more than 3 years, they enter the subchronic stage. For most of these patients, depression and somatic preoccupations become a way of life.

## A COGNITIVE CONCEPTUALIZATION OF CHRONIC PAIN

The physical limitations imposed by many chronic pain conditions block the continued validation of basic components of a sufferer's self-image (Gallagher & Wrobel, 1982; Violin, 1982). Many chronic pain patients have lost the ability to view themselves as sexual, or as independent and resourceful. Their pain-related limitations make it more likely that contrasting polarities of their self-image will be validated, so they begin to see themselves as nonsexual or sexually incapable, unresourceful, helpless, and dependent on others (Shealy, 1976; Skevington, 1983). Negative self-perceptions such as these are likely to produce thoughts of guilt and self-blame for failure to meet one's former standards, feelings of sadness about the loss of one's former functions, and anger about being incapable of gratifying one's former desires. The chronic pain sufferer is likely to develop the belief that it requires more effort than he or she has available to realize even some portion of his or her former goals. This belief can form the breeding ground for cognitions of hopelessness and helplessness (Seligman, 1975), feelings of discouragement, withdrawal behaviors, and may set the stage for the reinforcement of excessive reliance on significant others. As the individual comes to feel increasingly vulnerable due to a diminished evaluation of his or her coping resources, anxiety, discouragement, disappointment, guilt, self-blame, sadness, and anger are likely to activate depressogenic cognitions in a final common pathway of depression (Covington, 1982; Hendler, 1984; Lefebvre, 1981; Rosenstiel & Keefe, 1983).

Chronic pain sufferers appear to engage in specific patterns of cognitive distortion that form a "downward spiral" of negative, depressogenic thinking (Catalano, 1987; Lefebvre, 1981). These patterns of cognitive distortions have been described and catalogued by Beck and his colleagues (Beck, 1976; Beck, Rush, Shaw, & Emery, 1979; Burns, 1980; Freeman, 1987). In an effort to validate empirically clinical data collected by clinicians treating chronic pain patients, Lefebvre (1981) compared the occurrence of cognitive distortions in depressed low-back-pain patients with that of nondepressed low-back-pain patients, depressed nonpain patients, and a control group. Depressed low-back-pain patients evidenced a greater frequency of catastrophizing, overgeneralization, and selective abstraction than did nondepressed low-back patients. They also rated their pain intensity to be higher than did the nondepressed pain patients.

Lefebvre's study bore out that many pain patients tend to catastrophize about their condition by exaggerating the seriousness of the consequences they anticipate will result from their pain sensations. For example, one patient seen by the author became preoccupied with the question: "What if my back pain becomes so severe that I'll be bedridden permanently?" His catastrophic ruminations on the negative possibilities suggested by the "what-if" question led him to magnify his perceptions of threat and minimize his estimation of his own coping resources (Beck & Emery, 1985). This heightened his level of anxiety.

Many chronic pain sufferers also selectively focus on their pain signals to the exclusion of everything else. This usually exacerbates anxiety and pain and can result in a state of chronic invalidism as the individual ruminates about and becomes increasingly absorbed in his or her experience of physical deterioration (Sternbach, 1974, 1987).

A particularly dysfunctional pattern of cognitive appraisal involves the misattribution of causality for pain. This can work in either of two directions, leading the pain sufferer mistakenly to internalize or externalize the blame for his or her continuing pain. As an example of dysfunctional internalization, the author treated a low-back-pain patient who attributed his musculoskeletal dysfunction completely to his own "negligent and unhealthy" lifestyle and to his belief that he was an inherently weak person. In addition, he held the belief that he had already caused himself irreversible damage and concluded that his coping options were limited. As an example of dysfunctional externalization, the author saw a woman who believed that her rheumatoid arthritis was completely the result of a viral and autoimmune disorder. Her absolutistic "medical model" attributions led her to believe that there was nothing that she could do for her pain and fostered an excessive reliance on the medical system. In both cases, these patient's extreme, one-sided attributions sabotaged their potential sense of self-efficacy and undercut their motivation to cope more directly with their pain-related conditions.

The tendency to evaluate one's health status in absolute, black-and-white terms is also prevalent in many chronic pain sufferers. For example, a very health-conscious young woman who had developed low back problems told the author: "Now that I'm not totally healthy anymore, I'm a sick person. If I can't exercise as vigorously as I used to, then I will turn into a physical weakling."

In addition, two particularly dysfunctional distortions that probably are at the root of the sick-role behaviors and invalidism of many chronic pain patients are termed overgeneralization and negative prediction (Burns, 1980). *Overgeneralization* refers to the tendency to exaggerate one's limitations in one area to all areas of one's life. It often leads patients to make negative predictions by concluding arbitrarily that, because they are currently in pain, they will always be in pain. The health-conscious young woman mentioned previously added to her misery by predicting that, because she was currently limited in the amount of exercise she could tolerate, she would never be strong again and never be able to live the kind of life she wanted to live. She then took this prediction as an *a priori* fact. This created a sense of hopelessness and made her feel depressed. She then acted on her mistaken assumption and asked her mother to sell all of her exercise equipment, planned on giving up her career, and even anticipated rejection by her boyfriend.

Another cognitive distortion, termed *disqualifying the positive* refers to the tendency to "snatch defeat from the jaws of victory" (Freeman, 1987). Many chronic pain sufferers distort in this manner by frequently finding reasons to avoid giving themselves credit for successfully coping. Positive events are discounted and overshadowed by negative impressions. Such discounting reinforces the "downward spiral" of negative thinking, exacerbating anxiety and depression and prolonging distress.

One of the most insidious patterns of negative thinking involves the excessive use of *should* and *ought* statements. Most pain sufferers tell themselves that they should not have to suffer pain and that their situation ought not have happened to them. However, excessive absorption in this kind of thinking invariably leads to feelings of anger and resentment given the implication that life has been unfair and that life must not be unfair. This pattern of thinking is potentially the most destructive because by fueling rage and resentment, it has tremendously debilitating psychophysiological effects.

The chronic pain sufferer who has not obtained pain relief from any of his or her contacts with the health care system is likely to feel angry and resentful given cognitions such as "I should have been helped by now!" and "It's not fair that I continue to suffer and others don't have to suffer as I do." A downward spiral of *shoulds* and *shouldn't haves* is set up and repeatedly reinforced by each unsuccessful effort at obtaining pain relief. Anger and rage trigger the "fight-or-flight" stress response (Asterista, 1984) that further depletes the body of its energy reserves as physiological systems work in overdrive.

Given all of the foregoing and building on Beck's (1976) cognitive model of stress, chronic pain can be viewed as a psychophysiological stress disorder. That is, the individual fails to recover physiologically and psychologically long after the original physical stressors have abated. The pain is maintained by a reverberating circuit of dysfunctional thinking, misdirected selective attention, negative feeling states, and autonomic hyperarousal. The pain sufferer's constructions of the pain's causes and anticipated short- and long-term consequences are active, ongoing cognitive processes that include successive reappraisals of the pain, its effects, the risks involved, the individual's coping resources, and the probabilities of forestalling permanent damage and progressive deterioration.

Consistent with Beck's model of a stress reaction, the individual's cognitive structuring of pain forms the basis for how he or she copes. Psychophysiological stress reactions follow from intense arousal that the individual has no effective way of discharging (Asterista, 1984). For example, the individual might downplay his or her resources as too minimal for modulating the pain. If the individual perceives vital interests to be at stake (i.e., perceives high threat), then he or she is likely to make extreme, absolutistic appraisals of his or her condition and its implications. This is likely to result in cognitive interferences such as overpreoccupation with the pain, difficulties in concentrating on anything else, forgetfulness, and so on. These disruptions eventually impair the individual's self-efficacy and deplete his or her coping resources.

Effective therapy with this patient population requires that the multiple modalities disrupted by the chronic pain condition be addressed. Following the psychophysiological model of Melzack and Wall (1970), these modalities would include the cognitive-evaluative system, the emotional-motivational system, and the sensori-physiological system.

## PSYCHOLOGICAL MANAGEMENT OF CHRONIC PAIN

In recent years, clinicians have developed multimodal treatment packages to address the cognitive, affective, behavioral and sensoriphysiological dimensions of the chronic pain experience (Eimer, 1988; Holzman & Turk, 1986; Tollison, 1982; Turk *et al.*, 1983). There are a number of basic assumptions that underlie these intervention packages.

First, it is assumed that the central nervous system is selective in processing stimulus input (Melzack & Wall, 1970). Stimulus input is automatically screened before being centrally processed and brought to the focus of attention. The nervous system's capacities for screening sensory input and employing attention selectively make it possible to retrain patients to exert deliberate control over their attentional resources. In other words, patients can be taught to attend to stimulus sensations other than pain (Turk *et al.*, 1983).

A second basic assumption is that pain sufferers' cognitive interpretations of pain have a profound effect on the pain experience, as was underscored by the Beecher (1946) study.

A third assumption is that the chronic pain response is a maladaptive collection of overt and covert learned behaviors and therefore can be unlearned (Fordyce, 1976). Pain control is seen as a skill that can be learned, consolidated, and refined with practice (Turk *et al.*, 1983).

In some early work, Cautela (1977) built on these principles and developed a technique he termed *covert conditioning* for modifying pain behavior. The essence of covert conditioning is to teach the patient to yell the words *stop* and *relax* whenever he or she experiences pain. The overt verbalizations are gradually faded into covert verbalizations over repeated trials. The patient is also instructed to reinforce these self-verbalizations by imagining a pleasant, relaxing scene. He or she is instructed to repeat this three-part sequence until the pain subsides or is eliminated.

In order to build tolerance for future episodes of pain, trigger situations for pain are identified and the patient is asked to practice imagining himself or herself in these situations comfortable and pain free. This is then followed by distraction in the form of imagining a pleasant scene. Pain occurrences in actual situations are also counterconditioned by having the patient practice distraction from the ''real'' pain and imagine being in the same situation with no pain. This is then followed by imagining a reinforcing scene. The use of these procedures is bolstered by repetitive practice as well as by employing overt operant principles such as prohibiting the patient from complaining about the pain and instructing significant others to withdraw attention when and if the patient does complain.

Building on the integrative work of Meichenbaum (1977), Turk *et al.* (1983) have developed a comprehensive psychological pain management program grounded in Meichenbaum's stress inoculation training paradigm. Their program addresses the cognitive-evaluative, emotional-motivational, and sensoriphysiological dimensions of chronic pain.

Painful episodes are conceptualized as occurring over time in four phases: (1) the prodromal phase that is seen as the time when one prepares for the onset of pain; (2) the actual confrontation with painful sensations; (3) coping with intense feelings and sensations during the most difficult and stressful moments; and (4) after the worst moments have passed, reflecting on the experience and one's coping strategies.

Patients are taught techniques for coping with the pain during each phase of the pain episode. There are physical techniques such as progressive muscular relaxation and deep breathing for reducing sensory input, releasing muscle tension, and decreasing physiological arousal. There are cognitive techniques that include the use of coping statements and self-instructions for talking to oneself positively through each phase of the pain episode. There are also various attention-diverting strategies for distracting oneself from pain and refocusing on positive emotive imagery (Lazarus, 1977).

The attention-diverting strategies are categorized into those that simply involve shifting the focus of attention and those that involve the deliberate utilization of imagery. Examples of the first kind are focusing attention externally on physical characteristics of the environment and focusing attention internally such as on various thoughts unrelated to pain or directly on the part of the body experiencing intense sensations. The rationale for the latter strategy is to look at the pain sensations objectively and impassively in order to reduce catastrophizing and lower emotional arousal.

Examples of strategies involving the deliberate utilization of imagery are engaging in mental imagery incompatible with the experience of pain (e.g., imagining oneself in a pleasant place), reinterpreting the pain sensations as something other than pain, minimizing the sensations so as to alter one's perceptions of the pain (e.g., hypnotic imagery such as visualizing the affected body parts as numbed by Novocain or seeing the affected body parts as made of some artificial substance rendering them incapable of transmitting pain sensations), and imaginatively transforming the context in which the pain is experienced (e.g., picturing oneself as an athlete or hero who can endure or ignore the pain in the midst of the action).

In self-instructional training, the patient is coached to develop a "library" of self-statements to facilitate coping with each of the four phases of the pain episode. For example, in preparing for the pain episode, the patient is taught to tell himself or herself to view the situation as a solvable problem, to plan how he or she will deal with the pain, to review all the techniques that might be employed, and to remember to use anxiety as a reminder to focus on what needs to be done. For confronting the pain, the client is coached to remind himself or herself to do one thing at a time to avoid becoming overwhelmed, to relax and breathe deeply, to focus on coping and to use tension as a cue to relax and to stay on task. For confronting especially difficult moments when the pain sufferer feels unable to continue constructively, the patient is coached to tell himself or herself to continue focusing on the task, to refrain from catastrophizing, to accept some pain as inevitable, and to remember that he or she has a repertoire of strategies for keeping the pain under control.

Throughout each of the phases of the pain episode and at its termination, the patient is asked to evaluate his or her performance, to use negative feedback as a cue to try different coping strategies, and to use positive feedback as a cue to self-reinforce. Following Hamburg and Adams's (1967) work, Turk et al. (1983) gear their program toward promoting "satisfactory adjustment" through the enhancement of the patient's self-care behaviors. "Satisfactory adjustment" is defined as:

> Keeping distress within manageable limits, maintaining a sense of personal worth; restoring relations with significant other people and increasing the likelihood of working out a personally valued and socially acceptable situation after maximum physical recovery has been obtained. (p. 60)

Turk et al. assert that successful coping requires that the patient understand the nature of his or her disorder and the rationale for employing various coping behaviors. In addition, it is essential that the patient believe in the efficacy of available coping techniques, have the self-confidence to apply them, be capable of coping with depression and anxiety, have the ability to problem-solve, and make realistic attributions concerning limitations in the efficacy of his or her coping efforts.

Psychological techniques for pain control can be grouped into a few main categories. In working with pain patients, this author has coined the acronym "PADDS" for teaching a comprehensive self-management approach that "pads you against your pain."

The first letter, P, stands for "pacing." A number of authors have emphasized the importance of pain patients pacing themselves in their activities so that they do not exhaust themselves and deplete their resources (Eimer, 1987; Fordyce, 1976; Sternbach, 1987; Tollison, 1982). Pacing oneself also means listening to the body's pain signals and learning to discriminate when the body is calling out "uncle," given overexertion, and when the body is "crying wolf." The pain sufferer needs to know his or her own physical limitations. It needs to be communicated that it is unfortunate, but realistically, the pain sufferer has some limitations that others may not have and that the patient may not have had in the past. Nevertheless, the important thing is to concentrate on abilities as opposed to disabilities (Tollison, 1982). Many chronic pain sufferers ruminate about activities they can no longer do rather than focusing on activities they can do.

The second letter, *A*, stands for "anxiety management." It is essential that pain sufferers learn some technique for reducing anxiety and producing the "relaxation response" (Benson, 1975). These include, among others, self-hypnosis, progressive muscle relaxation, deep breathing, autogenic training, meditation, yoga, and biofeedback. An excellent review of the major relaxation techniques is provided by Davis, Eshelman, and McKay (1982).

The third letter, *D*, stands for "distraction." As was discussed earlier, distraction capitalizes on the nervous system's capacity for selective attention. The basic idea is to block pain out by refocusing attention on something else. Various attention-diverting coping strategies were reviewed earlier in the discussion of the Turk *et al.* program.

The second *D* stands for "disputation of negative thoughts." The term *disputation* refers to a procedure for identifying automatic thoughts and underlying beliefs and then questioning their validity. Once cognitions are determined to be invalid, the next step is to alter or restructure them. Various authors (Beck *et al.*, 1979; Burns, 1980; Ellis, 1985; Freeman, 1987; McMullin, 1986) have catalogued and described strategies for cognitive disputation and restructuring. For heuristic purposes, these cognitive strategies may be seen as falling into five categories. The categories are uncovering strategies, hypothesis-testing strategies, reinterpretive strategies, problem-solving strategies, and cognitive rehearsal strategies.

Uncovering strategies would include clarification of the idiosyncratic meanings a patient places on events (Freeman, 1987), labeling cognitive distortions, tracing a patient's reasoning to the underlying schematic issues with the "downward arrow" technique (Burns, 1980), and helping a patient become aware of his or her worst fears.

Hypothesis-testing strategies would include questioning the evidence supporting particular beliefs and sorting out the probabilities of occurrence of patients' anticipated and feared consequences.

Reinterpretive strategies would include helping patients to learn the causal connections between their thoughts, feelings, and behaviors; helping patients to modulate the extremity and intensity of their evaluations; helping patients more realistically to sort out what is and what is not controllable; and helping patients substitute adaptive cognitions for maladaptive ones.

Problem-solving strategies would include helping patients sort out coping options and alternatives and helping them to weigh the advantages and disadvantages of holding particular beliefs or behaving in certain ways.

Last, cognitive rehearsal strategies would include techniques for mentally practicing new ways of thinking, feeling, and behaving, role-playing techniques for practicing how to dispute dysfunctional cognitions effectively, and the experimental method for testing-out hypotheses.

The last letter, *S*, of the acronym PADDS stands for "stopping negative thoughts and images." Thought-stopping techniques were discussed previously. In summary, however, thought stopping might be conceptualized as a general category for interventions that involve cueing oneself to abort the flow of negative thoughts and images and to "change the channel" to an alternative flow of cognitions. In these terms, cognitive disputation and cognitive restructuring may be seen as "elegant" versions of thought stopping.

Cognitive techniques are not best employed in a rote or mechanical manner. Their clinical application with the pain patient requires sensitivity and clinical knowledge. Turk *et al.* (1983) assert:

> A spontaneous, flexible approach will help to establish an atmosphere of rapport, confidence, and alliance [p. 194]. . . . There is no substitute for the personal import of the trained therapist and there is no easy means of acquiring the sensitivity and judgment that are the fruits of experience (p. 195).

When psychotherapy is indicated for the pain patient, it is essential that the therapy be adapted to fit the patient rather than expecting the patient to adapt to fit the therapy (Lazarus, 1985). The remainder of the chapter will cover the parameters that need to be considered in the psychotherapeutic treatment of chronic pain patients by the cognitively oriented therapist. These parameters are dictated by the cognitive, behavioral, and affective commonalities among chronic pain patients who have had numerous unsuccessful and often iatrogenic contacts with the medical system. These patients provide the utmost challenge to the psychotherapist who is often their "court of last resort."

## STRATEGIES FOR BUILDING A THERAPEUTIC RELATIONSHIP

Initial sessions need to be devoted to assessing the patient and the patient's complaints and translating the presenting problems into cognitive and behavioral terms congruent with the implementation of a cognitive-behavioral treatment package. In effect, the patient needs to be socialized to a cognitive-behavioral coping skills model and prepared to accept the ideas that the therapist will present.

From the outset, the therapist needs to facilitate a free exchange of feelings, thoughts, and beliefs, so that misconceptions potentially destructive to developing a therapeutic alliance can be identified and corrected. For example, many chronic pain patients anticipate that their therapist will doubt the authenticity of their pain complaints (Covington, 1982). It is essential to examine the basis for such misconceptions and assure the patient that this is not the case. A thorough cognitive and behavioral assessment of the patient's pain during the initial therapeutic contacts focusing on factors that make the pain better and worse helps to communicate to the patient that his or her complaints are construed as valid.

In the following sections, strategies for promoting the development of a positive therapeutic relationship while assessing the patient, socializing the patient to the cognitive coping skills model, and dealing with various sources of patients' resistance to therapeutic change efforts will be discussed.

## INITIAL ASSESSMENT OF THE PATIENT

There are a number of excellent sources that present in detail specific categories of data that are relevant to conducting a comprehensive cognitive-behavioral assessment of the pain patient (Cinciripini & Floreen, 1983; Getto & Heaton, 1985; Holzman & Turk, 1986; Melzack, 1975; Tollison, 1986; Turk *et al.*, 1983). Only a brief listing of the categories will be given here.

These include the patient's medical and psychiatric treatment history, details about health status, characteristics of the pain (including information about location, onset, course, intensity, duration, frequency, and idiosyncratic characterizations of the symptoms), situations and activities that exacerbate the pain, situations and activities that relieve the pain, and associated physical and psychological complaints. It is important to inquire about the patient's personal theories of the pain's etiology, the idiosyncratic meanings that the patient assigns to the pain, the ways in which the symptoms place restrictions on the patient's life-style, health-related behaviors such as diet, exercise, and sleep patterns, previous and current coping strategies, and the reactions of significant others. It is also important to inquire about what the patient is willing to do to reduce his or her pain, how hard he or she is willing to work, and the ways in which the patient thinks things will be different when pain relief is attained.

## SOCIALIZING THE PATIENT TO THE COGNITIVE MODEL

Once an adequate assessment is conducted, the patient should be introduced to the conceptual framework underlying the cognitive-behavioral coping skills model. Following the psychophysiological "gate-control" model of Melzack and Wall (1970), pain is discussed as a complex phenomenon that results from the interaction of sensoriphysiological, motivational-emotional, and cognitive-evaluative modalities.

It is important that the therapist have a basic medical understanding of the nature of the underlying disorders or syndromes contributing to the patient's pain. Part of the therapist's role is to teach the patient basic biomechanical and physiological concepts of the bodily systems that are disordered. This is important as increased knowledge on the patient's part is facilitative of enhanced self-care behaviors. Following assessment and conceptual-educational phases, the patient is gradually introduced to various pain and stress management strategies and given homework assignments for practicing and consolidating new skills.

Unfortunately, as various authors have pointed out (Gallagher & Wrobel, 1982; Merskey, 1982; Violin, 1982), many chronic pain patients are not psychologically minded. They tend to complain about multiple symptoms, all usually equally severe, and to deny past and current life stressors that may have precipitated or that may be maintaining their pain (Covington, 1982). They also tend to deny psychological problems and often are not particularly motivated to work hard at learning coping skills given their depressed outlooks and perceptions of their limitations as overwhelming and insoluble. Therefore, the cognitive therapist's job early in the therapy is to socialize the patient to anticipate that multiple problems are each amenable to solution if they are broken down into more concrete tasks that can be approached one step at a time.

The patient's lack of awareness of life stressors can be dealt with by recommending that the patient keep a pain diary in which he or she records the connections between pain and different situational contexts. Once the patient begins to associate variations in pain with variations in situations, the next step is to teach the patient to identify automatic thoughts and feelings in those situations. These, too, can be recorded in the diary. Turk *et al.* (1983) provide a sample pain diary format. In addition, the Daily Record of Dysfunctional Thoughts (Beck *et al.*, 1979) provides a useful format for this activity. The therapist can eventually use the patient's diary entries to discuss the connections between activating situations, thoughts, feelings, and pain. This relationship is basic to the cognitive model of the emotional disorders (Beck, 1976) and to building a cognitive understanding of pain.

## SOURCES OF PATIENTS' RESISTANCES TO THERAPEUTIC CHANGE EFFORTS

During initial contacts, the therapist is likely to encounter a patient who is resistant to accepting the therapist's suggestions (DeGood, 1983; Pilowsky & Bassett, 1982). These resistances often manifest themselves in the patient's unwillingness to carry out assignments, in the patient's communication of an impatient and intolerant attitude toward the therapist's ministrations, and in the expression of anger and resentment toward the therapist. The therapist needs to address these resistances by first addressing the feelings and then examining with the patient the probable underlying cognitions and behavior patterns.

First of all, many pain patients, disgruntled by a track record of unsuccessful medical contacts, expect that the therapist will doubt the authenticity of their pain. Therefore, at the outset, the therapist must reassure the patient that he or she believes that the pain is real and not "all in the patient's head."

A mistaken belief that frequently underlies the aforementioned expectation is the notion of a mind–body duality. Mind and body are viewed as independent entities and often no connection is seen between the ways in which psychological stressors are handled and the body's reactions. This misconception needs to be corrected through education. The therapist needs to teach the patient about the reciprocal relationship between mind and body and about the ways in which thoughts and feelings affect and are affected by one's physical functions. Biofeedback is an excellent tool for helping patients to become more aware of their bodily functions and for teaching patients cognitive and imaginal strategies for regulating their bodily functions and controlling their pain (Basmajian, 1983; Schwartz, 1987). In addition to examining the ways in which the patient has been coping with pain, therapist and patient need to assess jointly the adequacy of the patient's coping skills in the domains of health habits, interpersonal relationships, work, habits, leisure activities, and personal expectations and goals.

As was mentioned earlier, chronic pain patients often present as angry and disillusioned. The pain sufferer has not gotten what he or she wants—pain relief. The health care system is seen as an adversary rather than as an ally. The therapist initially must be willing to tolerate the negative transference and countertransference that are likely to develop in the therapeutic relationship. It is often useful to allow the patient some time during initial sessions to ventilate about his or her journey through the health-care system. It is not wise during the initial contacts to attempt to dispute the patient's impressions. It is likely that the patient will react negatively to such attempts and jump to the conclusion that the therapist does not accept his or her reality. The patient is also apt to be hypersensitive to any indications that the therapist lacks sincerity or interest. In the face of the patient's hypersensitivity and hostility, it is necessary that the therapist show interest, concern, and communicate hope.

The therapist can acknowledge the patient's frustrations and relate similar experiences shared by other patients. However, it is important that the therapist eventually address the underlying beliefs or "beefs" that fuel the patient's anger. These are probably variants of the belief that it is terribly unfair that the patient has been stricken with enduring pain, whereas others who are less deserving (especially because they do not take good enough care of the patient!) are pain free. Commiserating with the patient about how unfair the world really is can go a long way in building rapport. The therapist needs to communicate that the patient has a right to be angry and that anger is understandable but that it may not be the best thing for the patient's pain. A useful phrase is the old saying that "living well is the best revenge." The patient has to come to the realization that ultimately he or she is punishing himself or herself by remaining angry.

The principle of moderation is also useful here for communicating the idea that a little anger is energizing and therefore adaptive but that excessive anger is immobilizing and worsens pain. Unfortunately, cognitions of helplessness and hopelessness maintain the patient's anger given the expectation that, because nothing has helped thus far, nothing will help. Therefore, the therapist needs to work gingerly to help the patient collect evidence contrary to these expectations of continued failure. One way of doing this is to persuade the patient to collaborate in setting up little experiments for evaluating the efficacy of different coping strategies.

A powerful cognitive strategy for countering hopelessness involves helping the patient to access his or her long-term memories and retrieve positive experience memories. The patient can be guided to create a lexicon of such memories that can then be accessed in "tight spots." Having such a growing "positive experience memory library" is also likely to orient the patient toward identifying positive experience opportunities for feeling good (Kall, 1986, 1987). The "bottom line" to be communicated to the patient is that living with chronic pain is unfortunate and often "just plain lousy." It would certainly be wonderful to be pain free. However, the patient would be better off if he or she makes the best of an unfortunate situation. The patient can learn to take advantage of the opportunities that having chronic pain affords for learning about his or her body and learning to listen to the body's signals.

Cognitions of hopelessness and helplessness arise in a breeding ground of catastrophic thinking that leads many pain sufferers to believe that their pain is horrible and the worse anyone has ever encountered. Such overexaggeration and catastrophizing needs to be addressed. The therapist should teach the patient how to dispute such thinking.

Given that many patients have been cognitively conditioned to believe that they must place either all or none of their reliance on the therapist to be "cured," the therapist needs to introduce the idea of "shades of gray" so that a middle ground can be discriminated. The therapist needs to utilize the developing "positive transference" in the service of teaching the patient self-management skills for relieving pain or at least making it more tolerable.

Pilowsky and Basset (1982) emphasize the necessity of making somatic interventions for building a positive therapeutic relationship. Their rationale is that the patient construes his or her discomfort primarily in somatosensory terms; therefore, if interventions are not made in this dimension, the patient is likely to doubt that the therapist believes in the authenticity of his or her pain. The author worked with a 44-year-old woman with cerebral palsy and crippling degenerative joint disease. He consulted on an ongoing basis with the patient's orthopedic physician, took an interest in helping the patient systematically reduce her reliance on analgesic medications, played an active role in helping the patient obtain orthopedic equipment, and adjusted the office arrangements in the clinic to accommodate the patient's unique needs.

The medication issue is an important one. Most pain patients become addicted to pain medications. Long-term use of analgesics, however, leads to the buildup of tolerance and to the occurrence of negative rebound effects (Covington, 1982; Tollison, 1986). Therefore, the therapist needs to negotiate with the patient a systematic program of medication monitoring and gradual reduction.

Another effective, nonthreatening somatic intervention is biofeedback-assisted relaxation training. Comprehensive treatments of this subject are available in other sources (Basmajian, 1983; Schwartz, 1987). The inclusion of biofeedback training in a multimodal cognitive-behavioral treatment program can help the patient learn to tune into and regulate bodily functions previously out of awareness. Concrete evidence from biofeedback instrumentation of positive changes in the patient's ability to self-regulate physiological functions can build the patient's overall sense of self-efficacy (Bandura, 1977) and help the patient fine-tune his or her control of the stress response. Biofeedback makes self-regulation training empirically based by providing technically precise data on a patient's progress in learning to lower sensory and physiological arousal and quiet the mind and body.

The therapist should also address the necessity of the patient's embarking on a graduated physical exercise program for increasing muscular strength and tone, joint flexibility, and range of motion. All of these variables are negatively correlated with pain. If the patient has already had exercises prescribed by his or her physician or physical therapist, then the psychotherapist ought to be aware of the kinds of exercises. If no exercises have been prescribed, then the therapist ought to make a judicious inquiry with the patient or with the patient's physician or physical therapist. The patient is likely to need remotivation periodically to keep exercising with the rationale that pain sufferers who exercise regularly experience less pain, suffering, and improved mood.

Some kind of training in self-hypnotic techniques is also frequently employed as part of a program of biofeedback-assisted relaxation and self-regulation training. Excellent guidelines for teaching self-hypnosis that are consistent with cognitive-behavioral principles are available in other sources (Catalano, 1987; Golden & Friedberg, 1986; Hilgard & Hilgard, 1983; Zilbergeld & Lazarus, 1987). Self-hypnosis can be utilized as a coping strategy for imaginatively transforming pain perceptions (Turk et al., 1983). Patients who learn the skills of self-hypnosis learn how to alter their pain experience by "reprogramming" their negative, dysfunctional self-suggestions and imagery in a state of "relaxed wakefulness." Negative self-talk is replaced by positive self-talk in a relaxed state when the patient is not thinking critically or analytically and is therefore more receptive to alternative ideas.

On the interpersonal front, the therapist needs to be on the lookout for "secondary gains" that might be maintaining the patient's sick-role behaviors and "down time" (Catalano, 1987; Fordyce, 1976). Many pain patients believe that love has to be earned through suffering and guilt and, on examination, report that they learned early in childhood that they could receive love and attention for being ill. As a consequence, pain often mysteriously becomes worse when certain people are around or are being discussed. In addition, many patients believe that they should be appreciated for all the suffering they endure due to their pain. Eventually, the therapist needs to discuss with the patient the secondary gains that appear to have resulted from being ill and that seem to lend certain advantages to remaining ill. The patient needs to be guided in examining the advantages and disadvantages of the sick role. It should be emphasized that secondary gains are likely to create primary losses. These primary losses need to be identified.

The ways in which pain behaviors prevent the patient from leading a happy life filled with positive experience opportunities need to be explored. The therapist's goal is to teach the patient more adaptive ways of being in control so that the patient can meet his or her own needs. Believing that one has available the resources to control one's experiences appears to mediate satisfactory adjustment in pain patients (Lefebvre, 1981; Rosenstiel & Keefe, 1983; Skevington, 1981).

In addition, on the interpersonal front, many patients believe that if they say "no," refuse another's request, or express anger, that rejection will follow. A behavioral and cognitive consequence is a habitual "biting of one's tongue" and holding on to feelings when one believes he or she has been treated unfairly. In such instances, assertiveness training is indicated (Lange & Jakubowski, 1976).

In many instances, marital or family systems interventions are indicated to resolve tensions stemming from the exacerbation of dysfunctional aspects of marital or family functioning. Many chronic pain sufferers complain that their mate does not really understand what they are going through and consequently is unwilling to accept their need to exercise, rest, or to not engage in certain activities. Ventilation by the pain sufferer is reported as being frequently met by sarcasm on the part of a mate or other family members. In both individual and marital or family sessions, the therapist ought to validate the fact that pain is likely to slow a person down and make the sufferer not feel like doing things. Family members need to be educated about what to reasonably expect from their family member with chronic pain. For example, it is likely to take the pain sufferer longer to engage in self-care activities. When family schedules are upset as a consequence, anger on the part of the other family members is a likely result.

There are some important principles for reharmonizing disturbed marital relationships in the chronic pain situation. These include the principle of moderation in ventilating or complaining, the principle of reciprocity or *quid pro quo,* and the principle of making expectations explicit.

The moderation principle refers to the importance of expressing feelings and lodging complaints, but in moderation. Too much complaining or nagging can reinforce pain-related dysfunctional behaviors. On the other hand, a taboo on expressing feelings or reactions in addition to making a relationship dysfunctional can also result in an increase in pain as interpersonal tensions find no outlets.

The principle of reciprocity refers to the importance of making compromises so that spouses do not feel exploited. A *quid pro quo* needs to be established with the therapist's help so that when something is given or a sacrifice is made by a spouse, something is received in return.

Last, the principle of explicit expectations refers to the necessity of avoiding "mind reading" by setting clear expectations for important roles and functions of each spouse and other family members. The therapist is often called upon to help family members vocalize unspoken, unmet, or misdirected expectations and air grievances and lingering resentments. It is often helpful to compose a contract signed by each family member that details central duties and obligations as well as "licenses and limits" for sick and well behaviors.

In the following section, principles will be presented for integrating the various therapeutic dimensions previously discussed into a cognitive approach to psychotherapy with the patient.

## PRINCIPLES OF COGNITIVE THERAPY FOR CHRONIC PAIN PATIENTS

Cognitive therapy is an integrative system of psychotherapy that is indicated in the treatment of a variety of psychiatric disorders where mistaken cognitive appraisals of reality and cognitive distortions play a significant role in maintaining or exacerbating the disorders (Beck, 1976; Beck & Emery, 1985; Beck *et al.,* 1979; Emery, Hollon, & Bedrosian, 1981).

Cognitive therapy is based on the cognitive model of emotional disorders (Beck, 1976; Guidano & Liotti, 1983) that holds that anxiety and depression are maintained by mistaken cognitive appraisals of the self, the world, and the future. Cognitive therapy is geared toward helping chronic pain patients correct the distorted cognitions that maintain their pain-related, dysfunctional emotions and behaviors. Following the principal tenets of the cognitive model, this should eventuate in relief from their symptoms of excessive anger, anxiety, and depression.

In standard applications of cognitive therapy with neurotically depressed and anxious patients (Beck & Emery, 1985; Beck *et al.,* 1979), the therapist works to keep therapy time-limited, the aim being to accomplish agreed-upon goals within an anticipated time period. Therapy is engineered for simplicity and concreteness. The therapist employs wise time-management strategies by setting agendas, focusing with the patient on manageable problems, maintaining a task-relevant orientation, assigning homework, and making ongoing assessments of the patient's progress. Effective cognitive therapy with chronic pain patients often requires a more extended time perspective. Although the cognitive therapist would be well advised to follow all of the aforementioned guidelines, the therapist should keep in mind that many chronic pain patients have occupied the sick role for a considerable length of time and have developed rigid beliefs that breed the kinds of resistances discussed previously. These beliefs breed hopelessness and mistrust of other people's intentions and reinforce the patient's despondency. Although the therapist needs to address these beliefs, therapeutic timing is essential. Effective cognitive therapy with chronic pain patients, as with all patients, requires that a sound therapeutic relationship be developed in order to build trust and a productive working alliance. However, as has been discussed, with chronic pain patients, more attention generally needs to be devoted to nurturing the relationship than is the case in doing standard cognitive therapy with neurotically depressed and anxious patients.

In cognitive therapy, the therapeutic relationship is built by collaboration between therapist and patient. The therapist aims to facilitate a team atmosphere wherein the therapist provides the structure and his expertise on problem solving. Given the team concept, collaboration does not have to be "50–50" (Freeman, 1987). The therapist and patient will vary in the percentage that one or the other is active versus passive. However, successful therapy with these patients requires high activity by the therapist and focused and relevant therapeutic interventions (Bellissimo & Tunks, 1982). The cognitive therapist needs to be aware of the power of self-perpetuated inquiry for helping the patient become aware of his or her thinking patterns and the connections between his or her thoughts and feelings. Therefore, whenever feasible, the cognitive therapist employs questions as leads in a Socratic dialogue.

> Good questions can establish structure, develop collaboration, clarify the patient's statements, awaken the patient's interest, build the therapeutic relationship, provide the therapist with essential information, open the patient's previously closed system of logic, develop his motivation to try out new behavior, help him to think in a new way about his problem and enhance the patient's observing self (Beck & Emery, 1985, p. 177).

Standard cognitive therapy is a structured therapy. The therapist directs the therapy with the assumption that the psychologically disordered patient needs to be lent more order and organization (Freeman, 1987). The therapist lends structure by setting agendas for each session in collaboration with the patient and helping the patient to keep focused on specific targets. The therapist helps the patient translate vague or overly complex complaints into more concrete terms amenable to change. In working with chronic pain patients, some modification of this principle often has to be made, especially in the early phases of therapy. As was mentioned earlier, the therapist has to be willing to allow the patient to complain and "ventilate" in order to give the patient the message that finally there is someone who accepts and understands him or her.

Nevertheless, cognitive therapy with chronic pain patients as with other types of patients still remains problem-oriented. This means that the therapist keeps the therapy relevant to identifying and solving problems. This is one of the ways the therapist lends the patient structure. Therapy moves from focusing on solvable here-and-now problems to helping the patient restructure old material in the present context, as well as in the context of planning for the future. The therapist strives to understand the patient's idiosyncratic conceptualization of his or her problems and from that point of shared understanding to develop problem-solving strategies collaboratively with the patient.

A central tenet to be emphasized is that cognitive therapy is based on an educational model. It is assumed that the best patient is an informed patient who understands each step in the therapy program. Also, it is held that often the intervention of choice is to provide the patient with information in order to correct misconceptions based on misinformation or a lack of knowledge. A major aspect of the therapist's role is to be a teacher of new skills and a provider of information (Turk et al., 1983). The ultimate educational goal of cognitive therapy, however, is to improve the patient's ability of learn from his or her experiences. Many pain patients continue to use coping strategies that are ineffective. Therefore effective cognitive therapy teaches the patient to take an experimental attitude, utilizing coping strategies as long as they work and discarding them when they do not.

In addition, the experimental attitude and the empirical approach is also applied to the patient's beliefs. The therapist treats each of his or her cognitions as hypotheses that need to be put to the test. In this vein, the therapist avoids making interpretations and instead shares hypotheses with the patient. Together as a team, therapist and patient conduct experiments to test their beliefs. Given the rigidity of long-held, repeatedly validated beliefs that many chronic pain patients have, the therapist has to move sensitively, being careful not to confront the patient's major resistances too soon or too forcefully. The therapist needs to model patience and persistence, and at appropriate times, when the patient is ready for inquiry, share hypotheses about the factors maintaining the patient's core dysfunctional beliefs. The therapist should always ask the patient for feedback regarding the plausibility of these hypotheses.

Although the optimal goal of cognitive therapy is to lead the patient to revise dysfunctional attitudes and beliefs, with many chronic pain patients this goal is not advisable. The therapist should know when to back off. It might be necessary for the therapist to examine his or her own dysfunctional attitudes or beliefs, if he or she is unable to slow the pace with the "resistant" patient. The therapist needs to apply behavioral shaping principles. Little adaptive changes will eventually add up to bigger adaptive changes, but if this does not happen, a little change for the better is still more advantageous than no change at all.

In standard cognitive therapy, homework is considered crucial to therapy's successful implementation. The bulk of the change process is seen to take place in between sessions when the patient has the opportunity to practice new ways of behaving and thinking and to test out his beliefs in problematic situations. With most chronic pain patients, the therapist needs to use clinical judgment in deciding whether to assign homework. Assigning homework too soon in the therapy program can put too much pressure on a patient who is hypersensitive to signs of failure and rejection, and who at this point more urgently needs to be listened to and understood. Homework might be more productive in the later phases of therapy after rapport is built, when the patient is ready to build up his or her repertoire of coping skills and reinforce his or her developing cognitions of self-competence.

One of the fundamental principles of cognitive therapy explained previously is the importance of engendering a collaborative relationship between the patient and the therapist. Collaboration requires that the patient trust the therapist. This requirement places a great deal of importance on the therapist's interpersonal skills, such as his or her capacity to show warmth, accurate empathy, and genuineness (Beck *et al.*, 1979). The essential feature of empathy is the ability to demonstrate an accurate understanding of the patient's cognitive and emotional perspective. Warmth is the quality of caring and interest in the patient conveyed by the therapist.

In working with chronic pain patients, warmth and empathy can be conveyed in the following ways: (1) The therapist demonstrates an accurate understanding of the patient's skepticism and pessimism and gives the patient permission to be skeptical and pessimistic. (2) The therapist communicates a belief in the reality of the patient's emotional and physical suffering, and in the possibility of attenuating it. (3) The therapist communicates the tentativeness and conditionality of everything. The therapist does not want to come on in a "gang-busting" or "bull-dozing" manner. He or she does not want to give the impression that he is out to chomp away at the patient's dysfunctional beliefs as in a "Pac-Man" model (Freeman, 1987). (4) The therapist, as soon as possible, focuses with the patient on any indications (e.g., statements, behaviors, shifts in the patient's affect) that the patient is dissatisfied with the therapy.

Adequate warmth and empathy are basic to developing a positive therapeutic relationship, and the relationship is the soil in which to implement active cognitive and behavioral interventions.

## CONCLUDING COMMENTS

This chapter has elaborated a cognitive approach to psychotherapy with chronic pain patients. Out of all of this, a unique tension or polarity can be identified that arises in the psychotherapeutic context. This is the fact that, on one hand, successful treatment requires a high level of therapist activity and relevance. Yet, on the other hand, patience is required to allow the patient to progress at his or her own pace especially in the initial phases of therapy. Appropriate timing of therapeutic interventions is a *sine qua non* for successful psychotherapy.

Chronic pain patients provide a challenge to the journeyman and master therapist alike. Balancing the opposing requirements of therapeutic activity with therapeutic patience necessitates that the therapist have available a wide array of techniques that can be employed when indicated. At the same time, however, the therapist needs to have a firm understanding of cognitive underpinnings of the patient's "resistances" in order to appreciate the patient's dilemmas and conflicts and to be able to communicate this understanding without threatening the patient's integrity. Although the therapeutic work is often very trying, the rewards are great. Most chronic pain patients have internalized the message from other health care professionals that nothing more can be done for their pain and that they must learn to live with it. Repeated contacts with a health care system that has let them down leaves these patients demoralized and depressed. Being in a position to understand their predicament and at the same time having available techniques for teaching them to lead more rewarding lives is a very heartwarming role to play as a therapist.

# REFERENCES

Asterista, M. (1984). *The physiology of stress.* New York: Human Sciences Press.

Bandura, A. (1977). Self-efficacy: Toward a unifying theory of behavioral change. *Psychological Review, 84,* 191–215.

Barber, J., & Adrian, C. (1982). (Eds.), *Psychological approaches to the management of pain.* New York: Brunner/Mazel Publishers.

Basmajian, J. V. (1983). *Biofeedback: Principles and practice for clinicians.* Baltimore: Williams & Wilkins.

Beck, A. T. (1976). *Cognitive therapy and the emotional disorders.* New York: International Universities Press.

Beck, A. T. (1984). *Cognitive approaches to stress.* In R. L. Woolfolk & P. M. Lehrer (Eds.), *Principles and practice of stress management* (pp. 255–305). New York: The Guilford Press.

Beck, A. T., & Emery, G. (1985). *Anxiety disorders and phobias: A cognitive perspective.* New York: Basic Books.

Beck, A. T., Rush, A. J., Shaw, B. F., & Emery, G. (1979). *Cognitive therapy of depression.* New York: Guilford.

Beecher, H. K. (1946). Pain in men wounded in battle. *Annals of Surgery, 123,* 96–105.

Bellissimo, A., & Tunks, E. (1984). *Chronic pain: The psycho-therapeutic spectrum.* New York: Praeger.

Burns, D. D. (1980). *Feeling good: The new mood therapy.* New York: Morrow.

Catalano, E. M. (1987). *The chronic pain control workbook: A step-by-step guide for coping with and overcoming your pain.* Oakland, CA: New Harbinger Publications.

Cautela, J. R. (1977). The use of covert conditioning in modifying pain behavior. *Journal of Behavior Therapy and Experimental Psychiatry, 8,* 45–52.

Cinciripini, P. M., & Floreen, A. (1983). Assessment of chronic pain behavior in a structured interview. *Journal of Psychosomatic Research, 27,* 117–123.

Covington, E. C. (1982). The management of chronic pain. In P. A. Keller & L. G. Ritt (Eds.), *Innovations in Clinical Practice: A source Book, Vol. 1* (pp. 126–140), Sarasota, FL: Professional Resource Exchange.

Davis, M., Eshelman, E. R., & McKay, M. (1982). The relaxation and stress reduction workbook. Oakland, CA: New Harbinger Publications.

DeGood, D. (1983). Reducing medical patients' reluctance to participate in psychological therapies: The initial session. *Professional Psychology: Research and Practice, 5,* 570–579.

Eimer, B. N. (1988). The chronic pain patient: Multimodal assessment and psychotherapy. *International Journal of Medical Psychotherapy, 1,* 23–40.

Ellis, A. (1985). *Overcoming resistance: Rational-emotive therapy with difficult clients.* New York: Springer Publishing Company.

Emery, G., Hollon, S. D., & Bedrosian, R. C. (Eds.). (1981). *New directions in cognitive therapy. A casebook.* New York: The Guilford Press.

Fordyce, W. E. (1976). *Behavioral methods for chronic pain and illness.* St. Louis: C. V. Mosby.

Freeman, A. (1987). Cognitive therapy: An overview. In A. Freeman & V. Greenwood (Eds.), *Cognitive therapy: Applications in psychiatric and medical settings.* New York: Human Sciences Press.

Gallagher, E. B., & Wrobel, S. (1982). The sick role and chronic pain. In R. Roy & E. Tunks (Eds.), *Chronic pain: Psychosocial factors in rehabilitation.* Baltimore: Williams & Wilkins.

Getto, C. J., & Heaton, R. K. (1985). Assessment of patients with chronic pain. In D. P. Swiercinsky (Ed.), *Testing adults: A reference guide for special psychodiagnostic assessments.* Kansas City: Test Corporation of America.

Golden, W. L., Dowd, E. T., & Friedberg, F. (1987). *Hynotherapy: A modern approach.* Elmsford, New York: Pergamon Press.

Guidanno, V. F., & Liotti, G. (1983). *Cognitive processes and emotional disorders. A structural approach to psychotherapy.* New York: The Guilford Press.

Hamberg, D. A., & Adams, J. E. (1967). A perspective on coping behavior: Seeking and utilizing information in major transitions. *Archives of General Psychiatry, 17,* 277–284.

Hendler, N. (1984). The chronic pain patient. In F. G. Guggenheim & M. F. Weiner (Eds.), *Manual of psychiatric consultation and emergency care.* New York: Jason Aronson.

Hilgard, E. R., & Hilgard, J. R. (1983). *Hypnosis in the relief of pain.* Los Altos, CA: William Kaufmann.

Holzman, A. D., & Turk, D. C. (1986). (Eds.). *Pain management: A handbook of psychological treatment approaches.* New York: Pergamon Press.

Kall, R. (1986). *The Kall Positive Experience Inventory.* Unpublished, copyrighted test. Bensalem, PA: Futurehealth.

Lange, A. J., & Jakubowski, P. (1976). *Responsible assertive behavior: Cognitive/behavioral procedures for trainers.* Champaign, IL: Research Press.

Lazarus, A. A. (1977). *In the mind's eye: The power of imagery for personal enrichment.* New York: Rawson Associates Publishers.

Lazarus, A. A. (1985). The specificity factor in psychotherapy. In A. A. Lazarus (Ed.), *Casebook of multimodal therapy* (pp. 200–205). New York: The Guilford Press.

Lefebvre, M. F. (1981). Cognitive distortions and cognitive errors in depressed psychiatric and low back pain patients. *Journal of Consulting and Clinical Psychology, 49,* 512–525.

McMullin, R. E. (1986). *Handbook of cognitive therapy techniques.* New York: W. W. Norton.

Meichenbaum, D. H. (1977). *Cognitive-behavior modification: An integrative approach.* New York: Plenum Press.

Melzack, R. (1975). The McGill Pain Questionnaire: Major properties and scoring methods. *Pain, 1,* 277–299.

Melzack, R. & Wall, P. (1970). Psychophysiology of pain. *International anesthesiology Clinic, 8,* 3–34.

Merskey, H. (1982). Body-mind dilemma in chronic pain. In R. Roy & E. Tunks (Eds.), *Chronic pain: Psychosocial factors in rehabilitation* (pp. 10–19). Baltimore: Williams & Wilkins.

Pilowsky, I., & Bassett, D. (1982). Individual dynamic psychotherapy for chronic pain. In R. Roy & E. Tunks (Eds.), *Chronic pain: Psychosocial factors in rehabilitation* (pp. 107–125). Baltimore: Williams & Wilkins.

Rosenstiel, A. K., & Keefe, F. J. (1983). The use of coping strategies in chronic low back pain patients: Relationship to patient characteristics and current adjustment. *Pain, 17,* 33–44.

Schwartz, M. S. (1987). *Biofeedback: A practitioner's guide.* New York: The Guilford Press.

Seligman, M. E. P. (1975). *Helplessness: On depression, development and death.* San Francisco: W. H. Freeman.

Shealy, C. N. (1976). *The pain game.* Berkeley, CA: Celestial Arts.

Skevington, S. (1983). Social cognitions, personality and chronic pain. *Journal of Psycho-Somatic Research, 27,* 421–428.

Sternbach, R. A. (1974). *Pain patients: Traits and treatment.* New York: Academic Press.

Sternbach, R. A. (1987). *Mastering pain: A twelve-step program for coping with chronic pain.* New York: G. P. Putnam's Sons.

Tollison, C. D. (1982). *Managing chronic pain: A patient's guide.* New York: Sterling Publishing Co.

Turk, D. C., Meichenbaum, D., & Genest, M. (1983). *Pain and behavioral medicine: A cognitive-behavioral perspective.* New York: Guilford Press.

Violin, A. (1982). The process involved in becoming a chronic pain patient. In R. Roy & E. Tunks (Eds.), *Chronic pain: Psychosocial factors in rehabilitation* (pp. 20–35). Baltimore: Williams & Wilkins.

Zilbergeld, B., & Lazarus, A. A. (1987). *Mind power: Getting what you want through mental training.* Boston: Little, Brown.

# 24

# Cognitive Therapy with the Elderly

MEYER D. GLANTZ

## INTRODUCTION

Historically, the elderly have constituted only a disproportionately small percentage of the psychotherapy patient population. Psychotherapists and health care providers, the elderly themselves, and their families have typically believed that psychotherapy for older adults is inappropriate, undesirable, and likely to be ineffective. The assumptions have typically been that the elderly's psychiatric problems are a consequence of their deteriorating physical condition, the natural concomitants of their many losses, or even the appropriate manifestations of their age-determined developmental or life stage. The stereotypes that health care providers have about the elderly have kept them from recommending and referring the elderly for mental health evaluation and psychotherapy; the stereotypes that the elderly have had about psychotherapy have contributed to their reluctance to consider psychotherapeutic interventions.

Recently there has been some change in these attitudes, at least among psychotherapists. Although some modifications in the approach and some age-specific knowledge and experience are necessary for successful psychotherapy with the elderly, older adults are generally excellent candidates for psychotherapy and for cognitive therapy in particular.

## PREVIOUS APPLICATIONS OF GERIATRIC COGNITIVE THERAPY

There is a small literature reporting the use of cognitive therapy with elderly patients. One of the earliest studies was conducted by Keller and Croake (1975). They used a rational-emotive "education" group approach stressing "teaching-learning" techniques in a design comparing 15 experimental with 15 waiting-list control elderly volunteers. The subjects were not identified patients or individuals with diagnosed psychological conditions. Pre–post test comparisons found significant declines for the intervention group on inventories measuring "irrational" ideas and anxiety.

MEYER D. GLANTZ • Private Practice, 6131 Executive Boulevard, Rockville, Maryland 20852; and Division of Clinical Research, National Institute of Drug Abuse, Rockville, Maryland 20857.

Meichenbaum developed an approach using self-instructional techniques to improve the problem-solving deficits and the self-control problems of children. Based on his experience, Meichenbaum (1974) proposed that this type of training paradigm could be used with some elderly individuals suffering from problem-solving difficulties and other age-related performance deficits. He hypothesized that teaching self-control verbalization, mediation, and rehearsal skills to some impaired elderly might help them to organize information, focus on relevant aspects of the problem, facilitate memory, enhance a positive, more confident attitude, help maintain task-relevant behaviors, and provide a means of coping with failure. Hussian and Lawrence (1981) found, in a study involving 36 depressed elderly nursing-home patients, that a group problem-solving training program based on the approach described by Goldfried and Davison (1976) could improve problem-solving ability and reduce depression. Hussian, (1987) discussed some of the issues and literature on the use of problem-solving training with institutionalized geriatric populations and concluded that therapists should expect "a relatively high rate of success."

Emery (1981) described some general guidelines and provided a discussion of some of the problems that may be involved in using cognitive therapy with the elderly. He referred to some treatment socialization and process issues and considered some of the specific age-group-related problems involved in treating older adults. He asserted that cognitive therapy is a "particularly attractive approach for working with the elderly" (p. 84). Taking a cognitive therapy perspective, Emery and Lesher (1982) described two personality variables, dependency and autonomy, that they believe have a significant influence on the causes, symptomatology, and treatment of the depressed elderly. In a discussion of the use of cognitive therapy with depressed elderly patients, Emery (1983) noted that many depressed elderly have negative views of themselves, the world and the future, and that "the relationship between negative thoughts and depression is compounded in the elderly because of age stereotypes." He described the role that physicians can play in helping the depressed elderly by providing accurate information, discriminating aging from depression-related symptoms, and by encouraging therapeutic activities and the minimizing of unpleasant activities. He also described some "typical thinking errors" associated with depression and some corrective exercises.

Based on a series of research studies, Fry (1984) concluded that "depression in the elderly is largely defined by a number of negative conditions such as rejection from and avoidance by others" (p. 27) and predisposing dysfunctional beliefs related to feelings of failure and helplessness and expectations concerning the probable reoccurrence of negative events. Fry also described the use of an individual therapy cognitive-behavioral treatment package that includes cognitive restructuring, cognitive and behavioral self-control techniques, cognitive monitoring and rehearsal procedures, fixed role therapy, relaxation training, and desensitization. A study of 28 nonpatient undiagnosed elderly community residents reported as having depressed affect and behavior showed that the treatment module significantly alleviated the subjects' depression and increased the frequency of positive talk and self-cognitions.

There are three large geriatric depression cognitive therapy research programs. The first is directed by Jarvik, Mintz, Steuer, and Gennen (1982). Reporting on the interim findings of a geriatric depression treatment study comparing the efficacy of a pharmacological intervention versus a cognitive-behavioral therapy group, a psychodynamic group, and a placebo group, Jarvik et al. (1982) found greatest improvement with the drug treatment and least with the placebo. Both psychotherapy groups showed approximately the same midrange level of symptom alleviation. The study had several serious methodological problems that the authors acknowledged, and the final results have not been made available. As part of a related study, Steuer and Hammen (1983), described four case studies and some of the issues and adaptations of a cognitive-behavioral group therapy for the depressed elderly. They considered the approach to be very promising with this population, and they asserted that age-related changes in intellectual functioning may slow the course of the therapy and increase the usefulness of the behavioral components with some patients. They also stated that the cultural and educational diversity of the population may impair group cohesiveness. Following up on this report, Steuer *et al.* (1984) described the results of a geriatric depression study that compared a cognitive-behavioral group therapy based on Beck's approach with a psychodynamic group therapy based on the approaches of Alexander, Grotjahn, and Yalom. A total of 33 moderately to severely depressed elderly began and 20 completed the 9-month course of therapy; patients were assigned to one of four groups, two using each approach. Both groups demonstrated clinically and statistically significant reductions in observer and self-report measures of depression; of the 20 patients who completed treatment, 40% went into remission, and 80% showed some improvement as indicated by Hamilton Depression Scale scores. Beck Depression Inventory (BDI) scores indicate that the cognitive-behavioral-treatment subjects experienced a greater reduction in depression, but no significant differences were detected with the other measures.

The second major cognitive therapy research program involving treatment of the elderly is the one conducted by Gallagher, Thompson, and their associates. The first of their reports (Gallagher & Thompson, 1982) was a study of the treatment of 30 elderly patients diagnosed as being in a current major depressive episode. Patients were randomly assigned to a cognitive therapy treatment (based on the approaches of Beck, Nush, Shaw, & Emery, 1979; Emery, 1981), a behavioral therapy treatment (using Lewinsohn's approach and described in Gallagher *et al.*, 1981) or a brief relational insight therapy (derived from Bellak and Small). All patients were seen in an individual therapy format. Based on observer and self-report ratings, patients in all three conditions showed significant and comparable improvement between the pre- and posttherapy assessments. However, data from the 1-year follow-up showed that the cognitive therapy and behavioral treatment subjects demonstrated greater improvement over time. The authors attributed this to the skills training of these therapies and the associated increase in self-perceived efficacy. Additional analysis of the data from this study (Gallagher & Thompson, 1983a) found for the nonendogenously depressed patients that, for all three treatment conditions, there was significant and durable improvement following therapy. When assessed posttherapy, 80% scored within the normal range on the Beck Depression Inventory, and none had relapsed into a diagnosable depression within the 1-year follow-up period. In contrast, one-third of the endogenous patients were noticably improved posttherapy, and only approximately half of the total had not relapsed by the 1-year follow-up. A discussion of some of the principles and issues involved in cognitive therapy with the elderly and a discussion of some of the preliminary data from this study can be found in Gallagher and Thompson (1983b).

In order to address some of the questions raised by the study, the researchers conducted a replication. Discussions of cognitive therapy and treatment of the elderly, some illustrative case studies, the methodological modifications, and some preliminary results are reported in Thompson and Gallagher (1984) and Thompson, Davies, Gallagher, and Krantz (1986). The major modifications for the replication included a larger sample of 91 patients, an increased number of sessions, the inclusion of a 6-week delayed treatment control condition, and the replacement of the insight-relational treatment condition with a brief psychodynamic psychotherapy (based on the approach of Horowitz & Kaltreider, 1979). Posttreatment results, reported in Thompson, Gallagher, and Breckenridge (1987), found no treatment condition differences but significant improvement on all measures for the subjects receiving psychotherapy; 52% of the treatment sample attained remission by termination, and an additional 18% showed significant improvement. Comparisons of treatment conditions at 6 weeks with the control condition indicated that improvement was attributable to the interventions.

Noting that resistance and failure to cooperate with treatment procedures often occur in the treatment of depressed elderly patients, Silven and Gallagher (1987) described a case study of resistance encountered in the cognitive-behavioral treatment of an elderly woman. They described the adaptations they made to enhance the efficacy of the treatment by strengthening the structure, focus, and patient participation in the therapy and the "turning point" in the therapy that occurred with the "successful challenging of an important cognition." Baum and Gallagher (1987) consider some of the issues related to psychotherapeutic treatment to facilitate preparation for death in terminally ill patients, and they recommend certain principles, including some guidelines, for the use of cognitive-behavioral therapy.

The third large research effort assessing the efficacy of cognitive therapy with depressed elderly is by Beutler, Yost, and their associates. The program of research is intended to develop the treatment for depressed geriatric patients and evaluate its effectiveness as an intervention to be used with and without psychopharmacological co-treatment. A preliminary effort, Chaisson, Beutler, Yost, and Allender (1984), involved determining whether nurse trainees and other mental health students and professionals could be successfully trained to a competency standard and then implement an effective course of cognitive group therapy treatment for depressed elderly. Eight of the 12 cognitive therapy trainees met the competency standard, but there was not a significant pre- to posttherapy change in depression scores for the 46 elderly patients. However, there was a significant correlation between the competency score of the therapist and the improvement of that therapist's assigned patients. This suggests that an important variable in successful geriatric cognitive therapy is the competency of the therapist.

The treatment manual used in the principle study being conducted by Beutler and his associates has been published (Yost, Beutler, Corbishley, & Allender, 1986). The therapy protocol uses a 20-session group treatment approach and "closely follows the structure outlined by Beck et al., 1979." (p. 11) Therapy is divided into four phases: (1) the preparation phase in which the therapist uses the information obtained during the screening to teach the patients what to expect during the therapy; (2) the identification and collaboration phase during which a collaborative relationship is established with the patient and problems conducive to change are identified; (3) the change phase during which the patient learns and practices a variety of techniques and skills; and (4) the consolidation/termination phased during which the patients consolidate and prepare for termination; primary foci of this stage are methods for expanding the patients' social network, stress inoculation, and learning techniques of self-evaluation. The protocol relies heavily on "lecturettes" (brief didactic presentations), monitoring assignments and skills development, behavioral mastery and graded task assignments, and reengagement in pleasurable activities.

A report of the principal study describes the treatment of 56 elderly adults with diagnoses of major unipolar depression (Beutler et al., 1987). Subjects were divided into four groups, receiving alprazolam pharmacotherapy, group cognitive therapy plus alprazolam medication, group cognitive therapy plus a placebo, or a placebo alone. Alprazolam is a psychoactive drug that has been advocated as an antidepressant for the elderly and that has compared favorably with tricyclic antidepressants. Patients treated with cognitive therapy showed significant improvement in subjective state and sleep efficiency measures. Cognitive therapy patients were also significantly less likely to terminate treatment prematurely. No significant differences related to medication assignment were detected. The treatment gains demonstrated by the cognitive therapy patients were maintained during the 12-week follow-up period. In a related effort, Scogin, Hamblin, and Beutler (1987) investigated the efficacy of cognitive bibliotherapy with 29 community dwelling moderately depressed elderly respondents to a newspaper announcement of a self-help program for depressed older adults. Participants were assigned to one of three conditions: (1) cognitive bibliotherapy treatment using Burns's *Feeling Good*; (2) a self-help presentation of cognitive therapy (Burns, 1980), an attention control bibliotherapy condition; or (3) a delayed treatment control. Significant treatment effects were observed on both self and observer ratings of depression at the postintervention assessment. A 1-month follow-up showed that the cognitive bibliotherapy effects had not deteriorated.

Although limited, the literature does demonstrate some important points. Psychotherapy with the elderly, and cognitive therapy in particular, can be an effective intervention, with favorable rates of success that are comparable to those achieved with younger populations. Even endogenously, long-term depressed elderly patients often can be helped. As is the case with younger patient populations, a major factor in many of the elderly patients' problems are maladaptive conceptualizations. Modifications of standard cognitive therapy approaches seem to be necessary with geriatric populations. This may include a greater emphasis on the amelioration of environmental and behavioral problems through therapist-supported patient activities. There is support for the use of cognitive therapy skills training to assist elderly patients to compensate for moderate memory and problem-solving difficulties. Although most of the clinical trials have been done with depressed geriatric patients, it is reasonable to assume that appropriately formulated cognitive therapy approaches could be similarly effective in alleviating other problems of elderly patients. In sum, the literature is strongly encouraging for the continuation of the development and evaluation of the use of cognitive therapy with the elderly.

## COMMON THEMES IN GERIATRIC COGNITIVE THERAPY

As shown in a National Council on the Aging (NCOA) national cross-sectional survey of adults, the problems that the elderly typically experience are not necessarily as severe as is believed by the general population and even by the elderly themselves (Harris, 1981). Old age can be and very frequently is a very fulfilling and satisfying period of life. In many cases, older adults have overcome or left behind the problems that plagued their earlier years, making their elder years the most enjoyable. Unfortunately, other elderly individuals face major environmental and personal problems and may continue to have the psychological problems that they had when they were younger, suffer from an exacerbation of those problems, incur a loss of their means of coping, or develop new difficulties. Many of the psychiatric problems are related to the losses, transitions, problems, and stresses common to old age. The segment of the elderly population suffering from any of these psychiatric problems constitutes the potential candidates for psychotherapy, and it is important to remember that these patients are being treated because of their problems and not because they are old. Many of the themes and problem foci involved in treatment of the elderly are the same as those encountered in the treatment of younger adult patients; there are almost no themes or problem foci that are unique to the elderly. However, there are a number of themes that are more commonly associated with the elderly and more prominent in the range of issues involved in geriatric psychotherapy. In many ways, these themes are the foundation of the distinct character of therapy with the elderly. Most of these themes and foci are based on the real and often unfortunate circumstances that are the frequent concomitants of old age. Following are some of the more common themes encountered in geriatric psychotherapy.

### PHYSICAL ILLNESS AND DISABILITY

Poor health and physical impairments are major problems affecting many elderly individuals. Even those who are not currently affected personally usually are concerned about their own future health prospects or have relatives and friends who are affected by poor health or impairments. Results from the 1984 National Health Interview Survey's (NHIS) Supplement on Aging (SOA) show that 32% of community-dwelling adults age 65 to 74 years and 33.2% of community-dwelling adults age 75 to 84 years were in fair to poor health, according to themselves or to the person most likely to know about them (Kovar, 1986a). Other 1984 SOA data show that for the noninstitutionalized adults 65 to 74 years, 14.4% had difficulty walking, 51% had arthritis or rheumatism, 33% had some difficulty hearing even if a hearing aid is used, and 24.7% had some vision trouble even if glasses are worn (Havlik, 1986). According to the NCOA study, 21% of the adults 65 and older reported themselves to be "very seriously personally affected" by poor health (Harris, 1981). Most elderly patients have at least one significant health problem. A health problem event can be an important factor in the etiology or exacerbation of psychiatric problems in the elderly (e.g., Phifer & Murrell, 1986).

As a theme and problem focus of geriatric psychotherapy, poor health and physical limitation can be involved in a variety of ways. Some elderly psychotherapy patients have great difficulty in adjusting to their medical problems and need practical assistance in dealing with their new limitations as well as help in coping with the related depression, anxiety, and/or anger that they feel. The prospect of becoming "blind, deaf, crippled, or senile" would be a devastating possibility for any adult. It is a reality or a real possibility for some elderly people. Many elder adults must cope with chronic pain, sensory loss, fatigue, memory deficits, motoric function replacements, or other chronic conditions. Some must cope with physical problems such as sexual dysfunction or incontinence that may cause feelings of humiliation and self-disparagement. A significant physical illness or disability often initiates the identification of oneself as being "old," fragile, mortal, at the end of one's life, vulnerable, and potentially subject to a long, slow period of physical deterioration and incapacity.

For some older adults, the onset of an illness or disability precipitates a sense of almost phobic insecurity, an erosion of self-image, or an obsessive preoccupation with health. Others experience a sense of a loss of control or feelings of helplessness and vulnerability. Physical illness and/or limitations may result in a loss of important activities, social contacts, sources of stimulation, enjoyment, pride, and self-perceived competence and independence. Even relatively minor reductions or impairments in function can have important consequences. For example, reductions in night vision and motor reflexes can preclude driving after dark. Dependence on assistance from others can lead to severe problems for those who greatly value their autonomy and independence as well as those who have difficulty in obtaining acceptable aid. Other adults may be subject to hypochondriasis or somatization; some adopt a "sick" role and become permanent patients with health concerns as their primary focus and activity. Many elderly must cope with the medical problems of their spouse and other relatives.

### Death and Dying

Related to the theme of health and impairment are themes focused on the nearness of death and a fear of the process of dying. Probably no other age group has a greater sense of the reality of their mortality than the elderly. Most measure their lives not only in terms of the years they have already lived out but also in terms of the number of years they think they have left to live (c.f. Neugarten, 1977); some count the anticipated number of remaining "healthy" years. Some depressed elderly become preoccupied with the anticipation of death and/or disability, and they adopt a "what's-the-point?" "I'm-just-waiting-to-die" attitude. Concern about death may include an end to having a "future" or a feeling of mourning for unattained dreams or unmet goals. One patient stated, "How can I be happy, the only thing I have to look forward to is dying. I've already lived longer than anyone else in my family. Wouldn't you be depressed if you knew you were going to die in the next 10 years?" Some elderly patients have strong fears associated with the process of dying. Older patients often report images of long, painful, and debilitating illnesses from which they do not recover. Fears of "wasting away until you die in a nursing home," "dying by inches in a hospital with tubes stuck in you," or "going senile and needing to be taken care of like a baby" are not uncommon. Anxiety about death often extends to concern about the loss of spouse and friends. Many elderly patients will have experienced such losses and may need assistance in coping with their grief and recovering their ability to function.

DIMINISHED ABILITIES AND DEPENDENCE

Also related to the theme of health are the themes of lost or reduced physical and intellective abilities and the often consequent dependence on others for assistance. Losses of ability are common in old age, and many elderly patients have difficulty in adjusting. Depression, anxiety, anger, lowered self-esteem, reduced confidence, diminished competency, and a withdrawal from activities may result. Some decrements, such as an increase in rigidity or a decrease in abstract and divergent thinking, memory, or problem-solving ability impair the individual's ability to overcome or compensate for other problems. Many elderly patients are too embarrassed or too discouraged to utilize or develop alternative means of accomplishing goals now unteachable by the means they previously relied on. Some develop a learned helplessness (cf. Miller, Rosellini, & Seligman, 1977) or find that the psychological coping strategies that they have previously relied on no longer function adequately or that they no longer have access to the resources, individuals, or domains of accomplishment and reinforcement that enabled them to cope and to feel competent and secure. In some cases, the problem is not a diminished ability but the failure to learn or develop a new needed skill. Finding their established skills to be obsolete, some elderly are too intimidated to even try to master the new needed skills. Some elderly patients have no activities or domains where they can satisfy their needs for mastery and competency.

With a loss in abilities often comes a need for assistance from others. Data from the 1984 NHIS Supplement On Aging show that 38.5% of the community dwelling adults in the 65 to 74 years age group and 38.8% in the 75 to 84 years age group reported at least partial physical limitation on their ability to perform their usual activities (Kovar, 1986a). The data for this noninstitutionalized sample also show that for adults age 65 to 74 years of age, 17.1% had difficulty with, and 6% received assistance with, one or more personal care activities, and 20.5% had difficulty with, and 16.1% received, assistance with one or more home management activities. For the group 75 to 84 years old, these percentages increase to 27.8% reporting difficulty and 11.9% receiving help with at least one personal care activity and 33% reporting difficulty and 27.6% receiving help with at least one home management activity (Dawson, Hendershot, & Fulton, 1987). NCOA data show that 14% of those 65 and older had very serious difficulty getting transportation to stores, health care, and recreation (Harris, 1981). Dependence on others can result in conflicts with the aid providers as well as the psychological difficulties associated with a deficit in the capacity to perform a basic previously available function.

SOCIAL NETWORK LOSSES

Almost all older adults must cope with the loss of important relationships in their lives; this may include loss of their spouse, their friends, and other relatives including their children. SOA data from 1984 show that 25% of community-dwelling adults age 65 to 74 years and 43.1% of community-dwelling adults age 75 to 84 years are widowed. The probability of living alone increases with age from 24.8% in the 65 to 74 years age group to 38.4% in the 75 to 84 years age group (Kovar, 1986a). Approximately 8 million adults 65 and older live alone. Of the community-dwelling adults 65 years and older living alone, 29% had no living children, and 28% had no living siblings. However, most had some family with whom they have relatively frequent contact and relatively few are completely socially isolated, often because they maintained contacts with others by means of the telephone. In the 2 weeks prior to the SOA assessment, 11% had not gotten together with, and 10% had not had telephone contact with family, friends, or neighbors (Kovar, 1986b). According to the NCOA data, 17% of adults 65 years and older reported that loneliness was a very serious problem for them (Harris, 1981). Social network losses mean a loss of caring, compassion, and companionship for many elderly patients. Social network losses usually mean losses in social supports that are likely to increase the individual's vulnerability to other stresses. Those who have lost a spouse may have lost an interdependent almost symbiotic relationship that spanned most of their adult lives. Many elderly patients need assistance in reconstructing their lives and in redeveloping a social network including initiating new friendships and intimate relationships.

## ROLE LOSS

Attendant to the transitions of old age are often changes in or losses of important roles. This may lead to the loss of a valued activity and access to an important domain of function and accomplishment that is a significant factor in the individual's self-esteem and identity. Also lost may be a sense of purpose, importance and being needed, a "place in the world," and an external source of structure and direction. Although the majority of elderly adults are able to develop new age and appropriate life-stage roles by themselves, some need assistance.

## DISENGAGEMENT AND REDUCED PLEASURE

The elderly are more likely than any other age group to have disengaged from people, concerns, activities and sources of reinforcement, stimulation, and pleasure. Some elderly patients develop a feeling of "not belonging" or of not being "part of the real world." NCOA data show that 14% of adults 65 years and older spent "a lot of time just doing nothing." They engaged in social and most types of recreational activities less than adults ages 18 to 64. Life satisfaction typically declines with increasing age (Harris, 1981). Whether disengagement is the product of losses, transitions, or more voluntary withdrawal, it is likely to be associated with psychological distress and difficulties. Elderly patients commonly report very few pleasurable activities. Psychotherapy for these patients must strongly support an increase in pleasurable activities and when appropriate, a reengagement in activities, concerns, and social networks.

## AGEISM AND LOW SELF-IMAGE

Some elderly adults have a low self-esteem that is a continuation of the self-image they held as younger adults. Other older adults develop or exacerbate a poor self-image due to the changes and problems associated with their circumstances. There are, however, some elderly who share the prejudices of younger "ageists" and associate old age with being useless, undesirable, unlovable, unwanted, obsolete, unattractive, incompetent, infirm, and defective. Some deny that they themselves are "really old" and may disdain their age peers and perhaps even their spouse. Many elderly individuals overestimate the age-related decrements in their level of function. Many also overattribute their problems to old age and to themselves rather than to environmental or other factors. Other elderly ageists may denigrate themselves and manifest a strong depression. They may adopt a self-defeating attitude that old age is a period of inevitable, irreversible loss and suffering, making little effort to overcome or compensate for their problems. One patient stated, "I'm old, I'm useless, and nobody wants me. I don't blame them, I wouldn't want me either." Some pessimistic anticipations may become self-fulfilling prophecies; for example, an elderly man who believes that he is unlovable and undesirable may withdraw from social contacts, lose the support of his social network, and become socially isolated. Although most elderly adults do not have such severe views of aging, a surprisingly high percentage of the elderly have more negative views of old age than appears warranted by the depiction of old age presented by research data (e.g., Harris, 1981). Aging is correlated with negative labels, and the elderly are particularly vulnerable to the effects of such labels (Rodin & Langer, 1980). Low self-esteem is a common problem among elderly patients and is integrally related to many of their psychiatric problems.

## CONFLICTS WITH FAMILY

Some elderly patients complain of problems with their children. Many of these intergenerational conflicts are the same as those reported by younger adults who are the parents of grown children. These may include the parents' belief that the children are not sufficiently respectful, attentive, or grateful, that they have not met the parents' expectations, desires, or needs, or that they continue to make too many demands for the parents' financial assistance, emotional support, or services such as child care. Other conflicts may center on the adult child's desire for seemingly rebellious self-determination and autonomy and the "heartbreaking" actions and decisions that result. As the adult child fights for adult status and independence, the elderly parent may suffer from the loss of the parental caretaking or authority role and may feel betrayed, rejected, and unappreciated. Ironically, some conflicts center on the child's complaint that the elderly person has abandoned the parental role and is not "acting their age," engaging in such "unacceptable" behavior as going back to school, dating younger people, or not doing their "job" as a grandparent.

Conflicts also can emerge when the elderly parent and the adult child "exchange roles." Both the children and the parents are often uncomfortable with or resentful about the exchange of provider/care giver and recipient roles. In those instances where the elderly parent is dependent on the adult child for practical and/or financial assistance, anger, a feeling of being intruded upon, a sense of inappropriateness, and/or feelings of inadequacy may be experienced by both parties. Some adult children think of their elderly parents as being less able to function than they actually are, and they overprotect and infantalyze them. It is not uncommon for the spouse of the adult child to feel resentment toward the elderly person, and this further increases the familial stress and conflict. As many more adults are surviving to much greater ages, an increasingly common situation is that of the young elderly adult whose frail elderly parent or parents are still alive. In all of these various situations, the conflicts must be addressed, and a new relationship must be negotiated between the parent and child.

Elderly married couples can experience severe conflicts related to their relationship. Some couples who "stayed together for the children's sake" no longer have a reason (or an excuse) for staying together. Couples who had very divergent lives may find they have difficulty when retirement, the children's leaving home, and problems such as ill health force them into each other's company. Because of a disparity in the ages of the husband and wife, a divergence in their health conditions, or a difference in the stages of their respective lives, older couples may find that they have very different interests, goals, and abilities. The necessity for caring for an ill or impaired spouse can also cause considerable conflict and resentment. Elderly couples are potentially subject to most of the problems that can affect younger couples, and some have had marital problems for much or most of the marriage and have never resolved them. Resolution of these marital and familial problems can be a critical component of the psychotherapy.

## ENVIRONMENTAL STRESSES

Many elderly patients report environmental stresses. Financial problems and concerns affect many elderly. Census data for 1980 (CHESS, 1982) show that 15.7% of all persons 65 years and older had incomes below the poverty level. According to the NCOA survey, 17% of the sample 65 years and older reported very serious problems related to not having enough money to live on, and 42% reported very serious concerns related to the cost of heating oil, gas, and electricity (Harris, 1981). Fear of crime was also a very serious concern reported by 25% of these respondents (Harris, 1981). Other social and cultural, environmental and technological, and bureaucratic and institutional problems and changes may present severe difficulties for some older adults. Some elderly have difficulty coping with the psychological stresses associated with these types of problems; this is particularly true of those who have impairments, poor health, or diminished coping abilities and resources. Partly due to health concerns and other problems and partly due to an attenuated sense of competence and efficacy, some elderly patients experience a feeling of vulnerability, a general loss of security. Depression, anxiety, anger, and self-isolative or idiosyncratic behavior may be concomitants.

### OTHER LIFE-STAGE PROBLEMS

There are many transitions and adjustments that are part of old age. A number of these may be enjoyable, being viewed positively by many elderly people, for example, retirement, moving to a new home, or becoming a grandparent. Any of the transitions may be problematic for at least some older adults. This is particularly true for those elderly also facing greater stresses with inadequate coping resources and for those elderly who are attempting to deal with irremediable, unanticipated, or unplanned-for transition problems or with distressing events that occur earlier than usually anticipated, such as a forced early retirement or the death of a spouse at a relatively young age (cf. Neugarten, 1977). Elderly patients may need assistance in adjusting to the transitions that they experience.

More than any other age period, old age is more likely to be a period of multiple and diverse losses and stresses. The multiplicative effect of these problems can be extremely distressing and overwhelming. Each problem is likely to compound and magnify the others, seriously reducing individuals' coping, problem-solving and compensating abilities and undermining their belief in their ability to improve their situation. One patient stated, "I've always had some big problem or other, but I could always handle it. Now, what with my arthritis and the wife being sick and all the rest of it, I've just about had it." Some elderly patients may be so overwhelmed or so depressed by their losses, physical problems, and stresses that, although they are not actively suicidal, they look forward to death. Elderly patients confronting numerous difficulties and/or incurring extensive loss of coping resources will need considerable aid in reestablishing a functional equilibrium.

## THE APPROPRIATENESS OF COGNITIVE THERAPY

As mentioned earlier, older adults demonstrating psychiatric problems are potential candidates for psychotherapy and for cognitive therapy in particular. Further, for those older adults who are appropriate candidates for psychotherapy, cognitive therapy is exceptionally well suited to and is most likely to be the psychotherapy of choice for this population. There are a number of reasons supporting this assertion, not the least of which is the author's experience that cognitive therapy is, in general, a highly effective and efficient intervention modality with a variety of patient populations and problems (e.g., Glantz, 1986). More specific to the elderly, cognitive therapy is stylistically more comfortable, reassuring, encouraging, and appropriately focused for the elderly. The approach is shorter term, active, directive, and interpersonally interactive. It is present-oriented as well as goal- and problem-oriented and allows goals to be broken down into manageable steps and facilitates the achievement of tangible results early in the course of therapy. These qualities make the modality more acceptable to the elderly and facilitate their participation and their accomplishments. The conceptualization emphasis of the approach is also particularly well matched to the needs of the elderly population.

Many of the problems that face older adults are strongly determined by maladaptive conceptualizations, beliefs, expectations, interpretations, attributions, role definitions, and values. Cognitive therapy is extremely effective at identifying and correcting maladaptive thought contents, making the approach particularly useful with elderly patients. Contrary to the stereotypes about the rigidity of the elderly, the author's experience is that elderly patients are not significantly more resistant to the consideration and adoption of alternative conceptualizations than are younger adult patients. Resolving the maladaptive conceptualizations utilized by elderly patients usually has a dramatic effect on their affect and level of functioning. These reconceptualizations, the patient's overall progress, and his or her involvement in the therapy are greatly facilitated by the strong behavioral component that cognitive therapy usually includes.

As described earlier, the elderly are likely to face many real physiological, environmental, and social problems that require direct action for amelioration. Elderly patients often have difficulty in actively dealing with these tangible problems, and they need encouragement and support for this. Cognitive therapy provides this and imparts a realistic sense of responsibility for dealing with one's own problems and a sense of one's true level of competence. The therapy teaches the necessary problem-solving, coping, and interpersonal skills. Patients are encouraged and are given the support required to make these behavioral/environmental changes. In treating elderly patients, it is commonly the case that interventions based on directives and support of behavioral environmental attempts are inadequate by themselves because the patients' maladaptive conceptualizations are implacable obstacles. A wide range of maladaptive conceptualizations are integral parts of the difficulties that most elderly patients have in confronting and ameliorating their "real-world" problems. These include low self-esteem, a belief in one's inability to cope, hopelessness, and self-attributed helplessness, distorted perceptions of the environment and interpersonal relations, misattributions of problem causes, assumptions that the state of being "old" involves inevitable loss of worth and pleasure, unrealistic standards, role loss, and confusion. The cognitive content and process focus of cognitive therapy makes it possible to remove the conceptualization barriers to, and facilitates the implementation of, behavioral/environmental interventions. The therapy also teaches, when needed, the conceptualization skills necessary to accurately appraise a problem, determine the extent to which it can be resolved and, if necessary, teaches a perspective enabling the patient to accept or adjust to those aspects that cannot be satisfactorily mitigated. This minimizes attempts that lead to predictable failures and also minimizes the loss of opportunities to have a successful impact on a problem. These conceptualization and behavioral aspects of cognitive therapy typically lead to patients developing an enhanced sense of competence and independence, a greater belief in their ability to cope with future problems, and an improved self-image. Patients become convinced that change, new possibilities, and an improvement in the quality of their life are possible and obtainable. All of these are particularly important for the elderly.

Last, the interactive nature of cognitive therapy provides an opportunity for the therapist to show the patient that he or she is valued and worth caring about and to demonstrate empathy, genuine respect, unconditional positive regard, and treatment of the patient as a full and responsible adult. Further, the therapist has a forum to demonstrate to patients that they can receive help in a collaborative relationship without incurring a demeaning dependence or loss of self-respect. Patients have the setting and support to discover that they can form new relationships and new types of relationships and can adopt new and satisfying roles. These features of cognitive therapy are also greatly facilitative in treating the elderly.

MEYER D. GLANTZ

As is the case with any special population, not all members of the elderly population demonstrating psychiatric problems are appropriate candidates for (cognitive) psychotherapy. The appropriateness of any given elderly potential patient must be determined on an individual basis. The first set of screening criteria are those that would generally be used with any adult population to determine the adult's appropriateness for psychotherapy. The second set of criteria are more specific to cognitive psychotherapy and to the elderly. Briefly stated, with cognitive therapy, change is primarily accomplished through four basic processes: (1) through directed behavioral experiences, "experiments," and changes in the environment and interpersonal relationships; (2) through the consideration and acceptance of alternative conceptualizations presented by or developed with the therapist; (3) through the correction of maladaptive thought (information) processes; and (4) through the monitoring and self-regulation of thoughts and habituated thought patterns. When appropriate, these processes are supplemented by the acquisition of new skills and information. A cognitive therapy patient must at least potentially have the intellectual capability to engage in these processes and the related activities and to have a reasonable possibility of accomplishing these goals. In general, these criteria will not exclude elderly patients with only mildly diminished intellective function, including general decrements as well as many focal decrements. For example, an elderly person who demonstrates a mild degree of memory loss or a minor diminution in abstract reasoning, even if somewhat greater than age-appropriate norms, is likely to be an acceptable candidate for cognitive therapy. For the most part, these sets of screening criteria will eliminate only those patients demonstrating a marked degree of intellectual decline or dementia; this would not include cases where the observed decrement in function is presumed to primarily be a product of the patient's depression or anxiety. The cognitive therapist should be prepared to assess, either informally or when necessary, formally, the intellective functioning of the prospective elderly patient and to formulate a differential diagnosis of the patient's problems. Although formal assessments are generally not needed to assess the cognitive sufficiency of the patient, an informal test of the person's ability and willingness to reconceptualize is helpful. It is recommended that during one of the initial sessions, the therapist offer an "easy," alternative, and more realistic point of view germane to the patient and relevant to some fairly unimportant matter. If the prospective patient is able and willing to at least consider the alternative perspective, this is usually a very encouraging indicator. None of the criteria described here are unique to screening the elderly. However, due to the increased intellective decrements associated with age and age-related physical conditions, greater attention must be given to screening elderly patients; compared to younger patients, a larger percentage of the elderly may not satisfy these criteria.

Related to the issue of screening criteria is the question of the age range of the psychotherapy candidates being considered here. People age at different rates and differ in their level of function at different ages; they also differ in the problems and supportive social and other resources available to them. For the most part, the author's primary geriatric treatment experience is with, and the cognitive therapy recommendations are for, the "young elderly." In general, the "young elderly" include older adults whose physical and mental functioning is relatively intact and complete; the term usually refers to adults 60 to 74 years of age. Often because of health or family losses, some adults age 55 to 59 experience problems and take on characteristics usually associated with older adults; some adults age 75 to 80, usually those with above-average health and more intact social networks, do not have, until this age, the experiences and problems typically associated with younger individuals. Adults meeting these descriptions who are also potential patients meeting the screening criteria described would be included in the therapy recommendations described here.

As is common with a special population, the basic therapy approach to be used must be altered in order to be most effective, given the particular characteristics and needs of that group. The author's experience and that of other therapists who have used cognitive therapy with older adults is that there are special themes and issues associated with the elderly and the therapy should be modified with patients of this age group. However, despite this, it is important to note that the majority of the problems to be dealt with and the majority of the strategies and techniques to be used in intervention with the elderly are those that are associated with cognitive therapy as it is commonly employed with younger adults. This chapter focuses on modifications of the therapy assuming that the reader is familiar with cognitive therapy and will place what is recommended here in the context of a "standard" approach. Therefore, the chapter does not devote attention to recommending the fundamental principles or techniques of cognitive therapy that do not need modification or a change in emphasis with elderly patients. It is assumed that the therapist is familiar with, and will employ, these basics of the modality without specific instruction to do so. This chapter does not describe a comprehensive therapy protocol but rather describes special issues and modifications and supplements to the standard cognitive therapy approach to facilitate its use with the elderly. These modifications are in accordance with two general phenomena. The first is related to the cohort characteristics and experiences of the particular age population.

COHORT CHARACTERISTICS

In general, the elderly are a very heterogeneous group due to the diversity of their cultural backgrounds, the variations in the courses of their lives, and differences in their rates of aging, their health, and their social and environmental circumstances. In many respects, the current elderly cohort is more heterogeneous as a group than are younger age groups. However, the adults who currently constitute the elderly population have experienced certain critical historical events, participated in the culture and internalized the cultural beliefs of certain decades, and have been affected by other strong developmental influences determined by their unique background, the period of time, and the particulars of the places in which they lived. For example, most of the current elderly cohort are older than most of the psychotherapies now being used to treat them. Their beliefs about psychotherapy were originally formed when stereotypes about mental illness and the experience and effectiveness of psychotherapy were very different from contemporary ones. Many older adults believe that psychotherapy is for "crazy" (psychotic) people or that psychological problems are the product of moral weakness. Some believe that the process of psychotherapy involves lying on a couch and talking about "dirty" (sexual) issues that are not really related to their problems or involves getting electric shocks if they do the wrong thing. Some believe that psychotherapy entails a well-meaning but irrelevant pep talk from a person who cannot really understand their problems. It is commonly the case that elderly patients think that psychotherapy is not effective in general or is at least very unlikely to help in their particular circumstance. The sentiment, "my problems are not mental, they are real," is often expressed by elderly patients. They often consider psychotherapy to be an invasion of their privacy and a threat to their "secrets" ("you don't air your dirty laundry in public"). They were usually raised to believe that adults do not share their feelings with or show "weakness" to a stranger and that an adult should not need to ask for help with his or her personal lives. They respect the authority of the "doctor" and are reluctant to discuss their discomfort and their doubts. Instead, they often withdraw and refuse to participate in psychotherapy. Those adults who are members of the current elderly cohort do not usually think of solving problems in terms of psychological solutions, and they are usually very resistant to seemingly "irrelevant" intrapsychic explorations. The elderly are also likely to be older than their psychotherapists. It is very common for an elderly patient to feel that his or her younger therapist does not and cannot understand what it is like to be old. A psychotherapist treating members of this cohort must be aware of the possibility that the elderly patient will have these beliefs about psychological problems and treatment and must be prepared to address them.

Similarly, the therapist must understand the patient's past and be prepared to deal with its influences and consequences. It is not enough for the therapist to "take a patient's history." The therapist must be a cultural anthropologist and a historian, at least somewhat knowledgeable about the history and the culture of the patient's cohort. For example, most of the adults who are currently elderly were strongly affected early in their lives by the economic depression of the 1930s and World War II. A therapist treating a member of this cohort must understand these events and their formative influences. It is more important for a therapist treating today's elderly to know about the golden days of radio and the early days of television than about MTV. As subsequent cohorts age, the historical and cultural information necessary to treat them will change, but the general principle will not.

## DEVELOPMENTAL/LIFE STAGE

The second general phenomenon determining the cognitive therapy modifications for use with the elderly relates to the older adults' developmental or life stage and its concomitants. During the elder years, physical, psychological, financial, social, and familial changes are typical. Although almost all of the circumstances that are associated with old age can happen to younger adults, they are much more likely to happen to any given elderly person, and that elderly person is much more likely to incur several of these circumstances. Just surviving for six to eight decades increases the chance that certain events will occur, and some of these phenomena are more a probable part of geriatric life. For example, loss of one's spouse and friends, ill health and disability, financial stress and fears of death and dying certainly occur to adults of all ages but not nearly as frequently as they occur with the elderly. Many of these problems are less likely to have a resolution or a remedy for an older adult. These types of phenomena must be understood and dealt with by the therapist treating the elderly. Unlike the cohort characteristics described before, these life-stage phenomena and circumstances will apply to younger cohorts as they reach their elder years.

## THERAPEUTIC STYLE

It is important to remember that the general goals and approach of cognitive therapy with the elderly are the same as they are for the treatment of younger adults. However, in consideration of the cohort and life-stage phenomena and based on the author's experience, a number of elderly appropriate modifications of cognitive therapy are recommended. Many of the modifications are related to the therapist's style of interaction with the patient. A therapeutic alliance is often harder to form with an older patient, and, for the reasons described before, elderly patients are often uncomfortable with psychotherapy and doubtful of its worth. Rogers (1957) has postulated six therapy conditions as being necessary and sufficient for successful psychotherapy. Without entering the controversy on the necessity or sufficiency of these characteristics, three of these conditions, those related to "attitudinal" characteristics of the therapist, are very important when treating the elderly. These characteristics are therapist genuineness, accurate empathy, and unconditional positive regard. This would include showing respect for the patient and the avoidance of a patronizing, infantalyzing, or condescending attitude. When treating an elderly patient, it is particularly necessary for therapists to demonstrate these characteristics to an even greater degree than with other age groups. The extent to which the therapist is successful in demonstrating these characteristics to the elderly patient will be a major determinant of the success the therapist will have in engaging the older patient in a working therapeutic relationship and in developing a strong therapeutic alliance. The formation of a strong therapeutic alliance and a comfortable working relationship are essential to effective psychotherapy with the elderly.

Related to this, the therapist should communicate the idea that the difficulties that the patient is experiencing are common among older adults and are neither unique to the patient nor horrible in their implications. Although showing an understanding of the reality and unpleasantness of the patient's experience, the therapist must place the experience in a realistic often more normalized perspective. It is often helpful to make the following kind of statement to the patient: "It is not that you are senile, crazy, or suffering from a severe mental disease, but you are not happy and things could be much better for you. Many people, including many adults your age have similar problems, and they are usually able to be helped by therapy. We will work together to accomplish this for you. During therapy, you will learn some new skills, get some information, confront, and overcome some specific problems and look at some things from a different point of view. This therapy has helped others to have a better life, and I am confident that it will help you." During the course of the therapy, it is helpful to periodically review the progress that the patient has made, to attribute those gains to the patient's work in therapy, and to reassure them that even greater progress is expected.

Having demonstrated an empathetic understanding of the patient's "real world" problems early in the therapy, it is helpful to show the patient that therapy can help ameliorate at least some of these problems. Therefore, it is usually a good idea to intensify the behavioral/environmental intervention component early in the therapy. If possible, the therapist should try to arrange for a behaviorally related subgoal to be identified and reached during the first four or five sessions. A therapy-related improvement in the patient's life, even if limited, greatly facilitates the patient's engagement, trust, and effort. For example, encouraging patients to reestablish contacts with old friends, to assertively state their feelings to someone, or even, if they are reclusive, to go to a movie or a social event is often enough of a change to make further improvement seem possible to the patients. Similarly important is ensuring that patients experience some improvement early in the course of therapy that is based on a reconceptualization. Other stylistic emphases are also helpful.

Elderly patients are usually more comfortable and responsive with therapists who are active and maintain an environment in the sessions, which is that of a moderately formal though warm and interactive discussion. Elderly patients typically do not like either a very passive or a highly directive style, and they resent being "pushed." They are uncomfortable with psychological assessments, confrontations, and an "interrogation" style of questioning. With many older patients, it is necessary to frequently refocus the topic of discussion, bringing the patient back to the topic being considered; this should be done in a nonconfrontational nonaccusative manner. It is usually helpful if therapeutic presentations to the patient are as concretely and briefly stated as possible, employing simple relevant analogies, and avoiding abstract, theoretical, or philosophical concepts. Didactic presentations of ideas such as alternative conceptualizations are usually less well received, whereas those developed with the therapist and based on the patient's experience are likely to be successful. When examples or cultural references are used, they should be ones that are familiar to the patient. Techniques that may seem "unnatural" to the patient, such as role playing, are more acceptable when they are introduced later in the course of the therapy. Techniques such as paradoxical intervention can be very effective with some patients but should be used sparingly in order not to disrupt the therapeutic alliance and the patient's faith and trust in the therapist. Last, the therapist must be more flexible when treating an elderly patient, being responsive to the needs of the patient. Examples of this would include varying the therapy plan to respond to the patient's immediate environmental problem, having session times that accommodate the patient's transportation, being more willing than with other patients to mediate with family and other professionals on behalf of the patient, or having a telephone therapy session when the elderly patient is unable to come into the office.

## PRAGMATIC LIFE-STAGE PROBLEMS

The next set of modifications and emphases are related to the greater number, severity, irreversibility, and incapacitating nature of the physiological, environmental, and social problems that often confront the elderly. The extent of these problems may require that a considerable amount of attention in the therapy sessions be devoted to these practical problems. Elderly patients may require a great deal of assistance in coping with these problems. Coping will entail ameliorating those problems that can be improved, adjusting emotionally and pragmatically to those that cannot, and discriminating one from the other. The therapist will need to be able to discriminate between physiologically based behavioral and psychological problems, psychosomatic, and hypochondriacal problems, and those problems that are psychological in nature and origin but have been somatized, presented as medical symptoms, or manifested as being similar to those produced by certain medical conditions. The therapist will also need to be familiar with psychological and behavioral symptoms that may be related to medication use and misuse.

In helping the elderly patient to cope with practical environmental problems, it is important for the therapist to be familiar with the wide range of resources and assistance that may be available to older adults. Many elderly adults lack important information (e.g., they may not know that there are electronic devices available that can summon medical assistance for a stricken person, making it more feasible for many medically at-risk older adults to live independently and more safely). Some elderly may have misconceptions. For example, they may believe that the mild memory losses they are experiencing are caused by Alzheimer's disease rather than being "normal" losses associated with senescence. Therapists treating the elderly must be prepared to deal with both types of information problems. Many otherwise healthy older adults experience some degree of intellective decrement. Common complaints include memory problems and a diminution of concentration and problem-solving ability in relation to new types of situations and problems. Compensating techniques based on behavioral and cognitive therapy strategies are usually quite successful in improving functioning in these areas, and therapists must be prepared to teach them. Some generally healthy "young" elderly have some difficulties with activities of daily living (ADL) that require therapeutic attention. There are many other special problems that frequently affect older adults and that the therapist must be prepared to assist the patient with. Examples of such problems include caring for an ailing or disabled spouse, adjusting to retirement, or learning to handle basic financial matters that previously had been managed by a now deceased spouse. Last, older adults often have problems that they are embarrassed about and are reluctant to disclose or deal with in therapy (e.g., incontinence, sexual dysfunction, ADL problems, sensory losses, etc.). Therapists treating the elderly must be skilled in eliciting older patients' reports and discussions of these problems. The therapist must also be vigilant to the possibilities of other types of problems that the patient themselves may not be clearly aware of but that may have serious behavioral consequences. Examples of this might include medication problems that cause memory and concentration impairments or a hearing loss that leads to paranoia, hostility, and/or withdrawal.

## TECHNIQUES

Other modifications for using cognitive therapy with the elderly are related to some of the foci and forms of the therapeutic techniques that are used. The adults who now constitute the elderly population are often predisposed to think of their problems in terms of a medical model, and they are often supported in this by their health care providers and families. This leads them to expect to be given a "pill" to be "cured," to have the "doctor" take responsibility and do the work necessary for the problem resolution and to pessimistically assume that if their problem does not have a medical cure, then, like old age, it cannot be ameliorated. They are also inclined to attribute many of their problems or their failures to deal with their losses and decrements in function as being appropriate given their advanced years; there is a tendency for people with this perspective to think of old age itself as being a degenerative disorder. In order for these patients to be able to address and ameliorate many of their problems, they must reconceptualize them in terms of a more psychological framework. As discussed earlier, elderly patients are often at least initially resistant to this. However, achieving the early session behavioral and reconceptualization "successes" described before can make a significant contribution to overcoming this resistance.

It has frequently been observed that the elderly are often the targets and victims of "ageism," age-related prejudice and discrimination. Unfortunately, elderly patients often subscribe to these prejudices themselves, and this exacerbates many of their problems and creates an additional barrier to their resolution. These elderly patients have watched their relatives, friends, and neighbors grow old, and they have come to believe that senescence is an inevitable and unpleasant decline made up of painful losses, increasing ill health and daily humiliations, ending only in death. They do not believe that old age can, despite its attendant problems, be an enjoyable and satisfactory time of life for most older adults. They both expect and accept their problems as being part of old age and therefore impossible to change. In order to help these patients, the therapist must demonstrate an empathetic understanding of the reality and painfulness of the patient's problems, acknowledging and validating their experience, whereas at the same time helping them to reconceptualize their situation to include a psychological perspective permitting the possibility of change and improvement. For the most part, the same overall cognitive therapy strategy that would be employed with a younger adult patient who has suffered a handicapping physical condition or other loss can be used with these patients. The therapist will attempt to communicate the following: "Your problem, the loss and the pain, is real. They must be accepted, minimized, and overcome when possible. They must not be allowed to destroy the good that is already in your life or the good possibilities of your future. You are not your disability, you are not alone, and you will have all of the help that you need. You can have a better and more satisfying life, if you fight for it." Behavioral/environmental and reconceptualization success will facilitate the acceptance of this perspective. When the elderly patient has accepted that his or her life can be worthwhile and satisfying, and has learned to focus on the specific problems and not just despair, blaming the general condition of old age, then the patient can work on and improve those specific problems and his or her adjustment to them. Therapists must adjust upward their expectations for the time and attention it may require to accomplish these goals with an older population. The type of patient just described is in contrast to another type who has so narrowly and obsessively focused on a specific loss or disability that he or she cannot adjust to it or gain any satisfaction from the other unimpaired aspects of their life. These patients must be helped to gain a broader perspective and, here again, the general cognitive therapy strategy that would be used with a younger patient is appropriate.

The psychological dysfunction of some depressed patients has been described in terms of a model of learned helplessness (Miller *et al.*, 1977). In this model of reactive depression, "previous exposure to uncontrollable aversive experiences interferes with escape and avoidance learning" that results in "deficits in response initiation and in association of reinforcement with responding" (pp. 104–105). This model has been hypothesized by some researchers to depict at least some cases of depression in the elderly. In terms of a more conceptualization-oriented model, multiple failure experiences lead some individuals to believe that they cannot be successful in overcoming or even having a positive impact on a domain or domains of problems. Construing themselves as incompetent and helpless, they become depressed. Believing that their future efforts will also be failures, they do not make attempts, thus creating a self-fulfilling prophecy that further increases their depression, their low self-esteem, and their feelings of impotence. This model is similar in many ways to Beck's postulated cognitive triad (negative views of the self, the environment and the future, Beck, 1976) that is presumed to be a major factor in adult depression, including depression among the elderly. It is hypothesized here that there is a related phenomenon that also plays a critical role in the psychological problems experienced by many of the elderly.

Many adults who have developed effective coping and pragmatic skills and strategies that enabled them to function successfully and satisfactorily discover that the life-stage transitions that they experience in old age render at least some of those skills and strategies ineffective. For example, retirees who previously coped with depression or loneliness by immersing themselves in their occupation or older adults who previously bolstered their self-esteem through the attraction of members of the opposite sex or through the exercise of authority over members of their family or another organization may no longer have these avenues accessible. Similarly, individuals who dealt with problems of financial management or home maintenance by turning the responsibility over to their spouse or adults who controlled their weight through exercise or their boredom through hobbies or sports may find that these methods are no longer available to them. It will be necessary for the therapist to assist these elderly patients in developing new and/or alternative skills and strategies. In some cases, the elderly patients will need to develop skills to cope with problems that they have never had to confront previously, for example, serious medical problems. Again the therapist will need to assist with the development of appropriate skills and strategies. Some patients will already have a skill that they need but that they are reluctant or unable to employ; for example, the patient might need "permission" to be assertive in asking questions of their physician. Therapists will need to give encouragement and a "license" in these cases.

In addition to the development of skills and strategies, therapists may also discover that they need to assist elderly patients in redeveloping the types of external structures that previously facilitated their functioning. As an illustration of this, many adults determine the schedules of their activities through the structure provided by their employment. They may go to work from 9 to 5 on weekdays, and, during these days, the job dictates what they will be doing during each hour. They engage in social contacts at lunch and coffee breaks and follow many of the "outside" activity recommendations made by their more active and imaginative co-workers. They may socialize with people from work and even arrange social contacts in response to the initiatives of co-workers. When they are not at work, they know that it is time to relax from being at work. Having retired, they may have difficulty knowing what to do or when to do things because there is no external structure to guide them.

Treatment of the elderly often involves the need for a greater emphasis on helping the patients to acknowledge and express their deeper feelings and thoughts. Elderly patients are often more disengaged from their negative affects and conceptualizations than their younger counterparts. Overcoming the denial and avoidance of these distressing emotions and frightening ideas allows them to be dealt with in therapy. Related to this, many elderly patients seem to have a consciously constricted range of affect. For some, it is as if they believe that it is not proper, or they do not have the right to express certain feelings, for example, that they do not have the right to be angry. Encouraging and giving "permission" for the patient to feel and express the full range of emotions is very beneficial. Some elderly patients mislabel their emotions. They may, for example, describe themselves as being depressed, although subsequent information indicates that they are in fact highly anxious or angry. Helping the patient to correctly label the feeling often facilitates the reconceptualization and behavioral changes necessary to overcome the negative affect. Similarly, some elderly patients mislabel their environmental or social problems. Examples might include elderly who state thay they have lost interest in socializing when they are ac!ually embarrassed about being incontinent or others who maintain that a lack of respect from their children makes them unwilling to visit them when they are really afraid to drive on the expressway to get there, or patients who claim to be opposed to an activity or service when in fact they cannot read, understand, or fill out the necessary forms. Correctly identifying and labeling these types of problcms is also an important early step in dealing with these types of issues.

Many older adults suffer a diminution or constriction of positive emotions. There are a number of possible reasons for this. Older individuals may no longer have access to or the capacity for the activities or experiences that were the source of their enjoyment or pride. They may be overwhelmed by the stresses and/or the negative affects they feel, their ill health, or other environmental problems that might be dominating their lives. They may have lost the spouse or other people who were an essential part of their feeling good and feeling love. In some cases, after a lifetime of hard work, pessimism, and worry, they may simply not know how to have a good time. For a variety of reasons, many elderly patients engage in relatively few pleasurable activities. The therapist must help these patients develop the expectation that they can have positive feelings, must assist them to overcome the maladaptive conceptualizations that are a barrier, and must facilitate the patients' participation in the activities and relationships that are likely to lead to the development of positive feelings. Patients must be strongly encouraged to engage in a broad range of pleasurable activities. A common obstacle is the feeling on the part of the elderly patient that his or her loss of a positive affect is attributable to an irremediable loss. It is unfortunately true that many of the losses common in old age are partly or even completely irreversible. The therapist must acknowledge the reality of the patients' situation and appropriately adjust the goals and the intervention time and attention in response to this. For example, in comparison to a younger widow, an older woman whose husband has died has a much smaller opportunity and probability of and a greater set of practical problems in reentering the social world and forming another romantic relationship. Therapists must make appropriate accomodations to reality. As mentioned, it is suggested that the therapist use the general cognitive therapy strategy that would be employed with a younger adult incurring a handicap. However, with elderly patients, there may a complex of losses that overwhelms and discourages them and prevents them from believing that their life can be satisfying and enjoyable. Sometimes even the alternatives and resources for compensation that would be available to a younger adult are lost or diminished for the older patient. Helping patients focus on and increase the positive affects and pleasurable activities that they do have will be critical to overcoming the patients' despair and enervation. Assisting the patient to maximize the positive feelings and activities that are possible and adjusting to the losses that are irremediable will be accomplished using the standard cognitive therapy strategies. However, as noted, therapists must take into account the frequently greater and more numerous problems confronting some elderly.

As discussed earlier, many elderly patients are uncomfortable with and uninformed about psychotherapy. For many, the closest analogous situation that they can relate to psychiatric treatment is that of going to see a physician. Not surprisingly, many come to psychotherapy with the same model of appropriate patient behavior that they bring to a medical practitioner. However, the patient behavior and expectations that are appropriate in a medical treatment situation are not appropriate and are often counterproductive in a psychiatric treatment situation. For this reason, it is often necessary to teach elderly patients about the process of psychotherapy and to inform them of the appropriate patient and therapist behaviors and expectations. The therapist must explain about the special rules, protections, and conditions of psychotherapy, showing the patient that many of the normal social rules, inhibitions, and dangers do not apply. The therapist must socialize older patients to the process of psychotherapy and introduce them to resolving problems with psychological solutions. As part of this, the therapist will often have to introduce the patient to a new type of interpersonal relationship, that of a collaboration that provides assistance to one of the participants without creating a state of dependency or loss of self or other respect. A collaborative relationship is an important component of the cognitive therapy approach, and the therapist will need to devote particular attention to developing such a relationship with an elderly patient.

A few other modifications of standard cognitive therapy protocols and changes in therapist expectations are often necessary. Cognitive therapy with the elderly may involve a larger number of sessions than does a comparable cognitive therapy intervention with a younger adult, and the pace and progress is often slower. This does not necessarily present any particular problem, but it is important for therapists to be aware of this in order to adjust the therapy protocol and their own expectations. It is sometimes more difficult to get the elderly patient to do therapy work between sessions, particularly if the between-session assignments are referred to as "homework" rather than "between-session therapy work." Persistence and encouragement usually suffice to overcome this resistance. Termination may be accomplished with less difficulty and concern by the patient if scheduling is tapered off rather than abruptly ending. It is recommended that during the posttermination year, two or three "check-in" sessions are planned.

Although the majority of therapeutic techniques that are used with the elderly are the same as those used with younger adults, there are a few that are relatively unique to the treatment of the elderly. One of the most useful of these is life review therapy that has been suggested by Butler (Butler, 1974; Lewis & Butler, 1974). Butler hypothesizes that the realization that one's death is approaching initiates a tendency for the return to consciousness of past experiences, particularly those involving unresolved conflicts. This reminiscence process is presumed to be a healthy one facilitating the resolution of past problems, the reorganization of one's life into a more satisfying perspective, the reintegration of one's life into the present, and the summation of one's life to produce a sense of accomplishment for oneself and a legacy for others. Life review therapy, which involves the production of an autobiography by the elderly patient, makes this normally spontaneous and unselective process into a more conscious, controlled, and effective one. The life review process also can be assisted by putting together scrapbooks, photo albums, and correspondence libraries, by tracing and recording family histories and genealogies, by recontacting family and friends, by making pilgrimages to important places from one's past, and by passing these records and information onto younger generations. From a cognitive therapy perspective, these activities can be very useful. Life review activities may serve a therapeutic purpose by helping elderly patients to form a satisfying perspective on their life, giving it a feeling of meaning and worth, by helping them to overcome some of their unresolved conflicts and to identify some of their neglected needs, and by helping them to develop a life-stage feasible role. It may also lead to a sense of accomplishment and pride and a recognition by the older adult that they have overcome seemingly insurmountable problems in the past. Elderly patients are often very surprised and pleased by their family's response to their life review activities as the family is likely to demonstrate an increased interest in the elderly person and their life. The life review activities usually provide a focus for mutually satisfying conversation and shared activities with the elderly relative. Through their interest in the product of the life review, the family show that they still value the elderly person and believe that he or she has something worthwhile to offer. For almost all patients, this technique is a useful supplement rather than a primary intervention. Based on the author's experience, this technique should not be employed with patients who resist a review of their past or who have had very unpleasant or very psychologically or socially dysfunctional lives.

Although it is important to consider the modifications of cognitive therapy that are recommended for treatment of the elderly, it is also important to note that, despite the discomfort that many patients and some therapists have in dealing with certain issues, the inclusion of these sensitive issues as potential therapeutic considerations should not be altered. The first such issue is the need for marital therapy. The elderly are appropriate candidates for couples or marital therapy and are, generally, very responsive. The second issue involves sexual dysfunction. Although great attention must be paid to the confounding medical and medication related issues, the elderly are also appropriate and responsive candidates for sex therapy. The third issue relates to suicide. As a population, the elderly are at great risk for suicide, and when there is a risk for suicide, a targeted intervention is necessary and can be effective. In dealing with all of these issues, it is probable that the therapist will need to elicit information that problems exist and will need to overcome some resistance on the part of the patient to discuss and work on these problems. Elderly patients may also be having conflicts or other problems with their families, particularly with their children. In resolving these problems, it is often very helpful to have the patient invite the family for family therapy sessions.

### THERAPIST QUALIFICATIONS

Treating a special population usually requires that the therapist have special qualifications, and this applies to the treatment of the elderly. The first requirement is that the therapist is competent and experienced in the use of cognitive therapy. Second is the requirement that the therapist is knowledgeable about gerontology, including both healthy aging and common patterns of pathology, and be informed about the cohort characteristics of the age population. The third requirement is that the therapist must be comfortable with elderly people, not being subject to any ageist prejudices. The therapist's own fears about old age, death, dying, irremediable dependency, and disability as well as any problems that therapists might have in their relationship with their own parents must be controlled and separated from the therapeutic activity so as not to interfere with the objectivity necessary for effective therapy.

## CONCLUSION

Although some modifications and special emphases are necessary, cognitive therapy can be a highly appropriate and a very effective intervention for the elderly. It is not possible to describe in a single chapter all of the issues related to the use of cognitive therapy with the elderly; however, the major principles and considerations have been described. Therapists and health care providers are strongly encouraged to consider older adults as appropriate candidates for psychotherapy, and psychotherapists are encouraged to employ a cognitive therapy approach.

ACKNOWLEDGMENTS. The author would like to thank Linda Gerson, Ellen Nannis, and Larry Beutler for their helpful comments on this chapter.

## REFERENCES

Baum, D., & Gallagher, D. (1987). Case studies of psychotherapy with dying persons. *Clinical Gerontologist, 7,* 41–50.
Beck, A. (1976). *Cognitive therapy and the emotional disorders.* New York: International Universities Press.
Beck, A., Rush, J., Shaw, B., & Emery, G. (1979). *Cognitive therapy of depression.* New York: Guilford Press.
Beutler, L., Scogin, F., Kirkish, P., Schretlen, D., Corbishley, A., Hamblin, D., Meredith, K., Potter, R., Bamford, C., & Levenson, A. (1987). Group cognitive therapy and alprazolam in the treatment of depression in older adults. *Journal of Consulting and Clinical Psychology, 55,* 550–556.

Burns, D. (1980). *Feeling good*. New York: New American Library.

Butler, R. (1974). Successful aging and the role of the life review. *Journal of the American Geriatrics society, 22*, 529–535.

Chaisson, G., Beutler, L., Yost, E., & Allender, J. (1984). Treating the depressed elderly. *Journal of Psychosocial Nursing, 22*, 25–30.

CHESS (Centers for Health Education and Social Systems Studies). (1982). Current Population Reports, Series P-60, No. 133. In U.S. Bureau of the Census, *Statistical Abstract of the United States: 1982–1983 (103d ed.)*. Washington, DC: U.S. Government Printing Office.

Dawson, D., Hendershot, G., & Fulton, J. (1987). Aging in the eighties: Functional limitations in individuals age 65 years and over. *Advance Data From Vital and Health Statistics, No. 133*. Hyattsville, MD: National Center for Health Statistics.

Emery, G. (1981). Cognitive therapy with the elderly. In G. Emery, S. Hollon, & R. Bedrosian (Eds.), *New directions in cognitive therapy* (pp. 84–98). New York: Guilford Press.

Emery, G. (1983). Cognitive therapy of depression in the elderly. In T. Crook & G. Cohen (Eds.), *Physicians' guide to the diagnosis and treatment of depression in the elderly* (pp. 84–98). New Canaan, CT: M. Powley Assoc.

Emery, G., & Lesher, E. (1982). Treatment of depression in older adults: Personality considerations. *Psychotherapy: Theory, Research and Practice, 19*, 500–505.

Fry, P. (1984). Cognitive training and cognitive-behavioral variables in the treatment of depression in the elderly. *Clinical Gerontologist, 3*, 25–45.

Gallagher, D., & Thompson, L. (1982). Treatment of major depressive disorder in older adult outpatients with brief psychotherapies. *Psychotherapy: Theory, Research and Practice, 19*, 482–490.

Gallagher, D., & Thompson, L. (1983a). Effectiveness of psychotherapy for both endogenous and nonendogenous depression in older adult outpatients. *Journal of Gerontology, 38*, 707–712.

Gallagher, D., & Thompson, L. (1983b). Cognitive therapy for depression in the elderly: A promising model for treatment and research. In L. Breslau & M. Haug (Eds.), *Depression and aging: Causes, care and consequences* (pp. 168–192). New York: Springer Publishing Co.

Gallagher, D., Thompson, L., Baffa, G., Piatt, C., Ringering, L., & Stone, V. (1981). *Depression in the elderly: A behavioral treatment manual*. Los Angeles: University of Southern California Press.

Glantz, M. (1986). A cognitive behavioral approach to day hospital treatment of alcoholism. In A. Freeman and V. Greenwood (Eds.), *Cognitive therapy: Applications for psychiatric and medical settings* (pp. 51–68). New York: Human Sciences Press.

Goldfried, M., & Davison, G. (1976). *Clinical behavior therapy*. New York: Holt, Rinehart & Winston.

Horowitz, M., & Kaltreider, N. (1979). Brief therapy of the stress response syndrome. *Psychiatric Clinics of North America, 2*, 365–377.

Harris, L., & Associates. (1981). *Aging in the eighties: America in transition*. Washington, DC: National Council on the Aging.

Havlik, R. (1986). Aging in the eighties, impaired senses for sound and light in persons age 65 years and over; Preliminary data from the Supplement on Aging to the National Health Interview Survey, United States, January–June 1984. *Advance Data From Vital and Health Statistics*, No. 125. Hyattsville, MD: National Center for Health Statistics.

Hussian, R. (1987). Problem-solving training and institutionalized elderly patients. In A. Freeman & V. Greenwood (Eds.), *Cognitive therapy: Applications in psychiatric and medical settings* (pp. 199–212). New York: Human Sciences Press.

Hussian, R., & Lawrence, P. (1981). Social reinforcement of activity and problem-solving training in the treatment of depressed institutionalized elderly patients. *Cognitive Therapy and Research, 5*, 57–69.

Jarvik, L., Mintz, J., Steuer, J., & Gerner, R. (1982). Treating geriatric depression: A 26-week intermin analysis. *Journal of the American Geriatrics Society, 30*, 713–717.

Keller, J., & Croake, J. (1975). Effects of a program in rational thinking of anxieties in older persons. *Journal of Counseling Psychology, 22*, 54–57.

Kovar, M. (1986a). Aging in the eighties; Preliminary data from the Supplement on Aging to the National Health Interview Survey, United States, January–June 1984. *Advance Data From Vital and Health Statistics*, No. 115. Hyattsville, MD: National Center for Health Statistics.

Kovar, M. (1986b). Aging in the eighties, age 65 years and over and living alone, contacts with family, friends, and neighbors; Preliminary data from the Supplement on Aging to the National Health Interview Survey, United States, January–June 1984. *Advance Data From Vital and Health Statistics*, No. 116. Hyattsville, MD: National Center for Health Statistics.

Lewis, M., & Butler, R. (1974). Life-review therapy: Putting memories to work in individual and group psychotherapy. *Geriatrics, 29,* 165–173.

Meichenbaum, D. (1974). Self-instructional strategy training: A cognitive prosthesis for the aged. *Human Development, 17,* 273–280.

Miller, W., Rosellini, R., & Seligman, M. (1977). Learned helplessness and depression. In J. Maser & M. Seligman (Eds.), *Psychopathology: experimental models* (pp. 104–130). San Francisco: W. H. Freeman.

Neugarten, B. (1977). Personality and aging. In J. Birren & K. Schair (Eds.), *Handbook of the psychology of aging* (1st ed.; pp. 626–649). New York: Van Nostrand Reinhold.

Phifer, J., & Murrell, S. (1986). Etiologic factors in the onset of depressive symptoms in older adults. *Journal of Abnormal Psychology, 95,* 282–291.

Rodin, J., & Langer, E. (1980). Aging labels: The decline of control and the fall of self-esteem. *Journal of Social Issues, 36,* 12–29.

Rogers, C. (1957). The necessary and sufficient conditions of therapeutic personality change. *Journal of Consulting Psychology, 21,* 95–103.

Scogin, F., Hamblin, D., & Beutler, L. (1987). Bibliotherapy for depressed older adults: A self-help alternative. *The Gerontologist, 27,* 383–387.

Silven, D., & Gallagher, D. (1987). Resistance in cognitive-behavioral therapy: A case study. *Clinical Gerontologist, 6,* 75–78.

Steuer, J., & Hammen, C. (1983). Cognitive-behavioral group therapy for the depressed elderly: Issues and adaptions. *Cognitive Therapy and Research, 7,* 285–296.

Steuer, J., Mintz, J., Hammen, C., Hill, M., Jarvik, L., McCarley, T., Motoike, P., & Rosen, R. (1984). Cognitive-behavioral and psychodynamic group psychotherapy in treatment of geriatric depression. *Journal of Consulting and Clinical Psychology, 52,* 180–189.

Thompson, L., & Gallagher, D. (1984). Efficacy of psychotherapy in the treatment of late-life depression. *Advances in Behavior Research and Therapy, 6,* 127–139.

Thompson, L., Davies, R., Gallagher, D., & Krantz, S. (1986). Cognitive therapy with older adults. *Clinical Gerontologist, 5,* 245–279.

Thompson, L., Gallagher, D., & Breckenridge, J. (1987). Comparative effectiveness of psychotherapies for depressed elders. *Journal of Consulting and Clinical Psychology, 55,* 385–390.

Yost, E., Beutler, L., Corbishley, A., & Allender, J. (1986). *Group cognitive therapy: A treatment method for the depressed elderly.* New York: Pergamon.

# 25

# Cognitive-Behavioral Marital Therapy

NORMAN EPSTEIN AND DONALD H. BAUCOM

Cognitive-behavioral therapies were developed primarily as approaches to understanding and treating problems of individuals, such as depression (Beck, 1976; Beck, Rush, Shaw, & Emery, 1979), impulsive behavior (Meichenbaum, 1977; Watkins, 1977), anxiety (Beck, Emery, & Greenberg, 1985), anger (Novaco, 1975), and unassertiveness (Lange & Jakubowski, 1976). However, cognitive-behavioral principles and procedures increasingly have been extended to the treatment of problems in intimate interpersonal relationships, with a focus on modifying repetitive dysfunctional patterns of marital and family interactions.

There appear to be two major reasons for the current trend toward cognitive-behavioral intervention with relationship problems. First, when individuals seek therapy for the individually oriented problems typically treated with cognitive-behavioral therapies (e.g., depression, agoraphobia), the problems they present commonly include difficulties in their marital and family relationships. For example, research has indicated that depression and marital distress are positively correlated, that critical and overinvolved behavior by nondepressed spouses is associated with relapse of their depressed partners' symptoms, and that the presence of a supportive spouse tends to prevent relapse of depression (Birchler, 1986; Epstein, 1985a; Hooley, 1985: Weissman & Paykel, 1974). Similarly, marriages between agoraphobic individuals and their spouses tend to become increasingly hostile and distressed over time, and a mixture of protective and withdrawing behaviors by the partner commonly reinforces and heightens the phobic's anxiety (Friedman, 1987). Consequently, clinicians have sought ways of treating symptoms of individual psychopathology and aspects of marital and family problems concurrently. One recent approach has been to use cognitive and behavioral interventions based on a social learning paradigm (Bandura, 1977) to modify both the intra- and interpersonal problems (Arnow, Taylor, Agras, & Telch, 1985; Bedrosian, 1988; Birchler, 1986; Epstein, 1985a).

---

NORMAN EPSTEIN • Department of Family and Community Development, University of Maryland, College Park, Maryland 20742.    DONALD H. BAUCOM • Department of Psychology, University of North Carolina at Chapel Hill, Chapel Hill, North Carolina 27514.

Second, research on relationship problems has identified several types of cognitions (which we will describe in this chapter) that can influence marital and family interactions. A growing body of empirical evidence has indicated that spouses' levels of satisfaction with their marriages depend significantly on how they appraise the meanings of their partners' behaviors. Clinically, it is common to find that one person changes his or her behavior in a manner requested by the partner, only to hear that the partner still is dissatisfied and attributes the change to factors such as pressure from the therapist rather than to "real" self-motivation. Thus it has become clear that attempts to assess and modify distressing marital interactions need to take cognitive factors into account.

A basic premise of cognitive-behavioral marital therapy is that dysfunctional interactions between spouses are influenced by both (1) problematic behavioral patterns (e.g., aversive behavioral exchanges; poor communication, problem-solving, and conflict-resolution skills), and (2) cognitions that are either distorted (invalid) or inappropriate. Distress in a marriage, which includes a cognitive component of dissatisfaction with the relationship and an affective component that can be a mixture of emotions such as anger, depression, anxiety, and jealousy depends on the ways in which spouses act toward each other *and* the ways in which they interpret each other's actions.

This chapter describes the types of cognitions and behaviors commonly involved in marital dysfunction, methods for assessing them, and procedures for modifying them. Because cognitive-behavioral marital therapy is a recent development, its procedures often are based as much on theory, extensions of established individually oriented cognitive-behavioral approaches, and the clinical experiences of marital therapists as they are on empirical findings. As the concepts and practices of cognitive-behavioral marital therapy are described in this chapter, it will be noted whether or not they have been supported by research results.

## TYPES OF COGNITIONS IN MARITAL DYSFUNCTION

When spouses describe aspects of their marriages that they perceive as the sources of their dissatisfaction, most commonly they focus on the *events* that occur between themselves and their partners, rather than their thought processes concerning those events. However, marital researchers and therapists have identified several types of cognitions that potentially can shape an individual's responses to events in his or her marriage. Because people tend to accept their own thoughts as reflections of reality and do not question these cognitions (Beck *et al.*, 1979; Nisbett & Ross, 1980), often the task of the marital therapist is to help spouses differentiate between appropriate and inappropriate cognitions. The appropriateness of a cognition can refer to either (1) the degree to which it is a *valid* representation of a reality that can be evaluated objectively, or (2) the degree to which it is a *reasonable* standard or explanation for events occurring in a marriage when no objective criteria exist for determining the reality of the situation. Thus one could assess the validity of a man's thought, "My wife will not compromise with me about child-rearing practices," by observing her behavior during a series of problem-solving discussions between the spouses concerning that topic, whereas one can judge how reasonable it is for this man to live by a standard such as "a wife should *always* be willing to compromise her ideas if her husband disagrees with her."

A cognitive-behavioral approach to marital problems focuses on how spouses often process information about their relationships inappropriately, either deriving invalid conclusions about events, or evaluating those events according to unreasonable standards. A growing body of research on cognitive factors in individual psychopathology, on social cognition, and on cognitions associated with marital distress has provided support for this approach to understanding and treating marital dysfunction. Based on current theory and research, the

following five types of cognitions are believed to play roles in the development and maintenance of marital problems.

493

MARITAL THERAPY

## Assumptions and Standards

The terms *cognitive structures, knowledge structures,* and *schemata* have been used to describe an individual's internalized representations about rules or principles for categorizing objects, understanding the relationships among objects, solving problems, and taking actions toward achieving particular goals (Nisbett & Ross, 1980; Piaget, 1948; Seiler, 1984). Based on one's life experiences beginning in infancy, one develops increasingly complex concepts about the characteristics of objects (including people) and how one can relate to them. Once a cognitive structure (e.g., "parent," "teacher") has been established, it allows a person to understand and interact adaptively with events in his or her life. To the extent that an individual's cognitive structures are valid and reasonable representations of actual people and events, the individual enters new situations with a store of valuable information and does not need to learn about the situations by trial and error each time. Two major types of cognitive structures that appear to influence marital interaction are (1) *assumptions* about the nature of the world and about correlations among characteristics of objects and events, and (2) *standards* about how objects and events "should" be.

### Assumptions

Two types of assumptions that people develop about marriage are *personae* about the set of characteristics typical of someone in the role of "husband" or "wife" (or similar characteristics of roles in intimate nonmarital relationships) and *scripts* about how two members of a relationship interact with one another. A persona about a person in a particular role such as "husband" includes both a set of characteristics and a set of assumed correlations among those characteristics (Nisbett & Ross, 1980). For example, an individual may assume that the typical husband tends to be motivated to provide for his family financially, is caring, fairly nonexpressive concerning emotions, and dominant in family decision making. Furthermore, the individual may assume that the degrees to which husbands are caring and are motivated providers are highly correlated, whereas the correlation between caring and emotional expressiveness is low. Consequently, whenever this individual meets a person whom he or she classifies as a "husband," he or she will assume that the person has the previously mentioned characteristics to some degree. When he or she observes that a particular husband has high or low degrees of particular characteristics, inferences will be made about the degrees to which the husband has the other (unobserved) characteristics. For example, from seeing that the husband describes himself as working long hours so that his family can live comfortably, the observer with the preceding "husband" persona would make an inference that this man cares deeply about his family. Of course, in the absence of other information about the man, it is possible that this inference is faulty.

Thus Nisbett and Ross (1980) note that when an individual assigns another person or object to a category based on observed characteristics, he or she uses personae to make inferences about unseen characteristics. Unfortunately, such inferences are much more susceptible to errors when they concern people (whose characteristics are quite variable) than when they concern concrete objects such as species of trees. People commonly hold stereotyped preconceptions about degrees of correlation among characteristics of others, and these preconceptions can produce biased inferences about a particular individual. On the one hand, a person who holds the assumption that "the more a husband cares about his spouse, the more he expresses loving feelings to her" may be likely to attribute a lack of caring as the cause of her own husband's lack of expressiveness, especially if her "husband" persona does not include other characteristics that could be associated with unexpressiveness (e.g., shyness). On the other hand, the same assumption may lead this woman to have an expectancy (prediction) that another man she knows who is emotionally demonstrative would provide a more caring relationship for her than her husband does. Both the causal attribution and the expectancy are shaped by an assumption about a link between caring and expressiveness that may not hold for this particular husband and male friend.

*Scripts* concerning marriage and other intimate relationships include assumptions about *sequences of events* that occur between partners. For example, an individual's script for "a sexual experience with my spouse" might include the following sequence: "I wait until my spouse doesn't seem busy with other things; then I behave mildly affectionately [hugs and kisses]; then, if my spouse reciprocates those gestures, I verbally suggest that love-making would be nice; and then if my spouse agrees, I initiate more intimate touching. If my spouse does not respond positively at any point, I back off and make no further sexual advances." As is the case with personae, scripts can vary in how valid or reasonable they are as representations of intimate relationships in general or of an individual's own relationship in particular.

Invalid or unreasonable assumptions can produce dysfunctional responses to relationship problems. For example, Epstein and Eidelson (1981) found that the more that distressed spouses assumed that partners cannot change a relationship and that disagreement is destructive to a relationship, the more they preferred individual therapy over marital therapy and the less likely they were to expect that therapy would improve their marital problems. Eidelson and Epstein (1982) also found that distressed spouses held these two assumptions significantly more strongly than did nondistressed spouses.

### Standards

Whereas people make assumptions about the way close relationships *are,* they also commonly have standards about the characteristics that they think a partner or relationship *should* have. Such extreme standards have been labeled *irrational beliefs* by rational-emotive therapists (e.g., Dryden, 1985; Ellis, 1986). Rational-emotive therapists have noted how (a) an individual may hold an extreme standard about marriage that no relationship could meet, and (b) people commonly become distressed when they make very negative evaluations (e.g., "It's *awful!*") as their real-life relationships fail to meet such standards.

Standards are not necessarily dysfunctional, because people's preferences and their ethical and moral standards commonly serve as functional guidelines for conducting satisfying relationships with others. However, a person's standards can become dysfunctional if they become extreme (i.e., setting goals that cannot be met or leaving no room for exceptions to the rule). An extreme standard can produce significant distress about a close relationship even when the individual does not apply an extreme evaluation to its violation (Epstein, 1986). The person experiences an accumulation of disappointments, none of which involves evaluations such as "this is awful" or "I can't stand it," but each of which chips away at the person's sense of satisfaction with the relationship. Thus it is important to evaluate the degree to which a couple's marital distress is associated with extreme standards *per se* versus extreme evaluations of standards not being met.

Marital distress has been found to be more highly related to extreme assumptions and standards specifically related to aspects of close relationships than to assumptions and standards less directly relevant to day-to-day interactions between spouses. For example, Epstein and Eidelson (1981) found that spouses' marital distress and low involvement in marital therapy were more highly correlated with unrealistic assumptions and standards about intimate relationships than with irrational beliefs about individual functioning (e.g., basing one's self-worth on approval from others). Also, Jordan and McCormick (1987) found that unrealistic assumptions and standards about relationships were more highly correlated with general marital distress than were extreme standards about sexual relationships. Thus it is important to assess the specific content of each individual's assumptions and standards that might contribute to marital problems, especially those cognitive structures that involve views about how close relationships function.

## PERCEPTIONS, ATTRIBUTIONS, AND EXPECTANCIES

As noted before, spouses can become upset about each other's actions even when that behavior does not violate standards about how partners "should" behave, as long as the partner is perceived as failing to act as one prefers or enjoys. Consequently, an individual's *perceptions* about what events occur and *inferences* about the meanings of those events can produce marital distress if they create a view of the relationship that is more negative than is appropriate.

### Perceptions

In any situation, an individual is likely to notice only part of the wealth of information that is available. Cognitive theorists and clinicians (e.g., Kelly, 1955) have stressed that perception is an active rather than a passive process of receiving information and that the information that an individual notices is susceptible to selective attention (Beck *et al.*, 1979; Nisbett & Ross, 1980). The aspects of a situation that an individual notices are likely to depend on factors such as the individual's emotional state, his or her level of fatigue, prior experiences in similar situations, and preexisting cognitive structures (e.g., an individual's persona for "husband" or "wife"). For example, Weiss (1980) has suggested that the impact that one partner's message has on the other partner is determined more by the overall positive or negative feeling that the receiver of the message has for the sender than it is determined by the actual quality of the message. Thus, according to this concept of "sentiment override," a woman may send her husband what she and outside observers would agree is a constructive message (e.g., a suggestion that they cooperate with each other on a household task), but her husband might experience the message as negative if he already is generally dissatisfied with her or their relationship. Similarly, Beck and his associates (e.g., Beck *et al.*, 1979) have described how depressed individuals often make a cognitive error of "selective abstraction" in which they tend to notice negative aspects of situations and overlook positive ones. This process also has been noted by marital therapists (e.g., Jacobson & Margolin, 1979) who use the term *negative tracking* to describe how distressed spouses tend to pay selective attention to negative aspects of their interactions. Because spouses commonly are unaware that their perceptions of their marital interactions are incomplete and therefore biased, it is important that marital therapists identify possible biases in a couple's perceptions and help them become more objective observers of their own relationship. Procedures for accomplishing these goals are described later in this chapter.

### Attributions

It appears to be a natural human tendency for people to search for causal explanations of events that occur in their lives (Baucom, 1987). Attributions are people's explanations for the factors that have caused specific pleasant or unpleasant events, and such inferences seem to serve a number of functions for members of intimate relationships, such as increasing an individual's sense of understanding and control over complex events that occur in his or her marriage.

Attributions have been the cognitions most frequently studied by marital researchers

NORMAN EPSTEIN
and DONALD H.
BAUCOM .

(Baucom, 1987; Thompson & Snyder, 1986), and the attributions most commonly investigated have been the global/specific, stable/unstable, and internal/external dimensions derived from the learned helplessness theory of depression (Abramson, Seligman, & Teasdale, 1978). Use of these dimensions by marital researchers makes sense because of the many cognitive and behavioral similarities between marital dysfunction and depression, such as a sense of hopelessness and helplessness to change an unpleasant life situation, "tracking" of negative events, and communication and problem-solving skill deficits (Epstein, 1985a). An important attributional difference between depression and marital distress concerns "internal" attributions. These focus only on the self in the learned helplessness theory of depression (i.e., depressed people attribute their problems to internal characteristics of themselves, such as a lack of intelligence), but, in marital attributions, one must differentiate between causes that spouses see as internal to the self and those that they see as internal to their relationship (Baucom, 1987; Fincham, 1985). Distressed spouses tend to assign responsibility for marital problems to factors internal to their relationships but most often by blaming their partners. However, when a marriage includes a depressed member, it is fairly common for both spouses to view that individual as the cause of their relationship problems (Baucom, 1987).

In studies of marital attributions, the most consistent findings have been that distressed spouses see the causes of their partners' negative behaviors as more global and stable (i.e., traits) than do nondistressed spouses, but nondistressed spouses see *positive* partner behaviors as due to global and stable causes more than distressed spouses do. This pattern suggests that members of distressed couples attribute their problems to global, stable factors that offer little hope for improvement, and they tend to discount positive spouse behaviors as fleeting events. Even if distressed spouses are at least partly accurate in attributing their partners' unpleasant behaviors to traitlike characteristics, such a view has great potential to undermine any efforts toward improving relationships because it easily leads to a conclusion that the situation is hopeless.

Marital distress also has been found to be higher when individuals attribute their relationship problems to negative characteristics of their partners, such as negative or malicious intent, lack of love, blameworthiness, and selfish motivation (Epstein, Pretzer, & Fleming, 1987; Fincham, Beach, & Nelson, 1987; Fincham & Bradbury, 1987; Pretzer, Epstein, & Fleming, 1985). Fincham, Beach, and Nelson (1987) found that such attributions can be more highly associated with marital distress than are attributions concerning dimensions such as global/specific and stable/unstable. Thompson and Snyder (1986) reviewed the attribution research literature and concluded that it is important to assess a variety of attributions that spouses make about the causes of each other's behaviors.

The results of research on marital attributions suggest that therapists need to evaluate whether spouses are making inaccurate attributions about events in their relationships, which can: (1) intensify the impacts of negative partner behaviors; (2) lead them to discount positive acts; or (3) produce negative reactions to partner behaviors that are judged by the partner and outside observers as actually neutral or positive. If such attributions are inaccurate, the cognitive restructuring procedures described in this chapter can be applied. However, if the attributions appear to be well founded (e.g., an individual's partner in fact seems to be acting aversively due to malicious intent), other clinical interventions such as training both spouses in the use of more constructive conflict-resolution skills would be more appropriate.

*Expectancies*

Based on a variety of learning experiences, (e.g., first-hand life experiences; observing events in others' lives), people come to anticipate different consequences for alternative actions in certain situations; that is, they make predictions about what is likely to occur. They then behave in particular ways (and avoid behaving in other ways) so that they will be likely to produce desirable rather than undesirable outcomes (Bandura, 1977; Rotter, 1954). Two major types of such expectancies described by Bandura (1977) are *outcome expectancies* (an individual's predictions that particular actions will result in particular outcomes in certain situations) and *efficacy expectancies* (the person's estimates of the probabilities that he or she will be able to carry out those actions that would produce those outcomes). Concerning outcome expectancies, in intimate relationships such as a marriage, individuals develop many expectancies that take an "if–then" form. These can include predictions about: (1) how one's partner will react to one's actions (e.g., "If I disagree with him, he'll most likely criticize my opinion"); (2) how one will react to the partner's actions (e.g., "If he criticizes me, I'm sure that I'll lose my temper and yell"); and (3) outcomes of joint actions (e.g., "If we have verbal battles in front of our adolescent children, they will avoid being at home").

As is the case with attributions, expectancies are inferences that can vary in their accuracy. However, an individual who is in the process of making such predictions does not tend to differentiate between accurate and inaccurate expectancies, and faulty predictions may guide his or her behavior as much as the valid ones do. Doherty (1981a,b) has proposed that when members of intimate relationships have low efficacy expectancies (i.e., they do not believe that they have much chance of carrying out solutions to their relationship problems), regardless of whether or not these expectancies are accurate, these individuals are less likely to engage in collaborative attempts to resolve their problems.

Pretzer *et al.* (1985) found that the lower spouses' efficacy expectancies were regarding their abilities to solve their marital problems, the higher were their levels of marital distress, depression, and their tendencies to attribute relationship problems to negative characteristics of their partners (negative behavior, stable personality traits, malicious intent, and a lack of love). Such results are correlational and cannot determine the direction of causality (whether negative expectancies produce marital distress, whether distress produces negative expectancies, or whether some third factor produces both of them). However, the results do indicate that distressed couples often have quite negative expectancies, and it is likely that marital therapists will need to alter these if they are to have success in motivating spouses to put effort into therapeutic tasks intended to modify unpleasant aspects of their relationships.

Research on the roles of assumptions, standards, perceptions, attributions, and expectancies in marital dysfunction is still in an early stage. As noted earlier, most attention has been focused on attributions, and much more work is needed to clarify how each of the five types of cognitions influences how spouses interact with one another. Also, much more knowledge is needed about how the types of cognitions are interrelated (e.g., whether the long-standing assumptions one has about close relationships in fact determine the attributions and expectancies one forms in a new relationship). Nevertheless, it seems prudent that a cognitive-behavioral approach to marital therapy include assessment of all five types of cognitions and modification of any assumptions, standards, perceptions, attributions, and expectancies that are contributing to destructive and dissatisfying interactions between partners.

## TYPES OF BEHAVIORS IN MARITAL DYSFUNCTION

A substantial amount of research has been devoted to identifying specific behaviors that differentiate distressed from nondistressed couples. This focus on couples' behavioral interactions has been based on a social learning view that the overt behaviors and covert responses (e.g., cognitions) of two members of a relationship continuously interact in a pattern of mutual influence (Bandura, 1977) and that the quality of a relationship is determined by (1) the amounts of positive and negative behavior exchanged by the two parties, and (2) the degree to which the couple has adequate skills for communicating, solving problems, and resolving conflicts (cf. Stuart, 1980).

NORMAN EPSTEIN
and DONALD H.
BAUCOM

It has been found consistently that members of distressed couples exchange more negative verbal behaviors (e.g., putdowns, criticisms, disagreements) and more negative nonverbal behaviors (e.g., inattention, staccato voice) than nondistressed spouses (Bornstein & Bornstein, 1986; Schaap, 1984). Distressed couples also engage in more negative behavior (e.g., coercive acts and personal attacks) and less constructive behavior (e.g., offering a compromise) during problem-solving discussions than nondistressed couples. Although the results are not as consistent, compared to nondistressed spouses, distressed spouses also tend to exhibit fewer positive verbal behaviors (e.g., approval, agreement) and fewer positive nonverbal behaviors (e.g., smiles, tender voice) (Baucom & Adams, 1987).

Studies of interaction *sequences* between partners (Gottman, 1979; Raush, Barry, Hertel, & Swain, 1974; Revenstorf, Hahlweg, Schindler, & Vogel, 1984) have indicated that distressed couples are more likely than nondistressed couples to engage in behavioral patterns during problem solving that either fail to resolve, or even escalate, conflicts. For example, Revenstorf *et al.* (1984) describe a sequence of "problem escalation" in which each time one spouse makes a description of a problem, the other responds negatively, and a pattern of "distancing" in which positive communications by one spouse are followed by negative responses from the other. In general, interactions of distressed couples are characterized by more *negative reciprocity* (in which a negative response from one person produces a negative response from the other) than those of nondistressed couples (Billings, 1979; Gottman, Notarius, Markman, Banks, Yoppi, & Rubin, 1976; Margolin & Wampold, 1981; Raush *et al.*, 1974).

Based on the social learning model and the research findings described before, behaviorally oriented marital therapists have focused their treatments on the goals of: (1) decreasing negative behavioral exchanges between spouses, (2) increasing positive exchanges, (3) improving communication skills (especially those for self-expression and listening), and (4) building problem-solving and conflict-resolution skills. The basic principles and procedures of these interventions that are used in cognitive-behavioral marital therapy are described later in this chapter.

## THE ROLE OF EMOTION IN COGNITIVE-BEHAVIORAL MARITAL THERAPY

The focus on cognitions and behaviors in cognitive-behavioral marital therapy by no means reflects a lack of attention to emotions in intimate relationships. To the contrary, this approach includes an assumption that the pleasant and unpleasant emotions experienced by spouses constitute a major part of what makes a relationship satisfying or not. Intimate relationships such as marriage can elicit a wide range of types and intensities of emotions (e.g., anger, happiness, anxiety, euphoria, rage, depression, jealousy, contentment), and cognitive-behavioral marital therapists attempt to identify factors that are producing an excess of unpleasant emotions or a deficit of pleasant ones.

In the cognitive-behavioral model, to a significant degree, the emotional quality of a relationship is assumed to be a function of: (1) the proportions of pleasant and unpleasant behaviors exchanged by the partners, (2) the couple's proficiency with communication and problem-solving skills that allow them to resolve conflicts and maximize the degree to which each person attains his or her personal goals and desires in the relationship, and (3) cognitions that influence how positively or negatively partners experience their behavioral interactions.

This model also posits that emotional states can influence spouses' behaviors and cognitions. For example, emotions such as depression, anger, and anxiety (as well as positive emotions) can influence the perception of events and memories of past events in a relationship (see Bradbury and Fincham's, 1987, review for a summary of research in this area). Weiss's

(1980) concept of sentiment override is an example of how an individual's general feeling about a relationship can determine whether he or she perceives the partner's messages as positive or negative, regardless of the objective quality of those messages.

Although a cognitive-behavioral approach assumes that emotions, behaviors, and cognitions have reciprocal influences on one another as two people interact, the therapeutic interventions focus mostly on altering cognitions and behaviors that influence emotions. In contrast to the sets of well-developed interventions for modifying problematic cognitions and behaviors (drawn largely from established procedures of individual cognitive therapy and behavioral marital therapy), techniques for altering emotions directly are limited.* Consequently, the major interventions used in cognitive-behavioral marital therapy are: (1) *skill training* (e.g., training in the expression of emotions and thoughts, listening skills, and problem-solving skills); (2) *behavior exchange procedures* (e.g., contracting) to decrease the exchange of aversive behaviors and to increase positive exchanges; and (3) *cognitive restructuring* to alter invalid and unreasonable cognitions that produce or exacerbate distress. An exception to this strategy of focusing primarily on cognitions and behaviors is when chronic or severe emotional states (e.g., depression, anxiety) interfere with spouses' abilities to participate in cognitive and behavioral procedures. In such situations, direct modification of the emotions (e.g., pharmacotherapy, systematic desensitization of anxiety responses) may be pursued, either prior to or concurrently with cognitive-behavioral marital therapy.

## METHODS FOR ASSESSING PROBLEMATIC BEHAVIORS

The following is a description of the major goals and procedures for identifying the presence and absence of behaviors and behavior sequences that are contributing to a couple's marital distress. Because it is beyond the scope of this chapter to provide detailed descriptions of all the existing assessment instruments and the empirical evidence regarding their reliability and validity, the interested reader can consult excellent reviews such as those by Margolin and Jacobson (1981) and Weiss and Margolin (1977).

### INITIAL INTERVIEW(S)

In practice, the purposes of the initial interview(s) are to establish rapport with both members of a couple and to collect specific information about behaviors and cognitions that are influencing their relationship satisfaction. Because spouses commonly are more attuned to upsetting behaviors than to cognitions such as attributions and assumptions when they begin therapy, the initial sessions tend to focus more on behaviors than cognitions. The behavioral assessment easily can require 2 to 3 hours, which might be conducted in one extended session or over a few shorter weekly sessions. Some cognitive assessment (described in the next section) is likely to be conducted at this time as well, but for the purpose of clarity, the behavioral and cognitive aspects of assessment will be described separately in this chapter.

The initial assessment consists of four major phases: (1) a marital history to place current concerns in perspective; (2) identification of current concerns *and* relationship strengths; (3) an actual communication sample, wherein the couple holds one or more brief discussions as the

---

*Greenberg and Johnson (1986) have developed an emotionally focused approach to couples' therapy using experiential techniques drawn from gestalt and client-centered approaches. By helping spouses to become more aware of and to express emotions that typically are not shared with one another (especially fear and feelings of vulnerability), the therapist allows the couple to experience each other in new (more benign) ways and thereby motivates them to interact in new and more constructive ways. The process of therapy tends to focus on evoking feelings rather than changing them directly, and cognitive shifts (perceiving the self and the partner differently) are assumed to produce more satisfying behavioral interactions.

therapist observes their interaction pattern; and (4) a summary discussion in which the therapist provides the couple with detailed feedback about the behavioral and cognitive factors that appear to be contributing to their distress.

### Marital History

Asking a couple to describe the specific conditions under which they met provides a fairly nonthreatening way to ease them into talking about their relationship, and, for many couples, it is a pleasant experience recalling what were often exciting and even humorous events. The spouses' responses to a subsequent question about what initially attracted them to each other can serve a number of purposes. First, this continues a positive focus on the relationship; second, it provides information about qualities of each partner that, at least in the past, were reinforcing for the other; and third, it helps the therapist identify shifts that occurred over time in either the characteristics and behaviors of the partners *or* the ways in which the two people perceived those characteristics and behaviors (i.e., cognitive rather than behavioral changes). When a spouse's description of his or her partner's behavior over the course of their relationship reveals that the behavior has remained fairly consistent but that the meanings that these actions have for the former individual have shifted from positive to negative, it is likely that significant attention to cognitive factors in the relationship will be needed. In contrast, when an individual describes how specific changes in a partner's behaviors over time have been associated with the development of marital conflict, the behavioral interventions of cognitive-behavioral marital therapy are likely to be relevant.

The therapist continues the relationship history by asking the spouses to recount the events that occurred in their life together over the years (e.g., the decision to get married (if relevant), job changes, moves, births of children, serious illnesses) as well as how they interacted with each other as those events unfolded. The therapist might learn that the couple has had a chronic pattern of arguing with each other (suggesting an entrenched pattern that might be more difficult to alter), or it may become clear that the couple handled conflicts constructively until a major stressor such as unemployment disrupted their lives.

Posing a question to the couple about the circumstances surrounding their decision to get married can reveal factors that have had a lasting impact on the quality of the relationship. For example, when a couple decided to marry due to parental pressure, desire to escape from an unpleasant parental home, or an unplanned pregnancy, the spouses often have chronic nagging doubts about their own and each other's commitment to the relationship. Thus, the couple's responses to this question provide both behavioral and cognitive data.

The next major question posed during the marital history is when either member of the couple first became aware that their relationship was experiencing significant problems, what they did about it (e.g., approaching the partner to discuss it), and which strategies were and were not helpful. The couple's descriptions of this process provide information about how observant each tends to be about relationship events, what behaviors each defines as problematic, and the range and effectiveness of the couple's problem-solving skills.

A question about how and when the couple decided to seek assistance for their problems can reveal any differences in the two spouses' levels of motivation for therapy. It also is useful to ask about any past therapy experiences and each person's expectations about the nature of marital treatment. When spouses do not expect an active and structured approach to building behavioral and cognitive skills, the therapist is likely to need to socialize the couple into the cognitive-behavioral approach (e.g., by providing a theoretical rationale concerning the roles that behaviors and cognitions such as attributions play in relationship problems, describing the procedures, and emphasizing how experience and research have demonstated that structured interventions help break chronic dissatisfying patterns).

It is helpful to discuss each partner's concerns about their relationship individually, with the other partner just listening, in order to avoid arguments about the nature of the problems or about who is at fault. The therapist's goal is to clarify what behaviors are occurring or not occurring that concern each individual. Each spouse is instructed to be concrete and specific in describing behavioral excesses and deficits. It often is quite helpful to have the spouses complete a questionnaire that surveys such behaviors prior to this interview and then to review their responses during the interview, asking them to clarify what does or does not occur in their own relationship. Questionnaires that can be used in this manner are described next. Inventories that cover numerous behaviors have an advantage of providing a quicker and more comprehensive overview of a couple's concerns than normally is possible in an open-ended interview where the therapist merely asks the spouses what their concerns are.

The following are brief descriptions of the major self-report questionnaires available for assessing marital behaviors. For more detailed descriptions, see reviews by Margolin and Jacobson (1981) and Weiss and Margolin (1977).

The Areas-of-Change Questionnaire (Weiss, Hops, & Patterson, 1973) asks each spouse to rate each of 34 behaviors twice: (1) noting whether he or she would like the partner to behave more, less, or not change in each area of marital interaction, and (2) how much the respondent believes that the partner wants him or her to change in each area. The items cover areas such as housekeeping and meals, finances, communication, relatives, friends, sex, work habits, children, leisure time, and physical abuse. For each item, the respondent also rates whether or not the area is one of major importance for the relationship. The therapist also can use items rated as needing no change as data concerning strengths of the relationship. It is important to note that this scale assesses spouses' *perceptions* about marital behaviors, rather than actual behaviors that do or do not occur. This does not diminish its utility because, in a cognitive-behavioral approach, it is often such perceptions of behavior that become the targets of therapeutic interventions.

The Dyadic Adjustment Scale (DAS; Spanier, 1976) is a self-report inventory widely used as an index of overall marital adjustment. It reliably discriminates clinical from non-clinical couples and has been a sensitive measure of improvement in response to behavioral marital therapy. A factor analysis of its 32 items yielded four factors: (1) Dyadic Consensus (the degree to which the partners agree on matters of importance to the relationship); (2) Dyadic Cohesion (the degree to which the couple engages in activities together); (3) Dyadic Satisfaction (the degree to which each partner is satisfied with the relationship and committed to its continuance); and (4) Affectional Expression (the degree to which each spouse is satisfied with the couple's expression of affection and sex) (Spanier & Filsinger, 1983). The Consensus items can be used to supplement information from the Areas-of-Change Questionnaire, identifying how much the partners *agree* (at least overtly) about various areas.

Another inventory that is useful in identifying particular areas of marital discord is Snyder's (1979) Marital Satisfaction Inventory. This 280-item true/false inventory, which can be completed in approximately 30 minutes, includes scales for global distress and the areas of affective communication, problem-solving communication, time together, disagreement about finances, sexual dissatisfaction, role orientation, family history of distress, dissatisfaction with children, and conflict over child rearing. It is wise to supplement this and the other scales by asking spouses whether they have any areas of concern not covered by the questionnaire items.

In contrast to the previously mentioned inventories that ask respondents for summary evaluations of various areas of their relationships, the Spouse Observation Checklist (SOC; Weiss *et al.*, 1973) asks each spouse to record which of 408 specific behaviors occur in a particular 24-hour period. Each person focuses on their spouse's behaviors, as well as some joint behaviors (e.g., "We went jogging or bicycle riding"). The items have been grouped into 12 content areas (e.g., affection, companionship, consideration, child care and parenting), and the respondent indicates that a behavior occurred by checking it as either a pleasing or displeasing act for the 24-hour period. The SOC is a long scale, and some couples are unlikely to cooperate with Weiss and Perry's (1983) recommendation that a couple be asked to complete it each 24 hours for 2 weeks. It also is important to note that, as with other reports of behavior, spouse reports on the SOC are susceptible to subjective perceptual processes (e.g., "negative tracking"). Thus it is necessary to exercise caution in interpreting SOC data.

All of the previously mentioned scales assess frequencies rather than sequences of behavior between spouses, so it often is helpful to ask a couple to monitor and take notes about the sequence of behaviors, thoughts, and emotions that occur during an interaction at home that involves a distressing aspect of their relationship. For example, if they are dissatisfied with their sexual relationship, they could be asked to monitor who does what, feels what, and thinks what, *in the sequence that these occur,* the next time they have sex.

### Evaluation of Communication

Although one must be cautious in generalizing from a sample of a couple's communication during a session in a therapist's office, the interaction patterns that are revealed still can be quite useful in identifying targets for intervention, such as high rates of aversive behavior exchanges and unclear self-expression. It is preferable to obtain more than one sample of a couple's communication because research has indicated limited stability of behaviors from one day to another (e.g., Haynes, Follingstad, & Sullivan, 1979).

Consistent with the distinction between expressive skills and problem-solving skills, a couple typically is asked to have two discussions while the therapist observes: one focused on expressing feelings to one another and the other focused on producing a solution to a problem in their relationship. Although systematic behavioral coding systems such as the Marital Interaction Coding System (MICS-III; Weiss & Summers, 1983) and the Couples Interaction Scoring System (CISS; Gottman, 1979) have been used extensively in marital research, they are not practical for clinical practice because they require many hours of training for coders and many hours to code even a brief tape of couple interaction. However, if clinicians become familiar with these behavioral coding systems and apply them informally, they are likely to be more sensitive to problematic behaviors when observing their clients during therapy sessions.

When a therapist observes problematic behavior such as inadequate expression of feelings, he or she is faced with determining whether this is due to an actual skill deficit or whether the spouses have the necessary skills but have failed to use them in their relationship for some reason. One clue to this answer is whether the spouses behave in a more positive and effective manner with the therapist than with each other. Also, information about the marital history can reveal whether the couple behaved differently in the past. Finally, an assessment of the spouses' cognitions as they interact negatively with each other in sessions can reveal whether their behaviors may be due more to choice than to skill deficits.

Spouses' own ratings of the quality of their communication are important because these have been demonstrated to be highly predictive of marital adjustment several years later (Markman, 1979, 1981). Spouses can be asked to rate the impact of each other's messages after each message is sent (Gottman, Notarius, Gonso, & Markman, 1976); they can rate videotape replays of their prior conversations (Weiss, Wasserman, Wieder, & Summers, 1981); or they can complete communication inventories such as the Primary Communication Inventory (Navran, 1967) and the self-report form of the Verbal Problems Checklist (Chavez, Samuel, & Haynes, 1981) that provide summary impressions of marital communication. Detailed descriptions of marital communication measures are available in Baucom and Adams (1987).

The behavioral summary provided to the couple typically consists of a profile of their strengths and weaknesses, including their frequencies of positive and negative behaviors exchanged, the specific conflictual areas of the relationship, and their strengths and weaknesses in communication and problem-solving skills. This summary is combined with a summary of the assessment of cognitions affecting the relationship, which is described next.

## ASSESSMENT OF COGNITIONS

The major methods for assessing marital cognitions are self-report questionnaires, clinical interviews, and the monitoring of *in vivo* cognitions by the therapist or the spouses themselves during couple interactions.

### QUESTIONNAIRES

The development of standardized questionnaires that survey potentially problematic marital cognitions is in its early stages. Eidelson and Epstein's (1982) Relationship Belief Inventory (RBI) assesses five schemata or cognitive structures theoretically related to relationship problems. These include the assumptions that disagreement is destructive to a relationship, that partners cannot change an established relationship, and that systematic differences between the two sexes cause marital problems. The RBI also includes scales assessing the unrealistic standards that spouses should be able to read each other's mind and that one must be a perfect sexual partner. The RBI has exhibited good reliability, validity, and sensitivity to change due to marital therapy.

A number of self-report scales have been developed to assess attributions that spouses make for positive and negative events in their relationship. Baucom, Bell, and Duhe's (1982) Dyadic Attribution Style Inventory (DASI) asks each spouse to rate the causes of hypothetical marital events on global/specific, stable/unstable and internal/external dimensions. A similar instrument was constructed by Fincham and O'Leary (1983). Recent investigations such as Fincham (1985), Holtzworth-Munroe and Jacobson (1985) and Fincham, Beach, and Baucom (1987) have had spouses use similar scales to rate causes of actual rather than hypothetical events from their marital interactions. The attributional dimensions assessed have included locus (self, spouse, the relationship, and outside circumstances), global versus specific, degree of stability, the partner's negative attitude toward the respondent, and the extent to which the partner was worthy of blame for the specific marital problem. As noted earlier, the inclusion of attributional rating dimensions assessing characteristics of the partner such as negative motives and blameworthiness is important because Fincham, Beach, and Nelson (1987) found these to be more strongly associated with marital distress than were attributions derived from learned helplessness theory.

Pretzer *et al.*'s (1985) Marital Attitude Survey (MAS) assesses spouses' attributions for marital problems in general, rather than for specified behaviors. As noted by Fincham (1985), couples who enter therapy generally make such global attributions for their problems. The MAS includes subscales tapping the locus of problems (own personality, own behavior, partner's personality, partner's behavior) and subscales assessing negative characteristics attributed to the partner (malicious intent, lack of love). The MAS also includes two subscales assessing *expectancies:* efficacy expectancies (perceived ability of the couple to change their relationship) and outcome expectancies (expectancy of improvement in the relationship). The MAS has demonstrated good reliability and validity, and it has potential in clinical practice as a screening instrument for potentially problematic attributions. The MAS and the other questionnaires that were described earlier can be used to stimulate exploration of cognitions with a couple by examining the spouses' responses on an item-by-item basis.

## INTERVIEW PROCEDURES

Assumptions, standards, perceptions, attributions, and expectancies can be assessed during clinical interviews in a number of ways. First, the therapist can probe for standards directly by asking each spouse about the ways that he or she believes a relationship "should" be. In a similar manner, personae can be tapped by asking each spouse questions such as "When you think of the characteristics that a wife [husband] tends to have, what comes to mind?" Scripts can be assessed by having the individual relate the sequence of events that he or she assumes occurs in a certain type of situation (e.g., a sexual encounter between two people married for several years).

Second, when a spouse reports a distressing event that occurred with the partner in the recent or distant past, the therapist can inquire about (1) any thoughts that the person remembers having at the time (which are likely to become more unreliable memories over longer periods of time), and (2) the distressing meanings that the event has for the person now.

Often the first cognition that an individual reports is not the most upsetting or significant one. Consequently, the therapist can search for other relevant meanings that an event has for the person by asking a series of questions that have the form, "If that is so, then what does that mean to you?" Basic underlying assumptions and standards also can be identified by looking for common themes in the situations and associated cognitions that are distressing to a spouse. In general, all of the interview techniques used for identifying significant cognitions in individual cognitive therapy (Beck *et al.*, 1979) are applicable in marital assessment, but *conjoint* marital interviews also offer the invaluable opportunity to tap cognitions as they occur *in vivo* when the spouses are interacting with each other.

## ASSESSING COGNITIONS *IN VIVO*

When a therapist observes shifts in a spouse's mood or behavior as the partners are interacting with one another during a session, he or she then can interrupt the interaction and ask that individual about any thoughts that occurred at the point when his or her mood or behavior changed. This is likely to elicit relevant cognitions such as upsetting attributions and expectancies about the partner's behavior. It also may elicit direct statements of standards or assumptions (e.g., "I became angry when he said he wanted to spend more time with his friends because he shouldn't need to do that if we have a good marriage").

As is the case in individual cognitive therapy, spouses also can monitor and record their cognitions about ongoing marital interactions at home, using forms similar to the Daily Record of Dysfunctional Thoughts (Beck *et al.*, 1979) or more informal logs and diaries. The goal of such records is to capture the emotional and cognitive responses that each spouse has to the other's actions as soon and as accurately as possible, before time and other events obscure memory.

Recently, Holtzworth-Munroe and Jacobson (1985) and Stratton, Heard, Hanks, Munton, Brewin, and Davidson (1986) have developed coding systems for identifying attributions in couples' spontaneous conversations (e.g., noting causal conjunctives such as "because," "the reason that," and "due to"), and these systems may be of use to clinicians who wish to increase their ability to spot *in vivo* attributional activity during therapy sessions. This may at times allow the therapist to identify important cognitions without having to interrupt the ongoing interactions and inquire about the spouses' thoughts.

Based on a careful assessment of behavioral excesses and deficits, the behavioral components of cognitive-behavioral marital therapy involve (1) instructing spouses in ways of behaving less negatively and more positively with each other, and (2) training them in communication and problem-solving skills as needed. We often begin therapy with behavioral interventions because even small shifts in long-standing aversive exchanges can give distressed spouses hope that their relationship can be improved. Also, distressed spouses commonly enter therapy blaming each other for marital problems, and they can be resistant to examining their own cognitions as sources of difficulty until they perceive some change in their partners' negative behaviors.

## INCREASING POSITIVE AND DECREASING NEGATIVE BEHAVIOR EXCHANGES

Because many distressed spouses make little effort to behave nicely to their partners, one intervention strategy is simply to stress to them that they need to break this pattern and exchange more positive behaviors. It is not expected that this approach will have an impact on the complex issues facing most distressed couples, but it is intended to begin the process of having the couple think and act in ways intended to improve the general atmosphere of their relationship. Also, when there has been a long-standing "standoff" between the spouses, even small behavior changes can help each spouse recognize the other's efforts to improve the marriage.

One such technique is to have each spouse complete the Spouse Observation Checklist and then to ask each person to increase positives and decrease negatives by some percentage during the next week. A second strategy is to use "love days" (Weiss *et al.*, 1973) or "caring days" (Stuart, 1980), where partners are asked to alternate days and do something nice for the other person. They are asked to select positive behaviors that they realistically could continue in the future—acts of caring that will bring pleasure to the other person. For example, spouses who feel distant and typically spend little time together could be encouraged to select behaviors that would provide togetherness. The caring days technique is not likely to work if spouses cling to a belief that such special efforts should not be needed if a relationship is a good one, or if an angry spouse does not want to do nice things for the partner. In these circumstances, cognitive interventions often are needed to challenge unrealistic standards and other cognitions that block collaborative efforts to alter distressing interactions (e.g., "He doesn't deserve to be treated nicely"; "If I act positively toward her, she'll think there's no longer a problem between us"). Cognitive interventions often are needed when an individual's painful memories of how the partner treated him or her badly in the past leads the person to discount the partner's current positive acts and even to seek revenge.

*Behavioral contracts* are a more structured approach to changing the positives and negatives exchanged by a couple. In *quid pro quo* contracts, each spouse agrees to do specified positive things requested by the partner in return for the other doing specified positive things. In *good faith contracts,* each person agrees to perform positive behaviors requested by the partner and receives rewards of his or her own choosing for doing so. In other words, each person is rewarded for complying with the contract no matter what the other does.

Stuart (1980) uses much less formal agreements called *wholistic contracts,* which involve no contingencies. Each spouse lists 10 to 20 desired partner behaviors, and the partner agrees to do some unspecified number of these some time during the next week. The sense of choice and freedom involved in this approach is appealing for many spouses. The more legalistic forms of contracts can lead some individuals to discount their partners' positive behaviors with attributions such as "she only did it because she wanted me to do things for her."

NORMAN EPSTEIN
and DONALD H.
BAUCOM

In cognitive-behavioral marital therapy, communication problems are seen as excesses and deficits in specific types of behaviors, and the goal of therapy is to teach couples skills for more effective and constructive communication. Such skill training is intended not only to remediate present problems but also to give couples tools for preventing future problems.

The basic strategies for teaching communication skills are those typical of behavioral skill training: instruction, modeling, behavioral rehearsal, and feedback (Epstein, 1985b). The therapist provides detailed, concrete instructions to spouses about desirable and undesirable communication behaviors, using minilectures or written handouts. Models of good communication and poor communication can be provided by the therapist demonstrating them or by using videotaped examples when available. Having the couple rehearse the new behaviors during therapy sessions until they have mastered them is the crucial component of the cognitive-behavioral approach. As the spouses practice the skills, the therapist provides detailed feedback about behaviors that they are performing well and those that need to be altered. Thus, the therapist serves as a teacher and coach in this approach.

### Emotional Expressiveness Training

The expressive and empathic listening skills developed by Guerney (1977) are taught in order to clarify messages sent between spouses, increase a couple's sense of control over confusing marital interactions, and increase feelings of mutual respect between the partners.

Spouses are taught to take turns operating in expressive and listener modes, with specific guidelines for each mode. The expresser is to state his or her thoughts and emotions subjectively (not as absolute truth), to be as brief and specific as possible, to include any positive feelings he or she may have about the partner or situation, and to express him- or herself in a manner that conveys caring and empathy about the impact that the statements may have on the listener. The empathic listener is to attempt to place himself or herself in the partner's position and sense what the partner is thinking and feeling, to communicate accurate understanding of the partner's experience, and to convey acceptance of the partner's right to his or her thoughts and feelings. The listener's communication to the expresser should include acceptance through voice tone, facial expressions, and posture as well as concise restatements and summaries of the partner's most important thoughts and feelings. The guidelines for empathic listening include injunctions against asking questions (except for clarification), expressing one's own views, interpreting or changing the meaning of a partner's statements, offering solutions, or expressing judgments of what the partner has said.

Couples typically are asked to practice these skills first with benign topics, so that strong negative emotions do not disrupt their learning. If a couple feels very impatient to move quickly to "hot" topics, the therapist may decide to permit this but be much more active in coaching the spouses so that the experience is a successful one for them. Details about the guidelines for the expresser and listener modes, procedures for teaching spouses how to switch modes effectively, and guidelines for teaching couples all of these skills are provided by Guerney (1977).

### Other Communication Skills

Although there is no consensus among marital therapists concerning the most important communication skills, the following are commonly included in a cognitive-behavioral approach. These are taught as generally important but also as prerequisites to good problem-solving (which is described later).

Spouses are taught to use "I" statements and are discouraged from mind-reading or speaking for the other person. They are encouraged to make direct statements of their desires, rather than inhibiting such expressions. They are instructed to acknowledge their own contributions to marital problems and discouraged from blaming the other person. Other guidelines taught for good communication include not interrupting the partner, not trying to establish the "truth" regarding issues about which the spouses disagree, not using extreme terms such as "always" and "never," not sidetracking to other topics, acknowledging positives in the partner and relationship, focusing on the present rather than the past when engaged in problem solving, not applying trait labels to one's partner, avoiding "power plays" by using assertive rather than aggressive (coercive) messages, and avoiding guilt-induction messages (e.g., "If you really loved me . . ."). Additional behaviors that acknowledge a partner include eye contact, head nods, avoiding messages that "disqualify" the partner (e.g., "You don't know what you are talking about," "You must be too tired; you aren't making good sense"). The therapist uses instruction, modeling, behavior rehearsal, and feedback to help spouses become proficient in following these communication guidelines.

## PROBLEM-SOLVING TRAINING

Some marital therapists (e.g., Hahlweg, Schindler, Revenstorf, & Brengelmann, 1984, combine emotional expressiveness communication and problem-solving communication, but we tend to keep them separate in order to minimize the chance that expression of strong feelings might disrupt the cognitive processes involved in generating and agreeing on solutions to significant relationship problems. Once a couple has mastered both types of communication, we give them opportunities to integrate them.

The following are the problem-solving steps taught to couples:

1. Spouses are taught to make a clear, specific *statement of the problem,* in terms of behaviors that are occurring or not occurring that are of concern to them. Complex problems should be broken down into several more specific problems that can be solved one at a time. Blaming can be minimized if problems are stated as *joint* issues in which both parties are involved.
2. When both spouses state their willingness to discuss a problem as stated, the couple is to *consider alternative solutions.* Alternative approaches to this step are (a) having the couple evaluate each solution as it is proposed or (b) asking the couple to "brainstorm" a list of solutions without evaluating any of them until the list is complete. The second approach may be more feasible when spouses are sensitive to negative evaluations by their partners and might be inhibited rather than creative in thinking of possible solutions. Therapists may need to help couples combine aspects of two or more solutions in order to devise a compromise solution acceptable to both partners.
3. In *adopting a final solution,* spouses are asked to restate the proposal and reflect on whether it is a feasible one that they will be comfortable carrying out once they leave the therapist's office. The therapist "walks them through" the solution, helping them anticipate circumstances that may require them to alter the plan.
4. The couple then is asked to *select a trial period* for implementing their solution. Because spouses may have devised solutions quite different from their usual ways of behaving, a trial period allows them to propose a new solution after that period if the original one does not work well for him or her. A time-limited trial also can reduce spouses' fears of change, and it provides a built-in time for reviewing the effectiveness of the solution. It is important for the therapist to be sure that the solution is evaluated as planned, so that modifications can be made if needed. A spouse's lack of compliance with an agreed-upon solution must be explored in order to determine whether it

is due to an inappropriate solution (e.g., one for which the person lacks relevant skills) or due to cognitive/motivational factors (e.g., the person does not want to comply because he or she is angry at the partner about other issues).

The preceding is an outline of the steps involved in problem-solving training. More detail can be found in sources such as Bornstein & Bornstein (1986) and Jacobson and Margolin (1979).

# MODIFICATION OF PROBLEMATIC COGNITIONS

When an individual's perceptions, attributions, and expectancies about events in his or her marriage appear to be valid and his or her assumptions and standards about relationships seem reasonable, the focus of marital therapy is likely to be on modifying behavioral aspects of the couple's interactions such as problem-solving skills. However, when the evidence indicates the presence of inappropriate cognitions, cognitive restructuring procedures are used to develop more appropriate information processing.

## TEACHING COUPLES ABOUT THE COGNITIVE MODEL

Even when the cognitive-behavioral marital therapist's approach to testing the validity and reasonableness of cognitions makes intuitive sense to clients, in practice many spouses find the techniques foreign to their way of dealing with their thoughts. Some other clients may find the idea of questioning one's thoughts repugnant. Consequently, it is important for the therapist to spend some time socializing each couple into this approach by providing a reasonable rationale. Such a rationale is likely to be more compelling if the therapist can use material presented by spouses during their assessment interviews to illustrate how cognitions influence the emotional and behavioral responses that one has to one's partner. For example, when one man described how he "knew" his wife was angry at him for getting home late—because she left all the lights out in the house except the one in their bedroom—the therapist was able to explore with him how this attribution led him to enter the house already angry at his wife and to pick a fight with her. Once the potential for cognitive distortion has been demonstrated, many spouses are more willing to test their cognitions. This is especially the case if the therapist stresses that he or she does not assume that spouses have inappropriate thoughts consistently but wants to catch any such instances that *might* occur.

As is the case with behavioral interventions, the therapist acts as a teacher and coach in helping spouses develop skills for identifying problems in their own thinking and modifying them. Didactic presentations, modeling, and coaching of the spouses as they practice these skills are standard procedures. The therapist models the same type of collaborative relationship with the spouses (e.g., exploring alternatives to a cognition with an individual rather than debating with the person about its validity) as he or she expects them to have with each other.

## COGNITIVE RESTRUCTURING PROCEDURES

We tend to begin cognitive restructuring by building spouses' skills for monitoring their own stream-of-consciousness thoughts ("automatic thoughts" in Beck's model). The initial goal is to increase the couple's awareness of *any* thoughts and visual images that are associated with their emotional and behavioral responses to each other. Techniques for achieving this goal include asking about spouses' cognitions when their moods and behaviors shift during couple interactions and having each person keep logs of cognitions associated with distressing interactions at home.

Next, couples are given definitions and descriptions of perceptions, attributions, expectancies, assumptions, and standards as well as explanations of how these can influence marital problems. Each spouse is coached in identifying instances of each type of cognition in his or her ongoing thoughts. Many individuals are not as aware of their basic assumptions and standards as they are of their perceptions, attributions, and expectancies, perhaps because the schemata tend to be more global and because stream-of-consciousness thoughts can be logical extensions of schemata rather than statements of the schemata themselves. For example, the thought ''she's so self-centered!'' may be an extension of a belief that caring, sensitive spouses can read each other's minds. Consequently, at times it is necessary for the therapist to help a spouse identify repetitive themes in automatic thoughts that occur across a variety of distressing marital interactions in order to deduce the person's underlying assumption or standard.

*Reduction of perceptual errors,* especially when spouses notice only part of the information available during their interactions, can be facilitated by instructing and coaching them in being more systematic and thorough ''scanners.'' This can be done by (a) providing video and audiotape playback of couple interactions to test the spouses' memories, (b) asking spouses to keep logs of daily events at home using an unstructured diary format or a structured inventory such as the Spouse Observation Checklist described earlier, and (c) training the couple in expressive and empathic listening skills that focus their attention on the messages that they exchange.

The appropriateness of the *attributions* and *expectancies* that a spouse makes based on perceptual data can be tested through *logical analysis.* Using Socratic questioning (see Beck *et al.,* 1979), the therapist guides the client toward evaluating the logic or illogic of his or her inferences. For example, one therapist asked a man who attributed his recent erectile dysfunction to a lack of effort whether it made sense to him that men tend to get erections by deciding that it is the appropriate time for one and concentrating on doing so. The client was able to see that sexual arousal tends to follow from stimulating thoughts and that concentrating on arousal is likely to be a distraction from sexual stimuli.

Another form of logical analysis involves coaching a spouse in thinking of *alternative explanations* for an event, in order to evaluate whether the individual's attribution or expectancy is the most accurate or reasonable inference.

Logical analysis also can be used to evaluate the degree to which an assumption or standard ''makes sense.'' For example, one man who examined the logic of his assumption that overt disagreement between spouses is destructive to their relationship concluded that the assumption did not take into account that expressions of disagreement actually may deepen each person's understanding of the other's basic needs and values.

The validity or reasonableness of a cognition also can be tested by *gathering evidence* from a number of sources. The types of evidence that are most credible tend to vary from one person to another. First, a spouse may be asked to recount details of *past experiences,* with the present partner and in other relationships, that bear on the accuracy of a cognition. Past experiences commonly provide exceptions to thoughts involving absolute (e.g., ''always'' or ''never'') descriptions of events.

Evidence also can be gathered from *in vivo marital interactions* during sessions or at home. For example, a therapist can play back a tape of a couple's argument so that each spouse can better see his or her own contribution to the aversive interaction and thus blame the other person less for it. Spouses also can provide each other immediate feedback about inferences that they make about one another. For example, when one spouse concludes that ''he didn't answer my question because he didn't care how I felt,'' the partner might respond that his silence was due to strong guilt feelings about the injustices that his wife said he had committed. Written logs and diaries of events and their associated cognitions that occur at home also are sources of evidence about the validity of cognitions such as attributions. For example, a man's attribution that "she likes to spend time by herself because she is tired of living with me" might be challenged by a record that indicates that his wife exhibited pleasure during a number of their shared activities but tended to want solitude whenever she had a stressful day at work. Identification of discrepancies in two spouses' cognitions listed in written logs concerning shared experiences also can illustrate how personal inferences are subjective and how there usually are alternative inferences possible for most marital events.

Negative trait attributions also can be challenged with information gathered from the marital history interview. Abrahms (personal communication, 1985) has described a "flip–flop" phenomenon in which a partner's behavioral characteristic initially is attributed to a desirable trait (e.g., self-confidence) but later is attributed to a negative trait (e.g., snobbishness). Challenging negative trait attributions is easier when the therapist can help the individual see that neither the original nor the subsequent trait label is likely to be a complete explanation of the partner's behavior. Spouses then may be more able to see that most behaviors have both positive and negative qualities and that changes over time in what one finds pleasing may be due to changes in one's own interpretations rather than changes in a partner's personality.

A final source of evidence regarding cognitions is the use of *behavioral experiments,* in which spouses interact in a planned manner and monitor the outcome (e.g., to see whether an individual's expectancy of how his partner will respond to his assertive behavior is accurate).

Therapists also can assist spouses in *assessing the utility* of assumptions and standards by coaching them in listing the advantages and disadvantages of adhering to a particular schema. For example, a woman who held the assumption that "becoming close to another person results in being controlled by that person" was able to list several advantages of living by that assumption (e.g., keeping a distance from people helps one avoid a number of hurts and disappointments), but she also listed a number of significant disadvantages (e.g., one misses a sense of intimacy and opportunities to share one's personal concerns with another person). Spouses can help each other complete such lists of advantages and disadvantages during therapy sessions. When a spouse decides that it would be desirable to reduce the disadvantages of an assumption or standard, the therapist (and the partner) can assist in devising a revised schema that retains the positive philosophy of the original but is more reasonable. For example, the preceding assumption might be revised to be "becoming close to another person affords opportunities to share experiences and provide mutual support, but one also can retain one's own identity by pursuing one's own interests, values, and some independent time as well." Such a revised assumption will become more believable if the individual sets up behavioral experiments to test its validity in daily living.

## SUMMARY

Cognitive-behavioral marital therapy draws upon the principles and procedures of cognitive therapy and behavioral marital therapy and combines them in order to alter patterns in which negative interaction between two spouses is shaped by exchanges of dysfunctional behavior and by faulty information processing that increases the aversiveness that each person experiences from the other's actions. In treating distressed couples, it is important that the therapist be attuned to the uniqueness of each couple without preconceptions regarding the cause of marital distress for particular individuals. Thus some spouses need great assistance in expressing emotions, but others evidence deficits in problem-solving skills. Some spouses do cling to extreme and dysfunctional beliefs or standards, whereas unwarranted expectancies or predictions are the cognitions requiring intervention for other spouses. Many couples have a multitude of such cognitive and behavioral problems. It is the richness and multifaceted focus on a number of types of behaviors and cognitions that make cognitive-behavioral marital therapy a challenge for the clinician and a treatment approach with great promise for addressing a wide range of marital problems.

# REFERENCES

Abramson, L. Y., Seligman, M. E. P., & Teasdale, J. D. (1978). Learned helplessness in humans: Critique and reformulation. *Journal of Abnormal Psychology, 87,* 49–74.

Arnow, B. A., Taylor, C. B., Agras, W. S., & Telch, M. J. (1985). Enhancing agoraphobia treatment outcome by changing couple communication patterns. *Behavior Therapy, 16,* 452–467.

Bandura, A. (1977). *Social learning theory.* Englewood Cliffs, NJ: Prentice-Hall.

Baucom, D. H. (1987). Attributions in distressed relations: How can we explain them? In S. Duck & D. Perlman (Eds.), *Heterosexual relations, marriage and divorce* (pp. 177–206). London: Sage.

Baucom, D. H., & Adams, A. (1987). Assessing communication in marital interaction. In K. D. O'Leary (Ed.), *Assessment of marital discord* (pp. 139–182). Hillsdale, NJ: Lawrence Erlbaum.

Baucom, D. H., Bell, W. G., & Duhe, A. D. (1982, November). *The measurement of couples' attributions for positive and negative dyadic interactions.* Paper presented at the annual meeting of the Association for Advancement of Behavior Therapy, Los Angeles.

Beck, A. T. (1976). *Cognitive therapy and the emotional disorders.* New York: International Universities Press.

Beck, A. T., Emery, G., & Greenberg, R. L. (1985). *Anxiety disorders and phobias: A cognitive perspective.* New York: Basic Books.

Beck, A. T., Rush, A. J., Shaw, B. F., & Emery, G. (1979). *Cognitive therapy of depression.* New York: Guilford Press.

Bedrosian, R. C. (1988). Treating depression and suicidal wishes within the family context. In N. Epstein, S. E. Schlesinger, & W. Dryden (Eds.), *Cognitive-behavioral therapy with families* (pp. 292–324). New York: Brunner/Mazel.

Billings, A. (1979). Conflict resolution in distressed and nondistressed married couples. *Journal of Consulting and Clinical Psychology, 47,* 368–376.

Birchler, G. R. (1986). Alleviating depression with "marital" intervention. *Journal of Psychotherapy and the Family, 2*(3/4), 101–116.

Bornstein, P. H., & Bornstein, M. T. (1986). *Marital therapy: A behavioral-communications approach.* New York: Pergamon Press.

Bradbury, T. N., & Fincham, F. D. (1987). Affect and cognition in close relationships: Towards an integrative model. *Cognition and Emotion, 1*(1), 59–87.

Chavez, R. E., Samuel, V., & Haynes, S. N. (1981, November). *Validity of the Verbal Problems Checklist.* Paper presented at the annual meeting of the Association for Advancement of Behavior Therapy, Toronto.

Doherty, W. J. (1981a). Cognitive processes in intimate conflict: I. Extending attribution theory. *The American Journal of Family Therapy, 9*(1), 1–13.

Doherty, W. J. (1981b). Cognitive processes in intimate conflict: II. Efficacy and learned helplessness. *The American Journal of Family Therapy, 9*(2), 35–44.

Dryden, W. (1985). Marital therapy: The rational-emotive approach. In W. Dryden (Ed.), *Marital therapy in Britain* (Vol. 1; pp. 195–221). London: Harper & Row.

Eidelson, R. J., & Epstein, N. (1982). Cognition and relationship maladjustment: Development of a measure of dysfunctional relationship beliefs. *Journal of Consulting and Clinical Psychology, 50,* 715–720.

Ellis, A. (1986). Rational-emotive therapy (RET) applied to relationship therapy. *Journal of Rational-Emotive Therapy, 4,* 4–21.

Epstein, N. (1985a). Depression and marital dysfunction: Cognitive and behavioral linkages. *International Journal of Mental Health, 13*(3-4), 86–104.

Epstein, N. (1985b). Structured approaches to couples' adjustment. In L. L'Abate & M. A. Milan (Eds.), *Handbook of social skills training and research* (pp. 477–505). Wiley.

Epstein, N. (1986). Cognitive marital therapy: Multi-level assessment and intervention. *Journal of Rational-Emotive Therapy, 4,* 68–81.

Epstein, N., & Eidelson, R. J. (1981). Unrealistic beliefs of clinical couples: Their relationship to expectations, goals and satisfaction. *The American Journal of Family Therapy, 9*(4), 13–22.

Epstein, N., Pretzer, J. L., & Fleming, B. (1987). The role of cognitive appraisal in self reports of marital communication. *Behavior Therapy, 18*, 51–69.

Fincham, F. (1985). Attribution processes in distressed and nondistressed couples: II. Responsibility for marital problems. *Journal of Abnormal Psychology, 94*, 183–190.

Fincham, F., & Bradbury, T. N. (1987). Cognitive processes and conflict in close relationships: An attribution-efficacy model. *Journal of Personality and Social Psychology, 53*, 1106–1118.

Fincham, F., & O'Leary, K. D. (1983). Causal inferences for spouse behavior in maritally distressed and nondistressed couples. *Journal of Social and Clinical Psychology, 1*, 42–57.

Fincham, F., Beach, S. R. H., & Baucom, D. H. (1987). Attribution processes in distressed and nondistressed couples: 4. Self-partner attribution differences. *Journal of Personality and Social Psychology, 52*, 739–748.

Fincham, F., Beach, S. R. H., & Nelson, G. (1987). Attribution processes in distressed and nondistressed couples: 3. Causal and responsibility attributions for spouse behavior. *Cognitive Therapy and Research, 11*, 71–86.

Friedman, S. (1987). Technical considerations in the behavioral-marital treatment of agoraphobia. *The American Journal of Family Therapy, 15*, 111–122.

Gottman, J. M. (1979). *Marital interaction.* New York: Academic Press.

Gottman, J. M., Notarius, C., Gonso, J., & Markman, H. (1976). *A couple's guide to communication.* Champaign, IL: Research Press.

Gottman, J. M., Notarius, C., Markman, H., Bank, S., Yoppi, B., & Rubin, M. E. (1976). Behavior exchange theory and marital decision making. *Journal of Personality and Social Psychology, 34*, 14–24.

Greenberg, L. S., & Johnson, S. M. (1986). Emotionally focused couples therapy. In N. S. Jacobson & A. S. Gurman (Eds.), *Clinical handbook of marital therapy* (pp. 253–276). New York: Guilford Press.

Guerney, B. G., Jr. (1977). *Relationship enhancement.* San Francisco: Jossey-Bass.

Hahlweg, K., Schindler, L., Revenstorf, D., & Brengelmann, J. C. (1984). The Munich marital therapy study. In K. Hahlweg & N. S. Jacobson (Eds.), *Marital interaction: Analysis and modification* (pp. 3–26). New York: Guilford Press.

Haynes, S. N., Follingstad, D. R., & Sullivan, J. C. (1979). Assessment of marital satisfaction and interaction. *Journal of Consulting and Clinical Psychology, 47*, 789–791.

Holtzworth-Munroe, A., & Jacobson, N. S. (1985). Causal attributions of married couples: When do they search for causes? What do they conclude when they do? *Journal of Personality and Social Psychology, 48*, 1398–1412.

Hooley, J. M. (1985). Expressed emotion: A review of the critical literature. *Clinical Psychology Review, 5*, 119–139.

Jacobson, N. S., & Margolin, G. (1979). *Marital therapy: Strategies based on social learning and behavior exchange principles.* New York: Brunner/Mazel.

Jordan, T., & McCormick, N. B. (1987, April). *The role of sex beliefs in intimate relationships.* Paper presented at the annual meeting of the American Association of Sex Educators, Counselors and Therapists, New York.

Kelly, G. A. (1955). *The psychology of personal constructs.* New York: Norton.

Lange, A. J., & Jakubowski, P. (1976). *Responsible assertive behavior: Cognitive/behavioral procedures for trainers.* Champaign, IL: Research Press.

Markman, H. J. (1979). The application of a behavioral model of marriage in predicting relationship satisfaction of couples planning marriage. *Journal of Consulting and Clinical Psychology, 47*, 743–749.

Markman, H. J., (1981). The prediction of marital distress: A five-year follow-up. *Journal of Consulting and Clinical Psychology, 49*, 760–762.

Margolin, G., & Jacobson, N. S. (1981). Assessment of marital dysfunction. In M. Hersen & A. S. Bellack (Eds.), *Behavioral assessment: A practical handbook* (pp. 389–426). Elmsford, NY: Pergamon Press.

Margolin, G., & Wampold, B. (1981). Sequential analysis of conflict and accord in distressed and nondistressed marital partners. *Journal of Consulting and Clinical Psychology, 49*, 554–567.

Meichenbaum, D. H. (1977). *Cognitive-behavior modification: An integrative approach.* New York: Plenum Press.

Navran, L. (1967). Communication and adjustment in marriage. *Family Process, 6*, 173–184.

Nisbett, R., & Ross, L. (1980). *Human inference: Strategies and shortcomings of social judgment.* Englewood Cliffs, NJ: Prentice-Hall.

Novaco, R. (1975). *Anger control: The development and evaluation of an experimental treatment.* Lexington, MA: Heath.

Piaget, J. (1948). *The moral judgment of the child*. Glencoe, IL: Free Press.

Pretzer, J. L., Epstein, N., & Fleming, B. (1985). *The Marital Attitude Survey: A measure of dysfunctional attributions and expectancies*. Unpublished manuscript.

Raush, H. L., Barry, W. A., Hertel, R. K., & Swain, M. A. (1974). *Communication, conflict and marriage*. San Francisco: Jossey-Bass.

Revenstorf, D., Hahlweg, K., Schindler, L., & Vogel, B. (1984). Interaction analysis of marital conflict. In K. Hahlweg & N. S. Jacobson (Eds.), *Marital interaction: Analysis and modification* (pp. 159–181). New York: Guilford Press.

Rotter, J. B. (1954). *Social learning and clinical psychology*. Englewood Cliffs, NJ: Prentice-Hall.

Schaap, C. (1984). A comparison of the interaction of distressed and nondistressed married couples in a laboratory situation: Literature survey, methodological issues, and an empirical investigation. In K. Hahlweg & N. S. Jacobson (Eds.), *Marital interaction: Analysis and modification* (pp. 133–158). New York: Guilford Press.

Seiler, T. B. (1984). Developmental cognitive theory, personality, and therapy. In N. Hoffmann (Ed.), *Foundations of cognitive therapy: Theoretical methods and practical applications* (pp. 11–49). New York: Plenum Press.

Snyder, D. K. (1979). *Marital Satisfaction Inventory*. Los Angeles: Western Psychological Services.

Spanier, G. B. (1976). Measuring dyadic adjustment: New scales for assessing the quality of marriage and similar dyads. *Journal of Marriage and the Family, 38,* 15–28.

Spanier, G. B., & Filsinger, E. E. (1983). The Dyadic Adjustment Scale. In E. E. Filsinger (Ed.), *Marriage and family assessment* (pp. 155–168). Beverly Hills, CA: Sage.

Stratton, P., Heard, D., Hanks, H. G. I., Munton, A. G., Brewin, C. R., & Davidson, C. (1986). Coding causal beliefs in natural discourse. *British Journal of Social Psychology, 25,* 299–313.

Stuart, R. B. (1980). *Helping couples change: A social learning approach to marital therapy*. New York: Guilford Press.

Thompson, J. S., & Snyder, D. K. (1986). Attribution theory in intimate relationships: A methodological review. *The American Journal of Family Therapy, 14,* 123–138.

Watkins, J. T. (1977) The rational-emotive dynamics of impulsive disorders. In A. Ellis & R. Grieger (Eds.), *Handbook of rational-emotive therapy* (pp. 135–152). New York: Springer.

Weiss, R. L. (1980). Strategic behavioral marital therapy: Toward a model for assessment and intervention. In J. P. Vincent (Ed.), *Advances in family intervention, assessment and theory* (Vol. 1, pp. 229–271). Greenwich, CT: JAI Press.

Weiss, R. L., & Margolin, G. (1977). Assessment of marital conflict and accord. In A. R. Ciminero, K. D. Calhoun, & H. E. Adams (Eds.), *Handbook of behavioral assessment* (pp. 555–602). New York: Wiley.

Weiss, R. L., & Perry, B. A. (1983). The Spouse Observation Checklist: Development and clinical applications. In E. E. Filsinger (Ed.), *Marriage and family assessment* (pp. 65–84). Beverly Hills, CA: Sage.

Weiss, R. L., & Summers, K. J. (1983). Marital Interaction Coding System—III. In E. E. Filsinger (Ed.), *Marriage and family assessment* (pp. 85–116). Beverly Hills, CA: Sage.

Weiss, R. L., Hops, H., & Patterson, G. R. (1973). A framework for conceptualizing marital conflict, a technology for altering it, some data for evaluating it. In L. A. Hamerlynck, L. C. Handy, & E. J. Mash (Eds.), *Behavior change: Methodology, concepts, and practice* (pp. 309–342). Champaign, IL: Research Press.

Weiss, R. L., Wasserman, D. A., Wieder, G. R., & Summers, K. (1981, November). *Subjective and objective evaluation of marital conflict: Couples versus the Establishment*. Paper presented at the annual meeting of the Association for Advancement of Behavior Therapy, Toronto.

Weissman, M. M., & Paykel, E. S. (1974). *The depressed woman: A study of social relationships*. Chicago: University of Chicago Press.

# 26

# Cognitive Therapy with Children

RAYMOND DiGIUSEPPE

Recently, cognitive-behavior therapy has become the zeitgeist in psychotherapy. Despite this trend, the cognitive orientation has been slow to filter down to interventions with children. The majority of practitioners working with children use behavioral psychodynamic family-systems approaches to treatment. As a result, children are viewed as passive recipients of external influences. Although it is true that children are often dependent on others for much of their physical needs, cognitive theory would challenge the notion that children have no influence over their own emotional reactions and that their emotional disturbance is only the result of systemic variables or reward contingencies. Although such factors are obviously important in shaping children's psychological development, cognitions can be viewed as the mediational variables by which these external factors (family systems and behavioral contingencies) have their effect. One can change children's behavior by restructuring systems or by rearranging contingencies or, more directly and perhaps more efficiently, by attempting to change the child's cognitions directly.

As with adults, cognition theories would hypothesize that children's disturbed emotions are largely generated by their beliefs (Ellis, 1962, 1976, 1977, and 1979). Irrational ideas and distortions of reality are likely to create anger, anxiety, and depression in children just as they do with adults. In fact, because children are children—immature, less sophisticated, and less educated—one might expect them to make more cognitive errors than adults and to become upset more easily.

There has been considerable research on the role of cognitions in causing emotions in adults. However, researchers have failed to perform similar types of investigations with youngsters. Less evidence exists to support cognitive-behavior hypotheses with children. Although there is a great deal of literature on the cognitive intellectual development of children, research on the role of cognitions in children's social and emotional development is small by comparison (Urbain & Kendall, 1980). However, several studies have indicated that the cognitive constructs developed by Beck (1976) and Ellis (1962) can be measured in children and are correlated with measures of emotional disturbance (Bernard, 1988; Leitenberg, Yost & Carroll-Wilson 1986).

---

RAYMOND DiGIUSEPPE • Institute for Rational-Emotive Therapy, New York, New York 10021.

Many therapists can accept the notion that children's thoughts lead to their emotions on a theoretical level, yet they are skeptical that one can implement change by direct attempts to manipulate children's cognitions. It may be helpful here to remember Piaget's stages of cognitive development. According to Piaget, children enter the stage of concrete operations around the age of 7 or 8. The next, and final, stage of development, formal operations, occurs in adolescence. However, Piaget pointed out that many adults never reach the stage of formal operations. They remain in concrete operations for the remainder of their lives, the same stage they entered when they were 7 or 8. One is left with the startling conclusion that many an adult client is in the same Piagetian stage of cognitive development as a fourth-grader. One could argue, then, that children are capable of many of the logical processes necessary to participating in and benefiting from cognitive disputing. Children who have not yet reached the stage of concrete operations undoubtedly have a difficult time with logic and the disputing modes of cognitive therapy. However, such children can benefit from other types of cognitive interventions, such as verbal self-instruction or training in the solving of social problems, which do not require the logical manipulation of thoughts; in fact there is growing evidence that children and adolescents can understand the principles of rational-emotive (see Vernon, 1983, for a review) and Beck's cognitive therapy (Garber, Deal, & Parke, 1986).

Factor analytic studies of child psychopathology have consistently found two broad factors that account for most childhood emotional and behavior problems. Disorders are described or either internalized, overcontrolled, withdrawn, or as externalized, undercontrolled, and over active. The overwhelming majority of the theoretical research and clinical literature in cognitive behavior therapy focuses on the treatment of externalized disorders. These disorders are very dissimilar, and the problems and procedures of treatment are very different. The material presented in this chapter will focus primarily on internalized disorders.

## THEORETICAL ASSUMPTIONS

Cognitive-behavioral psychotherapies share similar views concerning the role of thinking in human emotion and behavior. We briefly describe three cognitive theories of maladjustment that have direct and practical implications for the treatment of childhood disorders. The distinctions between emotional and practical problems as well as rational and irrational beliefs are elaborated.

### COGNITIVE CONCEPTUALIZATION OF EMOTIONAL DISORDERS

Ellis (1962) has provided his now-famous ABC model to help clients grasp the role of their thoughts in causing emotional disturbance. Wessler and Wessler (1980) have recently expanded the ABC model to help therapists to a fuller understanding of these complex psychological events. At the start of every emotional event, a stimulus is presented to the child:

Step 1: Stimuli are then sensed by the person's eyes, ears, sense of smell, touch, and so forth.

Step 2: Sensory neurons process the stimuli and transmit them to the CNS.

Step 3: Not all sensations enter consciousness. Some are filtered out, and others are perceived. Perception is Step 3. Perception, however, is not an exact replication of reality. Perceptions consist of equal parts of information provided by the senses and information provided by the brain (Neisser, 1967). At this point, all information is organized, categorized, and defined. Perception is as much a peripheral as a CNS function.

Step 4: People usually do not stop thinking after they have perceived information. In most cases, they attempt to extract more information than is present in the perception, so some interpretations or inferences are likely to follow perceptions.

Step 5: Humans are not just passive processors of information. Inferences and conclusions usually have some further meaning associated with them. Conclusions and inferences may vary in their importance to an individual. Almost all inferences are evaluated either positively or negatively in relation to the person's life. This appraisal or evaluation lead to action tendencies or behavioral response sets that are learned.

Step 6: According to rational-emotive therapy, affect or emotion follows appraisal. We feel happy or sad or mad at Step 6, after we have appraised something as being beneficial, threatening, and the like.

Step 7: Emotional states are not separate psychological phenomena. Emotions have evolved as part of the flight–fight mechanism and exist primarily to motivate adaptive behavior. Therefore, emotions usually include not only the reactions of the autonomic nervous system and the phenomenological sensations, but action tendencies or behavioral response sets that are learned.

Step 8: Responses, once they are made, usually have some impact on the external world. This effect can be desirable or undesirable, and feedback of our action tendencies serves as a reward to strengthen or extinguish a response set.

Elements of the emotional episode are: (1) stimulus; (2) sensation; (3) perception; (4) inference; (5) appraisal; (6) affect; (7) action tendency; and (8) feedback.

Of these eight steps, cognitive theory focuses on Steps 4 and 5 as causes for disturbed affect at Step 6. Emotional disturbance develops because of one or two types of cognitive errors: empirical distortions of reality that occur at Step 4 (inferences) and exaggerated and distorted appraisals of inferences at Step 5.

Let us take a hypothetical clinical example to explain how these two cognitions operate. Harry, an 11-year-old, has moved to a new neighborhood and has not met new friends. While he sits in the neighborhood playground, the other children are running about. He feels frightened. As he sees the other children coming, Harry thinks, ''they'll never like me, they'll think I'm not very good at these games, and they won't play with me no matter what I do.'' Harry has drawn these inferences about the other children's behaviors. In fact, they are predictions about what might happen but never actually has happened. Inferences alone are not sufficient to arouse fear. Some children, although not Harry, might be perfectly happy to sit by themselves and read books, but Harry appraises this situation quite negatively and catastrophizes: ''It's awful that I don't have anyone to play with.'' ''I must be a jerk if they won't play with me.''

## SOCIAL PROBLEM-SOLVING VIEW OF MALADJUSTMENT

Most cognitive therapists (i.e., Beck & Ellis) focus on the presence of maladaptive, illogical, antiempirical, and irrational cognitions. Other cognitive theorists have taken a different perspective and see emotional disturbance as resulting from a deficit in the cognitions that are usually present in well-functioning children. Spivack, Platt, and Shure (1976) have identified several interpersonal cognitive problem-solving skills. Their research focused on developing psychometric measures of these skills and correlating them with psychopathology. So far, their research has been impressive, and they have identified several skills in solving social problems that consistently distinguish psychopathological from normal populations. The most important skill they have uncovered is alternative-solution thinking (i.e., the number of different solutions that a child can generate to solve a specific practical problem). The second most important skill, consequential thinking, measures children's ability to predict the social consequences or results of their actions. Once children can generate alternatives and predict sequences, the next skills that seem to be important are the ability to anticipate problems and the implementation of a solution to plan around them. Spivak and his colleagues have termed these "means–end thinking."

There is a growing body of research to suggest that attempts to teach children interpersonal, cognitive problem-solving skills can lead to reduced emotional upset and more adaptive behavior (Kendall & Branswell, 1985; Urbain & Kendall, 1980). Interpersonal, cognitive problem-solving skills can be effective for several reasons. Problem solving could occur after the inferences, the appraisals, or the affect. Effective problem solvers may experience disturbed affect less often because: (1) they distract themselves from the appraisal and thereby lift affect—as long as one is thinking about how to go about solving a problem, one is less likely to be entertaining catastrophizing ideas and therefore to become upset; (2) social problem solving may bring about solutions to change the activating event and thereby eliminate the problem in the first place; and (3) thinking of alternative solutions may help one change one's appraisal of a negative event. People who believe they have options may be less likely to view events as awful or catastrophic.

## OVERVIEW OF COURSE OF THERAPY

There are four discernible stages in applying cognitive-behavioral approaches with children: (1) rapport building; (2) assessment; (3) skill acquisition; and (4) practice and application. We have already alluded to the necessity of building a relationship with a young client to maximize the likelihood that the child will be open about thoughts and actions. To facilitate self-disclosure, three strategies have been recommended:

1. Don't be all business. If your initial expectations are too high, the child may find the sessions aversive and then just not talk to you. Allow the child some time to get acquainted with you through play and off-task conversation. Shaping can be used to develop the self-disclosure and on-task conversation required in therapy.
2. Always be honest with the child. Children are more cautious than adults, probably because they are more vulnerable. They appear to be sensitive to deception, which they use as a measure of a person's trustworthiness.
3. Go easily and carefully on the questions. Children do not trust those who try to give them "the third degree" (DiGiuseppe, 1981, p. 56)

Waters (1982) indicated that self-disclosure can be learned quite effectively if the practitioner (1) is a good model for self-disclosure; (2) accepts whatever the child says without putting her or him down; and (3) reinforces the child for disclosing.

There are two distinct sets of skills taught during skill acquisition: emotional problem-solving skills and practical problem-solving skills (see Waters, 1982). Teaching children to solve their own emotional problems involves their initially understanding and expressing their emotions. Techniques for building emotional awareness have been discussed in the problem assessment section. Children begin to understand that there is a difference between helpful and hurtful feelings, that feelings come from thoughts, and that their thoughts control their feelings. A second step taken in emotional problem solving is teaching the relationship between thoughts and feeling.

Interpersonal cognitive problem-solving training may be the most appropriate treatment with certain children. Some children are not severely upset when they misbehave. They do not experience disturbed affect and do not appear to have irrational beliefs. Such children may think rationally and may manifest appropriate affect but behave in a self-destructive or anti-social manner because they do not have an adequate alternative response. This repertoire deficit might exist because of poor modeling or poor training. Children who do have irrational beliefs at the appraisal stage and who do have disturbed affect may still fail to behave appropriately (once they have changed their irrational beliefs and reduced their affect) because of the same limited repertoire at the action potential level. Here, interpersonal cognitive problem-solving skills may be a very important component of a comprehensive treatment plan. Many disturbed children have irrational beliefs, disturbed affect, and a limited action potential with few alternative adjusted responses. Thus, the comprehensive child therapist would be best advised to make sure that he or she teaches skills in solving both emotional and practical problems.

The final stage of therapy, practice and application, involves the practitioner's helping the young client to practice his or her newly acquired skills in problem situations at home and in school. In seeking to foster generalization, the child is given a variety of homework assignments.

## EMOTIONAL AND PRACTICAL PROBLEM SOLVING

In order to help the therapist clarify the goals of treatment, it is helpful to distinguish between emotional and practical problems. Emotional problems are generated by self-defeating and goal-defeating belief systems and are characterized by extremely uncomfortable, disturbed emotions. Practical problems are realistic difficulties or aversive stimuli in the environment resulting in unsatisfactory situations, which one desires to change.

In children, common emotional difficulties include anger, anxiety, and self-downing (depression), and practical problems are not having enough friends, getting into fights, being teased and not knowing what to do, and the like. It is frequently but not always the case that practical problems are accompanied by emotional problems and that, indeed, emotional problems often originate in practical problems.

Many therapists attempt to alleviate children's problems by removing the presenting problem. This may help temporarily, but it does not teach the child to develop cognitive coping skills that can be used when similar practical problems arise again.

By way of example, let us see the variety of ways of helping Harry, who has no friends. There are several ways. The first would be to play camp counselor and introduce Harry to new friends. This would be very helpful to Harry, and he would probably greatly appreciate it. However, it would not help Harry to learn to cope with fearful situations. This approach is the practical solution. Practical solutions change the stimuli or activating event. Although they are often effective in changing children's specific emotional episodes, they are palliative. Practical solutions assume that the child cannot learn to deal with the adversity on her or his own. Carried to extremes, it could become a self-fulfilling prophecy because the child would get no practice in solving emotional problems.

A second strategy to help Harry is to reduce his anxiety. There are two primary ways to teach a young client to resolve emotional difficulties. At the inferential stage in Wessler and Wessler's model, Harry believes that the other children will never like him. How does he know this to be true? He did not try to meet them. He most probably has had other friends in other places. Few kids in his past have actively disliked him. One could go on eliciting from Harry reasons that the other children would not like him and put these to the empirical test. If Harry became convinced that the other children would like him if he introduced himself, there would be no reason for him to be fearful. He might then attempt to behave differently and actively initiate social contact. We call this the empirical solution because it attempts to test empirically the truth of inferential thinking by collecting data. Harry is probably distorting reality in believing that the children would have such a negative view of him, and the therapist could show Harry how his thinking in this manner is untrue. The empirical solution deals with changing Harry's emotional reaction to the situation. However, it is an inelegant solution because it challenges the inferences and not the appraisal. Harry's inferences could be true—if not this time, maybe the next. Suppose that, in his next move, he encounters children who dislike him for his race, creed, color, or any other characteristic. No amount of empirical challenging may change his emotional devastation at being disliked if the other children's negative prejudice against him is real.

The philosophical solution challenges the appraisal, the evaluation, or the meaning that a person applies to the inferences and conclusions he or she draws. In this way, Harry can learn to reduce his anxiety in this situation and other similar situations that may occur. We would help him to come to the conclusion that it is not awful if others don't like him. Even if he would rather play with them, he can go about his business, do the next most enjoyable thing, and not catastrophize. If Harry believes that it would not be terrible if the other children did not like him, he might also take the risk of asking them to play with him because the stakes would be lowered considerably for rejection.

### RATIONAL AND IRRATIONAL BELIEFS

Underlying the appraisals that a person applies to inferences and conclusions is what Ellis has referred to as the person's "belief system," which is composed of both rational and irrational beliefs. This is as much the case with children and adolescents as it is with adults. Rational beliefs (and appraisals) tend to be consistent with objective reality, are expressed conditionally and relativistically, and lead to self-enhancing emotions and goal-directed behaviors. Irrational beliefs are generally distortions of reality, are expressed unconditionally and absolutistically, and lead to inappropriate feeling that often block goal attainment. Major categories of irrational beliefs include demandingness, awfulizing, and self-downing. The common irrational beliefs of children include (adapted from Waters, 1982):

1. It's awful if others don't like me.
2. I'm bad if I make a mistake.
3. Everything should go my way; and I should always get what I want.
4. Things should come easily to me.
5. The world should be fair, and bad people should be punished.
6. I shouldn't show my feelings.
7. Adults should be perfect.
8. There's only one right answer.
9. I must win.
10. I shouldn't have to wait for anything.

# SPECIAL CONSIDERATIONS WITH CHILDREN

Cognitive-behavior therapies were initiated, refined, and practiced on adult clients. Most of the books, research articles, clinical literature, and folklore focus almost exclusively on treating various adult populations. This section deals with some of the differences with children. The topics covered include defining expectations and developing rapport, language, developmental limitations, assessment, teaching critical thinking skills, and disputing strategies.

### EXPECTATIONS

Few children understand what psychotherapy is about. They have some notion that a psychologist is a person who "helps" people, but outside of this, most of their notions are negative. Many children believe that our profession treats "crazy people" and therefore that being at our office is a stigma. The other model that children have for us is the school psychologist. Often, they perceive this role as a disciplinary one. What kind of children get sent to the school psychologist in your district?

Besides not knowing about the process of psychotherapy, many children arrive at our offices with no awareness of why they have come. Their parents have not discussed it with them. Children are unlikely to become collaborators in a process they do not understand. Our first job is to explain to them what we do, who we help, how we help. After such an explanation, the child should have a problem-solving set and hopefully a positive schema for the profession, as well as no negative stereotypes.

## RAPPORT

Self-disclosure is a prerequisite for any verbal psychotherapy. Children are less likely than adults to self-disclose to therapists because they desire help. For most children, a warm, accepting relationship is probably a necessity before they will honestly tell how they feel or think. With children, and especially with adolescents, rapport becomes much more important before starting therapy. I do not mean to imply that rapport is curative in and of itself with children but that it is more desirable to attain self-disclosure and to convince them to listen so that the therapist's interventions can have an effect.

Although reflection has been the primary strategy by which therapists have developed rapport, reflection is not the only way. Another strategy is honest, direct questions that communicate a commitment to help. Children are quite sensitive to dishonesty, and they generally respond well to people who are open and who trust them. Many therapists ask children questions when they already know the answer (e.g., after the mother has called to inform the therapist that money is missing from her pocketbook, the therapist's first inquiry is "were there any problems at home this week?" or "did you do anything wrong?" Children are not stupid, and they are likely to see a trap. They may be reluctant to disclose their misdeeds. So they usually respond to inquiries about their misdeeds with "No, I didn't do anything," or "No, there are no problems." Here the therapist has set up a situation in which the child is most likely to lie. Once the child has lied, the therapist is placed in the difficult situation of revealing a lie before it can be discussed. Exposing the child's lie impacts negatively on rapport. To avoid such situations, it is better to confront children honestly with the facts as you know them and then to ask for their opinion or interpretation of the events.

Another strategy to help foster rapport is to discuss with the child how therapy can achieve ends that the child desires, rather than focusing on the goals of the parents and teachers. Because children are not self-referred and they may not always have the goals of the significant others in their lives, it may be particularly important to show children how they can benefit from therapy before they will be willing to participate. Some goals of therapy that children desire may be: (1) to lessen the degree of parental anger and yelling, (2) to develop more predictable rules within the family so that life does not appear arbitrary, or (3) to attain some major rewards they are seeking, such as a larger allowance, staying out later, or a home video game. The therapist may then act as the child's agent in negotiating for these items when contracting for appropriate behavior. An additional strategy is to help shift some of the responsibility for the problem and referral away from the child. A child may feel outnumbered if there is a group of adults trying to induce change. By focusing on how the parent's behavior may contribute to the child's problems or how the parents' upset exaggerates the problem, one diffuses responsibility away fron the child and may form an alliance with the child.

## CONSEQUENCES AND ALTERNATIVES

Cognitive therapy is a process whereby a client's irrational beliefs and erroneous inferences are challenged and attempts are made to substitute more rational alternative ways of thinking. This approach to therapy makes sense only if one has prerequisite assumptions about the nature or emotional disturbance. The first assumption seems somewhat obvious. It is the idea that the client's affect or behavior is negative, disturbed, self-destructive, and better changed. The second assumption is that the negative, disturbed emotions can be replaced with alternative nondisturbing, non-self-destructive, *albeit unpleasant,* affective states. A third is that faulty beliefs create the disturbed affect in the first place. Given these prerequisite assumptions, it logically follows that disputing one's cognitions would be helpful. If these assumptions are not made, however, a client might find disputing a critical, unpleasant process and either drop out of therapy or become extremely uncooperative.

Children usually do not recognize that their behaviors or emotional states have a negative impact on their lives. Nor are they necessarily aware that there are *alternative* ways to act or feel. Most adult clients have a headstart on children in this way. Because adults are usually self-referred, they usually recognize that their actions and emotions are self-defeating and that the therapist can help them develop alternative ways of feeling and acting. If they did not believe this, they probably would not have come in the first place. Children are almost never self-referred. Therefore, it is suggested that the initial stages of treatment be exclusively devoted to an *evaluation* of children's affect and emotions and behaviors and to helping them see that these negative consequences that are avoidable. Focusing on the consequences of the child's present *modus operandi* is the first treatment step.

Children usually have limited schemata for emotional reactions. They may conceptualize feelings as bipolar dichotomous constructs (i.e., happy/mad or glad/sad). It would be quite unlikely for a child to work with a therapist to change mad to only annoyed when her brother pulls her hair if she has no schema to incorporate the latter emotion. Schachter (1966) has demonstrated that social expectations play a large role in a person's emotional experiences. Social cues and private interpretations determine what emotions a person reports to experience when aroused by injections of adrenaline. DiGiuseppe (1986) argues for an extension of Schachter's theory and suggests that cognitions drawn from external cues influence not only the types of emotions but also the *intensity or degree* of emotions as well. Many disturbed children appear to believe that their intense fear or depression is either a desirable or a necessary reaction to certain events. Aggressive adolescents commonly report the desirability of becoming fighting mad at taunts by their peers in order to preserve their reputation. In many cases, children report that they have no options. They believe their disturbed emotions are the way a person should or must feel. Children probably develop beliefs concerning their emotional responses by modeling or direct reinforcement from their parents or families. In many families, the parents respond in the same exaggerated ways as their children do, so that the child may have never seen an alternative response. The parents may show a wider range of emotional reactions, but they may never expect this range of their children and fail to directly teach them alternatives.

In summary, *before one can proceed to identifying and disputing irrational beliefs, one must first agree on a goal. The child must see that a change in his/her emotional state or behaviors is desirable. After the child agrees that change is desirable, it might be necessary to expand the child's schemata concerning emotional reactions so that the goal is within his or her frame of reference.* This expansion can be accomplished through modeling, imagery, stories, parables, and discussions of TV characters who play out different emotional reactions.

Evaluating the consequences of the child's emotional reactions and developing a wider range of perceived, possible emotional reactions is likely to be an important and lengthy step in therapy. Once children perceive that their affect and action tendencies are self-defeating and conceptualize alternative ways of responding both emotionally and behaviorally, they will be more willing to enter into a discussion of how their thinking causes their emotions, and they will be more likely to participate in the disputing and not to see it as an attempt to be critical of them. The therapist is advised not to assume that these two initial steps in therapy will be achieved instantaneously. It may take a number of sessions to explore these issues before the child becomes convinced of them.

Children may also lack a vocabulary for expressing emotions. Even if they do possess a schema for a wide degree of emotional reactions to problems, they might not have the words to express these differences. If they do not have the wide range of alternative emotional reactions mentioned in the preceding sections, along with teaching the emotions themselves it is desirable to provide children with a vocabulary for easily expressing the emotions.

The lack of a vocabulary for expressing subtleties in emotional reaction may partly be a result of the structure of the English language. The common use of words to define emotion is rather vague and imprecise. People frequently use affective words in idiosyncratic ways. One child's *fear* may be another's *panic* or a third's *concern*. It is also helpful to check out what the child means by emotional words behaviorally, physiologically, and phenomenologically. Setting definitions of emotional words helps to prevent confusion as the sessions progress. One helpful suggestion is to use Wolpe's (1973) SUD scale (subjective units of discomfort) to describe the child's present emotional state and to provide a numerical rating that indicates the intensity of an emotion. In this way, children learn that affects can be named along a continuum and that their own emotional states can be compared with the desired goal of the treatment. Thus, a child may talk about becoming angry at a SUD 4. If this numerical system appears undesirable to the therapist, she or he can set a specific vocabulary to try to describe the different intensities of emotional states.

## DEVELOPMENTAL LIMITATIONS

Cognitive-behavior therapists are just beginning to take into account the child's cognitive-developmental status in selecting appropriate cognitive assessment and intervention procedures (Cohen & Schleser, 1984). Armed with the knowledge that basic learning processes and abilities (e.g., attention, memory, verbal mediation, and cognitive strategies) appear to develop progressively over the childhood period, child-oriented practitioners have, in the past few years, begun to question the role of different developmental characteristics in determining the efficacy of cognitive-behavioral intervention (e.g., Cohen & Myers, 1983). The main work in this area has been in determining whether children's level of cognitive development influences their capacity to profit from self-instructional training (Meichenbaum, 1977), which is introduced at different levels of complexity employing different teaching formats. Schleser, Meyers, and Cohen (1981) suggested that pre-concrete-operational children may not have achieved a sufficient level of metacognitive development to profit from verbal self-instruction that employs directed discovery rather than direct expository methods. The related research of Cohen and Meyers (1983) seems to indicate that preoperational children are unable to spontaneously generate cognitive self-guiding strategies.

Piaget states that it is only when children are in the formal operational period (approximately 12 years and older) that they are generally capable of the type of hypotheticodeductive reasoning we believe is a necessary prerequisite for the disputational examination of irrational beliefs. In line with this proposition, Bernard and Joyce (1984) have proposed that many children do not have the capacity to: (1) recognize their general irrational beliefs *when it is presented as a hypothetical proposition,* and (2) rationally restate beliefs.

We know from Piaget and others (e.g., Flavell, 1977) that children between the approximate ages of 7 and 11 structure their world in an empirical and inductive manner. As a consequence, basic insights, concepts, and beliefs are taught to children *through intensive analyses of specific situations.* Concrete examples and teaching illustrations are the rule. The section of this chapter that deals with treatment will illustrate how disputational strategies can be modified for use with younger populations.

When working with very young children (under 7 years old), we are especially cognizant of their difficulty in taking the perspective of others (egocentrism) and considering more than one relevant dimension at a time. As children during this period rely heavily on perceptual analysis rather than conceptual inference (Morris & Cohen, 1982), it is best to deemphasize extensive discussion and analysis of irrational concepts and, instead, rely on the child's more advanced capacity for dealing with iconic representation and employ a great many concrete and simple materials (pictures, diagrams, stories) that young children can readily learn from.

Developmental work in verbal mediation (e.g., Flavell, Beach, & Chinsky, 1966) indicates that children between the ages of 6 and 9 who fail to spontaneously produce functional self-guiding verbal mediators may learn to do so from instruction. Therefore, one can spend a great deal of time with younger children teaching them through a variety of different techniques what to think and how to spontaneously use rational self-talk in problem situations.

Children, especially at the earlier developmental levels, are active learners and that knowledge acquisition is facilitated by "doing" and "seeing" as much as by "hearing." The use of pictures and stories, which may serve as imaginal mnemonic aids, may also enhance the experiential aspect of the learning episode.

## ASSESSMENT

Good assessment is invaluable in designing a cognitive-behavioral treatment program for children. Its importance as an initial step, and, as an ongoing factor, it cannot be overstated. Parents often do not provide complete information or even all the problems of a child when treatment begins. They may withhold mention of family conflicts simply because they do not see a connection between the discord and the child's problems. Or, they may feel too guilty, perhaps too embarrassed, to bring up parts of the child's behavior. On the child's part, the self-disclosure so vital to the assessment stage may not be sufficiently present in the personal repertoire to allow for speaking openly. Thus, months may go by before a therapist learns that a child is encopretic or school-phobic or that the father and the child do not speak to each other.

The optimal product of assessment, then, is a flexible conceptualization of the child's problem, that is, one that can change when new information presents itself. This approach sensitizes the therapist to incorporate treatment strategies as indicated. In addition, an ongoing assessment process quite naturally underscores successes achieved during treatment. Now its usefulness has doubled—it is further motivating the parents and the child; and even tripled—it is providing quality-control information to the therapist.

## UNTANGLING THE REFERRAL

Children are often unwilling consumers of mental-health services. They arrive for therapy because they are viewed as disturbed by someone else or disturbing to someone else. The manner of referral often seems hostile or, at best, unpleasant to the child. If left unattended, it will have a braking effect on collaboration with the therapist.

The first question a therapist would do well to ask is, "Do you know and understand the reason for the visit?" Many children report not knowing why they have come to my office. Some think, because they are coming to a doctor's office, it is for some sort of a checkup. Others see themselves as crazy, or bad. They reason: Bad kids in class are sent to the school psychologist, or on television "shrinks" only help crazy people. The initial task for the cognitive-behavior therapist then is to dispel these misconceptions and replace them with accurate information. Explanations about the role of the therapist and the process of therapy need not be complicated. I have found the simpler my presentation, the more likely it will be accepted. Note that first a problem-solving tone is set, and second, the participants' roles are clearly defined. The child is not misled into thinking the therapist is another friend to play with. Such deceptions are unfortunately common, and although not done with malice, a tragic result could be the eventual loss of the child's trust.

Problem ownership may present another difficulty stemming from the nature of the referral. The therapist must decide exactly who has the problem. Perhaps it is not the child at all! In situations where the problem lies outside the child, the therapist can be caught between changing what the adults wish or changing what appears to be in the best interest of the child, that is, changing the adults. In either case, I have experienced considerable difficulty convincing the "grownups" to change. It might be easier to change the behavior the parents or school identified as deviant. However, to do so could have had Iatrogenic consequences for the child. For example if the child perceived his/her behavior as normal and his/her parents' behavior as oppressive and was correct, then action by the therapist to change the child could undermine the child's correct cognitions and teach him or her an incorrect view of reality. The bottom line for the therapist then is: Who is my client? Is it the parents who pay my bill? The school that sends me referrals? Or, the child? Failure to always identify the child as one's primary client will prevent one from challenging parents and schools when their views of the child are erroneous and detrimental.

## DATA FOCUS

The following areas are recommended for inquiry in a thorough cognitive-behavioral assessment of children's problems. Not all this information needs to be assessed before an intervention is started. The more that is attained, however the greater the likelihood the therapist will design an effective treatment program.

### Specificity

The first task is to specify the target behavior. Referrals for children often include vague comments, such as "acts out in school" or "has temper tantrums." Therapists are urged to get a clear description of exactly what behaviors comprise the complaint. Thus, "acting out in school" can be redefined as, the child gets out of his or her seat, talks to other children, makes paper airplanes, daydreams at least half of the time. "Has temper tantrums" may mean that the child cries, stamps his or her feet, throws whatever is nearby, yells at the top of his or her lungs.

Once the target behavior is thoroughly detailed, its frequency must be accurately monitored. It is equally important to identify what eliciting stimuli precede the target behavior as well as the consequences that the behavior itself elicits. For example, the child begins to cry when his or her wishes are thwarted, and, at the tantrum stage, the parents capitulate. Each target behavior may be maintained by independent cognitive and environmental factors. Specificity allows a more precise matching of techniques to problems and situations.

In assessing behavior, therapists are advised to seek information from as many persons as possible, especially if the problem includes behavior outside the home. When the referral involves a school-related problem, information obtained from parents, obviously secondhand, is far less useful than reporting by those who directly observed the behavior.

### Functional Cognitive Analysis

A functional cognitive analysis as described by Meichenbaum (1977) is the next step. Just exactly what thoughts are in the child's head as the target behavior is being performed? Are there self-statements? Images? Does the child guide the behavior by language? Keep in mind, too, that the absence of reported self-statements can be as important as the presence of maladaptive ones. Children with impulse-control problems may lack self-instructions as a mediator of inhibition responses (Kendall & Braswell, 1985). Anxiety and depressive disorders may exist because the child has no coping self-statements to help deal with provoking incidents (Meichenbaum, 1977).

## Social Problem-Solving Skills

Therapists are advised to assess early each child's interpersonal problem-solving skills as these frequently figure in children's emotional adjustments. Research has identified two social problem-solving skills as most important in maintaining adjustment: (1) alternative solution thinking, or the ability to generate a number of solutions to a social problem, and (2) consequential thinking, or the ability to predict the social consequences of one's behavior (Spivack & Shure, 1975). Given the importance of these skills and the usefulness of problem-solving therapy techniques in the reduction of children's behavior disorders, this area should be assessed for a full picture of the child's cognitive functioning.

The skills in question can be assessed by having the child make up stories, as in the Thematic Apperception Test. As a problem arises in a story, the therapist asks what solutions the child can think of to solve it. The child's responses will indicate the degree of alternative solution thinking. Consequential thinking skills can be elicited at a point where people in the story interact. Now the therapists asks the child to speculate on the reactions of the people involved. Apart from storytelling techniques, questions eliciting alternative solutions and consequential thinking can quite easily be put to the child during discussions of specific problems.

## Distortions of Reality

During assessment, therapists should also be watchful for distorted perceptions of reality, statements the child makes about him- or herself or others that reflect unrealistic or incorrect views of the world. Errors in logic such as arbitrary inference, selective abstraction, or overgeneralization (Beck, 1976) are quite common in a child's thinking. This category of cognitive distortions would include statements that are contradicted by available data—for example, "My Mother doesn't love me," "I'm stupid," "None of the other children play with me," and "No one will ever like me."

## Irrational Beliefs

The assessment is not complete without investigation of the child's evaluation of personal experiences. What do the eliciting stimuli mean to the child? What value do the consequences of the behavior have? What importance does the child attach to events and people? Are these evaluations logical and rational or excessive? Note that cognitive distortions of this type do not involve thoughts that can be challenged or disputed on empirical grounds. These types of errors would fall under Beck's description of minimization/maximization errors of thinking or Ellis's irrational beliefs. In both conceptualizations, such distortions reflect an exaggeration of the importance of certain elements for the child.

No evidence indicates which of the previously mentioned factors are most important in the development or maintenance of various childhood behaviors or which are best stressed in treatment design. Research has focused on each of the five areas independently, and there has been little, if any, collaborative or contrasting research. My hypothesis, borrowed from Lazarus (1976), is that the more modalities a therapist investigates and subsequently works in, the greater the chance for attaining behavior change and the longer lasting that change. Also, by acquiring data on all modalities, the therapist can determine which modalities have deficits.

As a reading of Ellis (1976, 1977, & 1979, & 1985), Beck (Beck, Rush, Shaw, Emery, 1979) and Meichenbaum (1977), and others (Dryden & Golden 1986) reveals, cognitive therapies usually rely on a combination of cognitive restructuring, behavioral problem solving, and emotive and imagery techniques to achieve effective therapy. In the remainder of the chapter we will focus on such comprehensive approach to therapy.

### BEHAVIORAL COMPONENTS

Because children are not self-referred, are likely to be less motivated for change, and are less responsible, it is incorrect to assume that they will carry out their behavioral assignments alone. However, their parents are usually willing to cooperate and can be enlisted to help structure the behavioral components of therapy. In almost all cases, except where the parents are uncooperative, one can use a behavioral modification program to reinforce the desired target behaviors. Whether the emotional problem is fear, depression, or anger, the parents can provide structured, systematic rewards for the nonoccurrence of the target behaviors and for behaviors that are incompatible with the target behavior, or they can provide response costs when the target behavior does occur. Behavioral programs that reward or penalize behavior may not only help children to behave better but may also help them to become more motivated to cooperate with the therapist and learn cognitive strategies to control their emotions and to internalize behavioral gains.

Remembering again that children are not self-referred, it may be helpful for us to go into a little more detail about how the construction of behavior and reinforcement systems motivates children to learn control of their emotional reactions. Self-referred adults who are anxious not only experience fear, but they are also in conflict (Dollard & Miller, 1950). Let us take the example of a young man, Fred, frightened of approaching women. Fred seeks therapy because he wants to find a lover. He is in an approach–avoidance conflict. Suppose he thinks that it would be awful and terrible if women rejected him; as a result, he experiences fright and avoids women, especially those he would like to date. On the other hand, he has a great desire to meet women for sex, romance, and companionship. It is this conflict that causes discomfort and motivates Fred to seek therapy. If, for some reason, Fred did not desire female companionship, he might still fear rejection by women; yet, under such circumstances, he would experience little discomfort from this fear. The fear would not be stopping him from achieving any desired goals. It would be quite easy for him to avoid women altogether. His anxiety would be limited to those situations in which he was forced to be in the company of women and was unable to avoid them. If you review your own case load, you may find that most of those who are self-referred are in one of Dollard and Miller's (1950) classic conflicts: approach/avoidance, avoidance/avoidance, or approach/approach. Conflict, then, causes most of the pain. Without the conflict, a person can easily avoid the feared stimuli. Discomfort arises only when people are forced to be in the presence of the feared stimuli and cannot escape, as in Fred's case. For example, the author has a dreadful fear of alligators. He does not wish to date them or seek their company in any way. Because he does not seek alligators, and there are none in his native Long Island, the fear never strikes him, except on those rare occasions when he visits the Bronx zoo. If, however, he developed a fondness for alligators, he might wish to be in their company. Experiencing this fear when he attempts to do so would cause him discomfort, and it is this approach/avoidance that may bring him to the therapist's office. Other types of conflicts operate in a similar way.

Children's fears often provide them no conflict:

> A case of school phobia is a good illustration. Karen experienced extreme panic whenever called on in class to give an answer. As a result, she did not wish to attend school. She developed stomach pains and had a few days off, and the illness seemed to

linger. Her mother, realizing that the ailment was more than an upset stomach, kept Karen home and felt sorry for her daughter when she realized the extent of Karen's emotional reaction to school. Karen was allowed to stay home and experienced no response cost for this behavior. During school hours, Karen watched TV, played alone, or listened to her records. After school, she met friends and joined in their activities. Not a bad life! Karen felt no desire to attend school and was not interested in any of the rewards that this institution dispensed. Why should she want to change? She listened carefully to a discussion of how thoughts caused feelings and how her catastrophizing about making mistakes caused her to feel frightened. She agreed. However, this is as far as we got. There was no conflict and therefore no motivation for her to overcome her fear. Disputing was out of the question. After a few sessions with Karen's mother, we succeeded in lessening her sympathy for Karen's fear. We then set out the following rules. Karen was denied access to her TV and stereo whenever absent from school. She was not allowed to join her peers unless she attended class that day. Once these rules were in effect, Karen was more willing to start disputing those irrational beliefs that she had identified earlier and was now willing to attend school and control her anxiety, with the procedures we had used. Once she was inside school, there was really no reason for Karen to attempt to raise her hand and answer questions, and she continued to make excuses to avoid answering questions when called on. We had made some progress, but the lack of any continued motivation stalled treatment. At this point, a reinforcement system was provided for answering in class. The teacher sent home daily feedback on the number of questions Karen attempted to answer. For each question, she was allotted a certain degree of money. Although this reinforcement did not help Karen to overcome her problems completely and she still experienced fear, again she was more interested in discussing her irrational beliefs and in attempting to overcome them because she wanted the money.

Behavioral incentives may provide the motivation for children to attempt to search for alternative strategies to overcome their emotional reactions. Although behavioral approaches to fear have achieved some success, it has not been the total improvement that one would expect. A cognitive-behavioral program, though, may be more successful. The behavioral incentives provide the motivation to change, and the cognitive interventions help to foster that change and to reduce the fear.

## THE IMPORTANCE OF PREREQUISITE CRITICAL THINKING SKILLS

Cognitive therapies are concerned primarily with epistemology, the philosophical study of knowledge. Therapists always ask clients, ''How do you know that what you are thinking is accurate?'' Disputing assumes that the client and the therapist share criteria for determining the truth or falsity of a statement. Many children have failed to develop critical thinking skills. Even if they have developed critical thinking skills and logic about the objective world, they may not have transferred these logical manipulations to the intrapersonal or interpersonal realm. As a result, they may have separate epistemologies for judging objective data and psychologically interpersonal statements. Children often have quite simple personal epistemologies. They may believe that things are true, just because they think they are true. Or just because they think them. Or because Mommy or Daddy says that they are true. Or because some other people think they are true, and, for adolescents, because their peers think they are true. All of these philosophical positions can get one into trouble.

Before attempting to dispute a child's irrational beliefs and automatic thoughts, it is a good idea to check out whether he or she can tell the differences among facts, opinions, and hypotheses, and to ascertain if he or she can follow logical arguments in verifying statements or in discovering illogic. If they are like most adults, children may find it easier to be logical about external matters and may find it easy to believe that all automatic negative thoughts are true because they have thought them. The idea of examining and questioning one's thoughts about private, personal issues may be new to many young clients. It may be best to start teaching these skills by modeling and parable rather than by first challenging their irrational creations. One strategy is to present the irrational ideas of other clients when one has helped and to talk about how their errors were spotted and how they learned to challenge them. It may also help to talk about the therapist's own irrationalities and how he or she tested these out and discovered that they were false.

### COGNITIVE STRATEGIES

Many cognitive therapists try to help their clients reach the elegant solution and to realize that even if life's events are bad, they need not upset themselves and can appraise these events less negatively. In working with children, this is still our goal; however, it is less often accomplished. Ellis has commented many times that not all clients reach the elegant solution, and some appear particularly resistant no matter how hard they try. Children are less likely to reach this goal because of their inability to handle the degree of abstraction necessary. When the elegant solution appears unreachable with a child, there are three alternative solutions:

1. To change the child's appraisal of the one particular activating event about which she or he is upset
2. To change the child's inferences when distortions of reality precede negative appraisals and disturbed effect. This approach is easier than elegant disputing because the empirical solution is more concrete.
3. To settle for verbal self-instruction that guides the child toward nonupsetting emotional responses and more adaptive behavior. This approach requires no disputing of the child's cognitions, but it does require an overriding cognition that directs the child to react differently. It is likely to be successful for a single stimulus or a narrow set of stimuli.

## INCORRECT INFERENCES: A CAUTIONARY NOTE

As noted before, the empirical solution to emotional problems is often the easiest for children to grasp. Because of this ease, it is the strategy taken for many child therapists. A caveat is in order. A serious problem can arise in using the empirical solution when the child gets upset about the behavior of significant-other adults, as children so frequently do. Children are apt to become upset when they believe that important adults in their lives do not love them, behave unfairly, or display serious personality disturbances. I have noticed a disturbing tendency on the part of child therapists to assume that the child incorrectly perceives such events. Rather than assuming that the child may be correct ("Let's suppose you're right, but why is that so awful?" as Albert Ellis so often says) and pursuing the elegant solution, the therapist sticks to the empirical disputing even when the data indicate that the child is correct. Many therapists do this because they believe that the realization that their parents are uncaring, unfair, or disturbed may be too much for the child to bear. Such a realization, they believe, would present an insurmountable obstacle to the child's emotional health. Although children may be more likely to produce cognitive distortions and incorrect inference, it also has been my clinical experience that their automatic thoughts are more often corroborated by an empirical analysis. Possibly because children cannot escape many problems that confront them, their perceptions of danger may be more real.

Some children correctly perceive that they have verifiable adversity in their lives. Uncaring, capricious, and disturbed parents exist. They are not only characters in Grimms' fairy tales. Therapists are often unwilling to pursue the elegant solution in such cases because they believe that it must be awful to live in such a situation. Empirical solutions for the children of these parents are unlikely to help and are likely at best to lead to reduced rapport because the child will know that the therapist cannot or will not help. At the worst, the therapist may succeed and leave the child feeling temporarily better, but with some distortions about love, fairness, and authority. Another therapeutic intervention often tried in such cases is to provide the child with a supportive relationship, again, temporarily making the child feel better. According to rational-emotive therapy, this strategy is merely palliative and leads to no permanent resolution. When children's adversity is verified by the therapist, it may be best to seek the elegant solution. Children may be more resilient than we believe, and at least, we may do them no harm.

Children often have negative perceptions about their parents that are emotionally charged. Unless the therapist shows a willingness to entertain these ideas and acceptance of the child for thinking them and speaking about them, in the true sense of collaborative empiricism, it is unlikely that the child will be open with the therapist. Some therapists may feel frightened about confirming the child's ideas about the parent, or they may feel that discussing the parents' behavior when the child is referred is risky. Other therapists have often told me that the discussion of such situations would be too traumatic for a child to face. I maintain that an openness and willingness to discuss such issues will get to the true irrational beliefs that are often upsetting to children and to the true evaluations that they make.

## COGNITIVE STRATEGIES

Beck (1976) and Ellis (1976, 1985) have focused on two types of cognitions that lead to emotional disturbances. Simply put, the first consists of distorted perceptions of reality, and the second, of evaluations about that perceived reality. When a client erroneously exaggerates the probability of occurrence and the degree of aversiveness, emotional disturbance will occur. For example, 8-year-old Linda sadly reports that the other children do not like or want to play with her. Linda's perception of her peers' feelings and behaviors may or may not be true. Compounding it destructively, though, is Linda's further belief that she needs the other youngsters' approval and that it is indeed terrible when they dislike her. The overall cognitive set is disastrous; the result is a depressed child.

Ellis (1977) recommends a twofold challenge of such beliefs. The first set of beliefs can be disputed by asking Linda to engage in empirical analysis. Together Linda and the therapist can design a simple experiment to measure how children respond toward her after she asks them to play. The therapist has led the client to challenge that a specific event has occurred or will occur. The experiment will either support, weaken, or discredit entirely Linda's notion of being ostracized by the other children. Ellis labels this type of disputing *empirical* or *inelegant*.

It is important here, not only if the experiment seems to support Linda's perception of peer rejection but also when such a perception is partially or completely discredited, for therapist and client to continue on the second set of beliefs—the assumption that the event is so terrible. This challenged by what Ellis calls philosophical or elegant disputing.

A third therapeutic strategy exists: Teach young clients problem-solving skills (alternative solutions) so that they come to believe they can avoid or cope with the event. In the case of Linda, I helped her think of alternative strategies to make new friends as well as accurately predict the outcome of these attempts.

No experimental evidence exists to prove which of these strategies or combination thereof is most successful. My own clinical experience suggests it is best to start with the simpler strategies, problem solving and empirical disputing, even though the remaining strategy, elegant disputing, may be more prophylactic. The first two strategies usually provided more rapid symptom relief. The third, challenging basic philosophical assumptions, is difficult with children because of their less developed reasoning ability. Two recent cases serve as examples.

Curt, an articulate 12-year-old, was referred because of his difficulty with peer relations at school. Specifically, he became involved in a fight whenever he was teased. A cognitive assessment revealed that, immediately after a taunt was tossed at him, Curt thought, "This kid doesn't like me—no one likes me—it's terrible not to have any friends." With the degree of aversiveness so exaggerated, Curt could match no other response to the teasing than a swing at his tormentors. He failed to conceptualize that this reaction only worsened his popularity.

The primary strategy was to teach Curt to develop a plan before fighting. First, he was to list the consequences of fighting. He would get in trouble, possible be hurt, probably become more unpopular. Then he was helped to consider other responses and to imagine their consequences. He could ignore the behavior, or he could retort with a similar comment. Once equipped with situation-specific responses, Curt was led to challenge the idea that teasing meant someone didn't like you. He was asked to observe the behavior of other children and found that children tease each other frequently. The idea that someone doesn't like you is the same as no one will like you was also empirically challenged. Curt and the therapist drew a diagram of the friendships in his class. In the model, some children had a more elaborate network of chums than others, but no child came up a total isolate.

This treatment plan produced rapid behavior change. Well aware that 12-year-olds have an exaggerated belief in the need for approval, I avoided elegant disputing. No attempt was made to challenge Curt's belief that it was terrible not to be liked. Attacking this belief would have required considerable more time and effort. In my opinion, the strategy would have been appropriate only if for some reason Curt could expect a great deal of unavoidable social rejection in the future.

Paul, a 10-year-old, displayed temper tantrums, specifically, yelling and arguing with his parents. A behavioral analysis revealed these behaviors occurred whenever his parents discussed an issue about which they held differing opinions, even if their disagreement was amicable. A cognitive analysis revealed Paul held two troublesome beliefs: first, that disagreement leads to divorce; and second, that he could not survive if his parents separated.

I asked Paul to set up an experiment to test his hypothesis that disagreement leads to divorce. He was willing to do so, and we designed a questionnaire for this purpose. Paul polled his teacher and principal, several storekeepers, a police officer, and others about whether they decided to divorce everytime they argued with their spouses. Paul found that disagreements were common in marriage and rarely resulted in divorce. His symptoms ceased.

This strategy would not have provided Paul with the coping skills if his parents did divorce but that possibility was remote in this case. Most children strongly believe they need both parents. Although this may not be true, it is a chore to change such a pernicious cultural belief. When a more practical strategy exists, it would be inefficient to spend time providing Paul with coping skills for an event that was unlikely.

There are times, however, when children are faced with unchangeable, unavoidable events that are undeniably aversive. In such cases, the problem-solving or empirical disputing strategies will provide little relief, and the best tactic is helping the child assess and accept the degree of risk or loss. Such a situation typically arises when significant others behave uncaringly toward a child. Some therapists try to protect the child from this awareness. Their therapeutic strategies may involve helping the child see the good qualities in the significant other or providing the child with a substitute relationship with the therapist. The cognitive therapist would reject these tactics and be concerned that the child perceive the situation accurately and develop coping strategies to deal with the stress.

The following case may illustrate this point. Junior was a 10-year-old boy referred by his school because he ran away from home and had been threatening suicide. In the initial session, Junior said he wanted to die because nobody cared about him, especially his stepfather. Junior and I began to discuss the definition of caring, and I asked him to describe how one could tell whether or not a person cared about you. Then I asked him to consider the people in his life and apply his criteria to each. In the course of a lengthy discussion, Junior was able to compile a list of 12 people who cared for him. Junior's mood improved dramatically during this session. After reviewing the names he had written, however, again Junior became morose: his stepfather was not on the list.

I focused the next discussion on the stepfather and asked Junior to apply his criteria to him. The stepfather failed to meet Junior's expectations. He spent more time with Junior's siblings and at times said he loved his own son more. The therapist asked Junior to monitor his stepfather's behavior in the following days to verify whether or not it met the criteria. Several attempts were made to reach the stepfather, but he refused to come in and discuss the issue.

At the next session, Junior reported that his stepfather had indeed failed to meet the criteria, and Junior drew the inevitable conclusion that Dad did not care for him. The therapist then focused on evaluation of this fact. The therapist was able to show Junior that he didn't really need more caring behavior from his stepfather and that life could be happy with such a deficit. This point was discussed in the subsequent sessions with the resultant lifting of Junior's depression and an improvement in his behavior at school and home.

# CONCLUSION

This chapter has outlined some of the ways cognitive therapy can be applied to the emotional problems of children. Although this approach is new and little experimental support for its effectiveness exists, it appears to be successful enough to warrant optimism and continued investigation. Many problems exist in translating cognitive techniques to use with children. The largest of these difficulties seems to be the therapist's underestimation of the child's abilities to reason. I have found that children can indeed think about their thinking. My hope is that we as therapists can help them think more clearly.

# REFERENCES

Beck, A. T. (1976). *Cognitive therapy and the emotional disorders*. New York International Universities Press.

Beck, A. T. Rush, A. J., Shaw, B. F., & Emery, G. (1979). *Cognitive therapy of depression*. New York: Guilford Press.

Bernard, M. E. (1981). Private thought in rational-emotive psychotherapy. *Cognitive Therapy and Research, 5*, 125–142.

Bernard, M. E., (August 1988). *The Child and Adolescent Scale of Irrationality*. Paper presented at the 24th International Congress of Psychology, Sydney.

Bernard, M. E., & Joyce, M. R. (1984). *Rational-emotive therapy with children and adolescents*. New York: Wiley.

Cohen, R., & Meyers, A. W. (1983). Cognitive development and self-instruction interventions. In B. Gholson & T. L. Rosenthal (Eds.), *Applications of cognitive development theory* (pp. 104–132). New York: Academic Press.

Cohen, R., & Schlesar, R. (1984) Cognitive development and clinical intervention. In A. W. Meyer & W. E. Craighead, (Eds.), *Cognitive behavior therapy with children* (pp. 45–68). New York: Plenum Press.

DiGiuseppe, R. A. (1981). Cognitive therapy with children. In G. Emery, S. D. Hollon, & R. C. Bedrosian (Eds.), *New directions in cognitive therapy* (pp. 50–67). New York: Guilford Press.

DiGiuseppe, R. A., & Bernard, M. E. (1983). Principles of assessment and methods of treatment with children. In A. Ellis & M. E. Bernard (Eds.). *Rational-emotive approaches to problems of childhood*. New York: Plenum Press.

Dollard, J., & Miller, N. E. (1950). *Personality and psychotherapy*. New York: McGraw-Hill.

Dryden, W., & Golden, W. (1986). *Cognitive-behavioral approaches to psychotherapy,* London: Harper & Row.

Ellis, A. (1962). *Reason and emotion in psychotherapy*. New York: Lyle Stuart.

Ellis, A. (1976). *Humanistic psychotherapy*. New York: McGraw-Hill Paperback.

Ellis, A. (1977). Rejoinder: Elegant and inelegant RET. The Counseling Psychologist, 7(1), 73–82.

Ellis, A. (1979). The theory of rational-emotional therapy. In A. Ellis & J. M. Whiteley (Eds.), *Theoretical and empirical foundations of rational-emotive therapy* (pp. 45–65). Monterey, CA: Brooks/Cole.

Ellis, A. (1985). *Overcoming resistance: Rational-emotive therapy with difficult clients*. New York: Springer.

Flavel, J. H. (1977). *Cognitive development*. Englewood-Cliffs, NJ: Prentice-Hall.

Flavell, J., Beach, D., & Chinsky, J. (1966). Spontaneous verbal rehearsal in a memory task as a function of age. *Child Development, 37,* 283–99.

Garber, J., Deal, S., & Parke, C. (1986, November) *The Coping with Depression pamphlet revised for adolescents: Comprehensibility and acceptability.* Paper presented at the annual meeting of the Association for the Advancement of Behavior Therapy. Chicago.

Kendall, P. C., & Braswell, L. (1985). *Cognitive behavioral therapy for Impulsive Children* New York: Guilford.

Lazarus, A. (1976). *Multimodal behavior therapy*. New York: Springer.

Leitenberg, H., Yost, L., Carroll-Wilson, M. (1986). Negative cognitive errors in children: Questionaire development, normative data, and comparison between children with and without self reported symptoms of depression, low self esteem and evaluation anxicty. *Journal of Consulting and Clinical Psychology, 5,* 528–536.

Meichenbaum, D. (1977). *Cognitive behavior modification*. New York: Plenum Press.

Morris, C. W., & Cohen, R. (1982). Cognitive considerations in cognitive behavior modification. *School Psychological Review, 11,* 14–20.

Neisser, U. (1967). *Cognitive psychology*. New York: Appleton-Century-Crofts.

Reese, H. (1962). Verbal mediation as a function of age. *Psychological Bulletin, 59,* 502–509.

Schacter, S. (1966). The interaction of cognitive and physiological determinants of emotional statee. In C. D. Spielberger (Ed.), *Anxiety and behavior* (pp. 193–224). New York: Academic Press.

Schleser, R., Meyers, A., & Cohen, R. (1981). Generalizations of self-instructions: Effects of general versus specific content, active rehearsal, and cognitive level. *Child Development, 52,* 335–340.

Spivack, G., & Shure, M. (1975). *The social adjustment of young children*. San Francisco: Jossey-Bass.

Spivack, G., Platt, S., & Shure, M. (1976). *The problem-solving approach to adjustment*. San Francisco: Jossey-Bass.

Urbain, E. S., & Kendall, P. C. (1980). Review of social-cognitive problem-solving interactions with children. *Psychological Bulletin, 88,* 109–143.

Vernon, A. (1983). Rational-emotive education. In A. Ellis & M. Bernard (Eds.), *Rational-emotive approaches to the problems of childhood*. New York: Plenum.

Waters, V. (1982). Therapies for children: Rational-emotive therapy. In C. R. Reynolds & T. B. Gutkin (Eds.), *Handbook of school psychology* (pp. 570–579). New York: Wiley.

Wessler, R., & Wessler, R. (1980). *Principles and practice of rational-emotive therapy*. San Francisco: Jose-Bassey.

Wolpe, J. (1973). *The practice of behavior therapy*. New York: Pergamon.

# 27

# Enhancing Cognitive Therapy with Women

## Denise Davis and Christine Padesky

In considering the array of therapeutic approaches available today, cognitive therapy offers some special advantages for women. The theory and practice of cognitive therapy appear to be especially harmonious with the feminist philosophy of advancing the rights and status of women (Farrell & Davis, 1986). Dealing with women clients does not mean that the fundamentals of cognitive therapy need to be substantially revised. However, cognitive therapists attempting to understand their clients' idiosyncratic, internal reality may enhance this understanding by considering the context of gender. Just as it is clearly a mistake to overgeneralize research findings based only on a male sample, so it is a mistake in clinical practice to assume male and female experiences and beliefs are identical. Therapists are becoming more sophisticated in applying cognitive therapy with special populations, as demonstrated by this volume. Recognizing women as a population in cognitive therapy involves consideration of the importance of gender and a willingness to explore the ways in which a woman's thoughts are influenced by her social realities.

## CONCEPTUAL ISSUES

Research has shown that gender is an important variable that can differentiate how individuals react in a situation, how they present themselves, how they appraise themselves, and how they are viewed by others (Deaux, 1984). One's identity as a male or female does influence the development and organization of other schemas (Markus, Crane, Bernstein, & Siladi, 1982). The information that is processed into schemas as a result of one's experiences in the world can profoundly differ on the basis of gender. Although certain experiences may not be completely unique to the lives of women, it is extremely important to recognize that

Denise Davis • Department of Psychiatry, Vanderbilt University, Nashville, Tennessee 37232. Christine Padesky • Center for Cognitive Therapy, Newport Beach, California 92660.

women occupy what Elaine Blechman (1984) and others (e.g., Schaef, 1985) have termed a separate social reality.

In Blechman's view, this distinct and separate reality typically includes a high degree of structure that encourages dependence on others and devalues instrumental competence. Women are taught to expect someone else to look after their well-being, according to Blechman. Then at critical times, such as when a woman is abused, becomes divorced, or ages, women are faced with a contradictory reality in which social support is withdrawn. In addition, these critical experiences for women may not even be acknowledged as important or worthy of attention. For instance, stressful life events measures typically do not include traumatic events experienced by women such as rape, battering, abortion, or miscarriage (Solomon & Rothblum, 1986).

Resick (1985) discusses women's reality in terms of a double bind of femininity. According to Resick, women must choose between social support or personal adaptation. Traditional femininity elicits more social acceptance and relationship maintenance, yet it also incorporates more behavioral deficits, lower self-esteem, and more characteristics labeled *unhealthy* or *neurotic*. Thus certain content areas merit added attention because of relevance to women's lives, and the process of women's experience also needs to be addressed in terms of its impact upon cognitive and affective organization.

Dealing with gender as an important variable in therapy requires some awareness of the treatment philosophy advocated by feminists for overcoming the damaging effects of a paternalistic system. This philosophy is outlined by Brown and Liss-Levinson (1981) as compatible with all systems except orthodox Freudian psychoanalysis. Gilbert (1980) summarizes the feminist approach to psychotherapy as revolving around two major principles: (1) therapy relationship egalitarianism, and (2) the perspective that personal experience is political.

Therapy relationship egalitarianism clearly overlaps with the spirit and letter of cognitive therapy. From a feminist perspective, this means fostering a consumer attitude in the client and orienting her to the process of therapy, discussing options, diagnoses, and reports. It means encouraging and answering her questions. It also means demystifying therapy, disclaiming the position of all-powerful authority, and encouraging personal power in the client by encouraging her to choose problems for the session agenda. Therapists foster personal power in clients by providing them with access to information and resources such as books, services, or adjunctive referrals. Feminists also advocate egalitarianism through selective self-disclosure and modeling by the therapist.

Cognitive therapists may recognize these and other expressions of relationship egalitarianism as fundamental to their system of therapy. What therapists may not have realized is the degree of importance this holds for women clients, and how much difficulty a woman client may have with something that a man may take for granted. For example, a woman client may be reluctant to ask questions about the therapist's background or choice of methods out of fear of offending the therapist or because she believes that her own capacity to evaluate the situation is inevitably inadequate or inferior to the therapist's authority. It may not occur to her that she does have the capacity to compare therapists and choose among them.

The second principle of feminist treatment philosophy outlined by Gilbert (1980), ''the personal is political,'' refers to recognition of the broader social and political systems within which both the client and the therapist must operate. In doing this, therapists are aware of their own values and attitudes, acknowledge the impact of sex role socialization and work to validate female experiences by incorporating content of importance to women. This is compatible with the social learning theory base of cognitive therapy but may require more concentrated attention to specific topics relevant to the life experiences of women.

In the rest of this chapter, we will propose a conceptual framework for therapeutic work with issues of socialization, and we will provide an overview of some content areas of particular concern to women. This is by no means an exhaustive list or a review of the literature. It is a synopsis of issues that affect women in cognitive therapy, and it is intended to broaden the awareness and the effectiveness of cognitive therapists working with women. Our statements regarding women should not be misconstrued as sweeping generalizations about all women but rather be viewed as working hypotheses for the cognitive therapist.

## CULTURAL CONTEXT

Within the context of being a woman, there clearly are culturally relevant variables that influence the woman's view of herself and her world. Although gender is a highly potent variable, women as a group still encompass much heterogeneity. Social context variables may be useful in further understanding of the variability among women. We propose a four dimensional conceptualization as a framework for sorting out additional cultural influences. The dimensions of ethnic or racial heritage, socioeconomic status, religious or spiritual affiliation, and sex role values each can help to characterize the individual woman's belief system.

For example, in assessment one can ask how the woman's perspective is influenced by her racial origins, her past and present economic status, her religious background, and her identification with masculine and feminine roles. Therapists can also use this as an opportunity to evaluate their own reactions to their client that may be based on cultural beliefs and could influence the therapy process. For example, do they tend to discredit or dislike poor or unattractive ("unfeminine") women?

A conceptualization of different cultural dimensions can provide a means to explore collaboratively the woman's beliefs as they have been shaped by her broader social connections. Understanding culturally based schemas within the therapist as well as the client also can help to delineate desirable treatment goals. In addition, this process begins to address the feminist goal of bringing society into treatment with the individual (Gilbert, 1980; Klein, 1976).

The degree to which a woman client sees her own belief system as in harmony with others in her world can be an important therapeutic issue. At times when the woman sees her thoughts and assumptions as discordant with those of her culture (be it ethnic, socioeconomic, religious, or sex role), she may be vulnerable to concluding that she is somehow flawed or bad, and she suffers a loss of self-esteem. In these instances, it may be useful to explore the idea of stereotyping. She may be falling victim to her own or others' notions that persons within a certain cultural context should necessarily demonstrate a specific set of characteristics or beliefs. This seems to be an overgeneralization that could potentially be reattributed to the automatic human tendency to simplify people and ideas by lumping them into catagories.

The specific thoughts or beliefs with which the woman finds herself at odds can also be reinterpreted as characteristic of some of the cultural group but not necessarily the only defining characteristic.

> An example is provided by a 30-year-old woman of Greek descent, Mara, whose family had labeled her as a "black sheep" because she had not followed the path of early marriage to a respectable Greek man, as a "good Greek girl should." Instead, she chose a career in business, moved away from home, dated a variety of men, and wore what her family considered to be an "unfeminine" short hairstyle. At the same time, Mara was still actively involved in the Greek community and with her friends and relatives who had followed a more stereotypic path in their early adulthood. Mara felt angry and alienated from her parents and inadequate within herself because she did not fit within her culture's definition of what was appropriate for women. In this case, her ethnic background reinforced certain sex role values that were inconsistent with her life experiences.
>
> Mara was able to reduce her distress with this inconsistency by focusing on

several ways in which she remained connected and involved in the Greek community and by recognizing that, by and large, her Greek peers accepted her and at times envied her life-style and freedom. She was able to reattribute the conflict to her parents and to separate herself from their belief that "she should already be married to a nice Greek man." Most important, she recognized that membership in her ethnic group involved many components, some of which she acquired through birth and some of which she learned through shared experiences, and these did not depend solely upon her conforming to the sex role stereotypes of that group.

Therapists are cautioned to be aware of their own tendency to attribute beliefs and behaviors to their women clients on the basis of their own cultural stereotypes. Doing so could constitute a form of "countertransference" in cognitive therapy.

Carolyn was a woman who experienced this several times in therapy, with female as well as male therapists. An obese, never-married mother of a 16-year-old daughter: she had only held one brief unskilled job prior to the birth of her child. For most of her adult life, she had existed as a "welfare mother." Her physical appearance suggested the life-style of a "bag lady," but she did maintain an apartment for herself and her daughter. For several years, she had been treated at a mental health clinic, primarily with medication, for agoraphobia and depression. A clinical social worker treating her daughter at another clinic referred Carolyn to a vocational rehabilitation program and to a women's cognitive therapy group.

In group, Carolyn worked on altering the beliefs that she "couldn't learn, couldn't openly express her feelings, and was inferior to other people". As she began to openly express her feelings in the group, she asked for suggestions on how to handle angry feelings toward her current therapist who had evaluated her as lacking progress and had interpreted this as a passive wish to be rescued by a man. The group suggested that she discuss these feelings with her therapist, and, if she still felt uncomfortable, she could claim her right to seek a new therapist.

Carolyn initiated new treatment relationships twice, but she felt uncomfortable and criticized by both therapists. The therapists viewed Carolyn as uncooperative and untreatable. Carolyn sought individual therapy again as she was attempting to make the transition out of her year-long vocational rehabilitation program. Her therapist evaluated her physical presentation (which was greatly improved but still reflected an obese woman with shabby clothing), her history, and previous therapeutic contacts and recommended that she give up on the idea of working and allow herself to go on disability payments from the government.

Consultation between the group and individual therapist revealed that the individual therapist did harbor the thoughts that Carolyn could not learn and probably could not function adequately in any type of paid labor situation. The evidence to support that evaluation was primarily from previous therapists' opinions and from observing Carolyn's lack of economic advancement. We speculate that Carolyn's low socioeconomic status and her lack of traditionally feminine physical attractiveness may have elicited reactions from others, including her individual therapists, that reflected a mixture of assumptions regarding a lack of value and motivation.

Her lack of culturally defined feminine attractiveness may have played an important role in blocking her access to the traditional female means of improving her economic status through marriage. Carolyn's physical appearance may also have been the most powerful factor in eliciting devaluing reactions from others, because being unattractive is more inconsistent and unacceptable to the female sex role than being poor or stupid. The therapists also appeared to have endorsed Carolyn's own all-or-nothing belief that she "couldn't learn." Luckily, she had come to challenge and replace this belief on her own. She had evidence that she could indeed learn, and she very strongly wished to hold a job and improve her economic situation. But she was faced with the dilemma of challenging and replacing the therapists who probably had dysfunctional assumptions about her!

## SUMMARY

Gender is regarded as an important variable in cognitive therapy because it can differentiate a social reality with rules, beliefs, and conclusions unique to the lives of women. Further distinction of the heterogeneity among women may be assisted by conceptualization of other sociocultural variables, such as the four-dimensional model proposed before. These considerations can serve as tools for the psychotherapist endeavoring to pinpoint and alter dysfunctional thought processes and belief systems. Specifically, therapists can recognize a line of thinking that has been shaped within in certain culture, and they can recognize that discordance with the beliefs of one's cultural reference group can be a source of distress. Therapists can also benefit from being sensitized to their own reactions as reflective of certain cultural expectations or values. It is especially important to consider how the therapist's choice of interventions or goals might be influenced by his or her own stereotypic expectations based on race, religion, socioeconomic status, or sex role. Culturally influenced beliefs can thus be sources of information for both client and therapist.

# CONTENT ISSUES

Our experience with women clients has suggested that there are a variety of content areas in which it is important to delineate the woman's view of herself and her functioning in the world. These can be broadly grouped into areas of physical experience and social living experience. The following sections highlight women's perspectives in processing information for each of these areas.

## PHYSICAL EXPERIENCES

A woman's identity and personal worth in the world have long been linked with her physical attractiveness and physical functioning. The Judeo-Christian tradition has historically equated women with matters of the flesh. Some attitudes developed by this philosophical tradition have, unfortunately, been quite negative, wherein female attributes and functions are regarded as dirty and evil. Access to economic security and power has been traditionally available to women only through the roles of wife and mother, and competition for those roles has been based to a large degree upon physical beauty and reproductive capacity.

An important function of the women's movement has been to expand a woman's range of options so that biology is no longer considered the fixed determinant of women's destiny. Nevertheless, a woman's biological attributes and functions continue to be prominant dimensions in determining her social worth. How a woman views the characteristics of her body and its functioning has a strong influence on conclusions she draws about herself in general.

Cognitive distortions in the areas of body image and body functioning are an important component of several major disorders that tend to affect a disproportionate number of women (e.g., eating disorders, anxiety disorders). Adjustment to major changes in body image such as a mastectomy and the experience of female bodily functions (menstruation, pregnancy, childbirth, lactation) may also involve certain cognitive distortions.

### Physical Image

Anyone who has worked with an anorectic woman is familiar with the profound body image distortion that takes place when an emaciated individual is convinced that she is fat.

Varying kinds of distortions may be evident for other women, whether or not they suffer from a major symptomatic disorder, as they struggle to reconcile their own physical self-image with the ideal image endorsed by the external culture. Socioeconomic status and ethnic or racial background can modify this image to a certain degree. However, those features that may distinguish an ethnic or racial background can be interpreted by the woman as further evidence that she is outside the mainstream ideal.

> Maria was a young, American woman of Syrian descent who reported feeling self-conscious and unattractive for as long as she could remember. Her dark complexion, dark hair and tendency toward hirsutism were viewed by her as devastating flaws that would render her as forever ugly and undesirable. Even though she was married, her husband's endorsement of her attractiveness was not powerful enough to overcome the evidence that she had accumulated over the years regarding the differences between herself and what other men and women regarded as attractive.
>
> After marriage, Maria became anxious about keeping her husband and focused her energy upon being a good wife by cooking tremendous meals. In the process, she also soothed her anxiety and self-doubt by overeating. Her sense of desperation about herself in general climbed with her increasing weight. She allowed her participation in the world to narrow as she felt more physically unattractive and therefore worthless. When she finally came to therapy, she reported that her ''whole life was on hold until she could lose weight.''
>
> It was very difficult for Maria to accept the idea that her whole life did not have to hinge upon her physical status. Gradually, she was able to reevaluate physical parts of herself, to view previously devalued features as acceptable or even attractive. It took a long series of graduated steps for Maria to activate various parts of her life such as friendships and work without the security that she imagined would come with physical perfection. In this respect, Maria was like many women who hold the expectation that an ideal physical self will guarantee happiness, security, and acceptance by others. Actual messages from significant others may reinforce a woman's notion that she should work harder to fit the image that others desire in her.

Many women expend enormous amounts of time, energy, and money in an attempt to conform to a socially reinforced physical image. In some instances, additional energy is devoted to self-criticism for deviations from an ideal image. Even women who achieve an ''ideal'' physical image never have continuous or complete payoffs for this effort. Rage, anxiety, frustration, and despair may result. For example, one woman who suffered through numerous diets to reach the ''ideal'' weight of 120 desired by her husband, became enraged when he next asked her to have breast augmentation surgery.

A real physical loss such as a disabling injury or disease presents a special challenge to a woman's ability to overcome long-standing cultural messages and to differentiate her physical self from her overall personal worth. Because of the close link between physical attractiveness and self-worth, some women are also apt to experience the aging process as one of loss and diminishing self-esteem. Thus, cognitive interventions may need to focus on altering the magnified importance of narrowly defined physical attributes, revaluing other personal attributes, and moving away from dependence on the approval of others because the culture tends to endorse some clearly dysfunctional standards for women.

### Physical Function

Dysfunctional ideas about body functioning are evident in a number of symptomatic disorders. A fear of various body sensations is characteristic among agoraphobics (Chambless, Caputo, Bright, & Gallagher, 1984). Body sensations or changes may provide a trigger for anxiety-laden thoughts that escalate into panic (Beck, Emery, & Greenberg, 1985). Difficulties with body functions are also a fundamental component of eating disorders and sexual dysfunctions.

From a cognitive perspective, common dysfunctional thoughts about body functioning often center around fears of losing control, of doing something publicly unacceptable, of appearing less than perfect, of something being terribly wrong with the body, or of not really being able to influence body functions via thoughts or behavior. It is not unusual to see two extremes in clinical presentation—that of a hyperawareness of any notable body sensation with corresponding hyperconcern over the potential meaning of that sensation or an overall disassociation from ongoing body sensations and a lack of awareness of body functions.

Men as well as women may be subject to developing these attitudes. However, girls do undergo a socialization process that emphasizes appearance and self-control and restraint in physical activity. And, as previously noted, physical appearance and function have a great impact upon a woman's sense of social worth. Dealing with a woman's dysfunctional thoughts about her body functioning may be enhanced by recognizing the social and cultural reinforcement of the dysfunctional process. Women may need assistance in recognizing, interpreting, and becoming comfortable with the active nature of their body sensations and functions. Developing a cognitive and behavioral harmony with her bodily energies requires that a woman be willing to accept herself, diminish the priority of perceived social approval, and engage in physically self-nurturing activity.

Four areas of body functioning merit special consideration for their specificity to the female gender. These include menstruation, pregnancy, childbirth, and lactation. Some clues to potential maladaptive cognition can be gleaned from considering prevailing attitudes toward these functions. Rarely are any of these publicly considered to be physically exhilarating endeavors. At best, one should tolerate and get through them as best one can. Menstruation is "the curse" or "the rag." Pregnancy is associated with discomfort, confinement, and loss of physical desirability. Childbirth means agony and pain. Breast milk is something to "dry up" in favor of a bottle or solid foods.

Cognitive therapists, both in and out of their professional roles in health or mental health care systems, can recognize the value in adopting more positive attitudes toward these female bodily functions. These physical experiences can be reevaluated as challenges that offer the opportunity for mastery, pleasure, and appreciation. Women may be prone to doubt their ability to meet a physical challenge, even if they do possess the necessary capability. Cognitive therapists can work directly with clients and with other health care providers (e.g., nurses, obstetricians) to sort out the cognitive distortions that stand in the way of a woman's sense of well-being or free choice regarding these events. Some examples of common distortions might include "I hate having a period. Menstration is always painful" or "I'll lose my figure and become ugly if I get pregnant" or "I can't stand the pain of childbirth" or "I'm not capable of nursing a baby."

Sexual expression is an area where physical functioning can be complicated by social interaction. Men and women need to overcome the sexual double standard that has generally held that good or nice women are not interested in sex. A woman's traditional sexual role has been to be receptive to the man's needs, making sure that he is pleased and satisfied. Women frequently grapple with assumptions about their sexuality that have a moralistic value judgment attached such as, "It is wrong for me to want or enjoy sex." Such a notion can be countered with permission to be sexual—"It's OK for me to want or enjoy my sexuality."

Redefining sexuality as incorporating a broad range of behaviors, beyond just penis-in-vagina intercourse, can be a great help to a woman attempting to change her view of herself as a sexual person. Hugging, caressing, and kissing are sometimes more permissible activities that can help the woman through a transition of seeing sexuality as an acceptable part of herself. Because they may view their role as more of a waiting gatekeeper for sex, many women will have difficulty taking an active role in initiating sexual activity. Again, a broadened range of what is labeled as *sexual behavior* may be of some assistance.

Focusing her awareness on her own wants and needs is another crucial aspect of increasing a woman's sexual initiative (see Barbach, 1975; Heiman, LoPiccolo, & LoPiccolo, 1976). An important cognitive component in this process is the woman's testing of the feasibility and acceptability of making requests on her own behalf. Besides identifying within herself what she might want sexually, she still needs to test whether she actually can ask for it and whether or not she is likely to obtain positive results by asking. It is important to appreciate how difficult it may be for a woman to want and seek anything for herself without feeling guilty or in violation of her feminine role, especially if that something is sexual gratification. Lack of a general behavioral repertoire for seeking on one's own behalf can make the process very clumsy. Significant others may have habituated to the woman's characteristic self-sacrifice, and they may not readily reinforce her attempts to change that behavior. Therapists are cautioned to help women avoid premature conclusions that they cannot ask for what they want or get their needs met.

Several underlying beliefs consistently reemerge across the various areas of physically linked experiences. First is that physical appearances are more important than physical functions. Physical functions are viewed as a source of embarrassment, devaluation, or loss of control. There also is the prevalent belief that it is wrong, bad, or unimportant for a woman to place a priority on nurturing or pleasuring her physical self, except in the interest of making herself more attractive to others. At the same time, a very potent but dysfunctional belief holds that perfection in physical appearance is the key to love, acceptance, pleasure, and enduring self-worth. Alternatives may be developed along the lines of increasing views that accept and value various female physical functions and deemphasize narrow definitions of attractiveness.

## SOCIAL LIVING EXPERIENCES

Experiences within interpersonal relationships constitute a second major area of influence in the development of a woman's schemas. Recent feminist works in the area of women's development highlight interpersonal attachments as fundamental to a woman's self-concept (Surrey, 1983), moral development (Gilligan, 1982), and cognitive organization (Belenky, Clinchy, Goldberger, & Tarule, 1986). Thus, we will consider problematic cognitions from a variety of vantage points in social living.

### Living Alone

Because women are often defined in terms of relationship roles (e.g., wife, mother, daughter), it is not surprising that single life is difficult for many women to accept as a normal and even advantageous lifestyle. And yet many women do live alone—either by choice, because of an absence of suitable partner, or due to divorce or death of a partner. Women who lose their partner due to divorce or death are often particularly vulnerable to the stresses of adapting to life alone. In addition to contending with grief, they also may be living alone for the first time in their life because many women move directly from parents' home to a coupled living arrangement.

Although some women fear life alone, this can be an opportunity for tremendous positive, personal change. For many women, this is the first time in their life they can learn to nurture themselves, to expand independent problem-solving skills, to enjoy time alone, and to value their own identity separate from meeting others' needs. Cognitive therapists can assist women by helping them formulate living alone as a valuable life status rather than as a problem condition to be alleviated as soon as possible.

Primakoff (1983) has described many of the general issues facing people who live alone.

She outlines a cognitive-behavioral group treatment program that helps clients: (1) make a committment to a relationship with themselves, just as one would commit to a love relationship, (2) seek out and pursue the positive opportunities afforded by living alone, and (3) identify the deficits of this lifestyle so systematic solutions for these can be devised (p. 298).

Many people confuse living alone with loneliness. Loneliness has been defined as

the unpleasant experience that occurs when a person's network of social relations is deficient in some important way, either quantitatively or qualitatively. (Perlman & Peplau, 1981, p. 31)

This comparison between the relationships one has and the relationships that are missed is strongly influenced by gender roles. Women are particularly prone to feel lonely living alone to the degree they accept the cultural bias that women are defined by their family or marital relationships.

Common beliefs that reflect this cultural viewpoint are "I am nothing without a man in my life," "It's selfish to only be concerned with my own wishes," and "I can't enjoy myself alone." Although these attitudes do not seem unusual for women, the gender bias is made startlingly clear if a man is imagined to make these statements. Men are expected to have a positive individual self-identity, to take care of themselves, and to manage time alone comfortably.

Cultural pressures for women to be in relationships, to turn to others for protection, and to focus their own energies on taking care of the needs of others often lead women to hold attitudes that make it difficult for them to imagine a happy single life. In addition, culturally normative behaviors make many women economically vulnerable to life alone. Many women now in their 40s and older have not had recent job experience, and so, living alone can bring financial hardship. Even younger women may be hampered by sex bias in salaries for women.

Linda, age 33, found herself contemplating living alone when she decided to separate from her husband of 15 years. As much as she was dissatisfied with her marriage, Linda was terrified to file for divorce because she was convinced she could not live alone. Her thoughts were "I won't know how to take care of things," "I'll be too lonely," and "It's not fair to leave him—he needs me."

Linda could not imagine living alone because she had never done so. She was convinced she would be constantly unhappy and face problems she would not know how to solve. A review of her history as both daughter and wife helped remind her of the many competencies she had both in home upkeep and in taking care of hew own feelings. In fact, one of the reasons she was leaving her husband was because he was oblivious to her emotional needs.

After testing her various negative beliefs about living alone and divorce, the therapist questioned Linda about the positive aspects of living alone. Linda was startled by the concept. The therapist proposed Linda arrange a few days at home alone to see what it was like. Linda was able to take a few days vacation and spend time at home alone while her husband was at work. The therapist gave Linda various assignments in self nurturance such as reading in the sun, taking a bubble bath, and working in her garden. These days were so nice Linda began to look forward to many aspects of living alone. This balanced view eased her anxiety enough that she was able to begin solving some of the realistic problems she would face.

For many women, assignments in self-nurturance are difficult. Women who strongly believe their only role in life is to take care of others may feel guilty or selfish when assigned to focus on themselves. It may be initially helpful to present a model that self-care is a prerequisite of other care. Women often know very well the physical and emotional toll spent in always attending to the needs of others. Often these women come to therapy for depression or stress-related disorders that interfere with their caretaking obligations. They may have an easier time with self-nurturance assignments if the goal is to regain their balance so they can help others again, as a sort of healing.

Once a woman has begun taking care of herself, the therapist may have an easier time getting her to examine schemas that "others always come first." These schemas can easily fit with schemas such as "I am unimportant." If left unexamined in therapy, women clients holding these beliefs are often bound to repeat patterns of self-neglect. An experience of living alone, whether for a few weeks or a lifetime, can provide an ideal opportunity for women to learn to value themselves and take care of their own needs.

## Relationships

Whether living alone or with someone else, most women will have important relationships in their life. Epstein (1983) and Abrams (1983) have addressed issues of cognitive therapy with couples. Burns (1985) has identified many of the beliefs and behaviors that can interfere with dating relationships.

There are a number of relationship issues that are frequent topics in cognitive therapy with women. These include nurturing others at the expense of self-nurturance (described before), difficulties with anger and assertion, conflict resolution strategies, and the importance of friendships outside of a primary relationship.

In relationships with men, women often assume near total responsibility for making the relationship work. From the third grade on, girls show greater ability to correctly identify the emotions of others compared with boys (Rosenthal, Hall, Dimatteo, Rogers, & Archer, 1979). This greater attunement to others is assumed to be a result of differential sex-role socialization rather than a genetic sex difference. A cross-cultural study by Beatrice and John Whiting (1975) found that girls showed more nurturance than boys by offering help and support. Women are socialized to notice feelings and relationship problems and then to solve them. Tavris and Wade (1984) note that "empathy is related to power . . . a less powerful person might learn to read the more powerful person's signals as a matter of self-preservation" (p. 61).

A goal of cognitive therapy with heterosexual couples can be to increase the man's awareness and sensitivity to relationship problems and his partner's feelings. This can be done by exercises in therapy and at home where each partner listens and then identifies the feelings and concerns of the other. Also, the man can be held responsible for making sure the couple sets aside time for the homework. If successful, the man may begin to share the emotional monitoring of the relationship and also give the woman's feelings equal recognition and importance.

Some women also take too much responsibility for relationship management in friendships. In some cases, women may be too accomodating, refusing to set limits on the demands of the friendship or to state personal preferences as to how the friends spend time. These assertion problems are common and can be treated by standard cognitive therapy techniques (Lange & Jakubowski, 1976).

Common underlying schemas for women in assertion situations include "I don't have a right to push my opinions on others" and "It's better to please others and selfish to please myself." For many women, their developmental history includes subtle cultural and familial messages that have supported the notion that women are less important than men. For instance, one client recalled that her father set aside a college fund for each child: $5,000 for her and $10,000 for each of her brothers. Another client reported that when her large family attended a private parochial school, the book fees for the boys were waived whereas the girls were required to scrub school bathrooms in exchange for their book fees.

Often in the course of therapy, women become angry when these issues are identified. It is important the therapist allow the client to experience her anger without prematurely testing the validity of all her angry feelings. A period of anger can be an important stage of identity change (Burtle, 1985).

At the same time, it is important the client be encouraged not to dump all her angry feelings on the one or two important men in her life. It can be helpful to remind her that, just as it has taken her years to recognize these troublesome patterns, it will take some time for others in her life to understand new perspectives on relationship roles. Therapy sessions that include important people in her life may help facilitate cognitive changes in her personal social system.

In some cases, the anger that can arise from reevaluating relationships will provide the energy to make major life changes.

> For example, Maria, age 48, had been in a very unsatisfactory marriage for nearly 20 years. She wanted to leave her husband who had battered her severely during this time. She was frightened to leave him and did not have confidence she could make it on her own. Her own family did not believe in divorce, and there was little sympathy for her battering situation because this was the norm in her family network. Central to Maria's difficulties in deciding to leave her husband were doubts about her ability to survive on her own. The anger she began to experience in therapy provided the energy she needed to take the risk of leaving him. Her anger gave voice to her own needs and rights to assert those needs.

In less dramatic cases as well, anger is often a preliminary stage for women who could improve the quality of their relationships by learning to recognize their wishes and assertively express them. Assertion skills can additionally help women learn to practice effective, non-destructive methods for conflict resolution. Many women either try to avoid conflict or influence relationship decisions through indirect means. A review of research on gender and social influence hypothesized that men are more influential than women because men are more likely to have higher status roles in society (Eagly, 1983). This viewpoint was supported by a series of experiments in which gender, status, and influence were examined (Eagly & Wood, 1982). Learning more direct methods of conflict resolution will add flexibility to women's relationships and can provide a basis for better communication with partners. At the same time, Eagly's research suggests women may need help changing their schemas of self-worth and status before they are comfortable employing new skills of assertion.

Because women are often in role relationships where the expectation is that they please or take care of others (e.g., childcare, pink collar professions), many do not have social support for or experience in the assertion of their own needs. Therefore, in addition to assertion instruction for women clients, it is often necessary to include couples or family counseling to help the relationship system adapt to and accept new assertion behavior. Assertion groups for women are also very helpful in providing a social support network for this change in interaction style.

Beliefs that her needs are less important than those of others or thoughts such as "It's not nice to put myself first" can inhibit women from practicing assertion skills even once they have been learned. Therefore, it is critical that cognitive therapists look for these underlying schemas and help women reevaluate these culturally predominant sex biases.

Finally, balancing the needs of multiple relationships is of concern for many women in therapy. Whether the client is a single mother balancing motherhood with dating or a woman in a committed relationship who also has or wants committed friendships, many women feel "caught in the middle." Cognitive therapy can be very helpful in resolving these dilemmas.

First, recognizing and valuing her own multiple relationship needs (including time for herself alone) can help a woman combat whatever guilty thoughts accompany her relationships. Common guilt thoughts include "It's not fair to leave the kids with a baby-sitter when I work all week." "I should feel happy just being with him." "I never seem to have time. If I were a good friend, I'd see her more often.

Next, it can relieve pressure for the client to communicate clearly with the important people in her life about her needs and to find out what relationship needs they have. Many women are startled to find out their partners do not mind them taking time alone or with other friends. Many friends are understanding of time limitations or a need for greater or lesser intimacy. Children can be supportive of parents' time away if communication replaces guilt. Practicing the communication and assertion skills she has learned in all her relationships can help women achieve a more comfortable balance among partner, children, and friends.

### Parenting Roles

Our culture has a long tradition of endorsing the belief that parenting and child care are primarily a woman's responsibility. Dad's role is that of breadwinner, and Mom's role is seeing to the day-to-day needs of the children. Parenting provides the most accessible source of influence and accomplishment for a large number of women. Many women are able to meet this challenge without major distress. However, mothers, particularly those with small children, constitute a group that is likely to suffer personal discomfort or mental stress (Gove, 1979).

Stressful aspects of this role that could account for the high levels of personal discomfort include low prestige, lack of power, and few contingent rewards (Gove, 1980; Horowitz, 1982). There are several potential factors involved in parenting stress among women that could be addressed with cognitive therapy. Women may have a tendency to equate their total personal worth with their performance in a caretaking role. This can become further complicated by an overgeneralization of the caretaking role so that the mother interprets any emotional or behavioral problem in the child as being ''her fault.''

This distorted belief may even be reinforced by significant others in the environment, including mental health professionals who attribute an astounding array of child psychopathology to inadequacies in the mother (Caplan & Hall-MacQuorcodale, 1985). This guilty, overresponsible view of herself greatly increases the likelihood a woman will conclude she is an inferior mother and, therefore, an unworthy person. Recognizing other potential sources of influence such as other family members and family circumstances or developmental demands can help the mother gain perspective on her sense of total responsibility. Criteria for success or failure in the role of a parent are also quite difficult to define and can be subject to overly global, all-or-nothing distortions.

Although a mother may acknowledge that other people and circumstances influence her child, she often still must confront a reality in which she is designated to provide most of the effort in day-to-day child-rearing responsibilities. The continuous, round-the-clock nature of these demands can limit a woman's access to other activities and thereby increase the likelihood that she views her personal value solely in terms of child rearing. Child care demands can also combine with demands of paid employment so that the mother feels she can not adequately meet the requirements of either role, much less take time for herself. Cognitive and behavioral interventions that assist the woman in structuring her access to other sources of mastery and pleasure and help her move toward these activities without guilt may be crucial to her well-being.

Gina, a 35-year-old mother of an infant girl and a preadolesent boy, experienced a severe exacerbation of a long-standing tendency toward generalized anxiety and panic after she quit her job as a nurse for that of a homemaker. Gina's husband was immersed in running his business and considered all matters of the home and family as delegated to Gina. He would not commit himself to even occasional appointments for child care, suggesting instead that Gina call upon his mother for that help.

Feeling overwhelmed by the daily demands of homemaking and cut off from the previous gratification that she had found through interacting with adults and pursuing athletic endeavors, Gina felt frustrated, unhappy, anxious, angry, and guilty for not totally loving the role of homemaker. Her own sisters were unsupportive because they covetously viewed her situation as an economic luxury to which they were not privileged. Thus, Gina thought that planning time out for herself was selfish and unacceptable because it meant "neglecting" her responsibilities as a mother or being ungrateful for her privileges.

In addition, asking others for help meant, as it does to so many women, that she was making demands rather than taking care of the other person. This violates a very deeply held belief that femininity is defined by nurturance and caring for others. In Gina's belief system, asking too much of others also meant that they would reject and abandon her. By identifying and testing these assumptions, Gina was able to seek assistance from a variety of resources without devaluing herself for doing so. For instance, she arranged for her daughter to attend day care while she went to exercise at a health club. She also began to see a connection between her anxiety about being abandoned and her relative lack of attention to self-nurturing activity.

When it comes to exercising authority in the parental role, women are placed in a double bind by their female socialization. Being kind, understanding, and sensitive to the feelings of their children can be difficult to reconcile with the need to confidently decide upon limits, make demands, and enforce rules. Mothers may manifest either passivity or authoritarianism, or they may vacillate between these two extremes.

In severe cases, the mother's problem with assuming authority may result in actual abuse or neglect of her child. These instances are also quite likely to be complicated by the mother's having had abusive parental models, not having had any model of authoritative parenting, and lacking adequate nurturing as a child and as a parent. Providing access to information about child development and basic behavior management principles is one important strategy for helping women to be more confident and successful as parents.

In addition to having adequate information, mothers may need to address their own cognitive sources of discomfort with parental authority. Sophia, the mother of a 4-year-old girl and a 7-year-old boy, sought assistance for dealing with problems of noncompliance and tantrums in her children. When it became apparent that Sophia was quite passive in enforcing limits with her children, several dysfunctional assumptions were revealed. Sophia believed that in order to raise happy children, she had to make them happy by always immediately gratifying their requests. If she said no to them, she felt guilty and afraid they would reject her. In addition, she believed that the children were the best authorities on how their needs should be met. It was clear to her that her parental authority was malfunctioning in some way, but she did not feel comfortable changing her behavior until she addressed her beliefs about parental limit setting. She was willing and even relieved to institute some more firm limits as part of an experiment to test her children's longer range responses. Although she needed structure and support in carrying out this experiment, she did find that her children were more responsive if she set clearer limits for their behavior.

Other dysfunctional assumptions include the belief that effective parents always get children to agree with their limits. This can set a mother up for an endless round of bargaining, negotiating, and giving in. Or she may believe that it just is not "nice" to be firm or decisive. The results of such distortions all too often are demanding children and a mother who feels manipulated, neglected, and resentful.

If authoritarianism is the problem, the mother may have perfectionistic goals for the way that her children should behave. She may believe that she is personally responsible for controlling their behavior at all times, and, in turn, she may expect her children to have an adult level of self-control. She may be overly invested in external social appearances and conformity and therefore vigilant about the kind of image that her children present. Or she may be systematically channeling anger down a path of least resistance and picking on the only people who are actually subordinate to her.

The most difficult and, unfortunately, probably the most common problem occurs when the mother fluctuates between authoritarianism and passivity. In any case, she may seek help due to feelings of resentment, frustration, guilt, and generally being out of control. Therapists can enhance their efforts to detect and adjust the woman's problematic attitudes toward parenting by focusing on authority as a problem. In therapy, women may need assistance in recognizing and learning the skills involved in exercising power and authority. Therapists may point out how a woman's socialization not only fails to groom her with the necessary skills for assuming authority but also provides her with rules for living (e.g., defer to the wishes of others) that can sabotage her pleasure and effectiveness as an authoritative parent.

Cognitive factors of a slightly different sort may affect a woman's adjustment when she assumes the stepparent role. One prominent area of difficulty involves idealistic expectations regarding the ability of the stepfamily to function as a "normal" nuclear family. In this, the woman may believe that she should feel the love and bonding with her stepchildren that she has or would have felt with her own biological offspring. She may expect benevolent love or at least appreciation and gratitude from her stepchildren. She may expect her spouse to somehow make it all work so that they can live happily ever after as a family.

The reality is more likely to fall far short of these and other expectations. A stepmother may have to use considerable effort to even like her stepchildren. If she has children of her own from a previous marriage, or from the current marriage, the contrast in her feelings may be quite dramatic and inconsistent with her ideal self-image as a consistent and fair mother. Her stepchildren may be indifferent, competitive, contemptuous, or even frankly rude toward her. She may have to contend with severe financial limitations, difficult custody arrangements, and an angry ex-wife. Her spouse may criticize or limit her attempts to discipline the children, whereas, at the same time, expecting her to assume all of the responsibilities traditionally held by the mother in the family. Add to this the difficulties that a woman might encounter in effectively exercising authority, and it becomes easy to understand why a woman might cite stepparenting as the most difficult task she's ever undertaken.

The social reality for a female stepparent incorporates the traditional woman's responsibility of maintaining the emotional well-being of the family as well as overcoming the mistrust cast upon her by the fabled image of a "wicked" stepmother. Individual cognitive interventions that emphasize the development of realistic expectations and limited goals are clearly indicated. At the same time, it is very important for the woman to allow other family members to take responsibility for their own emotional well-being. It may, at times, be desirable to include a family format for addressing these difficulties in cognitive therapy.

*Lesbianism*

Women who identify as lesbian come to therapy for the same issues described throughout this chapter. In addition, depending upon her age, the length of time she has identified as a lesbian, and her sociocultural environment, a number of issues unique to her lesbian status might be a focus in therapy.

In a largely homophobic society, achieving a positive lesbian identity may be difficult for some women due to negative attitudes they may have learned. It is important for therapists working with lesbian clients to familiarize themselves with the myths and realities of lesbian relationships and lesbian culture. The American Psychological Association (APA) publishes a bibliography of responsible writings on lesbian and gay issues (APA, 1985).

For instance, some therapists may not be aware that the Kinsey *et al.* report (1953) estimated that 28% of adult women in the United States experienced attraction to other women. Kinsey and his colleagues estimated that at least 12% of adult women had at least one sexual experience with another woman (pp. 474–475). Contrary to myth, most women who identify as lesbian have had prior romantic/sexual relationships with men (Peplau, Cochran, Rook, & Padesky, 1978). Lesbianism is not caused by poor relationships with parents, fear or hatred of men, chemical imbalances, or masculinity (Storms, 1983). Some lesbians hold the view they were "born lesbian," and others feel they made a choice to love women or one particular woman.

Woman in lesbian relationships report high degrees of satisfaction with these relationships (Peplau, Padesky, & Hamilton, 1983). However, a lesbian client may have difficulty reconciling her positive feelings for women with the negative attitudes she may encounter in her family and the culture at large. In fact, some of her own self-schemata may be negative, due to early socialization toward a poor view of lesbian relationships. A cognitive therapist can help a lesbian client develop a positive self-identity by helping her identify and evaluate her own homophobic beliefs and later by helping her cope better with negative attitudes held by others (Padesky, 1989). When possible, it is helpful if she can take some action to change prejudiced biases held by others, including those in her broader community.

A positive self-identity does not protect lesbians from the special social pressures they may face. Many clients may want help figuring out solutions to some of these dilemmas: expectations at work and in the neighborhood that she is dating men, parental expectations at holidays that she be with them without her lover, what and when to tell her children; how to meet other lesbians; and decisions about how open she will be about her partner preference.

Cognitive therapy can provide a useful framework for the lesbian client by helping her to clarify and test her own beliefs and values about these issues.

> For example, Mariko, age 43, entered her first lesbian relationship when her two sons were 12 and 16 years old. Her parents had raised her in a traditional Japanese family, and she and her husband had raised their sons with a mix of American and Japanese standards. When Mariko left her husband, she had decided her sons would be best cared for by living primarily with their father. This had been a painful decision for her to make. As her relationship with her lover continued and deepened, Mariko wanted to tell her sons but felt unsure if it was the right thing to do.
>
> Her therapist helped Mariko evaluate her sons' capacity to understand and deal with the information about her lesbianism. In addition, she had to consider the potential legal implications of revealing her lesbianism to her family in case she or the boys wanted her to have primary custody at some point in the future. There is legal precedent for denial of custody if the mother is lesbian.
>
> Over time, Mariko was able to talk with her sons and other, more receptive family members about her lesbian relationship, telling some it was a close friendship and others that is was a love relationship. It was also important to Mariko that her lover understand and share some of her family's Japanese traditions. In this way, she was able to reconcile her life with her sons and her new lesbian lifestyle.

## Work

When the role of "worker" is considered, women's social reality clearly diverges from men's in several major respects. This difference is illustrated by the various qualifications that are used in reference to working women that are not typically used when referring to men. There is an interesting paradox in noting that we usually say women work "outside the home." But if a woman works as a homemaker, then she "doesn't work." Work is an area where there is a strong tradition of a division of labor. When work-related problems are the focus of treatment, cognitive therapists are advised to consider incorporating the feminist principle of recognizing negative social realities that contribute to women's difficulties.

A full-time homemaker of today may need considerable assistance in emotionally resolving feelings of guilt and inferiority that stem from thoughts such as ''I must bring in a paycheck in order to be worthwhile'' or ''I am depriving my family by not working'' or ''I'm not very capable or intelligent.'' Although these and similar thoughts reflect problematic attitudes, they are also logical reactions to living in a culture that values achievement and economic status over relationships.

Therapeutic interventions can provide an alternative by reevaluating the homemaker's activities and assigning value by some means other than dollar remuneration. An evaluation of the fair market value of her services may also be of some use to the homemaker, but this cannot factor in the intangible worth of her unique love and commitment. At the same time, homemakers may need support in claiming their right to a portion of their family income. Women who continue to believe that ''it's his money because he earned it'' may be subjecting themselves to maladaptive passivity and dependence. Such attitudes can lead to extremes of guilty self-deprivation or to irresponsible spending.

Homemakers can increase their own sense of value within the family by identifying and altering those attitudes and behaviors that sabotage their self-esteem. At the same time, it is important to recognize that our cultural values do have an impact. Although the culture is shaped by broader factors that are beyond individual control, such as economics, population growth, and technology, individuals can have a small, reciprocal influence, at least in their own day-to-day life.

For women in the paid labor force, there are also clear cultural barriers that can intertwine with individual cognitive distortions. There is much documented evidence that jobs populated primarily by women are typically assigned lower pay and status and less recognition and advancement. For women, there is sexism in obvious and subtle ways, possible sexual harassment, gender isolation, especially at advancing levels, and very little institutional support for the demands of childbearing and family life.

Obviously, if a woman focuses her attention primarily on these barriers, she is apt to become depressed. At the same time, her personal well-being is affected by how she defines such problems as they personally affect her and what reasonable action she takes to create more suitable circumstances. Therapists can encourage women to explore possibilities for higher pay or status jobs, keeping in mind that it may be difficult for a woman to seek something on her own behalf without guilt or awkwardness. On the other hand, a woman's lack of advancement may realistically be attributable to limited opportunities rather than a lack of effort or initiative.

Therapists can also be alert to helping women separate their relational strivings from their achievement strivings. Wanting to be liked or to avoid conflict at all costs can be quite dysfunctional in a work setting, yet it may be hard for a woman to put these relational strivings in perspective. ''I should always be nice and accommodating'' is a widely held belief that can be very incompatible with the demands of the workplace. The personal toll of this belief can range from exploitation and burnout to sexual harrassment. Susan, a secretary in treatment, revealed that she had been doing most of the work in her office in order to ''cover'' for the other secretary who seemed incapable of doing the designated work. Despite doing the work of two, Susan had not received a raise in over 7 years. She had not confronted either of these situations because she did not want to create conflict or hard feelings or risk the possibility that someone might dislike her for seeking recognition.

In addition to individual strategies, it is important to note the feminist principle of bringing society into therapy with women. From a cognitive perspective, this could mean changing some underlying attitudes and rules of our culture in order to resolve problems faced by working women. The attitudes to be changed are those that reflect a devaluation of work done by women. For example, one therapist brought a client's supervisor into therapy sessions and focused on solving the communication patterns that made her feel put down. Therapists can also encourage clients to begin or join groups to help improve work conditions for women or to become involved in political or legislative efforts towards specific social changes.

*Victimization*

Although most women do not come to therapy identifying themselves as victims, in the course of therapy, many women identify past or present victimization experiences that contribute to their problems. These include sexual harassment, rape, incest, and domestic violence.

Survivors of physical, sexual, or emotional violence can benefit from learning to transform the guilt, depression, self-blame, and avoidance that may follow these traumata into self-understanding, support, anger, and social/personal action (cf. NiCarthy, 1986; Nicarthy, Merriman, & Coffman, 1984; Sprei, 1987; Walker, 1979). For women who are repeating the abusive pattern in their current relationships, there will be a need to identify and change schemata of the self and relationships. Case examples illustrate two types of situations.

Janet, age 19, was victim of a date rape 2 years before she began therapy for depression. In the therapy, she gradually revealed to the therapist that her depression had begun after this rape experience. With the therapist, she tested out her various automatic thoughts about the meaning of this rape: "No nice guy will want me now." "It was all my fault—I must have wanted this to happen." "The only way to avoid this from happening again is not to date."

Using the methods of cognitive therapy, Janet evaluated these beliefs and saw that they were not true. She was able to identify what she would do differently in future dating situations. She also recognized that, even if she did all the "right" things, she could never completely eliminate the risk of rape because it was not her action. Janet was able to grieve over her experience once she freed herself from guilt and blame. She then took steps to tell a few close friends about the experience, called the male student who had raped her and let him know how harmful this had been and how angry she felt, and joined a women's support group on campus. By the end of therapy, Janet had resumed dating, was no longer depressed, and felt proud that she could speak out with other students to help them understand the violence of date rape.

Another young woman, Beth, had been the victim of incest by her father for 9 years. She blamed herself for the sexual molestation that began at age 5 and intercourse that began at age 10. She had very negative schemata about herself ("I'm bad and deserve to be abused"), relationships ("People will hurt me. All men are interested in is sex"), and her future ("I'll always feel bad").

Beth had learned to "cope" with her father's sexual abuse by passive dissociation whenever he approached her (i.e., she would become silent, physically passive, and try to block all feelings until he was finished). When Beth began dating in her late teens and 20s, she continued this pattern of behavior whenever the boys and men she dated began to touch or kiss her. Several men and boys were sexually involved with Beth, and she experienced each of these as rapes.

With Beth, the therapy work took much longer and involved a reexamination of her beliefs about incest, her father, and herself. There are several excellent reviews of therapy with incest survivors (cf. Courtois & Sprei, 1987; Herman & Hirschman, 1977), so those issues will not be reviewed here. Cognitive therapy approaches are extremely helpful for women who have survived incest, although cognitive therapists working with these types of problems should also be well-grounded in the incest/rape literature (cf. Finkelhor, 1979; Meiselman, 1978) so client experiences can be evaluated in the context of normative responses. As with all posttraumatic stress reactions, women who survive sexual violence may appear very pathological until the victimization experience is revealed and understood by the therapist. Many "pathological" patterns are actually attempts to cope with unusual traumata. Beth was able to reexamine and change extremely negative schemata about herself and relationships over the course of several years of therapy.

These case examples have emphasized sexual victimization of women because these are common but very traumatic experiences. As many as one-third of all women (Kohn, 1987; Tavris & Wade, 1984, p. 28) are sexually assaulted in their lifetime. Recent research on date rape (Tavris & Wade, 1984) shows that young men frequently interpret women's friendliness or dress as sexual invitation even when a woman states clearly she is not interested in sex. These types of data are important for cognitive therapists working with both women and men in therapy so we can do our part to help clients not misinterpret data, especially when misinterpretation of data may be the cultural norm.

### Midlife and Beyond

As women age, there are changes in roles, relationships, and the experience of self that can be interpreted in a variety of ways. For some women, the years after children leave home are an opportunity to spend more time on personal interests. For others, it is a time of loss and emptiness. Physical aging can be experienced as a series of losses or as a transformation of life. Cognitive therapy has been shown to be an effective therapy for older adults (Thompsen & Gallagher, 1987). Beutler (1987) and his colleagues (Yost, Beutler, Corbishley, & Allender, 1986) have recommended methods for conducting cognitive therapy groups with older adults.

It is helpful for clients concerned with aging issues to make realistic appraisals of losses, whereas, at the same time, adopting a focus on which possibilities exist for the present and future. For example, one woman came to therapy following a stroke. She was quite depressed because she could no longer cook, garden, or dress herself. With the help of therapy, she discovered new activities that brought her joy, including assembling historical scrapbooks for her grandchildren.

Among the very old, a disproportionate number are women. Therefore, although most men spend their older years with a spouse, most women spend their older years without a life partner. According to a recent Census Bureau report, 41% of older women live alone (Horn & Meer, 1987). The earlier section in this chapter on learning to live alone is very applicable for these women.

In their overview of the lives of the elderly, Horn and Meer report that fewer than 1% of older people say they would prefer living with their children. However, they also summarize a Travelers Insurance Company survey that found 28% of their employees older than age 30 directly cared for an older relative in some way for an average of 10 hours per week. According to Horn and Meer,

> "Women, who are more often caregivers, spent an average of 16 hours, and men 5 hours per week. One group, 8% of the sample, spent a heroic 35 hours per week, the equivalent of a second job, providing such care. (p. 89)

Because women are the most likely to provide care for elderly parents, these responsibilities and the feelings that accompany them are discussed frequently with therapists. The additional closeness that comes from caring for an aging parent can be bittersweet in the case of a daughter and parent who have shared a positive relationship throughout life. The daughter may feel anticipatory grief as she watches her parent become older and shares in the losses of friends and function in the parent's life.

On the other hand, the role of caretaker can be especially difficult in families where familial beliefs, emotions, and behaviors have been a source of conflict or emotional distress over the years. In these cases, the caretaker may feel anger and resentment at other family members who may avoid contact with, and responsibility for, the aging parent. In addition, there is the daily stress of learning to be assertive and understanding with a parent who may have very different beliefs and behavior patterns than the daughter.

Standard cognitive therapy techniques can help adult children caring for parents sort out feelings of guilt, anger, grief, and anxiety. In addition, an overview of the family history can help a client question expectations that most caregiving should be done by one child in the family. A shift in duties can protect one family member from becoming overburdened relative to the others. All adult children and the parents may need help in testing the validity of their beliefs about other family members and also help in finding creative solutions to problems.

## SPECIAL CONSIDERATIONS IN THERAPEUTIC TECHNIQUE

### GROUP THERAPY

Group therapy can be a powerful forum for assisting women in their development of more functional beliefs, emotional expression, and behavioral skills. Standard cognitive therapy groups (Hollon & Evans, 1983; Yost *et al.,* 1986) can be modified with some of the characteristics of women's support groups (Brody, 1987) to emphasize social support ingredients, especially for change issues that may not receive sufficient social support outside a therapy format (cf. NiCarthy *et al.,* 1984, on groups for abused women; Whalen & Wolfe, 1983, on sexual enhancement groups for women).

Group therapy has some advantages compared with individual treatment. For example, depressed group members will have distorted views of themselves but fairly accurate views of other group members. Therefore, depressed members can help by pointing out cognitive distortions others have about themselves. In the process, these members begin to understand the idea of cognitive distortion more quickly than they might in individual therapy. Groups also provide an immediate social opportunity for practice of new behaviors and emotional expression.

In addition, women in groups can help each other see patterns that are not only personal but also sociocultural. For example, one group of depressed women notes that they all lacked pleasant activities in their week. At first, they blamed this on themselves, "I must want to be depressed." Then they noted that they all worked, cared for children in the evening, and did cleaning and laundry on weekends. As they shifted the focus from self-blame to cultural norms that they be "supermoms," the women began to feel somewhat better. This new view allowed them to begin problem-solving ways to build pleasure into their lives. The solutions they reached were different for each woman, but each was able to transform the problem from personal blame to a social problem. This change in perspective expanded the range of solutions available. Ultimate solutions including getting help from others (partners or children), modifying standards of performance, and forming child care cooperatives with other women.

In addition to standard cognitive therapy group themes, therapy groups with women often include techniques to enhance an awareness of feelings and expression of affect. Assertion rights, especially the right to have feelings of anger, may be emphasized. Group members can be encouraged to practice assertion in the group by assisting other group members to stay on task. For example, one group member may act as timekeeper, and she can be encouraged to explore her cognitions related to putting limits on other group members.

### SUPERVISION ISSUES

Several different models for cognitive therapy supervision have been presented (Childress & Burns, 1983; Moorey & Burns, 1983; Whalen, 1987). As with the therapy, supervision is best when it is collaborative and when the supervisees are engaged via Socratic questioning and role playing to examine their beliefs and behaviors regarding the therapeutic interaction.

Several areas of supervision are of importance relative to issues discussed in this chapter: transference and countertransference issues with same-sex and opposite-sex therapist, therapist sex role assumptions and beliefs, therapist cultural awareness and sensitivity, and issues of dependency and client empowerment.

Therapist assumptions and beliefs about women, sex roles, and different cultures are certainly important topics for supervision because these therapist cognitions can have a profound influence on the therapy. A supervisor can assist the therapist by asking her or him to identify the beliefs and assumptions that they hold about women, men, sex roles, parenting, lesbians, racial or ethnic groups, religions, or other aspects relevant for particular clients. Then the supervisee can be asked to identify how these beliefs might influence the therapy process.

This analysis is often enhanced within group supervision because supervisees have the benefit of hearing a variety of opinions and beliefs. Of course, the supervisor will be more effective if she or he is well aware of cultural myths and realities and also is able to create an accepting environment where supervisees do not feel attacked for expressing and struggling with biased beliefs.

Testing out culturally influenced beliefs in supervision can provide a model for how the supervisees can do this with clients. It is important for supervisees to become comfortable working within diverse cultural beliefs systems. For example, a young feminist therapist felt it was "wrong" for her Persian client to wear a veil. The therapist decided this "patriarchal custom" was the primary cause of the client's depression. Her supervisor was able to help her acknowledge that not all Persian women who dressed traditionally were depressed. The therapist realized her biases against certain aspects of Persian culture were impeding her ability to listen to the client's idiosyncratic story. The therapist decided to ask the client to explain the meaning of her dress and customs. This new therapeutic stance enhanced rapport, and they then were able to begin to understand the woman's depression.

Of course, part of cultural sensitivity involves developing an awareness of community resources and using these as adjuncts to the therapy. Examples of important community resources are churches, temples, gay and lesbian community groups, parent groups, singles clubs, women's organizations, and classes or clubs coordinated by different ethnic groups in the community.

One supervisee was assigned a client who had grown up in Israel. She came to therapy for panic disorder and a lifetime of generalized anxiety. The therapist attributed the anxiety to interactions with her highly critical and hypochondriacal father. The supervisor suggested the therapist ask the client for more details about her childhood in Israel. The client described bombing raids that terrified her and separations from her parents during wartime confusion. Once the therapist understood the truly traumatic circumstances of the client's childhood, client and therapist were better able to design a successful therapy protocol.

Culturally dominant sex role expectations in our culture can play an important part in transference and countertransference reactions. These may vary, according to the sex of the therapist. Female therapists may be expected to be feminist, even though they may not be so. Some traditional female clients who are homemakers may have thoughts that their working therapist is critical of them for staying at home. Indeed, some female therapists may be very critical of their female clients for acting "dependent" or "passive" in their lives. It is important that female therapists not assume their life experience or values are the same as their female clients. Female therapists can try to elicit transference thoughts from their clients when appropriate. For example, one client was embarrassed to tell her female therapist that she gave up a promotion at work due to performance anxiety because she felt her seemingly self-assured therapist would be disappointed in her.

Male therapists working with female clients need to be alert for subtle sex role pressures that may limit therapy effectiveness. A supervisor noted that many female clients working with one male therapist brought him food and presents. Several clients could be heard teasing him in the hallways after sessions. This behavior was brought up for analysis in supervision. At first the therapist could not see any problem. He felt secure that he was not flirting with these women. The supervisor pointed out that they might be flirting with him or following the female socialization pattern of "taking care of others" rather than allowing themselves to be the focus of help. The therapist agreed to pay closer attention to these therapy relationships.

After several weeks, he recognized that he had gotten hooked into sex role stereotyped behavior with several women. In two cases, he played the role of "protector," rescuing the women from uncomfortable feelings through reassurance rather than helping them learn to cope via collaborative empiricism. He was able to see how this dynamic fit their histories of turning to a strong man to take care of them and his tendency to see women as vulnerable. He recognized that the cognitive therapy goal of helping them learn to take care of themselves was being sabotaged by this interaction no matter how positive it felt for both him and the clients.

In another case, this same male therapist noted an older woman client had adopted a mother role with him—bringing him food and even trying to find him a girlfriend. This interaction fit her pattern of nurturing others rather than herself. Fortunately, once he saw the interactional pattern, this therapist was able to address these issues with these clients. As therapist and clients worked together to relate in more therapeutic rather than sex role stereotyped ways, these transference/countertransference issues provided powerful learning opportunities for all involved.

## CONCLUSION

Enhancing cognitive therapy with women requires that gender be recognized as an important variable that interacts with social realities and cognitive schemata. In the process of conducting cognitive therapy with women, therapists have an opportunity to enhance the well-being of women by fostering egalitarianism in the therapy relationship, by recognizing the impact of cultural socialization, and by validating female experiences through attention to relevant content areas.

Case examples cited in the context of supervision issues illustrate the importance of not fostering dependency with women clients. One of the strengths of cognitive therapy is that it helps empower clients by teaching them to help themselves. This goal is particularly important for women because many aspects of socialization hamper a woman's confidence in her ability to care for herself. Cognitive therapists can use their awareness of this fact to be alert for indications of negative self-schemata in women clients.

Although there are many variations, most of these negative beliefs center around distortions in the woman's views of her value, importance, capability, and responsibility vis-à-vis other people. An important theme in the therapeutic development of alternatives is helping the women to incorporate self-nurturing as an acceptable part of a female repertoire. At the same time, multiple relationship needs are accepted, valued, and integrated with self-nurturing strategies. The processes of cognitive therapy can thus provide a powerful transformational tool for women of diverse cultural backgrounds and for therapists stretching their own conceptions of client possibilities.

## REFERENCES

Abrams, J. (1983). Cognitive-behavioral strategies to induce and enhance a collaborative set in distressed couples. In A. Freeman (Ed.), *Cognitive therapy in couples and groups* (pp. 125–155). New York: Plenum Press.

556

DENISE DAVIS and
CHRISTINE PADESKY

American Psychological Association. (1985). *A selected bibliography of lesbian and gay concerns in psychology: An affirmative perspective*. Washington, DC: Author.

Barbach, L. (1975). *For yourself: The fulfillment of female sexuality*. New York: Doubleday.

Beck, A., Emery, G., & Greenberg, R. (1985). *Anxiety disorders and phobias*. New York: Basic Books.

Belenky, M., Clinchy, B., Goldberger, N., & Tarule, J. (1986). *Women's ways of knowing*. New York: Basic Books.

Beutler, L. (1987, Winter). The application of CT in groups of older adults. *International Cognitive Therapy Newsletter*. pp. 3, 5. (Available from Center for Cognitive Therapy, 1101 Dove Street, Suite 240, Newport Beach, CA 92660.)

Blechman, E. (1984). Women's behavior in a man's world: Sex differences in competence. In E. Blechman (Ed.), *Behavior modification with women*. (pp. 3–33) New York: Guilford.

Brody, C. (Ed.). (1987). *Women's therapy groups: Paradigms of feminist treatment*. New York: Springer Publishing Company.

Brown, L., & Liss-Levinson, N. (1981). Feminist therapy I. In R. Corsini (Ed.), *Handbook of innovative psychotherapies*. (pp. 229–314). New York: Wiley.

Burns, D. (1985). *Intimate connections*. New York: New American Library.

Burtle, V. (1985). Therapeutic anger in women. In L. Rosewater & L. Walker (Eds.), *Handbook of female therapy: Women's issues in psychotherapy* (pp. 71–79). New York: Springer Publishing Company.

Caplan, P., & Hall-McCorquodale, I. (1985). Mother-blaming in major clinical journals. *American Journal of Orthopsychiatry. 55*(3), 345–353.

Chambless, D., Caputo, C. G., Bright, P., & Gallagher, R. (1984). Assessment of fear of fear in agoraphobics: The Body Sensations Questionnaire and the Agoraphobic Cognitions Questionnaire. *Journal of Consulting and Clinical Psychology, 52,* 1090–1097.

Childress, A., & Burns, D. (1983). A group supervision model in cognitive therapy training. In A. Freeman (Ed.), *Cognitive therapy with couples and groups* (pp. 323–335). New York: Plenum Press.

Courtois, C., & Sprei, J. (1988). Retrospective incest therapy for women. In L. Walker (Ed.), *A handbook on sexual abuse of children: Assessment and treatment issues* (pp. 270–308). New York: Springer Publishing Company.

Deaux, K. (1984). From individual differences to social catagories: Analysis of a decade's research on gender. *American Psychologist, 39,* 105–116.

Eagly, A. (1983). Gender and social influence: A social psychological analysis. *American Psychologist, 38,* 971–981.

Eagly, A., & Wood, W. (1982). Inferred sex differences in status as a determinant of gender stereotypes about social influence. *Journal of Personality and Social Psychology, 43,* 915–928.

Epstein, N. (1983). Cognitive therapy with couples. In A. Freeman (Ed.), *Cognitive therapy with couples and groups* (pp. 107–123). New York: Plenum Press.

Farrell, J., & Davis, D. (1986). *Feminist perspective in cognitive-behavioral psychotherapy*. Unpublished manuscript.

Finkelhor, D. (1979). *Sexually victimized children*. New York: The Free Press.

Gilbert, L. (1980). Feminist therapy. In A. Brodsky and R. Hare-Mustin (Eds.), *Women and Psychotherapy* (pp. 245–265). New York: Guilford.

Gilligan, C. (1982). *In a different voice: Psychological theory and women's development*. Cambridge, MA: Harvard University Press.

Gove, W. (1979). Sex, marital status, psychiatric treatment: A research note. *Social Forces,* 89–93.

Gove, W. (1980). Mental illness and psychiatric treatment among women. *Psychology of Women Quarterly, 4,* 345–362.

Heiman, J., LoPiccolo, L., & LoPiccolo, J. (1976). *Becoming orgasmic: A sexual growth program for women*. Englewood Cliffs, NJ: Prentice-Hall.

Herman, J., & Hirschman, L. (1977). Father-daughter incest. *Signs, 2,* 735–756.

Hollon, S., & Evans, M. (1983). Cognitive therapy for depression in a group format. In A. Freeman (Ed.), *Cognitive therapy with couples and groups* (pp. 11–41). New York: Plenum Press.

Horn, J., & Meer, J. (1987, May). The vintage years. *Psychology Today,* pp. 77, 80–84, 89–90.

Horowitz, A. (1982). Sex-role expectations, power, and psychological distress. *Sex Roles, 8,* 607–623.

Kinsey, A., Pomeroy, W., Martin, C., & Gebhard, P. (1953). *Sexual behavior in the human female*. Philadelphia: Sanders.

Klein, M. (1976). Feminist concepts of therapy outcome. *Psychotherapy: Theory, Research and Practice, 13(1),* 89–95.

Kohn, A. (1987, February). Shattered innocence. *Psychology Today,* pp. 54–58.

Lange, A., & Jakubowski, P. (1976). *Responsible assertive behavior: Cognitive/behavioral procedures for trainers.* Champaign, IL: Research Press.

Markus, H., Crane, M., Bernstein, S., & Siladi, M. (1982). Self-schemas and gender. *Journal of Personality and Social Psychology, 42,* 38–50.

Meiselman, K. (1978). *Incest,* San Francisco: Jossey-Bass.

Moorey, S., & Burns, D. (1983). The apprenticeship model: Training in cognitive therapy by participation. In A. Freeman (Ed.), *Cognitive therapy with couples and groups* (pp. 303–321). New York: Plenum Press.

NiCarthy, G. (1986). *Getting free: A handbook for women in abusive relationships.* Seattle, WA: The Seal Press.

NiCarthy, G., Merriman, K. & Coffman, S. (1984). *Talking it out: A guide to groups for abused women.* Seattle, WA: The Seal Press.

Padesky, C. (1989). Attaining and maintaining positive lesbian self-identity: A cognitive therapy approach. *Women & Therapy, 8,* 145–156.

Peplau, L. A., Cochran, S., Rook, K. & Padesky, C. (1978). Loving women: Attachment and autonomy in lesbian relationships. *The Journal of Social Issues, 34,* 7–27.

Peplau, L. A., Padesky, C., & Hamilton, M. (1983). Satisfaction in lesbian relationships. *Journal of Homosexuality, 8,* 23–35.

Perlman, D., & Peplau, L. A. (1981). Toward a social psychology of loneliness. In R. Gilmour & S. Duck (Eds.), *Personal relationships: 3. Personal relationships in disorder* (pp. 31–56). London: Academic Press.

Primakoff, L. (1983). One's company: two's a crowd: Skills in living alone groups. In A. Freeman (Ed.), *Cognitive therapy with couples and groups* (pp. 261–301). New York: Plenum Press.

Resick, P. (1985). Sex role considerations for the behavior therapist. In M. Hersen & A. Bellack (Eds.), *Handbook of clinical behavior therapy with adults.* New York: Plenum Press.

Rosenthal, R., Hall, J., Dimatteo, M., Rogers, P., & Archer, D. (1979). *Sensitivity to non-verbal communication: The PONS test.* Baltimore: Johns Hopkins University Press.

Schaef, A. (1985). *Women's reality.* Minneapolis: Winston Press.

Solomon, L., & Rothblum, E. (1986). Stress, coping, and social support in women. *The Behavior Therapist, 9,* (10), 199–204.

Sprei, J. (1987). Group treatment of adult women incest survivors. In C. Broody (Ed.), *Women's therapy groups: Paradigms of feminist treatment* (pp. 198–216). New York: Springer Publishing Company.

Storms, M. (1983). *Development of sexual orientation.* Washington, DC: American Psychological Association, Office of Social and Ethical Responsibility.

Surrey, J. (1983). The relational self in women: Clinical implications. *Work in Progress,* No. 82-02, Wellesley College.

Tavris, C., & Wade, C. (1984). *The longest war: Sex differences in perspective* (2nd ed.). New York: Harcourt Brace Jovanovich.

Thompson, L., & Gallagher, D. (1987, Winter). The efficacy of individual cognitive and behavioral therapies for late-life depression. *International Cognitive Therapy Newsletter,* pp. 3, 6–8, 10. (Available from Center for Cognitive Therapy, 1101 Dove Street, Suite 240, Newport Beach, CA 92660.)

Walker, L. (1979). *The battered woman.* New York: Harper & Row.

Whalen, S. (1987, Summer). Supervision training in cognitive therapy: Part II. *International Cognitive Therapy Newsletter,* pp. 2, 5. (Available from Center for Cognitive Therapy, 1101 Dove Street, Suite 240, Newport Beach, CA 92660).

Whalen, S. & Wolfe, J. (1983). Sexual enhancement groups for women. Kin A. Freeman (Ed.). *Cognitive therapy with couples and groups* (pp. 221–260). New York: Plenum Press.

Whiting, B., & Whiting, J. (1975). *Children of six cultures. A psychocultural analysis.* Cambridge, MA: Harvard University Press.

Yost, E. B., Beutler, L., Corbishley, M. & Allender, J. (1986). *Group cognitive therapy: A treatment approach for older adults.* New York: Pergamon Press.

# 28

# Cognitive Group Therapy

RICHARD L. WESSLER AND SHEENAH HANKIN-WESSLER

## INTRODUCTION

In this chapter, we describe three broadly defined approaches to cognitive group therapy: (1) a structured psychoeducational approach, (2) a problem-solving approach, and (3) an experiential-affective approach. None of these approaches needs to be used exclusively or to the exclusion of the others, and they may be used in flexible combinations depending upon clients' characteristics and the setting in which the therapist works. Regardless of approach, the focus in cognitive group therapy is upon the individual rather than upon the group or upon relationships that develop among members of the group (including the therapist).

Group therapy, even more than individual therapy, provides opportunities for observing clients' interactions and making comments about them. Goldfried (1980) identifies two common features of all verbal psychotherapies: corrective emotional experiences and direct feedback about clients' behavior. The group process provides material and the group setting a forum in which both the leader and members can give useful information about clients' belief systems and behaviors, especially social behaviors. These observations can be valuable when changes are contemplated. A woman who complained that she was only approached by men who treated her as though she were immediately available sexually was surprised by feedback she received from the group about her overtly flirtatious manner and appearance. Using their feedback and information about new venues where she might meet more suitable men, she was able in subsequent group sessions to practice her new image and to rehearse new introductory conversations with two or three male members of the therapy group.

Groups provide a setting in which members can make plans for having novel and corrective emotional experiences and can observe their own behavior and receive feedback about it. A therapy group is an ideal setting for this to occur in that it provides an environment of perceived safety—a small, unusual version of the often-feared outside world.

In the pages that follow, we discuss the role of the therapist, therapeutic alliance,

RICHARD L. WESSLER AND SHEENAH HANKIN-WESSLER • Cognitive Therapy Associates, 103 East 86th Street, and Pace University, New York, New York 10128.

RICHARD L.
WESSLER and
SHEENAH HANKIN-
WESSLER

assessment, three approaches to group therapy, and applications and limitations of cognitive group therapy.

# RESPONSIBILITIES OF THE THERAPIST

The task of the cognitive group therapist varies, depending upon which of the three approaches is used. There are obvious differences among teaching mental health principles to a group to people (who then have the task of applying them to their individual concerns), solving practical and psychological problems presented by individuals, and using methods more often associated with humanistic-experiential therapies to raise affect, gain insight, and formulate individual plans of action that aim to promote changes in behavior, affect, and personality. In addition to procedural differences, there are differences in theoretical assumptions and in what information about each group member the therapist attends to.

Cognitive group therapy is based partly on an educational model rather than a medical, emotional release, relationship, or conditioning model of psychotherapy. The use of an educational model is typical of those cognitive approaches Mahoney and Gabriel (1987) classified as rationalistic, that is, they assume that incorrect descriptions of and inferences about reality are the sources of emotional disturbance. For example, fear results when one mistakenly describes a situation as dangerous and depression when one incorrectly infers a situation to be hopeless. The correcting of misconceptions is assumed to be necessary for lasting change to occur, and the principal change technique is the presenting of new or corrective information. As Raimy (1975) stated:

> If those ideas or conceptions of a client or patient which are relevant to his psychological problems can be changed in the direction of greater accuracy where his reality is concerned, his maladjustments are likely to be eliminated. (p. 7)

A rationalistic approach usually assumes that behavior and emotion are direct results of cognitive processing. To say the same idea differently, cognitions are seen as mediators between stimulus events and psychological responses. This assumption in part determines the task of the therapist:

> Therapists begin by helping their clients to find the thoughts, belief, or schemata that are causing their negative emotions and behaviors . . . [and then help] clients to change their irrational beliefs from those that are unrealistic and harmful to those that are more rational and useful. (McMullin, 1986, p. xv)

A different view of the therapist's task comes from what Mahoney and Gabriel called a constructivistic position or one in which people create rather than recreate reality. In the rationalistic position, the human is likened to a camera, which, when properly focused and in the right light, records an accurate though miniature picture of reality. The constructivistic position draws an analogy between the mind and an artist who creates a unique version of reality on paper or canvas, a creation that may be nonrepresentational but whose accuracy is taken for granted by the artist. The question to be answered in the rationalistic position has to do with the accuracy of one's depiction of reality, but, in the constructivist position, the question has to do with the usefulness of one's portrayal of reality. The task of the therapist is to help each person develop less problematic and more useful cognitions about self, others, and the world.

Cognitive psychotherapy is also partly based on an attitude-change model (Wessler & Wessler, 1980; Wessler 1983). In social psychology, attitudes are typically defined as having three components (knowledge, affect, and action) in a mutually interdependent relationship. One of these, the affective component, is virtually synonymous with attitude and consists of appraisals, cognitive evaluations, or simply "hot" cognitions. Several contemporary theories of emotion assign a crucial role to appraisals or evaluative cognitions (Arnold, 1960; Beck, 1976; Lazarus & Folkman, 1984; Plutchik, 1980). Information giving has little effect on these hot cognitions, for they are implicated with affect rather than knowledge, and they are rooted in attitudinal processes rather than evidence and logic. The therapist's task is one of persuasion rather than education. There is nothing quite so persuasive as personal experience. People tend to adjust their appraisals to fit what they have done or to fit what they have learned, or both.

Thus far, we have distinguished among descriptive and inferential (or cold) cognitions and evaluative (or hot) cognitions and related these distinctions to the task of the therapist. There are two other types of cognitions that influence what the cognitive group therapist does.

One distinction is between conscious and nonconscious cognitions. The use of the term *nonconscious* should not be understood in a Freudian sense, with its emphasis on hidden motives and ego-protecting mechanisms. Cognitions may be nonconscious in the sense that they lie outside one's awareness and have not been labeled or verbalized (Guidano & Liotti, 1983). Contemporary cognitive psychology has come to accept a significantly less conscious version of human functioning, one that takes nonconscious processes as standard (Kihlstrom, 1987). Cognitive psychotherapy has postulated the existence of, and worked with, nonconscious processes in the form of irrational beliefs (Wessler, 1983), automatic thoughts (Beck, 1976), cognitive structures (Meichenbaum, 1977), and personal rules of living (Wessler & Hankin-Wessler, 1986). Experimental evidence for nonconscious algorithms (i.e., stored routines for the processing of social information) has been compiled by Lewicki (1986) and clinical implications discussed by Wessler (1988).

The therapist's task, except when functioning as an educator, is to identify an individual's nonconscious processes. This can be done by taking an "as-if" attitude: One can say that the client acts "as if" he or she were following some nonconscious algorithm or holds a particular belief or cognition. The therapist must be able to cite evidence to support the "as-if" statement. Feedback from other group members can add further support for the therapist's inference, and group members themselves can offer speculations about each other's nonconscious cognitions.

The final category of cognitions is decisions about one's behavior. These are special cognitions in which the probable outcomes of one's actions are weighed (Janis, 1983). Of special therapeutic importance are decisions to think and act in ways that are inconsistent with one's affective states, for example, acting in spite of anxiety in order to demonstrate self-efficacy and to bring about changes in one's self-conceived competence (Bandura, 1977). In addition to thinking about one's actions (instead of mindlessly repeating them), it is possible and often desirable to use self-instructional statements to help carry out one's decisions to act differently (Meichenbaum, 1977). Self-instructional statements not only guide the person to act differently, but they can encourage by expressly noting what new affective consequences are likely to result from carrying out one's decision. The therapist's task, especially in problem-solving groups, is to help clients to reach decisions and to help them implement their decisions.

## THERAPIST AS LEADER

Skillful and inventive leadership can result in the group being much "larger than life," in that feared stimuli, either internal or external, can be introduced in the group members' experiences, and normal anxiety-reducing avoidance and escape from such situations can be overcome. A member of a therapy group may test out different ways of behaving and begin to experience and reevaluate the cognitive structures that are the predictors of human behavior. Between group sessions, a member can continue to build on his or her experiences by

RICHARD L.
WESSLER and
SHEENAH HANKIN-
WESSLER

undertaking carefully planned homework assignments. The therapist and group members can provide modeling and direct feedback on his or her in-group behavior, proposed homework assignments, and how they were carried out.

The authors attempt in their groups to mirror and exaggerate the real world by creating a dynamic atmosphere in which a variety of different opportunities and unexpected situations are presented. We help members to work on their presenting concerns and conscious disturbances. We also attempt to help them uncover their nonconscious algorithms. We agree with Lazarus (1981) that images that a person creates are often the direct cause of emotional disturbance and that many streams of images are nonconscious thoughts outside one's awareness. By the use of imagery and guided fantasy, we attempt to raise affect, which helps clarify clients' cognitions and to illustrate vividly the interrelation of cognition, affect, and behavior (Greenberg & Safran, 1987). We also attempt to create for the group members situations in which they may have new experiences. The members, as a result of this experience, become more motivated in their attempts to change and develop more commitment, which will increase the attractiveness of the chosen course of action.

The leader of a therapy group is a therapist who has the task of providing structure for group experiences and problem-solving efforts. The group members are clients who have the task of furnishing content for each session. The leader is not a facilitator who merely creates conditions for positive growth potentials to become fulfilled nor a member of the group and thus free to probe his or her own problems or socialize with clients outside the therapy sessions. The therapist is a professional with the ethical responsibilities of a professional in the psychological counseling and therapy field.

The therapist takes an active role in each session unless he or she deliberately chooses to withdraw from the discussion and act as a coach rather than teacher–therapist. The therapist manages each session to insure that no one or two people dominate it, that no one becomes disruptive, and that antitherapeutic statements and actions by group members are not allowed to influence other group members in a detrimental way. The management of the group discussion can be done diplomatically and the discussion steered into productive areas rather than allowed to wander aimlessly.

When the therapist acts as a coach, the group members are responsible for solving personal problems presented by a focal client, processing a group experience, and applying the therapeutic model in a helpful manner. If the group does not stick with its task or does it poorly, the therapist can intervene. Because group members are likely to propose practical solutions without attempting to work on psychological difficulties or cognitions, the therapist should remain alert and actively involved in this discussion even when silent.

The therapist also has responsibility for emotional-expressive interactions within the group. Although cognitive therapy groups are primarily task oriented, they are not exclusively so. Personal and interpersonal concerns are not uncommon in the course of a discussion, unless the therapist takes a highly didactic, therapist-focused approach to the conduct of group therapy.

The process of group therapy requires attention to the dynamics of the therapy group. The individual is the focus of change, and dynamics are important insofar as they affect the individual's thinking, feelings, and actions. The norms of the group, its communication patterns, and emerging leadership roles can be used therapeutically, or they can encourage continued maladaptive thinking, emoting, and acting. There is a risk that group members may reach a tacit agreement (group norm) not to confront each other or to offer only practical problem-solving suggestions or substitute commiseration for help in order to protect themselves from shameful feelings. An experienced leader–therapist will recognize such actions, comment on them, and try to prevent their recurrence.

Cohesiveness of group members, which is a usual prerequisite for the development of group norms, is allowed, promoted, or discouraged, depending on whether therapeutic aims of individual group members are helped or hindered by group cohesiveness. It is not a primary aim in cognitive group therapy, but, if used wisely, cohesiveness can significantly facilitate the therapeutic process.

Wessler and Wessler (1980) have discussed the general clinical and counseling skills possessed by professionals who most effectively learn to do cognitive psychotherapy. These include skill at assessing clients' problems (including defensive maneuvers that work against change), ability to empathize with clients, knowledge about monitoring the relevant aspects of the interactions between therapist and client, willingness to work actively and directively with clients and to provide structure for sessions, and having the flexibility to vary one's approach in order to fit each client's individuality.

Psychotherapy resembles surgery more than it resembles medicine. Successful outcomes in surgery depend on both the procedure *and* the practitioner. Just as the skill of the practitioner interacts with the procedures he or she employs, so the "bedside manner" of the practitioner and the confidence it inspires in the patient interacts with procedures. Flexibility is the byword of the effective therapist. Practicing clinicians can seldom afford the luxury of a "pure" approach. A well-constructed treatment plan can more fully meet the challenges of the client's problems.

A qualified leader is a member of the psychological, counseling, social work, psychiatric, or closely allied professions, for example, nursing, or the clergy. The leader is, therefore, bound by the ethical code of his or her respective profession and subject to its discipline. Leaders should not knowingly harm clients, should keep privileged information confidential, and should avoid such unethical practices as sexual contact with clients.

In addition, the therapist has the responsibility to assure that group members conduct themselves according to ethical standards. The therapist should prevent any harmful actions or statements made by group members, and, if harm is done, to try to correct it. The confidentiality of group discussions should be stressed; client breaches of confidentiality should be met with warnings followed by expulsion from the group for a repeated violation.

The therapist may also see individuals from the group for private sessions. Individual sessions may supplement group sessions for clients with pressing problems or acute disturbances. Group sessions may also supplement individual sessions for clients with interpersonal and social problems. Clients who initially appear suitable for group therapy but later prove otherwise might be referred for individual sessions, or for medication, and even hospitalization. Clients' acceptance of such referrals can be made a condition for remaining in the group or for rejoining it at a later time.

## THERAPEUTIC ALLIANCE

There is no assumption that any special relationship must be established between therapist and client or therapist, client, and other group members. However, as Dryden (1984) has noted, for treatment to proceed, a sound therapeutic alliance between the group leader and members should exist. In order to establish an effective therapeutic alliance, the client probably has to perceive the therapist as credible and accepting of the client as a person. The literature on attitude change and persuasion (Zimbardo, Ebbeson, & Maslach, 1977) and on effective counseling (Janis, 1983) supports this notion. Perceptions of credibility are promoted when the therapist shows expertise and trustworthiness. A confident manner and belief is what he or she does tend to communicate expertise as do educational degrees and professional reputation and recognition.

The therapist provides a model for the group. In order to be seen as trustworthy, the leader will try to build warm, empathetic relationships with group members and to create an atmosphere in which clients' improvement and welfare are seen as goals of therapy. Clients develop when the therapist is perceived as genuinely interested in helping them and not in meeting his or her own views of what constitutes change.

There are many other therapist variables that can color clients' perceptions. A leader who is energetic, highly motivated, and appropriately enthusiastic will help to encourage optimism among group members. Credibility is promoted when clients feel understood by their therapist. Good diagnostic skills seem essential to good understanding, including understanding what the client does not know.

The therapeutic alliance is important for another reason that is quite unrelated to any presumed curative aspects of the relationship. Therapist characteristics that are irrelevant to clients' beliefs probably influence the acceptance of alternative ways of thinking. This point is supported by studies of attitude change (Strong & Claiborn, 1982). In other words, clients may change their minds for reasons other than evidence and logic. Clients may believe a therapist because they like him or her, or reject statements because they do not feel positively toward the person making them. If the individual does not like, respect, or trust group members and therapist, the chances of helping are greatly reduced.

The reduction of defensive communication is an important goal in therapy. We prefer to confront this issue directly and help convince group members that, by disclosing personal information and thus risking criticism and rejection, they cannot only survive but live better. "Who believes that 'keeping oneself to oneself' is a good idea", "Is it better to be polite or honest?" are questions that usually afford lively discussions. Often the emotional consequences of living by such rigid norms and values are revealed.

In many approaches to group psychotherapy, leaders, or rather "facilitators," attempt to develop a warm, loving, supportive climate in which people can trust each other because the approach assumes that such a climate is in itself therapeutic. The authors share the view that such a climate is not therapeutic by itself, but we believe that a warm, loving, supportive climate can promote conditions by which other therapeutic interventions can prove effective.

It may be desirable, and at times necessary, to encourage people to reveal facts about themselves and to trust each other, but it is seldom necessary to continue this practice for very long. *Trust* is a term that is regularly raised in the early stages of group therapy. The so-called need for trust is often overemphasized and requires clarification. Logically, some group members may refuse to trust the group and refuse to reveal intimate details about themselves because they could easily be disadvantaged by others' having knowledge of some privileged communication. Dissatisfied employees and unfaithful spouses come into this category. There is no guarantee that group members will not reveal secrets; despite careful security screening, the CIA regularly experiences such leakage. No promises of confidentiality can be made and invariably kept—and this is the definition of trust in this case. However, the therapist can firmly request that no group business be discussed outside the group setting and can show how this is unhelpful.

More often, personal information is withheld for psychological rather than practical reasons. The experiencing of guilt and shame may lead to avoidance reactions. Skeletons that are silently concealed in closets are especially hard to exorcise. Here the therapist would best concentrate on the maladaptive cognitions that relate to these emotions. "I don't trust the group; if I confess that I sleep around they will say I am promiscuous, and I will be sexually harassed as a result," one young woman claimed. The therapist focused on the clients' rigid rules of living, which in this case include ideas such as "It is wrong to enjoy sex and be sexually active. I am a hypocrite for thinking it is wrong and then doing it anyway. If men know that a woman likes sex and is available, they will treat her like a whore." Each of these statements is extremely evaluative in tone. The dissuasive tactics employed in this example included helping the woman adopt a more self-accepting and less critical self-attitude for choosing (and choice is emphasized) to act in certain ways. Later, through assertiveness training, the woman learned to refuse unwanted sexual overtures.

Fear of psychological attack is yet another problem that hovers around the shaky trust issue. Some clients fear revealing their personal problems because they suspect that there might be some undiscovered psychological cause for their disturbance—that their difficulties may be much more serious than anyone has yet declared. They fear having their fears confirmed and expect they will suffer at the hands of other people. Of course, there is nothing to trust other people with, in a very important sense, as psychological reactions result from their own cognitions and symbolic representations of reality, not from other people's words. The group members might more usefully ask, "Can I trust this therapist and these other people to help me with my problems? Do they have the necessary skills and information?" This issue, which seems much more realistic, is rarely mentioned in therapy groups.

## ASSESSMENT ISSUES

Cognitive group therapy begins with an assessment of each person's problems. This individual assessment occurs prior to the formation of a group or the person's joining an already established group. Persons who cannot participate effectively due to the severity of pathology, tendencies to dominate discussions, excessive withdrawal and silence, or other disqualifying behaviors can thus be screened out and referred for other forms of treatment.

Assessment includes inventorying the person's main cognitions, appraisals, emotional difficulties, and patterns of behavior, and their interrelations. Physical and demographic data are needed as well. A convenient way to collect such information is to use the Life History Questionnaire (Lazarus, 1981) or some similar form supplemented with an individual interview.

Assessment of DSM-III-R Axis-I conditions may be done in a clinical interview with or without additional information provided by psychological tests. The use of the Beck Depression Inventory (BDI) is common in cognitive group therapy for depression; Hollon and Shaw (1979) recommended its routine use during each meeting of the therapy group. Other measures used in individual therapy can be used in group therapy with equal confidence.

The authors also recommend that DSM-III-R Axis-II conditions be assessed. Disordered features of the personality are a barrier to therapeutic change, and, in an unknown number of cases, account for the failure of therapy to attain success. Depressed persons who show strong features of borderline personality disorder (a common subtype of borderline personality disorder) are unlikely to benefit from group therapy and can be expected to impede the progress of other group members. When anxiety and depression do not improve during a 3- or 4-month period, or when a client voluntarily stays in treatment after Axis-I symptoms have improved, the therapist, knowingly or not, has begun to deal with the personality (Wessler, 1988; Millon, 1981).

The assessment of borderline and other personality disorders may be done in a clinical interview, using DSM-III-R criteria as a guide for making the assessment. Scales developed by Millon (1981) are valuable, especially for therapists who are not familiar with the diagnosis of the disorders of personality.

Therapists, unless they are working with homogeneous populations, should assess the cultural backgrounds of potential group members. Group members need to understand each other, just as the therapist needs to understand the norms and values of each group member and the cultural source of these norms and values (Sue, 1981). The "stiff-upper-lip WASP" seems unemotional in contrast to the colorful and often histrionic expressions of Hispanic peoples. Increasing numbers of immigrants to America come from non-Western European countries, a fact that underscores both the challenge to therapists and the importance of cultural factors to therapy.

Assessment also involves an understanding of clients' cognitive appraisals and patterns of behavior, as the therapeutic process must begin here. Other nonpsychological problems are usually revealed in this procedure; it is convenient to think of clients as having practical problems of living and psychological disturbances about those practical problems. Direct assessment methods involve the therapist and group members in an active dialogue with the focal client. They ask questions, probe answers, offer comments, and test hypotheses inferred from a focal client's self-reports of thoughts, feelings, and actions, as well as his or her behavior in the group.

## PSYCHOEDUCATIONAL APPROACH

The term *psychoeducational* refers here to approaches that have teaching as their primary objective, with little or no attention given to the individual problems or concerns of each group member. Typically, psychoeducational approaches are time-limited and highly structured. Psychoeducation groups might meet for as little as 1 or 2 sessions, or for as many as 15. Group members might be a passive audience for lectures supplemented with audiovisual materials or enter into limited discussions with one or more group leaders.

Psychoeducational groups usually emphasize self-help and furnish information each participant can use in a self-administered program of personal growth and development. They rely on suggested or assigned readings of popular self-help books, for example, Burns's *Feeling Good* and Ellis and Harper's *A New Guide to Rational Living*.

Written and behavioral homework might be assigned, especially if the group meets more than once or twice. These assignments can be discussed during group meetings, or in the case of written homework, reviewed later by the leader to check on each person's understanding of the concepts and principles that have been presented. Written homework consists of forms and schedules filled out by participants between sessions. These forms include self-inventories of cognitions, records of attempts at change, self-monitoring of progress on a target problem, and other materials used in individual cognitive therapy. Sank and Shaffer (1984) compiled a number of useful forms to be used in psychoeducational groups, along with a structured curriculum for teaching and applying cognitive therapy concepts and principles.

Psychoeducational approaches can be useful when dealing with large groups or when the participants cannot make a commitment to a lengthy series of therapy sessions. They are efficient means of teaching a lot of information in a relatively short amount of time. And, they are systematic if the sessions are well-structured and well-planned so that vital information is not omitted.

The limitations of psychoeducational approaches are the same as those of other self-help efforts. Books, tape recordings, lectures, and written homework can produce only limited results for their audience for several reasons. First, they do not and cannot deal with nonconscious cognitions, and thus an important source of influence on behavior and emotion is inaccessible. Second, they deal in generalities, not with the idiosyncratic cognitions of the individual. Third, they may present correct principles that the individual nevertheless finds confusing to apply appropriately. Fourth, they assume that the individual is highly motivated—Sank and Shaffer (1984) recommended the *screening out* of those persons who lack motivation to work on their problems—thus the person who does not take the time or trouble to start or continue the self-help program will not be helped much if at all. Fifth, psychoeducational groups are limited to self-counseling and therefore are inappropriate for moderately and severely disturbed persons (i.e., persons who meet DSM-III criteria for an anxiety or affective disorder).

## PROBLEM-SOLVING GROUPS

Problem-solving groups may have educational aspects about them, but these are secondary to the main objective of working on each individual's practical and psychological problems. The principles of cognitive therapy are usually taught so that group members can participate effectively, especially in the self-monitoring efforts that are as much a part of cognitive group therapy as of individual therapy. Most of the formal teaching occurs during the early sessions in the life of the group. Hollon and Shaw (1979) presented a schedule for group cognitive therapy that includes an explicit presentation of cognitive theory during the first session, using examples furnished by group members.

In many respects, problem-solving groups resemble multiple individual therapy. Each individual receives attention from the therapist (and from other group members) but gets less time than in individual therapy. Group members get experience helping each other, learning from others' successful and unsuccessful attempts to use cognitive theory, and vicariously learn about their own problems by witnessing other members struggle with theirs. Written and behavioral homework is used as it is in individual therapy.

Problem-solving groups may be time-limited or open-ended. Hollon and Shaw's schedule covered a 12-week period, but longer or shorter periods may be used. Time-limited groups typically take a particular diagnosis (e.g., dysthymic disorder) or theme (e.g., social skills training) as their focus. The outline or format of each session and of the series of sessions is fixed in advance, but the content varies, depending upon the individual problems, concerns, and practical considerations presented by each participant. Thus, the agenda for each session is determined by the concerns of the group members just as the client contributes to the agenda in individual cognitive therapy. A time-limited group tends to encourage clients to actively work on their problems, to seek corrective experiences rather than additional insights.

Open-ended groups have no time limit, are usually heterogeneous with respect to theme or diagnoses, and may have many complete changes of personnel in the course of their history. Agendas are determined each session, but there is no predetermined schedule of what topics to cover as there is in time limited groups. Presentations of theory may be done when new members are added and justified to established members as review, or new members can be oriented privately.

In an ongoing group with a personal problem-solving focus, discussions may become routine and predictable if there are fewer than six group members and little turnover in membership. On the other hand, if there are more than 12 in a group with a personal problem-solving format, it is difficult to include everyone, and there may be low or variable involvement. For some purposes, for example, in training for social skills deficits, it is wise to include members of both sexes because many problems of interpersonal anxiety involve relations with the opposite sex and unsegregated groups provide more realistic behavioral rehearsal possibilities. The length of session may vary and can be adapted to the purpose and size of the group. Weekly group meetings are probably typical, but less frequent meetings can be effective, especially when the therapist wants to provide ample time for group members to try out new behaviors and have corrective experiences.

The use of videotape recordings enhances behavioral rehearsals and is valuable for giving feedback to participants about their mannerism and style of self-presentation. Chalkboards and flipcharts can be used, especially if the therapeutic methods are educational, or the therapist wishes to record clients' cognitions (Covi, Roth, & Lipman, 1982; Hollon & Shaw, 1979; Sank & Shaffer, 1984).

Clients seem to benefit from audiotape recordings of portions of personal problem-solving sessions when they are the focal clients. Such tape recordings can be reviewed several times between sessions and seem especially helpful because clients do not retain in memory everything that has been said to and about them during a discussion. They might also record didactic portions of a therapy session. Tape recordings can readily lead to breaches of confidentiality, and clients should be cautioned not to play tapes for nongroup members that contain revelations made in the group session by anyone but themselves.

The following segment of a problem-solving group session illustrates the focal group member, the therapist, and other group members working together in a collaborative, thera-

RICHARD L.
WESSLER and
SHEENAH HANKIN-
WESSLER

peutic alliance. A range of cognitive and behavioral interventions is employed to aid the group process. Jane's problems are by no means solved, and there are many other areas she may choose to deal with as illustrated by the therapist's unstated hypotheses cited at the beginning of this annotation. She has provided a wealth of information, and it is the job of the therapist and the group to assist her toward her stated goal of reduced emotional disturbance. Other group members may gain by acting as co-therapists and by working covertly on their own related issues.

The client presents a problem of leaving her small daughter to return to college. The emotions she is experiencing are guilty anxiety, anger, and possibly depression.

Helped by other group members, the therapist sets out to gain further factual information to highlight the problem. The relationship between the client Jane and her daughter Linda is briefly explored. Facts about the college course and the involvement required are elicited. The client's predictions about what she anticipates will happen if she leaves her daughter are examined. The therapist then suggests a goal for the work to be undertaken by the group, and Jane agrees.

The therapist focuses on the guilt issues, although the cognitions leading to anxiety, anger, and suspected depression are hypothesized but not stated at this time. They are Jane's negative predictions about financial insecurity (marital problems are mentioned later) causing anxiety; Jane's personal rules of living regarding the extreme unfairness of the world to mothers and children leading to anger; and Jane's many negative thoughts about herself and the impact of separation from her child that are typical of depression.

The aim is to uncover Jane's cognitions that interface with guilt. "I think you have some very strong rules about mothers and children being together.") Jane supplies some information immediately when she expresses her strong disapproval of women who leave their children in order to study or work. Jane defines herself as a bad mother who is shirking her responsibility. Her depressive ideation about her past failure to have adequate money before having a child and her self-judgmental statement that she is disorganized are revealed. The therapist begins to raise questions about the client's rules—"I think you are making some very black predictions"—and supplies evidence for this statement. Other group members supply further evidence to support the therapist's words. The therapist embarks on an exercise combining imagery and time projection. The group is invited to join in the hope that they will have a reinforcing impact on Jane's personal rules of living by sharing their own experiences. The therapist relaxes the group and verbally paints a picture of the client and her daughter in two differing life situations. The client is asked to view herself and her child as they might be in 10 years time if the client chooses to remain as a full-time housewife and mother. The second imaginal scene is the same as the preceding one except that Jane is asked to add the role of working accountant and to internally speculate on the effects of this difference on herself and Linda. The exercise is then repeated, projecting an image 10 years hence, because in 20 years the much feared separation of Jane and Linda will almost inevitably have taken place.

After the exercise, Jane explains to the group the insights that she has gained from this new experience. She has reinforced her desire to become qualified and return to work and cannot predict any real differences in her image of her daughter if she does not remain with her full time. Also she sees the separation as happening whichever course of action she might choose.

The therapist suggests a homework assignment designed to build on Jane's experiences. Jane is asked to undertake a small research project to see if other women in a similar situation share her thoughts and feelings. She is asked to report her findings in the next group session. The therapist is very specific in order that the assignment is actually possible, clearly understood, and obviously relevant to the client's problem.

Jane is to ask several people certain questions in the hope that she will gain a broad spectrum of opinion. She is also asked to outline the kind of questions to be asked to check for relevance. Marge and David reinforce Jane in her effort by expressing interest, friendly disagreement, and enthusiasm.

JANE: I'm thinking about Linda—she's my little girl. Now that her baby days are over, I've decided to go back to college and leave her with a friend during the day. I dread leaving her. She cries when I do, and I feel really guilty.

DAVID: What made you decide to go back to school?

JANE: I've always felt insecure that I'm not really qualified to get a good job. If anything happened to my husband, I don't know how I'd manage to support Linda and myself. It's something I really have to do.

THERAPIST: Is the program of study full time?

JANE: Yes, it is. And it's just not designed for people like me. There's no evening classes in accounting. I think it's unfair that they don't think about women with children. I don't want to leave her at all.

MARGE: Oh, lots of people leave their children these days and go to school. I left my two little boys when they were quite small to go to school, and it worked out fine. Why are you feeling so guilty?

JANE: Oh, it's just that Linda has always been so close to me. She's our only child. She doesn't like to play with other children very much. She just follows me around the house and likes to be with me. We like to do things together. I'm sure she'd find it very difficult. I know I would. I'm just used to having her there all the time. I'm not happy even being away from her to come to this group.

MARGE: Well, you know she may find it difficult at first, but she will get used to it. I still don't know why you feel so guilty about that. It seems like something you want to do very much.

JANE: I just get this picture of her face. She always cries when I leave; I must say that she does settle down after a while. I just don't feel good about leaving her. I can't explain it anymore.

THERAPIST: I suspect you'd like to go back to college and feel somewhat less guilty. Let's see what we can do about that.

JANE: Yes, I feel like crying a bit now. It seems like such a big problem.

THERAPIST: I think you have some very strong rules about mothers and children being together, especially when they are so small. Could you tell me some more about that, Jane?

JANE: Yes, I don't like the ideas of mothers and children being apart. I think it's quite wrong. I really disapprove of these women who go out to work and leave their babies with other people. I feel sorry for the children. They don't grow up and know what a real mother and father are like.

DAVID: Well, you know, most fathers have to leave their children, have to go out and work, and do that all the time. I do that, and I have a very good relationship with my son. I think you're being too hard on yourself.

THERAPIST: I think a lot of people would share your ideas, Jane, but I think you hold them very strongly. Do you think that it's terrible for mothers and children to be separated at all? What degree of separation do you think is acceptable?

JANE: Well, I think when they're babies, they should be together all the time, but I suppose when they get big some degree of separation is inevitable. I just don't think I'm doing my job properly if I let someone else take care of her during the day.

MARGE: Do you know this person well? Is she caring?

JANE: Oh, yes. Of course. I wouldn't leave her with just anyone. I just don't think she can do as good a job as I can. I think Linda will miss me, and I think she won't forgive me for deserting her.

THERAPIST: We don't know about that, do we. That's really a guess. Most children forgive their mothers when they go to school. Do you forgive your mother for leaving you when you went to school?

JANE: I never thought of that. I never thought of that at all. I guess I must have. I hardly remember really starting school.

RICHARD L.
WESSLER and
SHEENAH HANKIN-
WESSLER

THERAPIST: Let's suppose Linda's a bit older and is looking back on her childhood. What might she say about you if you left her and went back to college?

JANE: She'll probably say that I deserted her and that I'm a bad mother. I didn't give her the love she needed. She'll probably grow up to be a difficult teenager and get back at me for deserting her.

DAVID: Don't you think "deserting her" is rather strong language for leaving her with someone while you go back to college during the day? I think you're still being very hard on yourself.

JANE: My relationship with Linda is so important to me that I'd hate to have anything upset it. I don't want her to dislike me. I really don't think I could stand it.

THERAPIST: Well, Jane, I think you're making some very black predictions about what might happen. Most of us were left by our mothers, and we don't seem angry about it. You don't seem angry at your own mother, either. Let's just stop for a moment and see what's going on here. What sort of things are you saying about yourself because you're planning this course of action?

JANE: Oh, I think I'm a bad mother. I don't think I should do that. Mothers shouldn't do that. I never did think so. I'm surprised I decided to do it. It's something I said I'd never do. I'm shirking my responsibilities to her. I don't think people should have children if they're going to leave them and go back to work, when they are so small. I really wanted to stay at home until she was about 11 or 12.

MARGE: You sound to me like you're trying to be too good a mother. You know, that kind of mothering can be bad, too.

JANE: I don't know what you mean. I don't see how taking too much care can mean being a bad mother.

THERAPIST: There are lots of different definitions of what a bad mother is. Your definition seems to be a very hard one. Do you really think you'll be a bad mother because you are making this decision?

JANE: Oh, yes. I really should have had more money before we had Linda. I should have worked longer so we wouldn't have this problem. I'm a disorganized person. I'm sick of that, and I'm really depressed about it.

THERAPIST: How are you depressing yourself, Jane?

JANE: Well, I suppose I'm doing that by thinking of what a bad person I am. How stupid and irresponsible! I'm always getting into scrapes like this!

THERAPIST: David's right. You're being very hard on yourself. If I had those ideas I'd be depressed, too. Come on, Jane, how can leaving your child with a responsible person make you into a stupid person?

MARGE: You really do look on the dark side. I mean, you don't really know that Linda's going to grow up to hate you.

JANE: Well, I suppose that's true. When we go around to my friend, Linda enjoys going there. She might, I suppose get used to it. She might not hate me, but I'll hate myself.

MARGE: Then, why do it? I don't know why you're putting yourself through this.

JANE: You know, Peter [Jane's husband] and I have had our troubles. We split up last year for 3 months. I've often wondered if we won't end up getting a divorce. It happened to my friend, you know. I'd be in a bad position then. He doesn't have much money—just his job. I'm not prepared to do anything, and I'd feel better if I had a college degree.

THERAPIST: In a perfect world, you'd be able to do all things easily. You'd be able to stay home with Linda and get a degree in accounting, the classes would be exactly at the time you want them. But it isn't that way, is it?

JANE: I wish it was! I get angry that it isn't a better place for mothers with children.

DAVID: I think you think it's worse for you than for anyone else. I don't see my children much except on weekends, and I'm so tired. I have to work so hard to make ends meet I hardly get to enjoy them at all. Yet, they don't hate me, and I certainly enjoy the time we do have together. That's the way the world is, you know.

MARGE: I think he's right. Have you thought about it this way: You're really making the best of the difficulties you face, by getting someone to look after your child while you go back to school. Why are you being so hard on yourself?

THERAPIST: I'd like to try something, Jane. I'd like you to sit back and relax; close your eyes and imagine something that's going to take place some time far into the future. Everyone else in the group can join in, too. Try and be Jane. Now, here's Jane, a young mother of 24, who's going back to college for the first time in several years. She's going to leave her child, and imagine her home with her child, making pastry, watching television, and talking. Stay with that thought for a minute. [Pause] I want you to make a magic leap. I want you to go 10 years into the future. Everybody come with us and be Jane. If you want to substitute your own children for Jane's, that's OK. Imagine, Jane, what you'll feel like 10 years in the future if you go on doing what you're doing now. Staying at home with Linda—she'll be 16 then—still doing things together, maybe going shopping, watching TV, and enjoying each other's company. What kind of person will you be if you've been a housewife all these years? What kind of person will your daughter become then? An active 16-year-old with friends of her own? [Pause] Right, Jane? Now substitute another image for a minute. You go back to college, and Linda stays with your friend. Imagine that you do get a degree and become an accountant. Imagine how your life will be different in 10 years time. What sorts of things do you think you will be doing? Some of the dreams and hopes that you must have had when you thought about getting some occupational skills. [Pause] And, how different will your daughter be? Will she still be the pretty 16-year-old, making friends, going to high school, and dating? What will be different? Which of those scenes gives you the most satisfaction? Stay with that thought for a minute. [Pause] Now, let's try another magic leap, 10 more years. Your little girl is a big woman now, of 26. She has a career, maybe traveling around the world—people travel so much these days. She'll not be at home with you anymore at 26. What will you be doing then? If you've chosen to be a housewife and a mother full time? [Pause] And again, change the scene: And let's see you as the working accountant. What satisfactions do you get from each of those scenes?

JANE: You know, it's really interesting. I've never thought of it like that before. I hadn't thought about it much at all. I hadn't thought of it much beyond going to college. I don't think I'd be satisfied just being a housewife all that time. I certainly always wanted to do something else as well. I like it, but I only have one child and don't plan to have any more. And, gosh, at 16, she's probably not going to want to stay home with me all the time. I'll be entirely different then. I realize now that I certainly do want to go back to college and get a degree, and I don't want to wait any longer. That's interesting. I do wish it were easier.

DAVID: I found it interesting, too. I hope I'll be retired in 10 years time. I was thinking, Jane, about you, though for the first time, as you were describing yourself becoming an accountant. I think it means a great deal to you, doesn't it?

MARGE: How did you see your little girl being different?

JANE: Well, it's funny. I only have one image of her, as this bright teenager. I really didn't think she'd be that much different. I can't really imagine that in all those years, she wouldn't get used to it. I think I might have exaggerated the situation.

THERAPIST: I've got a suggestion, Jane. I think you gained quite a lot of insight by that imagery exercise. Why don't we actually go out into the field and check out whether this sort of relationship is changed—when mothers and daughters don't spend so much time together. Do you know anyone who's gone back to college or gone back to work recently? With little girls or boys the same age as your daughter?

JANE: Oh, yes. There's plenty people in my apartment building. It's a young apartment block. Many of them go out to work.

THERAPIST: Well, let me suggest this idea. Why don't you ask them what they think. Have you ever discussed it with them?

JANE: No, not really. Because I've always gone around saying that I don't approve of mothers going out to work. I'd be a bit ashamed to say that I've changed my mind.

DAVID: So, you don't know what they think!

JANE: Well, I see the children. I don't suppose they look any different. I hadn't actually thought about it. I suppose I could ask. People do change their minds, and one or two of them are close friends of mine. I suppose I could ask them.

THERAPIST: What kinds of questions could you ask, Jane?

JANE: I could ask how difficult it was for them to leave their children. How they got along, and what the children thought about it.

THERAPIST: What might you discover?

JANE: You know, I really don't know.

MARGE: Well, it might be worth finding out. Because I didn't share your view of the situation.

JANE: That's true. No one here seemed to agree with me. I guess I'll do it.

THERAPIST: How many people will you ask before next week?

JANE: Well, I know four people I can think of immediately. Yes, I will ask them. I think I will ask them.

DAVID: I'll look forward to hearing what they say. I wonder whether they'll say what you think?

Cognitive methods may be employed as homework assignments, but we prefer experiential assignments. Clients are less likely to change long-held cognitions simply by deciding to do so. Better results can be achieved when the individual acts differently and witnesses at first hand the consequences of behavior (Bandura, 1977). A woman with a forceful personality believed that she had destroyed a close relationship by attempting to control the life of the partner who had rejected her. She predicted that she would always act this way and was depressed, seeing her future as empty and unrewarding. Her homework task was to attempt to test out her own hypothesis by issuing detailed instructions to several friends and colleagues and therefore effectively taking control of their lives. Some people resisted some of resisted some of her suggestions by not carrying out her instructions. Others would not do as they were told. Many laughed at her dictatorial manner. She discovered that she did not have magical powers of control and, at the same time, that few people actually rejected her totally for her efforts. After this experience, she modified her attitudes and felt less depressed.

We have found that these corrective experience activities are usually more effective when the client decides on the task to be undertaken. We prefer to increase motivation by asking clients to suggest assignments that they see as appropriate to the maladaptive rules of living that they are attempting to modify. If they cannot, we make suggestions and, in either case, negotiate an assignment both client and therapist can agree is likely to prove beneficial.

Often these assignments involve clients' acting in ways that they may regard as daring. To behave in a daring way usually involves "stepping out of character" (similar to Kelly's fixed-role procedure). This exercise is used with individuals, but all members of a therapy group can be asked to "step out of character" as well. The basic instructions are simple but can be elaborated and discussed with clients as needed: "For a short period of time act like the type of person you imagine you may like to be." A shy young man who envied his more assertive friends decided to ask several women in his office for a date. To his surprise, he actually did do so.

Most of the women refused his invitation but seemed unoffended by his request, and one of them agreed to go to a concert with him. He found that he was not uniformly rejected as he had feared. We think of "step out of character" as doing something positive and desirable for oneself and "shame attacking" as doing something negative—doing something one wants to do versus doing something generally recognized as socially unacceptable.

A difficulty that commonly occurs when clients claim that something is too hard, too difficult, or too inconvenient is that they may fail to carry out homework assignments. Most people want to change easily and comfortably. Others fear the discomfort they expect to experience in doing a difficult piece of homework. They desire to feel better *before* changing instead of changing *in order* to feel better. We ask clients to accept the fact that they can stand to be in tough situations, at least in the short term.

Client problems are then taken back to the drawing board in an attempt to uncover what the client fears. It is necessary, in fact critical, for the therapist and group members to attempt to understand the degree of the focal member's emotional response, which can lead to avoidance of a task. The prospect of a short shopping trip to a supermarket or attendance at a job interview may be simple stuff for some but a stimulus for terror and pervasive shame for others. The avoidance then becomes the focus for emotional understanding and cognitive intervention before the person can be expected to consider entering a threatening situation. We are as interested in why a person avoids certain tasks as we are in encouraging him or her to do them. Encouragement itself rarely suffices as an agent of change.

Cognitive and behavioral rehearsal within the group are techniques that can give the person psychological preparation to withstand anticipated attacks in the outside world. The young man who stepped out of character first rehearsed his dating techniques in the group to help him overcome his initial anxiety. He was encouraged to reevaluate his ideas about rejection (cognitive rehearsal). Behaviorally, he benefited from direct group feedback when he simulated dates with two of the female group members. Although this activity often has amusing results as the group gains enthusiasm for cognitive and behavioral rehearsal, the intent is serious. A group provides a unique pool of experience that can prove to be very influential— a safe, shallow pool where, under the caring vigilance of experienced supporters, a person may learn to swim and develop style before plunging into the deep end of the real world.

Cognitive and behavioral change can be strongly reinforced by informative group feedback. The therapist encourages group members to comment on each other's problems, to share common experiences, and to give appropriate advice and information. In a fast-moving, increasingly complex society, a therapy group can provide the kind of service that troubled people used to receive from parents, grandparents, priests, and peer groups.

Feedback does not provide rewards in itself. It can be very uncomfortable to be the focus of negative or even positive opinion. Reinforcement of one's performance often leads to reevaluation of failures and accomplishments and the setting of new goals. As the client attempts to act on new decisions and to observe the consequences, the group can provide an encouraging, motivating forum. Often the reactions of significant others to changes made outside the group can be unhelpful, perhaps because they dislodge long-standing patterns of interaction.

A husband whose marriage was "in trouble" decided, after receiving extensive feedback from other members of a group, to talk more openly with his wife. He told of his warm, loving feelings for her and of his fears that their marriage of 12 years seemed to be failing. His wife was confused by his new, unexpected behavior, and accused him of being weak. "You are having an affair and feeling guilty" was her angry response. He had decided to give up his new behavior when a woman in the group who had recently been divorced told him how much she respected his efforts and regretted that she and her former husband had not had intimate conversations. Other group members added their encouragement, and he decided to try again, this time prefacing his remarks with the information that he was seriously trying to improve their life together. Eventually, his wife began to respond more positively, and they talked about their problems and felt closer than they had for years. Feedback from the group gave this man new information that initially helped him to decide on a course of action and to test its effectiveness. When he did not receive the response he had hoped for, he retreated. Further feedback then encouraged him to modify his plan, give more complete information, and again strive to reach his subgoal—better communication with his wife. This decision paid off, and he had a basis on which to work for his ultimate goal—a happier, more rewarding marriage.

RICHARD L.
WESSLER and
SHEENAH HANKIN-
WESSLER

Direct methods can be effective ways to teach cognitive principles, but we often prefer to use indirect, experiential methods for this purpose. Our preference is based on the conviction that people assimilate new information better when they actively participate in the learning process rather than passively absorbing material through listening and reading. Indirect methods include exercises, games, and guided fantasies, each of which is specifically designed to raise certain issues. In the early stages of the group's existence, we use games and fantasies that illustrate connections between cognitive appraisals and resulting emotions. Later, the process of cognitive change is undertaken in guided group fantasy in which each member can work on his or her own problem areas and can afterwards process the experiences in the group.

Indirect methods also include the exploration of group relationships, an example of which is as follows:

Elizabeth continuously avoided confronting and contributing to discussions of Andrea's problems. Elizabeth perceived Andrea as unpleasant and authorative, misunderstanding Andrea's more open expression of feeling as a sign of her feeling superior to Elizabeth. Elizabeth came to recognize her misperceptions about Andrea and was surprised to discover that she felt the same way about her critical and domineering mother. This example illustrates the value of the group as opposed to one-on-one therapy for the recognition of personal rules of living and habitual emotional responses.

The rationale for employing a range of didactic and experiential techniques in group therapy is that we attempt to provide conditions in which members can have novel experiences and act differently within the group. A group is a forum of diverse experiences with the goal of personal change. Members can support each other in the commonly experienced anxiety about "loss of identity" that often prevents change. Such questions as "who will I be when and if I change?" can be addressed and responded to with personal experiences by other group members.

Here is an example of an exercise designed to produce quite strong and diverse emotional consequences (usually anxiety, guilt, shame, but sometimes joy). Defenses are exposed, and a new group can be introduced to the principle that thinking, especially strongly evaluative thinking, correlates with emotional experience and that a great deal of such thinking is automatically done without much awareness. A great deal of information can be quickly gained in an indirect and nonthreatening way. Humor acts to "loosen up" a tense, new group, and the subsequent processing of the exercise involves a large measure of self-disclosure. Many less responsive, reticent, and unassertive group members can respond more easily because everyone is involved in the process, and it is seen as an external game.

### THE TOOTHPASTE EXERCISE

The therapist begins by inducing an atmosphere of calm. He or she asks members to relax, to remove their shoes if they wish, and to close their eyes. Speaking quietly and slowly (those skilled in hypnosis use induction techniques), the therapist says, "You are all feeling relaxed. Check your bodies for tenseness. Does your neck hurt? Relax your tense stomach muscles and let your hands rest loosely in your lap. It has been a busy week, but it is over, and the weekend is here. You are invited to visit friends who live in the country. You have not seen them for a considerable time and do not remember them well. (Pause) All you really remember is their warmth and familiarity.

"You travel to their country house—choose your method of transport—drive your car or take a bus or train. Look at the countryside as it passes by—trees, fields, and hills. It is a calm, warm day, and you will soon arrive.

"You see the drive to their house. [Pause] And build a lovely house in your imagination. Fill in the door and the windows and sit in the garden of your choice. Watch it grow.

"The front door is welcoming and open. Go in. Pause in the beautiful hall. No one is there, but you feel relaxed and sense that your friends will return soon. Enter the living room. There is a large comfortable sofa—a tray of drinks and food—flowers, and perhaps a fire in the fireplace. Lovely china, silver, and furniture surround you. [Pause]

"Go upstairs. You know where the guest room is. Go in and look at the luxurious bed—the comfortable chairs. Walk to the windows and look at the beautiful garden. Next door is a magnificent bathroom. Furnish this room in the way you prefer. Perhaps mirrors, soft lights, warm towels, or a whirlpool bath and wooden furniture. Build your perfect bathroom. [Pause]

"Go to the washbasin. It is sparkling clean and a large, shining mirror faces you. [Pause] Lying on the basin is an extremely large new tube of toothpaste in its box. Take it out and feel it—it is new and unsqueezed. Hold it in your hand. Slowly remove the cap—unwind it carefully and place it on the basin. Taking your time, begin to squeeze the toothpaste all over the bathroom. Squeeze wherever you want to—walls, drapes, bath, mirrors, everywhere you want to. [There is a long pause while this image is created.]

"When the tube is completely empty, look around you carefully. Examine your feelings. What are you feeling now? When you are ready, leave your imagination and return to the group."

When everyone is ready, the therapist asks them to reveal what they are now experiencing. Some usually report anxiety, others anger, and some joy. Usually one or two people will have no particular feelings to report as they refused to engage in the imaginary toothpaste squeezing. Occasionally, someone reports refusing to enter the empty house! As discussion of feelings gains momentum, it soon becomes obvious to the group that it was *not* the imagined action of squeezing toothpaste over an imaginary room that led to the different reports of emotional responses. Each member appraised the event and drew an idiosyncratic conclusion. Some typical responses are:

"I am very anxious. I think my hosts will return and be very angry. They will never speak to me again."

"I am angry. You [the leader] forced me to defile that lovely room."

"I feel happy. I have always wanted to do something like that but never had the nerve."

"Depressed—that's what I feel. I was really enjoying my self but predictably it had to end badly—things always do."

"I have no particular feelings. I only squeezed the tube into the bathtub and washbasin. I cleaned it up immediately."

Further discussion may show people their defensiveness and self protectiveness.

"I simply couldn't do it—even though I know it wasn't a real situation."

"I blame you—you made me do it. I am not responsible for the mess."

Group members who had similar emotional experiences find that they had similar cognitions, whereas others might be surprised that some persons responded in ways that they would not have predicted. The task of the therapist at this point is to keep the discussion (which is often enthusiastic and spiked with humor) focused on the cognitive descriptions, inferences, and evaluations that occurred during the experience. Attempts to describe the house, the journey, and so forth are deferred for later enjoyment; although happiness and pleasure are important therapeutic goals, the therapist should maintain a professional, work-oriented atmosphere. "Is your reaction typical of the way you usually act when faced with a difficult task?" is a question to test how responses are generalized to other life situations.

This is but one example of the ways an imaginative and inventive group leader can use almost any exercise in the group. The art of the therapist is in processing the experience based on the specific purpose for which the exercise was designed.

One of the basic tenets of RET philosophy is Ellis's contention that humans cannot be judged or rated holistically because they behave badly. The behavior itself is subject to criticism, but the person is not a fool for acting foolishly (Wessler, 1983). Many group members present problems of anxiety and depression that result from their damning themselves totally for acting, or sometimes even thinking, in stupid and unrewarding ways. Such ideas lead to attempts to be perfect, further self-damning, and even more anxiety and depression for failing. The following exercise was conceived to demonstrate both the idea of human complexity and the illegitimacy of self-evaluation.

### THE PERSONAL COMPARISON EXERCISE

The chief participant can be a group member who has made some self-depreciating remark. The therapist points out that the client is globally denigrating himself and asks the group to join in a research project that will discover which of two group members is better, more valuable, and therefore to be preferred.

To set the scene, the therapist asks a third group member to process all the data collected, and—to promote group involvement—asks everyone to imagine that the room is completely wall-papered with graph paper for recording the results. The question, "Where shall we begin this research project?" is usually met with silence. "How about your jobs? John (the focal client), on a scale of 1 to 10, how well do you perform at work?"

JOHN: [after some thought]: "I'd say a four."

JANE: [The other group member]: "I'm a seven."

THERAPIST: "What's next? Let's see who is better at driving a car."

Other performance are measured and added to the list. Group members quickly get into the spirit of the exercise and make suggestions. The therapist endeavors to treat the topic in a more lighthearted manner, "Who is the better dancer?" (This question once resulted in an impromptu Charleston contest, with the remaining group members forming a dance contest committee.) After several activities have been measured, someone usually asks, "Where will this stop?" The therapist replies, "When we have measured everything in the universe that these two people can do and feed the data into our computer." Most group members quickly see they have embarked on an interesting, often amusing, but quite impossible task. Many clients have reported using this graphic illustration in real-life situations when they are attempting to measure themselves, usually negatively, against some other person.

The next exercise is a guided fantasy. The use of guided fantasy is economic. With a group of 10 participants, the time spent on an individual is necessarily limited, although vicarious learning may occur from listening to and attempting to help others. With these techniques, those who decide to participate are involved almost all of the time. They work internally on their concerns: Thus defensiveness and resistance, due especially to interpersonal fears, are reduced to a minimum. Only during the processing of the exercises are the participants asked individually to discuss the experience. It is important that adequate time be available for processing.

The leader evokes a peaceful atmosphere and encourages group members to relax in silence. Everyone is asked to look back into their memories and uncover some loss experience, for example, the end of a special relationship, a death of family member or close friend, a transition period in life when we move from one close group into a new situation from college friends to work, or perhaps leaving home or getting married. "Maybe the memory of a child, once so small, and now grown up and gone." The therapist asks the group to remember the face or faces of the person or people in their past and to recall some of the very special times that occurred then. "Remember both the quiet and hectic experiences, the laughter, tears, unique moments." Several minutes of silence are allowed for reflection.

"How did you feel about yourself at that time?"

"What plans were you making for the future?"

"Do you remember some of your wishes and expectations?"

"How many of your hopes were fulfilled?"

"This person or group of people no longer plays a central role in your life. What are your thoughts about that?"

Provide adequate time for the group to consider the questions and to answer them silently. A high degree of affective responsive often occurs at this time. Several group members may cry and others exhibit nonverbal behaviors that indicate anxiety, discomfort, sadness, and dejection.

The therapist asks questions that are intended to help members to become aware of their evaluative thinking:

"How has this loss affected your thinking?"

"What conclusions have you drawn from this experience?"

"How do you judge yourself, the person concerned, and yourself, as a result of what happened?"

Some typical appraisals that have emerged during the later processing of this exercise are:

"I'll never get over this loss—I can't stand it."

"I always fail in relationships and always will."

"I am a mean, spiteful person for treating him so poorly."

"People cannot be trusted and will always treat me badly."

The leader, at this point, has helped the group to generate enough material and now attempts to encourage members to reappraise their experiences. Group members usually make a decision to modify or change some of their descriptions, inferences, and evaluations with a resulting reduction in negative emotional responses. The fantasy, however, continues as follows:

"You are alone on a quiet, country road. It is warm, calm, and very beautiful. The road winds down a hillside. You see a slow, wide river and a bridge ahead of you. You are carrying a very large, very heavy suitcase. You are hot and tired. Your arm is hurting. Progress is slow and difficult. Finally, you make it to the apex of the bridge.

"Put down the case and rub your sore arm. Look at the river. The suitcase contains all your memories—everything—about the loss experience.

"In your pocket you have a small plastic shopping bag. Take it out. Open the huge suitcase and look at all the contents. Slowly and carefully select what you really want to keep from this huge store of memories. Be extremely selective. Ask yourself, 'Do I really want to keep this—do I need it?'

"The contents of the suitcase are many, yet the shopping bag is small. Some of the memories are unhappy. Remember them and choose to keep some of them, too. Slowly fill the plastic bag and then proceed to throw everything else into the river. Discard them and watch them slowly float away. Now, throw away the suitcase, too."

Allow several minutes for this procedure.

"When you are ready, pick up your plastic bag. Feel your arm. It no longer hurts. The bag is light. You can easily take it wherever you choose to go.

"Walk down the other side of the bridge. A narrow road curves away in front of you and merges with the horizon. This is the road to your future. How are you feeling now?"

At this point, the leader and group are ready to process the exercise. This begins with each group member relating his or her experience. The therapist reinforces the conceptual connections between cognitions and emotions and shows individuals how they respond more appropriately and functionally when they change or modify their descriptions, inferences, and evaluations. Some typical responses are:

"I realize that I only remembered the good times, and I also recognize that I didn't just behave badly. I do not need to cling to the past. I learned from it and now feel less guilty and more relaxed."

"From the group experience, I now realize that many others have had similar tough times. I am no different, and I was not singled out for this treatment. I feel relieved—less angry."

During the processing of the exercise, the therapist discusses reinforcing consequences. For example, persons who have remained depressed and guilty might reveal that they see these as suitable self-punishment for bad behavior. Someone with a personal rule of living that states "people are untrustworthy" might become aware that this is a defensive response designed to protect the believer from possible future rejection. Good processing of the group experience is the key to successful outcome. Typically, a lively and insightful discussion ensues in which the therapist has many different examples to use in order to aid the process of change.

The following exercise was designed to show the role of pervasive shame in emotional disturbance (Wessler, 1988). Shame describes the painful, negative feeling people have about who they are. Often these feelings are unconscious.

### THE MIRROR EXERCISE

The therapist, without prior announcement, provides a mirror, a full-length mirror of the type that is attached to closet doors and is readily available in department stores. Each group member is asked to spend 3 minutes looking at themselves in the mirror without comment. Then the person returns to his or her seat and is asked to describe who they see.

This exercise is usually greeted with strong affective response; typically some members are angry with the leader for not giving prior warning and exposing them to shame and perceived ridicule. Anger is a commonly held response to shame. Others will refuse to comment on who they see, passively angry with the exercise and stubborn in their refusal to face who they are. As the less self-conscious and self-critical members partake in the exercise, most will follow suit.

Discussions are highly emotional charged. Many personal rules of living are evoked. Here are some excerpts from several group sessions showing how this exercise evokes affect and cognitions.

JOANNE: I am so fat and ugly! Who could love me? I binged last night. I really hate myself.

DON: I can't believe what you're saying! You are young and attractive. Sure, you could use to lose 10 pounds or so, but so could I. My wife complains about her weight, too, but I still find her attractive.

JOANNE: Oh, you're just trying to be nice to me.

DON: [angrily] Are you saying that I'm not telling you the truth?

JOANNE: I get very embarrassed when people pay me compliments. In fact, I get angry.

THERAPIST: It seems to me, Jane, that you want to stay very much with your own ideas about yourself.

(Joanne is *ashamed* of her appearance and has a personal rule of living that states approximately, ''I am hateful and unlovable.'' She expresses *anger* and *anxiety* when asked to consider changing this rule.)

JACK: Look at this short, skinny wimp! How can I ever expect to be successful? I'm so non-descript everyone will overlook me.

THERAPIST: Who described you as nondescript?

JACK: My dad. I was so small, they all called me the family runt.

THERAPIST: Are you familiar with being inconspicuous and overlooked?

JACK: [crying] Oh, yes. I know how to play that role all right.

SEVERAL MEMBERS OF THE GROUP: [They intervened in different ways. The message was similar in content.] You feed into this system, Jack. It isn't true. You make it happen. What can you do to change?

(Jack, like, Joanne is also ashamed of his appearance and maintains a personal rule of living that ''short men are overlooked and therefore cannot be successful.'' When confronted with his own involvement in perpetuating his rule, he becomes *sad* and *depressed* as he acknowledges his role and thinks he cannot change.)

This exercise is particularly powerful in raising issues of self-value and self-hate and the maintenance of poor self-image. The emotion of shame, which is not always readily available to the client and therefore often unexpressed, is easily seen throughout this exercise. The exercise bears repeating at a later date as a self-report measure of self-perception.

The authors attempt to be inventive when working with groups and advocate the creation of new exercises that seem responsive to the concerns expressed by group members. The foregoing exercises should be taken as representative of our work, not a full description of it, as well as an encouragement to others to innovate whenever possible. Along with inventiveness, therapists should have flexibility. Flexibility can occur when the therapist is well informed, inventive, and imaginative, and it seems essential in order to effectively deal with a wide range of different people and problems. In turn, a diverse, creative atmosphere can encourage clients to become more flexible (and therefore less rigid) in their attitudes and more creative as they seek solutions to their personal problems.

## APPLICATIONS AND LIMITATIONS

The cognitively oriented psychotherapies assume that the correction of cognitions is the key to lasting outcomes. These approaches take the individual, not the group, as the focus. They can treat specific problems, for example, public-speaking anxiety and thus operate like behavior therapy. They can promote self-exploration and self-awareness and thus share a goal with psychodynamic and humanistic approaches. The cognitively oriented psychotherapies can utilize specific procedures developed within the context of other approaches to treatment to promote cognitive, emotional, and behavioral changes. Versatility in counseling a range of human problems is one of the outstanding strengths.

Like other forms of verbal psychotherapies, the cognitively oriented approaches are most easily employed with clients who want very much to change rather than simply to understand how their personalities developed according to some theory. Conditions for which verbal psychotherapy in general has not proved effective, for example, psychosis, antisocial personality, fall outside the scope of the cognitively oriented psychotherapies.

Group therapy has additional limitations. Very disturbed clients, those who refuse to participate in group proceedings, and those who require a great deal of personal attention would benefit more from individual therapy sessions. On the other hand, for certain clients, group treatment is better than individual treatment. Many problems of living involve relations with other people, and therefore a group is an ideal setting in which to work on such problems.

The group can provide a phasing-out experience for clients who have been in individual therapy. Such clients may have begun to make important changes but require additional practice to complete the process. The group, if it is ongoing, can also be a place for clients to return when faced with new life crises.

The strengths and limitations of the cognitively oriented psychotherapies as approaches to treatment in individual sessions also apply to treatment in group sessions. The cognitively oriented psychotherapies taken as a whole have begun slowly to accumulate a sound, empirical base (Schwartz, 1982).

If one accepts an attitudinal account of neurotic disturbance and treatment, with the indirect support offered by several decades of research in attitude change and persuasion and by contemporary research into emotion, then a different form of research question emerges. Can attitudes and appraisals be influenced in dyads and in larger groups? The answer is yes, and meta-analyses of therapeutic processes, for example that of Strong and Claiborn (1982), furnish a rationale for cognitive-oriented psychotherapies to employ these tactics to bring about evaluative and other cognitive changes.

The process of cognitive group therapy varies greatly, from an educative position to the plethora of direct and indirect methods. The procedures are different, the goals are the same—to aid clients in their attempts to live more effectively in their own social environments.

# REFERENCES

Arnold, M. D. (1960). *Emotion and personality* (Vol. 1). New York: Columbia University Press.

Bandura, A. T. (1977). *Social learning theory.* Englewood Cliffs, NJ: Prentice-Hall.

Beck, A. T. (1976). *Cognitive therapy and the emotional disorders.* New York: International Universities Press.

Covi, L., Roth, D., & Lipman, R. S. (1982). Cognitive group psychotherapy of depression: The close-ended group. *American Journal of Psychotherapy, 36,* 459–469.

Dryden, W. (1984). *Rational-emotive therapy: Fundamentals and innovations.* London: Croom Helm.

Goldfried, W. (1980). Toward the delineation of therapeutic change principles. *American Psychologist, 35,* 991–999.

Greenberg, L. S., & Safran, J. D. (1987). *Emotion in psychotherapy: Affect, cognition, and the process of change.* New York: Guilford.

Guidano, V. F., & Liotti, G. (1983). *Cognitive processes and emotional disorders.* New York: Guilford Press.

Hollon, S. D., & Shaw, B. F. (1979). Group cognitive therapy for depressed patients. In A. T. Beck, A. J. Rush, B. F. Shaw, & G. Emery (Eds.), *Cognitive therapy of depression* (pp. 328–353). New York: Guilford Press.

Janis, I. L. (1983). *Short-term counseling: Guidelines based on recent research.* New Haven: Yale University Press.

Kihstrom, J. F. (1987). The cognitive unconscious. *Science, 237,* 1445–1452.

Lazarus, A. A. (1981). *The practice of multimodal therapy.* New York: McGraw-Hill.

Lazarus, R. S., & Folkman, S. (1984). *Stress, appraisal, and coping.* New York: Springer.

Lewicki, P. (1986). *Nonconscious social information processing.* Orlando, FL: Academic Press.

McMullin, R. E. (1986). *Handbook of cognitive therapy techniques.* New York: Norton.

Mahoney, M. J., & Gabriel, T. J. (1987). Psychotherapy and cognitive sciences: An evolving alliance. *Journal of Cognitive Psychotherapy: An International Quarterly, 1,* 39–59.

Meichenbaum, D. H. (1977). *Cognitive-behavior modification.* New York: Plenum Press.

Millon, T. (1981). *Disorders of personality.* New York: Wiley.

Plutchik, R. (1980). *Emotion: A psychoevolutionary synthesis.* New York: Harper & Row.

Raimy, V. (1975). *Misunderstandings of the self.* San Francisco: Jossey-Bass.

Sank, L. I., & Shaffer, C. S. (1984). *A therapist's manual for cognitive behavior therapy in groups*. New York: Plenum Press.

Schwartz, R. M. (1982). Cognitive-behavior modification: A conceptual review. *Clinical Psychology Review, 2*, 267–283.

Sue, D. W. (1981). *Counseling the culturally different*. New York: Wiley.

Strong, S. R., & Claiborn, C. D. (1982). *Change through interaction*. New York: Wiley-Interscience.

Wessler, R. L. (1983). Rational-emotive therapy in groups. In A. Freeman (Ed.), *Cognitive therapy with couples and groups* (pp. 43–62). New York: Plenum Press.

Wessler, R. L. (1988). Affect and nonconscious processes in cognitive psychotherapy. In W. Dryden & P. Trowrer (Eds.), *Developments in cognitive psychotherapy* (pp. 23–40). London: Sage Publications.

Wessler, R. A., & Wessler, R. L. (1980). *The principles and practice of rational-emotive therapy*. San Francisco: Jossey-Bass.

Wessler, R. L., & Hankin-Wessler, S. W. R. (1986). Cognitive appraisal therapy (CAT). In W. Dryden & W. L. Golden (Eds.), *Cognitive-behavioural approaches to psychotherapy* (pp. 196–223). London: Harper and Row.

Zimbardo, P. G., Ebbesen, E. B., & Maslach, C. (1977). *Influencing attitudes and changing behavior*. (2nd ed.). New York: Random House.

# 29

# Cognitive Therapy with Inpatients

Wayne A. Bowers

## INTRODUCTION

The introduction of psychotropic medications in the 1950s and 1960s revolutionized inpatient treatment of emotional disorders, reducing the census of pyschiatric hospitals. During the late 1960s and early 1970s, the emphasis on long-term inpatient treatment changed to reflect the new philosophy of returning patients as quickly as possible to their home environment. This followed the creation of community-based treatment centers established during the Kennedy administration. The community mental health movement's attempt to limit hospitalization was made possible by advances in chemotherapy and psychosocial treatments.

Other approaches to inpatient care also began during this period. Therapeutic communities grew with patients given an active role in their own treatment and the running of their hospital unit. Behavioral programs also grew with emphasis on the token economy. Halfway houses and day-hospital treatment programs developed into integrated systems of modern treatment—combining medication and daily therapy without removing patients from their homes and reducing the stigma attached to psychiatric care.

In the 1970s and 1980s, advances in medications and psychosocial treatment of major psychiatric disorders (schizophrenia and depression) further reduced hospital stays. The philosophy of many psychiatric hospitals is to treat the acute symptoms, then release the patient for outpatient care with medication and/or therapy at home. Recent advances in psychosocial treatment of depression have shown that therapy can be as effective as medications for certain depressive disorders, and the combination of both may be more powerful in relief of symptoms and prevention of relapse in outpatients (Hollon & Beck, 1986).

Beck (1985) suggests that there are communalities between biological and psychological approaches to treating emotional disorders and that each theory focuses on a relative deficit of the positive components of experience. The common pathway seems to be in the change in cognitive processing with biological and psychotherapeutic treatment having an impact on these processes. It appears that, when there is a shift from negative to positive affect, there is a consequent shift in cognitive processing. The key to change consists of correcting the negative

Wayne A. Bowers • Department of Psychiatry, University of Iowa, Iowa City, Iowa 52242.

balance in cognitive processing (via medication, therapy, or both). The changes in the cognitive processes play an essential therapeutic role in each type of treatment.

An idea compatible to Beck's has been offered by Aksiskal and McKinney (1975). They assert that depression (or other emotional disorders) is more than a syndrome based on a single set of physiochemical variables. They strongly feel that depression "represents the feedback of three sets of variables at chemical, experiential, and behavioral levels." (p. 299). This allows for multiple causes to exist for one disorder.

> Once they arrive at the common pathway, this heterogeneous group shares a number of clinical features and symptoms such as cognitive distortions. (Askiskal & McKinney, 1975, p. 299)

These viewpoints reduce the multiplicity of theories into a more cogent view that offers many routes to the complex emotional, biological, behavioral, and cognitive processes of psychiatric disorders. Thus it makes clear why a wide range of treatments may help alleviate symptoms of various disorders.

## COGNITIVE THERAPY AND MEDICATION

The view that psychological or medical interventions have powerful effects on psychiatric disorders has led to combining various treatment modalities, especially in an inpatient setting. The combination of cognitive therapy and medication can treat the psychological and physical symptoms of psychiatric disorders. Reduction of physical symptoms (insomnia, impaired concentration, anxiety) can aid the psychotherapeutic process. Conversely, psychological improvement can enhance compliance with medication and reduce hopelessness. Long-term follow-up suggests superior outcome for the combination of cognitive therapy and medication with outpatients (Hollon, DeRubeis, Evans, Tauson, Wiemer, & Garvey, 1986). The same may be true of inpatients (Weissman, 1979; Wright, 1987). Weissman *et al.* (1979) found fewer dropouts from treatment with a combination of pharmacotherapy and interpersonal therapy than with either treatment alone.

Research on the combined use of cognitive therapy and medication suggests a positive effect from their combination. (Beck, Hollon, Young, Bedrosian, & Budnez, 1985; Blackburn, Bishop, Glen, Whalley, & Christie, 1981; Murphy, Simons, Wetzel, & Lustman, 1984). Independent studies reached remarkably similar conclusions and state that Cognitive Therapy (Beck, Rush, Shaw, & Emery, 1979) and antidepressant drugs each have a useful and powerful effect on depression. Using Cognitive Therapy and chemotherapy seems neither to add to nor detract from efficacy of either treatment, although there is speculation that the combination of the two may improve long-term stability. In any event, it would seem that cognitive therapy, whether alone or combined with medications, provides a viable option in the treatment of outpatients with primary, unipolar depression. These data along with the few studies made of inpatients suggest beneficial effects of combining cognitive therapy and medications.

## CLINICAL EXPERIENCE

Although cognitive therapy is best known through studies demonstrating its effectiveness with depressed outpatients (Hollon & Beck, 1986), there are reports of its increased use in other psychiatric inpatient settings. There is some literature on the application of this approach with psychiatric inpatients and other disorders resulting in hospitalization.

Glantz (1987) used the cognitive model in a day-hospital treatment program for alcoholics. This model is based on the idea that the basic characteristic of substance abuse of any kind is the reliance on the use of the drug as a primary coping mechanism. This use becomes abuse because it is based on maladaptive conceptualization processes developed early in life. From Glantz's perspective, the maladaptive conceptualizations play a crucial role in the etiology and maintenance of the disorder. In this treatment approach, the maladaptive conceptualizations are the primary target of the cognitive behavioral psychotherapy.

Glantz's treatment consists of two parts: (1) a cognitive behavior therapy group supplemented with individual cognitive behavior therapy, and (2) the entire daily hospital program of which the group and individual therapy are a part. During the early phase of treatment, the patients are introduced to the cognitive model and identify their particular psychopathology, maladaptive conceptualizations, and themes. An effort is made to help individual patients understand the negative consequences of their conceptualizations and themes and to show them alternatives and improvements that would result from altering their conceptualizations. At this stage, the primary goal of therapy is to teach generalized coping and reconceptualizing skills, going beyond the specific content of the problems dealt with in therapy. Patients are taught to substitute adaptive behavior rather than to simply stop maladaptive behavior such as drinking.

The treatment program involves group and individual therapy components. The group therapy relies on the development of a facilitative group emphasizing open interaction among the group members. Therefore, in addition to skills as cognitive therapists, the therapists who lead the groups must have some expertise in group interventions. Treatment goals for the individual patient are coordinated with the therapy protocol, and the therapists attempt to accomplish the scheduled group tasks for each therapy session while taking advantage of opportunities presented to advance therapeutic plans of individual patients. Groups meet twice weekly for 1½ to 2 hours, and patients are asked to commit to 2 months in the program. The co-therapists also function as the individual therapists for patients and meet with them at least once a week.

Patients who benefit from the therapy seem to have four characteristics in common: (1) they are motivated to change; (2) they accept the general cognitive-behavior model and its implications; (3) they feel that they have been able to exercise some degree of increased insight into and control of their conceptualizations; and (4) they have had some experience in which they benefited from reconceptualization and application of some of their newly acquired cognitive skills. Other factors in a successful outcome are an ability and willingness to engage in experiences that enhance the model such as role playing, reality testing, and guided exercises in self-monitoring. Glantz believes that cognitive therapy is a powerful intervention modality for alcoholics, and therapists who treat this patient population are encouraged to explore its potential.

Schrodt and Wright (1987) used Beck's Cognitive Therapy techniques developed for outpatient therapy in the creation of an adolescent psychiatric unit. They found that the active, goal-oriented, here-and-now focus of cognitive behavior therapy is well-suited for work with adolescents. The collaborative problem-solving approach of cognitive therapy helps to counter difficulties that adolescents can have in engaging in a working relationship with adult therapists. The egalitarian, empirical approach of cognitive-behavioral therapy encourages healthy skepticism. If the therapist can convey to the subject that his or her perception of a situation is but one possible alternative, and if the teenager can be encouraged to reciprocate by looking at his or her own thoughts with the came critical analysis, then collaborative empiricism can be attained.

Adolescence is the time when abstract thought and awareness of alternatives begin to occur, and Schrodt and Wright think cognitive behavior therapy can nurture this. Increased awareness of distorted or dysfunctional information processing may result from a variety of factors, including depression, cognitive immaturity, and substance abuse. Cognitive distortions are extremely common in hospitalized adolescents but are also rather common in normal teenagers. Schrodt and Wright think maturation of more rational and flexible modes of thinking is usually associated with an improvement in self-concept and self-esteem. Consequently, a goal of the treatment is to supplant immature and flawed reasoning with more mature cognitive processes.

Cognitive-behavioral therapy stresses the need for specificity in target symptoms and goal setting. Because of considerable family instability and ambivalence among families of hospitalized adolescents, cognitive therapy emphasizes eliciting and testing underlying assumptions and beliefs concerning the family. Treatment is most effective if the family, the adolescent, and the treatment team collaborate. Dysfunctional attitudes, cognitive distortions, and maladaptive behavior patterns within the system are treated by family therapy.

The process of cognitive therapy involves bringing automatic thoughts, schemas, and other cognitions into full awareness. Adolescents vary in their capacity for formal operations or, more specifically, in the capacity to think about thinking. Therefore, putting their thoughts into writing can help in the analysis of their perception of events and eventually testing or validating their own cognitions. This can help the adolescent gain an objective view of a situation that can lead to mastery as well as insight into particular dysfunctional and distorted perceptions.

Beyond the basic advantages of cognitive therapy with adolescents, Schrodt and Wright (1987) believe that this treatment has several unique characteristics that facilitate therapy with this difficult group. The collaborative-empirical working relationship helps to reduce oppositional behavior and destructive acting out. At the same time, normal adolescent cognitive development can be facilitated through psychotherapeutic encounters and other multiple learning experiences in the milieu, peer group, family, and school. An expanded sense of self-efficacy is supported by success in these activities.

Another inpatient population that may benefit from cognitive therapy is the chronic young adult patient. Greenwood (1987) developed a group model of treatment using cognitive therapy with individuals diagnosed primarily as schizophrenic. Three stages facilitate change among the group members: (1) securing the patient's involvement in treatment, (2) facilitating the patient's understanding of the cognitive therapy process, and (3) application of specific cognitive and behavioral techniques with the main goal of changing the patient's maladaptive perceptions and ideas.

Because of the psychotic nature of these patients' thinking, a variation in usual cognitive procedures is important. It cannot be assumed that the members in this type of group are motivated to seek treatment, believe that self-disclosure is acceptable, are capable of attending to and understanding the treatment, or that they can acquire the fundamental skills that are the focus of cognitive therapy. Greenwood suggests several treatment strategies to overcome these difficulties: (1) setting goals for each group; (2) using Cognitive Therapy principles to guide the therapist's behavior as a model for the group; (3) noting how the cognitive change that has been made occurred; and (4) awareness of specific techniques that have been successful so they may be used to their fullest potential.

The first stage of the group is to get patients to be involved. Given the intensity of social interactions, the guiding principle at the beginning of treatment is to create a trusting, emotionally supportive climate by achieving strong patient–therapist rapport. Two guidelines are followed: (1) overawareness that the patient is being understood, and (2) comments that reduce anxiety rather than increase it. Self-disclosure is one intervention that can facilitate participation. Communicating understanding and tolerance for the patient's self-defeating behavior seems to be essential for future collaboration. At all times the therapist must convey a cognitive view of the world.

The next objective of the group is to increase the patient's understanding of the cognitive therapy process and to create a working alliance focused on how problems can be solved. At this stage, the therapist needs to be more direct and didactic. This is accomplished by emphasizing the central role of thinking on the person's affect and behavior and encouraging self-attributions of internal causation.

At the third stage, the group is introduced to cognitive strategies and behavioral change. Successful ones were increasing awareness of cognitive errors such as selective abstraction, all-or-nothing thinking, catastrophizing, and faulty attribution. The focus of therapy should not be on the central pathology of the patients but on alerting them to the fact that they do distort events in a way that reinforces their avoidance tendencies and sense of worthlessness. When delusional material is presented, attempts are made to translate it into consensually validated interpersonal or intrapersonal concerns. It is essential to develop a realistic framework to gauge change. Greenwood cautions that this approach is an experimental one, but he believes that cognitive therapy offers a technical advantage with the young adult chronic patient. This advantage lies in repeated learning experiences to supplant distorted thinking and perceiving, through flexibility of interventions and the collaborative model with its emphasis on cognitions influencing behavior.

Cognitive-behavioral therapy has also been studied with a schizophrenic population (Meichenbaum, 1977). Meichenbaum and Cameron (1973) used self-instructional training (SIT) to help schizophrenics monitor their behavior and thinking. The schizophrenic patients were taught to become sensitive to interpersonal signals (facial and behavioral actions) from others that would imply to them that their behavior was "schizophrenic." The object was to help schizophrenic patients modify interpersonal and intrapersonal cues interpreted as psychotic. SIT helped patients increase appropriate attention to task by preventing internally distracting stimuli from interfering with target performance and by mediating generalization across tasks and situations. Meichenbaum and Cameron suggested SIT improved and maintained attentional, conceptual, and performance tasks among schizophrenic subjects. An attempt to replicate the findings of Meichenbaum and Cameron was unsuccessful. Margolis and Shemberg (1976), using a larger sample of schizophrenic subjects, were unable to show a significant difference in favor of SIT to increase attentional, conceptual, and language tasks. Although the use of SIT has shown promise in working with schizophrenic subjects, more research in the area is needed. However, Hollon and Beck (1986) suggest that little evidence exists "supporting any particular efficacy for the cognitive-behavioral interventions in the treatment of the schizophrenias." (p. 472).

Use of Cognitive Therapy has also been useful in general hospital settings. Modified cognitive therapy has been used with depressed, brain-damaged individuals. Hibbard, Gordon, Egelko, and Langer (1987) recommend use of more behavioral aspects of cognitive therapy during the early sessions and then shifting to cognitive interventions later as the person can

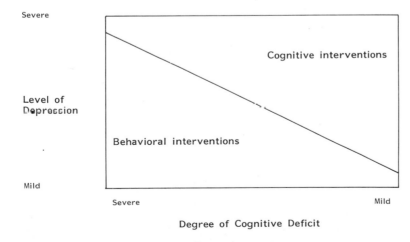

Degree of Cognitive Deficit

FIGURE 1

handle them. The greater the cognitive deficit, the greater the need for reliance on behavioral methods during the earlier stages of treatment and perhaps throughout later stages of treatment (see Figure 1).

Hibbard *et al.* suggest that most of the cognitive work can be done during the session—focusing on immediate distorted cognitions. When working with this population, there is a need to reduce the procedures to level of the patients' understanding. Further, the severity of the cognitive deficit may dictate the ratio of cognitive-behavioral interventions.

## RESEARCH STUDIES

A few studies detail use of cognitive therapy with depressed inpatients. Shaw (1980) used Cognitive Therapy with drug-free depressed patients hospitalized either for endocrine studies or nonresponsiveness to antidepressant medications. A total of 11 patients received Cognitive Therapy. At the end of their hospital stay (mean duration 8.1 weeks), 10 of the 11 patients showed significant improvement in depressive symptoms measured by the Beck Depression Inventory (Beck, Ward, Mendelson, Mock, & Erbaugh, 1961). BDI scores changed from an average of 29.8 at admission to an average of 15.6 at discharge. At 4- to 6-week follow-up, patients maintained their change in depressive symptoms with BDI scores being 13.5 on the average.

DeJong, Henrich, and Ferstal (1981) evaluated a cognitive-behavioral approach consisting of cognitive therapy and social skills training with depressed inpatients in a psychiatric hospital. Their program reduced symptoms of depression, improved social skills, and changed faulty thought patterns when compared to an unspecified treated control group. In follow-up, DeJong, Treiber, and Henrich (1986) studied 30 depressed inpatients divided into three equal groups. One group received cognitive-behavioral therapy, one group received only cognitive restructuring with no behavioral interventions, and one group was a wait-list control. Each treatment group received 5 to 6 weeks of their respective treatments. At the end of treatment, the cognitive-behavioral group equaled the cognitive restructuring group on observer-rated symptoms of depression, and both groups were better than the wait-list group. On self-report depressive measures (BDI, D-scale) the cognitive-behavioral group was superior to the cognitive restructuring group, and both were superior to the wait-list group. Decrease in cognitive and somatic symptoms was equal for all groups. Miller, Bishop, Norman, and Keitner (1985) compared cognitive therapy with medication against social skills with medication in 6 patients who had multiple depressive episodes, hospitalizations, and unsuccessful treatments. Treatment for both groups began in the hospital and continued on an outpatient basis for approximately 4 months. Therapy sessions were held 5 days a week during hospitalization and were scheduled for 16 weeks after discharge with total treatment lasting, on the average, 22 weeks. At the end of treatment, 4 of the 6 patients exhibited complete remission on measures of depressive symptoms. One subject in each group exhibited partial remission of symptoms but continued to show impairment in general functioning.

Bishop, Miller, Norman, Buda, and Foulke (1986) reported a case of psychotic depression treated with Cognitive Therapy. An intensive inpatient program consisting of 12 sessions of Cognitive Therapy and milieu therapy was used. At discharge, the patient reported significant decrease in depressive symptoms as measured by the BDI and the Hamilton Rating Scale for Depression (HRSD; Hamilton, 1960) and in negative thoughts common to depression as measured by the Automatic Thoughts Questionnaire (ATQ; Hollon & Kendall, 1980). Reduction in thoughts of suicide and an increase in the degree of belief in positive thoughts were also evident. These changes were sustained at 10- and 16-month follow-up without medication.

Wright, *et al.* (1987) reported on 38 hospitalized depressed patients treated with cognitive therapy and pharmacotherapy. After 4 weeks of treatment (three sessions per week), the mean Hamilton Rating Scale scores fell from 29.53 to 10.39.

Bowers (1988) compared nortriptyline against cognitive therapy plus nortriptyline and against relaxation plus nortriptyline with 30 depressed inpatients. Patients were assessed on five measures, three for symptoms of depression (BDI, HRSD, Hopelessness Scale; Beck, Weissman, Lester, & Trexler, 1974) and two assessing cognitions (ATQ and the Dysfunctional Attitude Scale; Weissman & Beck, 1979). The Cognitive Therapy plus medication and relaxation plus medication groups each received 12 sessions of their respective treatments on a daily basis. At discharge from the hospital (mean number of days 29.43), all three groups were significantly less depressed on self-report on all five dependent measures. However, the Cognitive Therapy plus medication and relaxation plus medication groups were significantly less depressed on self-report of depressive symptoms (BDI) and thoughts common to depression (ATQ) than the medication-alone group. Also, at discharge from the hospital, the Cognitive Therapy plus medication group had a significantly higher percentage of patients who were judged nondepressed on observer rating (HRSD) than the other two groups. Cognitive Therapy plus medication and the relaxation plus medication groups had significantly greater percentages of nondepressed patients on self-report (BDI < 7) than the medication-alone group.

Although a few studies attempt to address the issue of cognitive therapy with an inpatient population, there is little research that assesses what, if any, effect Cognitive Therapy will have on reduction of further episodes of depression.

## COGNITIVE THERAPY ON AN INPATIENT UNIT

### STRUCTURE OF THERAPY

The structure of cognitive therapy with inpatients is altered little from that used with outpatients. It is important to be flexible in the early stages of cognitive therapy and establish a good collaborative working relationship. Initial sessions are primarily behavioral in orientation. These sessions set the stage for cognitive interventions by establishing situations that generate cognitions. An emphasis on behavioral interventions is likely as the severity of symptoms is greater with inpatients. Beck (1976) also suggests that a focus on behavioral interventions is important with more severely disordered individuals. Graded task assignments and daily mood ratings are particularly important early stages in treatment. These help the therapist to establish a baseline for further work but also offer the patient immediate results that can motivate and encourage involvement. They can also reduce a patient's feeling of hopelessness. Behavioral assignments give the therapist time to fine-tune therapy and intervene early when assignments are not effective in reducing symptoms.

The move into more cognitive aspects of therapy follows smoothly from the behavioral interventions. Inpatient work offers the therapist the opportunity to look at automatic thoughts and assumptions when they are "hot"; that is, at a closer proximity to the time when the patient experiences them. Daily sessions offer almost immediate work on negative thoughts and cognitive distortions occurring in the hospital. Interventions can be more specific as the therapist can step in when problems arise whether within the individual or within their environment. Homework assignments can be fine-tuned as opportunities arise to work directly with the patient on the homework. The therapist may be able to watch interactions or set up role playing with other hospital staff.

The combination of cognitive therapy and medications can precipitate cognitive distortions about the usefulness of each treatment (Wright, 1987). A strict biological explanation undermines the usefulness of psychological interventions, and the patient may feel no need to understand the psychological aspects of the disorder. The patients may "wait for the medication to work," contributing little to their own treatment.

Putting medications on the therapy agenda offers the patient time to discuss fears and expectations about medications. The discussion can be used to combat distorted perceptions about medication and educate the patient about medication and therapy. This is an opportunity to acquire information important to the patient's medical care to transmit to the team psychiatrist. This is especially true when the primary therapist is not a physician or if the cognitive therapist meets with the patient more frequently than the physician.

> It is very important to know what positive or negative effects have been associated with a medication and then to use the information to make decisions about continuing or changing the pharmacotherapy regimen. (Wright, 1987)

An advantage of using cognitive therapy with inpatients is the chance to work *in vivo* with the patients. *In vivo* treatment allows the therapist to engage in the patients' phenomenological world and better understand their problems. Probing nonverbal cues can elicit automatic thoughts that help patients to be aware of those cues and challenge the automatic thoughts. Within the session itself, the therapist can help the patient to be more aware of thoughts that are missed by *post hoc* self-reports. The "here-and-now" of *in vivo* therapy facilitates identification of dysfunctional thoughts and uncovers the basic assumptions or schemata of the patient. Patient problem conceptualization can be more accurate when working with real-life situations. (Sacco, 1981).

*In vivo* work can help motivate inpatients for treatment. Simple tasks such as organizing a day or cleaning a room can demonstrate to patients how much they can be involved in their own treatment. Also, it can show the patients that thoughts do effect their feelings and behavior. Also, patients learn that tasks that seem overwhelming can be solved with simple interventions.

Working *in vivo* offers the therapist and patients immediate feedback into the patients' view of self, experiences, and future that contribute to reduced motivation. This can be accomplished by reducing fears through modeling positive behavior and working with immediate cognitions. This is particularly powerful with anxious and phobic patients (Sacco, 1981).

### CONTINUITY OF CARE

Admission to an inpatient unit can be very confusing for patients. Preexisting ideas or lack of information about cause and treatment for a particular disorder can contribute to dissatisfaction and possible impairment of a return to health. In order to provide an efficient treatment plan, coordination of all possible interventions is important. With emphasis on biological interventions and number of possible care givers, introduction of Cognitive Therapy can be just another intervention. Shaw (1981) and Perris *et al.* (1983) make several recommendations for instituting a comprehensive inpatient cognitive therapy treatment program:

1. *Establish weekly team meetings.* This will give all those involved in treatment a forum in which to assess progress, develop interventions, discuss problems, and coordinate or enhance the overall treatment package and develop continuity of care. This team would ideally be composed of the attending psychiatrist, cognitive therapist, primary nurse, adjunctive therapists, and psychiatric aide(s). Perris *et al.* (1987) suggests that these meetings be held as often as twice a week for 1 to 1½ hours.

2. *An extensive written treatment plan is essential.* The treatment plan should be shared with the patient and updated on a weekly basis. This will enhance consistency in the under-

standing of the patient's problem among the staff involved. It will also provide a smaller number of people to deal with in the event of development of negative cognitions by the staff (Shaw, 1981).

3. *Train the staff in cognitive therapy.* It is important to train as many of the treatment team in the theory and practice of cognitive therapy as possible. Continuous in-service training is most important to sustain continuity of care. If possible, work with an experienced and stable group of team members. It may be important to restrict the number of personnel working with the patient, thereby reducing confusion about treatment and enhancing continuity of care.

4. *The patient must understand the principles of cognitive therapy.* The patient's understanding of cognitive therapy will provide opportunities to practice on the unit what has been worked on during an individual session. Treatment plans tailored to the individual patient enhance interventions, increase continuity of care as an outpatient, and possibly reduce admissions (Perris *et al.*, 1987).

When working on an inpatient unit, one cannot assume that all involved will hold the same theoretical orientation. For a cognitive therapy program to be most successful, the therapy model must organize the treatment received by the patient. The conceptual framework of treatment, a crucial aspect of cognitive therapy, must be communicated to all staff. To foster the acceptance of cognitive therapy, the primary therapist must be able to determine issues to be worked on and (with the collaboration of the patient) to structure the therapy.

> Treatment must follow rational decisions about priorities followed by behavioral observations as part of the feedback system. Points to be stressed include: The need for clear communication of the treatment goals; the education of staff in the collaboration of cognitive data; the importance of central conceptualization; and the view of the patient as an active collaborator in the therapy (Shaw, 1981, p. 46).

Most inpatient psychiatric units follow a biological model in treating psychiatric disorders. The biological model is clearly not antithetic to the cognitive model. It is reasonable and often essential to combine the two approaches, particularly when working with more severely disordered individuals.

Another reason for the combination is the severity of pathology of individuals who are hospitalized. By the time a hospital stay is indicated, social and psychological as well as economic supports are often strained or eroded. A need to approach and treat all aspects of the disorder are important, and a combination of several interventions is warranted. In the event that medications cannot be used or are contraindicated (i.e., cardiac problems, religious beliefs, pregnancy), cognitive therapy could be used alone.

Although the ideal is to have both medications and the cognitive therapy administered by the same person, this is seldom the case. The most common treatment is for a physician to prescribe the medication and a nonmedical therapist administer the cognitive therapy (i.e., psychologist, nurse, social worker).

The inpatient must balance different therapists (orientation, frequency, and length of contact) and integrate this into his or her own perspective on the disorder. Consequently, the relationship of each member of the treatment team directly affects the patient. Problems within the working relationship of the physician and the cognitive therapist detract from treatment. Acceptance and understanding of differing treatment modalities is a must for successful treatment. Wright (1987) states that:

> The pharmacotherapist and the psychotherapist should know each other quite well, work together on virtually a daily basis, have a good fundamental understanding of both treatments, communicate freely with one another, and agree on a clear model for combined treatment that can be communicated to the patient. They should also be able to adjust their treatment techniques as the therapy proceeds based on shared information and mutual agreement. (p. 42)

When using cognitive therapy on an inpatient basis, there must be some adaptation of the model developed for outpatients. Outpatients commonly receive 12 to 25 sessions over a 4- to 6-month period. With inpatients, it may be realistic to assume a 3- to 6-week stay. Therefore, the number of therapy sessions needed to see effective change is not known. There are no established guidelines for the number of sessions when treating inpatients, but the literature suggests that a minimum of 12 sessions is needed to effect change in symptoms. Bishop *et al.* (1986), Bowers (1988), and Wright *et al.* (1987) all saw significant change with 12 sessions. Miller *et al.* (1985) used 16 to 20 sessions when working with their group of inpatients. It is useful to attempt as many sessions as the patient can tolerate and to continue seeing him or her until the end of hospitalization.

Along with the number of sessions, frequency of sessions may also play an important role in change. Again, the literature has little to offer as guidance, but it would seem that meeting at least three times per week is a minimum (Wright *et al.*, 1987). Others (Bishop *et al.*, 1986; Bowers, 1988; Miller *et al.*, 1985) all met on a daily basis. Again, the frequency of sessions will depend on each individual patient, but more sessions may enhance outcome.

SUGGESTED GROUP COGNITIVE THERAPY WITH INPATIENTS

Group therapy approaches are widely used in inpatient settings. Activity groups focused on either individual or communal activities, medication groups offering an opportunity for patients to discuss medication-related issues, social skills groups both educative and experiential, or "process groups" purporting to deal with emotional issues are all commonplace in hospital settings. The utilization of communal or group treatments would seem to make use of one of the strengths of inpatient treatment, that is, the therapeutic community. Some patients are placed in groups because of the patient's need for a social milieu to discuss his or her problems. For others, the group experience is a transition point toward discharge. Finally, some patients are placed in groups so that the group members will say to the patient what the therapist feels he or she cannot or will not say, that is, "you are very demanding." Groups are used, however, for many reasons that are management-oriented rather than therapy-related, that is, keeping patients occupied, making optimal use of limited staff, unit meetings, or the training of new therapists.

The traditional therapy group takes a process focus, that is, offers an opportunity for patients to discuss conflicts, history, and dysfunctional thoughts and feelings. Given the open-ended format of most of these groups, patients often experience a lack of closure. New members are placed in the groups as they are admitted to the unit, and other members leave the group, often suddenly, as they are transferred or discharged. This creates difficulties for the therapist in terms of maintaining group cohesiveness and facilitating group process. Freeman (1987) has developed a theme-focused group approach for use in inpatient settings that effectively deals with most of the problems inherent in the inpatient group.

Frequent problems involve any or all of the following:

1. A new patient in the group is unaware of the issues being discussed by "older" group members. This causes the new member not to be able to participate fully in the group.
2. "Older" group members are often angered by the need to bring the newcomer up to date on the issues, problems, and cast of characters being discussed.
3. Patients move in and out of the group because of admission/discharge.
4. Not all patients are equally verbal or comfortable when speaking in front of a group.

5. The extemporaneous and spontaneous nature of group interaction is difficult (or virtually impossible) for some patients.
6. The more verbal patients often utilize larger segments of the group time (with the tacit agreement of the less verbal patient).
7. Certain patients tend to repeat the same, well-practiced, oft-repeated model that can be utilized or adapted to the setting and patient population. It has been used successfully in both inpatient, day-hospital, and outpatient settings. Freeman recommends the following:

1. Groups should be theme-focused rather than free-floating.
2. Homogeneity by age, severity, or diagnosis is ideal, though not essential.
3. Staff members can estimate average length of stay, number of group sessions possible within that length of stay, and possible session length.
4. Initially, staff members generate a list of topics for the group to discuss; patient input can be sought after the initial series of group meetings.
5. Homework can be assigned before and after each group.
6. Group members can prepare (or be helped to prepare) for the group meetings.
7. Structure and focus allow an effective modeling for patients whose thoughts are confused.
8. Groups would be run in continuing cycles.
9. Each group session would be self-contained with closure at the end of the session. Sessions would not be cumulative.

A member joining the group at Session 1 would be in the group through Session 12. A member joining the group at Session 7 would cycle through Sessions 8 to 12 and 1 to 6. This would allow members to enter and leave the group at various times. A group member staying in the hospital for more than the average stay would continue to cycle through the topics. A group member in the hospital for a shorter than average stay would still have a complete experience in that he or she would profit from the group sessions that he or she attends.

The group would operate in the following manner:

After the number of available group sessions are estimated by the staff, that is, average stay, 4 weeks; available sessions, 3 per week; available session length, 2 hours. This would allow for 12 sessions. The topics chosen by the staff might include:

| | | |
|---|---|---|
| Monday | 1. | Family problems |
| Tuesday | 2. | The stigma of being in a hospital |
| Thursday | 3. | Impulse or anger control |
| Monday | 4. | Work or career issues |
| Tuesday | 5. | Social skills training |
| Thursday | 6. | Family problems |
| Monday | 7. | Relationships and friendships |
| Tuesday | 8. | Impulse or anger control |
| Thursday | 9. | Fear of asking for what you want (assertion) |
| Monday | 10. | Coping with anxiety |
| Tuesday | 11. | Work issues |
| Thursday | 12. | Dealing with loss. |

The topic or theme list would be posted on the unit. Each member would be asked to prepare, in advance and in writing, two of his or her own problems related to the topic of the day and to bring the list to the session. New group members could be asked to prepare their topics before the start of the group. In the group, one of the group members will be asked to be secretary for the day and to write down on a blackboard the problems that are read off by the patients in a "go-around" at the start of the session. This establishes a group agenda. Given overlap of topics or themes, the therapist can combine issues. Every member could then have his or her problems discussed. Those patients less comfortable at public speaking can organize thoughts. Written notes brought to the session would be encouraged. The nonparticipating patient would gain a great deal from listening to the discussion of the others.

Homework relevant to the group work can be assigned subsequent to each session. Members who would like to repeat their practiced statements would be encouraged to contain their remarks until the appropriate day or to bring the issues up with their individual therapist.

## CONCLUSION

Cognitive Therapy offers many different applications to emotional problems or concurrent physical and emotional difficulties. Its applications range from inpatient psychiatric settings to more traditional medical settings. Starting cognitive therapy during the inpatient phase of treatment may shorten the amount of time an individual will spend as an outpatient. The cognitive model can offer a strong framework for change when dealing with more chronic problems. The format of treatment may be either group, individual, or both and can structure the whole inpatient stay when a unit is properly trained and implemented. The literature on depression and inpatients indicates that Cognitive Therapy is a very strong adjunct to current medical interventions. Guidelines for the use of Cognitive Therapy with inpatients are slowly developing with increased research. The potential for its use has yet to be tapped.

The inpatient stay is designed to return the individual to an adequate level of functioning and does not replace outpatient Cognitive Therapy. It is very important to facilitate the transition from inpatient to outpatient status. Early use of cognitive principles helps patients to feel that they are in control of their own treatment and can enhance outcome. For the staff of an inpatient unit, the cognitive model can also increase continuity of care, staff morale, and efficiency in delivering treatment.

Shaw (1981) stated that inpatient units where control is possible should receive attention from researchers. It is essential to begin well-controlled process and outcome studies of cognitive therapy (either alone or in combination with other treatments) in an inpatient setting. Research in the use of cognitive therapy on an inpatient basis will bring further understanding of Cognitive Therapy and those problems that it treats.

## REFERENCES

Akiskal, H. S., & McKinney, W. T. (1975). Overview of recent research in depression: Integration of ten conceptual models into a comprehensive clinical frame. *Archives of General Psychiatry, 32*(3), 285–305.

Beck, A. T. (1976). *Cognitive therapy and the emotional disorders.* New York: International Universities Press.

Beck, A. T. (1985). Cognitive therapy, behavior therapy, psychoanalysis, and pharmacotherapy: A cognitive continuum. In M. Mahoney & A. Freeman (Eds.), *Cognition and psychotherapy* (pp. 325–347). New York: Plenum Press.

Beck, A. T., Ward, C. H., Mendelson, M., Mock, J., & Erbaugh, J. (1961). An inventory for measuring depression. *Archives of General Psychiatry, 4,* 561–571.

Beck, A. T., Weissman, A., Lester, D., & Trexler, L. (1974). Measurement of pessimism: The Hopelessness Scale. *Journal of Consulting and Clinical Psychology, 42*(6), 861–865.

Beck, A. T., Rush, A. J., Shaw, B. F., & Emery, G. (1979). *Cognitive therapy of depression.* New York: Guilford Press.

Beck, A. T., Hollon, S. D., Young, J. E., Bedrosian, R. C., & Budenz, D. (1985). Treatment of depression with cognitive therapy and amitriptyline. *Archives of General Psychiatry, 42,* 142–148.

Bishop, S., Miller, I. V., Norman, W., Buda, M., & Foulke, M. (1986). Cognitive therapy of psychotic depression: A case report. *Psychotherapy, 23*(1), 167–173.

Blackburn, I. M., Bishop, S., Glen, I. M., Whalley, L. J., & Christie, J. E. (1981). The efficacy of cognitive therapy in depression: A treatment trial using cognitive therapy and pharmacotherapy, each alone and in combination. *British Journal of Psychiatry, 139*, 181–189.

Bowers, W. A. (1988). *A comparison of three therapeutic approaches to the treatment of depression with inpatients: Cognitive therapy plus medication, relaxation therapy plus medication.* Submitted for publication.

de Jong, R., Henrich, G., & Ferstal, R. (1981). A behavioral treatment programme for neurotic depression. *Behavior Analysis and Modification, 23*(1), 167–287.

de Jong, R., Treiber, R., & Henrich, G. (1986). Effectiveness of two psychological treatments for inpatients with severe and chronic depression. *Cognitive Therapy and Research, 10*(6), 645–663.

Emery, G., Hollon, S. D., & Bedrosian, R. C. (1981). *New direction in cognitive therapy.* New York: Guilford Press.

Freeman, A. (1987). *Group cognitive therapy model with inpatients.* Unpublished manuscript.

Glantz, M. D. (1987). Day hospital treatment of alcoholics. In A. Freeman & V. Greenwood (Eds.), *Cognitive therapy: Applications in psychiatric and medical settings* (pp. 51–68). New York: Human Sciences Press.

Greenwood, V. B. (1987). Cognitive therapy with the young adult chronic patient. In A. Freeman & V. Greenwood, (Eds.), *Cognitive therapy: Applications in psychiatric and medical settings* (pp. 103–116). New York: Human Sciences Press.

Hibbard, M. R., Gordon, W. A., Egelko, S., & Langer, K. (1987). Issues in the diagnosis and cognitive therapy of depression in brain-damaged individuals. In A. Freeman & V. Greenwood (Eds.), *Cognitive therapy: Applications in psychiatric and medical settings* (183–197). New York: Human Sciences Press.

Hamilton, M. (1960). A rating scale for depression. *Journal of Neurology, Neurosurgery, and Psychiatry, 23*, 56–62.

Hollan, S. D., & Kendall, P. (1980). Cognitive self-statements in depression: Development of an automatic thoughts questionnaire. *Cognitive Therapy and Research, 4*(4), 41–50.

Hollon, S. D., & Beck, A. T. (1986). Cognitive and cognitive-behavioral therapies. In S. L. Garfield & A. E. Bergin (Eds.), *Handbook of psychotherapy and behavior change, Vol. III* (pp. 443–482). New York John Wiley & Sons.

Hollon, S. D., DeRubeis, R. J., Evans, M. D., Tauson, V. B., Weimer, M. J., & Garvey, M. J. (1986). *Cognitive therapy, pharmacotherapy, and combined cognitive-pharmacotherapy in the treatment of depression: Differential outcome.* Unpublished manuscript. University of Minnesota and St. Paul-Ramsey Medical Center, Minneapolis-St. Paul, MN.

Margolis, R. B., & Shemberg, K. M. (1976). Cognitive self-instruction in process and reactive schizophrenics: A failure to replicate. *Behavior Therapy, 7*, 668–671.

Meichenbaum, D. (1977). *Cognitive-behavior modification: An integrative approach.* New York: Plenum Press.

Meichenbaum, D., & Cameron, R. (1973). Training schizophrenics to talk to themselves: A means of developing attentional controls. *Behavior Therapy, 4*, 515–534.

Miller, I. V., Bishop, S. D., Norman, W. H., & Keitner, G. I. (1985). Cognitive/behavioral therapy and pharmacotherapy with chronic, drug-refractory depressed inpatients: A note of optimism. *Behavioral Psychotherapy, 13*, 320–327.

Murphy, G. E., Simons, A. E., Wetzel, R. D., & Lustman, P. J. (1984). Cognitive therapy and pharmacotherapy: Singly and together in the treatment of depression. *Archives of General Psychiatry, 41*, 33–41.

Perris, C., Rodhe, K., Palm, A., Abelson, M., Hellgren, S., Livja, C., & Soderman, H. (1987). Fully integrated in- and outpatient services in a psychiatric sector: Implementation of a new model for the care of psychiatric patients favoring continuity of care. In A. Freeman & V. Greenwood (Eds.), *Cognitive therapy: Applications in psychiatric and medical settings* (pp. 117–131) New York: Human Sciences Press.

Rush, A. J., Beck, A. T., Kovacs, M., & Hollon, S. (1977). Comparative efficacy of cognitive therapy and pharmacotherapy in the treatment of depressed patients. *Cognitive Therapy and Research, 1*, 17–37.

Sacco, W. P. (1981). Cognitive therapy in-vivo. In G. Emery, S. D. Hollon, & R. C. Bedrosian (Eds.), *New directions in cognitive therapy* (pp. 271–287). New York: Guilford Press.

Schrodt, G. R., & Wright, J. H. (1987). Inpatient treatment of adolescents. In A. Freeman & V. Greenwood, (Eds.), *Cognitive therapy: Applications in psychiatric and medical settings* (pp. 69–82). New York: Human Sciences Press.

Shaw, B. F. (1980). *Predictors of successful outcome in cognitive therapy: A pilot study*. Paper presented at the First World Congress on Behavior Therapy, Jerusalem, Israel.

Shaw, B. F. (1981). Cognitive therapy with an inpatient population. In G. Emery, S. D. Hollon, & R. C. Bedrosian (Eds.), *New direction in cognitive therapy* (pp. 29–49). New York: Guilford Press.

Simons, A. D., Garfield, S. L., & Murphy, G. E. (1984). The process of change in cognitive therapy and pharmacotherapy for depression. *Archives of General Psychiatry, 41,* 45–51.

Weissman, A. N. (1979). *The Dysfunctional Attitudes Scale: A validation study*. Unpublished PhD dissertation, University of Pennsylvania.

Weissman, M. M., Prusoff, B. A., DiMascio, Å., Neu, C., Golkany, M., & Klerman, G. L. (1979). The efficacy of drugs and psychotherapy in the treatment of acute depressive episodes. *American Journal of Psychiatry, 136,* 555–558.

Wright, J. H. (1987). Cognitive therapy and medications as combined treatment. In A. Freeman & V. Greenwood (Eds.), *Cognitive therapy: Applications in psychiatric and medical settings* (pp. 36–50). New York: Human Sciences Press.

Wright, J. H., Barrett, C. L., Linder, L. H., Chase, S., Weinstein, G., & Hurst, H. (1987). Nortriptyline effects on cognition in depression, Unpublished manuscript.

# Epilogue: Synthesis and Prospects for the Future

Our goal in compiling this volume, as expressed in the title, was to make it as comprehensive a handbook as possible. In the pursuit of that goal, the volume has grown far beyond our original plans. Upon discussing our ideas with colleagues around the United States and in Europe, we added chapters that highlighted the application of Cognitive Therapy to new populations with clinical problems that previously had not been systematically treated within a cognitive behavioral mode. Having assumed a basic model, the various contributors have stretched the limits of that model beyond the treatment of depression or anxiety. The ingenuity and creativity of these new applications are noteworthy in that they expand Beck's model of Cognitive Therapy greatly while staying within the overiding theoretical framework. There is a "parochial eclecticism" that does not merely offer the reader an addition to his or her therapeutic bag of techniques, but rather encourages the mastery of a basic model, and then offers ways of expanding and modifying that model to best fit the needs of particular patients or patient types.

It is for this reason, that the first part of this volume is so important. It sets out the theoretical model that is then applied in the second part. If the reader has gone straight to the treatment section of this volume in an attempt to immediately acquire the techniques and skills necessary to treat the patient that he or she is seeing in the next hour, we think that it is important to go back and carefully review the theoretical basis for the Cognitive Therapy model so well set out by our contributors in Part I. For those readers who think that the technique alone is sufficient, we would offer the following anecdote. A story is told of the Jewish father who goes to see the Rabbi in a small Russian village with a complaint against his son. "Rabbi, my son wishes to become an atheist. What shall I do?" "Send him to me," said the Rabbi. The young man came to the Rabbi. The Rabbi asked him, "I am told that you wish to become an atheist. Is this true?" "Yes, Rabbi," replied the youth. "Young man, have you mastered the Torah?" "No, Rabbi," he replied. "Have you mastered the Talmud and the Mishnah?" "No, Rabbi." "Have you studied the mystical Cabbala?" Once again the response was "No." "Then," said the Rabbi, "you must first master the basic texts, before you choose to abandon them." The lesson holds true in the present context. It is essential to master the basic material before modifying it, ignoring it, or leaving it.

We hope that it is obvious that one does not become a skilled therapist in any model by reading any handbook. However, since Cognitive Therapy is a relatively new approach, there are many clinicians who are interested in Cognitive Therapy but who have not had access to

597

training programs. Freeman, Pretzer, Fleming, and Simon (1989) point out the variety of options available to the practitioner who wishes to develop or enhance skills in Cognitive Therapy. These include formal training, individual or group supervision, peer consultation, self-assessment, use of client feedback, and, of course, reading and study of relevant books and journals.

Formal training programs in Cognitive Therapy are now much more accessible to practicing therapists than has been the case in the past. At one time, persons interested in training had no recourse but to travel to Philadelphia to study with Beck and his colleagues, or to New York to study with Ellis and his colleagues. Currently, there are Cognitive Therapy programs that offer a variety of training options in many locations throughout the United States and Europe. We are aware of training programs that exist in Philadelphia, Atlanta, Cleveland, San Diego, Boston, Newport Beach, New York, Seattle, and Washington, D.C., in addition to programs in Stockholm and Umea (Sweden), Trondheim (Norway), Buenos Aires (Argentina), Santiago (Chile), and Copenhagen (Denmark). Ellis and his colleagues offer intensive short-term training programs at various sites. Workshops, institutes and seminars in Cognitive Therapy are also offered periodically at other locations sponsored by private agencies, hospitals, state or local associations, and at a number of national conventions. These include the American Psychological Association, American Psychiatric Association, and the Association for Advancement of Behavior Therapy. The annual convention of the Association for Advancement of Behavior Therapy (AABT) usually offers a number of workshops and preconvention institutes on Cognitive Therapy and, in addition, many of the papers and symposia presented at this convention are relevant to the theoretical basis and clinical applications of Cognitive Therapy.

Expert supervision is the most effective way to develop skill in the practice of Cognitive Therapy. Several models of supervision have been used in training cognitive therapists in addition to the traditional preceptor model in which supervisor and supervisee meet regularly to discuss the supervisee's experiences and problems with clients. Moorey and Burns (1983) describe an apprenticeship model of training in which the trainee works along with a more experienced therapist as a co-therapist and gradually takes increasing responsibility for conducting the therapy session as his or her skill grows. A second supervision model is the group supervision model described by Childress and Burns (1983).

By reviewing videotapes or audiotapes of therapy sessions or observing live therapy sessions, the supervisor can get a clearer picture of exactly what goes on in the therapy session and can provide the supervisee with valuable feedback. Role-playing of therapist–client interactions with the supervisor or another supervisee in a supervision group acting as the client can provide clinicians with valuable practice in executing interventions and an opportunity to experiment with alternative approaches to a particular problem. By reversing roles so that the supervisee plays the client and the supervisor plays the therapist, supervisees can learn from the therapist's example as well as gaining insight into the client's perspective. Finally, by framing conceptualizations of clients as hypotheses to be tested in subsequent therapy sessions, the supervisor and supervisee frequently can replace theoretical debates with data collection and avoid being misled by misconceptions.

Throughout supervision, the supervisor must be sensitive to therapeutic "blind spots" that the supervisee may have. Although the supervisor–supervisee relationship should not become psychotherapeutic, it may well be necessary to help the supervisee address some of his or her dysfunctional thoughts or beliefs in order to overcome his or her difficulty with certain types of problems or clients (Ellis, 1985).

Another valuable, though underutilized, option for developing skill in Cognitive Therapy is a regularly scheduled consultation group consisting of peers who are also interested in skill improvement. Although it might seem at first glance that consultation with peers who are no more expert than oneself would have little to offer, one does not have to be a superior player to be an excellent coach. Nonexpert peers can offer each other valuable feedback and support inasmuch as it is often possible to see the mistakes or problems of others before one becomes equally self-observant. Interested professionals can meet regularly to review a case presented with accompanying audiotape or videotape material or relevant readings. The case can then be discussed in terms of the case conceptualization, goals of the therapy, therapy process, and specific interventions. Suggestions can be made and follow-up offered from previous peer consultation/supervision sessions. An important focus in the sessions would be the specific therapist–client interactions or problem situations. In this regard we would advise the use of videotapes and role plays when possible.

When peer consultation is not available, a practitioner can greatly facilitate the development of his or her skills by regularly assessing his or her own progress as a cognitive therapist. The Cognitive Therapy Rating Scale developed by Young and Beck (1980) and revised by Freeman *et al.* (1989) provides an objective method of assessing the quality of a Cognitive Therapy session. When it is necessary for an individual to rely on self-assessment, it is important to record sessions and then complete the Cognitive Therapy Scale while reviewing the recording, as it is virtually impossible to accurately be a participant observer and then rate performance after the session. Self-assessment can also be done in a variety of other ways. The practice of maintaining complete session or progress notes and periodically reviewing them enables the therapist to obtain a clearer view of the process and progress of the therapy than is possible on an informal session-by-session basis. Charting progress by graphing the client's weekly scores on the Beck Depression Inventory and other relevant measures provides both client and therapist with valuable feedback regarding treatment progress or treatment problems. Finally, the therapist can identify and overcome many impediments to effective therapy by monitoring his or her own automatic thoughts and responding to them where necessary.

Many clients respond to therapy with intelligence, sensitivity, and integrity and can be an excellent source of feedback regarding the progress of therapy, the therapist–client relationship, the therapist's performance and, to some degree, therapist competence. Beck, Rush, Shaw, and Emery (1979) suggest that the therapist encourage client feedback throughout the session and explicitly invite client feedback at the beginning and end of each session. This feedback lets the therapist know whether he or she is understanding the client and can be particularly valuable in identifying problems in the therapist–client relationship before they disrupt therapy.

The literature in the cognitive-behavioral approaches is a rapidly growing one. The only practical way to keep abreast of new developments is to read widely. In addition to the new books which appear on a regular basis and the articles published in "mainstream" journals in psychology and psychiatry, two specialized journals are particularly valuable. *Cognitive Therapy and Research* (Plenum Press, New York) is a research-oriented journal which publishes many of the new empirical studies as well as a limited number of theoretical or clinically-oriented articles. *The Journal of Cognitive Psychotherapy: An International Quarterly* (Springer Press, New York) is oriented towards clinical practice and publishes clinical and theoretical papers as well as empirical papers which are clinically applicable.

It is important to remember that skill in therapy is not a static entity that is permanently engrained once it has been obtained. It is incumbent upon even the most skilled therapist to periodically assess his or her performance, to consult with colleagues regularly, and to keep abreast of new developments in this rapidly developing field.

This volume was difficult to end. New material is constantly being developed and published. The reader may have reached the Epilogue and wondered why we have excluded the work of a particular author, a particular orientation or the treatment of a particular patient group. The reason is simply that given the limits of space and time, we had to bring the volume to a close. Having said that, we offer the theoretical and clinical material in this volume as a beginning for the reader. Our hope is that the reader will integrate the treatment models discussed in this volume into his or her particular treatment focus and style. We encourage the reader to systematically introduce the cognitive behavioral model into his or her clinical practice. Having done that, we recommend that the reader evaluate the success and efficacy of the model, and make the necessary adjustments and modifications. We hope that the further extension of the cognitive therapy model will come from these therapeutic experiments of our readers, and that the next edition of this comprehensive handbook will include them.

## REFERENCES

Beck, A. T., Rush, A. J., Shaw, B. F., & Emery, G. (1979). *Cognitive therapy of depression*. New York: Guilford.

Childress, A. R., & Burns, D. (1983). The group supervision model in cognitive therapy training. In A. Freeman, *Cognitive therapy with couples and groups* (pp. 323–335). New York: Plenum Press.

Ellis, A. (1985). *Overcoming resistance: Rational Emotive Therapy with difficult clients*. New York: Springer.

Freeman, A., Pretzer, J., Fleming, B., & Simon, K. M. (1989). *Clinical applications of cognitive therapy*. New York: Plenum Press.

Moorey, S., & Burns, D. (1983). The apprenticeship model: Training in cognitive therapy by participation. In A. Freeman, *Cognitive therapy with couples and groups* (pp. 303–321). New York: Plenum Press.

Young, J., & Beck, A. T. (1980). *Cognitive therapy scale: Rating manual*. Unpublished manuscript. Philadelphia: Center for Cognitive Therapy.

# About the Authors

## HAL ARKOWITZ

Hal Arkowitz is an associate professor of psychology at the University of Arizona. He has published in the areas of social anxiety, depression, and psychotherapy. For the past few years, he has been working on the integration of behavioral and psychodynamic therapies, as represented by his book (co-edited with Stanley Messer) entitled *Psychoanalytic Therapy and Behavior Therapy: Is Integration Possible?* (Plenum, 1985). His most recent research centers on the development and empirical testing of an integrated behavioral-psychodynamic model of depression.

## DONALD H. BAUCOM

Donald H. Baucom is an associate professor of Psychology at the University of North Carolina at Chapel Hill. His research program is two-fold. One focus is on evaluating the effectiveness of various cognitive-behavioral intervention strategies with maritally distressed couples. The second focus is on basic research attempting to provide an understanding of the mechanisms of marital discord. His most recent work includes a marital-therapy outcome study exploring whether or not the effectiveness of behavioral marital therapy can be increased by the inclusion of additional cognitive and affective intervention techniques. He is presently co-authoring a book with Norman Epstein on cognitive-behavioral intervention strategies for maritally distressed couples.

## AARON T. BECK

Aaron T. Beck, M.D., is internationally known as "The Founder of Cognitive Therapy." Dr. Beck is considered one of the four most influential psychotherapists currently alive, and his groundbreaking monograph on cognitive therapy and depression is among the five most influential books of all time in psychotherapy.

Dr. Beck is University Professor of Psychiatry at the University of Pennsylvania School of Medicine and director of its Center for Cognitive Therapy. He is the author of over 200 scientific and scholarly articles and monographs, and of six books on depression, anxiety, suicide, and cognitive therapy. A former president of the Society for Psychotherapy Research,

601

he has received the Foundation Fund Prize for Research in Psychiatry of the American Psychiatric Association, the Paul Hoch Award of the American Psychopathological Association, and the Louis Dublin Award of the American Association of Suicidology. He received an honorary doctor of medical science degree from Brown University in 1982 and was elected a fellow of the Royal College of Psychiatrists in 1987.

## E. EDWARD BECKHAM

E. Edward Beckham is clinical psychologist and an assistant professor of psychiatry and behavioral sciences at the University of Oklahoma Health Sciences Center. He has been involved for the past 8 years in the NIMH Treatment of Depression Collaborative Research Program. He is co-editor of the *Handbook of Depression: Treatment, Assessment and Research,* and is co-author of two scales: the Cognitive Triad Inventory and the Coping Strategies Scale. His current research focuses on the role of individual differences in determining the outcome of psychotherapy for depression.

## LARRY E. BEUTLER

Larry E. Beutler is a professor of psychiatry and psychology, chief psychologist and director of clinical research in the Department of Psychiatry at the University of Arizona Health Sciences Center. He is an associate editor of the *Journal of Consulting and Clinical Psychology,* and has previously authored *Eclectic Psychotherapy: A Systematic Approach,* and co-authored *Group Cognitive Therapy: A Treatment Approach for Depressed Older Adults,* among other works. He is president of the Society for Psychotherapy Research, and currently directs the Affective Disorders Research Programs at the University of Arizona, Department of Psychiatry.

## MICHAEL D. BOLTWOOD

Michael D. Boltwood is currently a doctoral student in the Department of Counseling and Health Psychology at Stanford University. He has served as a clinical assistant professor of social work at the University of Washington and as co-principal investigator for the University of Washington Rehabilitation Study, which was a multidisciplinary study of the recovery of patients following a major burn injury. His current interests focus on health psychology, especially the relationship of emotions and cognitions to illness and health behaviors.

## WAYNE A. BOWERS

Wayne A. Bowers is clinical psychologist in the Department of Psychiatry at the University of Iowa. His research and theoretical work focus on the use of Cognitive Therapy with depression, anxiety, and eating disorders. He is currently researching Cognitive Therapy with social phobia, eating disorders, panic disorder, and depressed inpatients. Other research interests include change in cognitive process during Cognitive Therapy with anxiety and eating disorders. He is also responsible for the training of psychiatry residents in the use of Cognitive Therapy.

## JAMES C. COYNE

James C. Coyne is an associate professor of psychology in the Departments of Psychiatry and Family Practice at the University of Michigan Medical School. He is also a faculty associate at the Institute for Social Research in Ann Arbor, Michigan, and was a former director of research at the Mental Research Institute in Palo Alto. He is the editor of *Essential Papers on Depression* (New York University Press, 1986), and his article "The Role of Cognition in Depression" (*Psychological Bulletin*, 1983) was the single most cited article in the field of social sciences in that year. His research interests include depression, stress and coping, and marital and family factors in coping with chronic illness.

## DENISE DAVIS

Denise Davis is an assistant professor of clinical psychology in the Department of Psychiatry at Vanderbilt University School of Medicine. Her research, clinical practice, and teaching of psychology interns and psychiatry residents focuses on Cognitive Therapy and on disorders of high frequency among women, particularly anxiety and depression. Dr. Davis is co-authoring a book on cultural variables among women in cognitive therapy.

## RAYMOND DIGIUSEPPE

Raymond DiGiuseppe is an associate professor of psychology and director of the Graduate Program in School Psychology at St. John's University. In addition, he is director of Training and Research at the Institute for Rational-Emotive Therapy. He has co-authored *The Practitioner's Guide to Rational-Emotive Therapy, Rational-Emotive Therapy for Alcoholics and Substance Abusers, Rational-Emotive Couples Counseling*, and *Inside RET: A Critical Appraisal of the Theory and Therapy of Albert Ellis*. His clinical interest is the application of cognitive behavior therapies to children and adolescents.

## E. THOMAS DOWD

E. Thomas Dowd is a professor and director of counseling psychology training at Kent State University. He is a fellow of the American Psychological Association and a diplomate in counseling psychology of the American Board of Professional Psychology. He is co-editor of the *Journal of Cognitive Psychotherapy: An International Quarterly*. His areas of research interest are in Cognitive Therapy and paradoxical interventions.

## JANET SASSON EDGETTE

Janet Sasson Edgette is employed by The Devereux Foundation in the Philadelphia area, working with adolescents in a residential treatment setting. She is also associate director of the Milton H. Erickson Institute of Philadelphia and wrote "Tempest in a Teapot: Ethics and Erickson," published in the *Ericksonian Monographs, Number 5*.

## DAVID J. A. EDWARDS

David J. A. Edwards is a professor and head of the Department of Psychology at Rhodes University in South Africa, where he teaches Cognitive Therapy at the undergraduate level and in a professional clinical training program. He has published a number of journal articles on nonverbal behavior in social interaction, and on interracial attitudes and political identity. These include several cross-cultural studies. A recent paper on the application of guided imagery techniques to work with traumatic memories recently appeared in the *Journal of Cognitive Psychotherapy: An International Quarterly*. He also contributed a chapter entitled "Personality and Psychopathology" to a recently published introductory psychology text-book. His other teaching and research interests include the relationship between Cognitive Therapy and humanistic, existential, and phenomenological therapies, as well as transpersonal psychotherapy and community psychology.

## BRUCE N. EIMER

Bruce N. Eimer is clinical psychologist on staff in the Departments of Psychiatry and Rehabilitation medicine at Abington Memorial Hospital in Philadelphia. He also maintains a private practice specializing in the application of cognitive-behavioral treatments and hypnosis for teaching patients to cope more effectively with chronic illnesses. Dr. Eimer has published a number of papers in the areas of the psychological management of pain, psychotherapy, personality theory, psychological assessment for treatment planning, parenting issues, and children's social-cognitive development.

## ALBERT ELLIS

Albert Ellis is Executive Director of the Institute for Rational-Emotive Therapy in New York City. He is the founder of Rational-Emotive Therapy (RET) and is often called the grandfather of Cognitive-Behavioral Therapy (CBT). He is considered to be the most influential psychologist alive today. He has published more than 600 articles and more than 50 books, mainly on psychotherapy, love, marital and family relations, and sex therapy. His books include *Reason and Emotion in Psychotherapy, A New Guide to Rational Living* (with Robert A. Harper), *Overcoming Resistance: Rational-Emotive Therapy With Difficult Clients,* and *The Practice of Rational-Emotive Therapy* (with Windy Dryden). Ellis is a diplomate in clinical psychology of the American Board of Professional Psychology, a fellow of the American Psychological Association, and served as president of Divisions XII and XXIX of the American Psychological Association.

## NORMAN EPSTEIN

Norman Epstein is an associate professor in the Department of Family and Community Development at the University of Maryland, College Park. His research, theoretical work, and clinical practice focus on cognitive and behavioral factors that contribute to marital and family dysfunction. His books include *Depression in the Family* (co-edited with Arthur Freeman and Karen M. Simon) and the forthcoming volume *Cognitive-Behavioral Therapy with Families* (co-edited with Stephen E. Schlesinger and Windy Dryden). He is completing a book, *Cognitive-Behavioral Marital Therapy* (co-authored with Donald H. Baucom).

## ARTHUR FREEMAN

Arthur Freeman is a clinical associate professor of psychology in the Department of Psychiatry in the School of Medicine at the University of Pennsylvania, and Senior Supervisor at the Center for Cognitive Therapy at the University of Pennsylvania. He is a diplomate in clinical psychology of the American Board of Professional Psychology, a fellow in the Division of

Clinical Psychology of the American Psychological Association, and a fellow of the American Orthopsychiatric Association. Freeman has published a number of volumes in Cognitive Therapy including: *Cognitive Therapy with Couples and Groups; Cognition and Psychotherapy* (with M. J. Mahoney); *Cognitive Therapy: Applications in Psychiatric and Medical Settings* (with V. Greenwood); *Clinical Applications of Cognitive Therapy* (with J. Pretzer, B. Fleming, and K. M. Simon); *Cognitive Therapy of Suicidal Behavior: A Treatment Manual* (with M. Reinecke); *Depression in the Family* (with N. Epstein and K. M. Simon); and *Cognitive Therapy of Personality Disorders* (with Aaron T. Beck). His books have been translated into Spanish, Japanese, and Swedish. Freeman is also editor of the Behavior Therapist, and he has presented workshops in Cognitive Therapy in the United States, Scandanavia, South America, and Europe.

## MEYER D. GLANTZ

Meyer D. Glantz is the head of the Vulnerabilities Studies Program in the Division of Clinical Research at the National Institute on Drug Abuse. As part of his work there, he has written several articles investigating the misuse and abuse of drugs by the elderly. He is currently preparing an extended description of the use of Cognitive Therapy with the elderly. His clinical practice focuses on the development of Cognitive Therapy and its application to special populations. He has published several articles detailing a Cognitive Therapy protocol designed for use with alcoholics.

## JOEL O. GOLDBERG

Joel O. Goldberg is clinical psychologist at the Clarke Institute, and holds appointments in the Department of Psychiatry at the University of Toronto and in the Department of Psychology at York University. Dr. Goldberg is a practicum supervisor of doctoral candidates in assessment and therapy and has published articles on validation research with cognitive tasks and personality instruments.

## MARVIN R. GOLDFRIED

Marvin R. Goldfried is a professor of psychology and psychiatry at the State University of New York at Stony Brook. His current research involves investigation of the process of psychotherapeutic change as it occurs within different therapeutic orientations. He is co-author of *Clinical Behavior Therapy* (with Gerald C. Davison) and editor of *Converging Themes of Psychotherapy*. In addition to his teaching, research, and supervision, he maintains a limited private practice in New York City.

## LESLIE S. GREENBERG

Leslie S. Greenberg is a professor of psychology at York University. His research focuses on the process of change in psychotherapy and the role of emotion in change. He has co-authored *Patterns of Change: Intensive Analysis of Psychotherapeutic Process* (with L. Rice), *The Psychotherapeutic Process: A Research Handbook* (with W. Pinsof), *Emotion in Psychotherapy* (with J. Safron), and *Emotionally Focused Therapy for Couples* (with S. Johnson). Dr. Greenberg is currently interested in the integration of different approaches to the treatment of individuals, couples, and families.

# PAUL D. GUEST

Paul D. Guest is a staff psychologist at Patton State Hospital, where he is involved in providing direct services for severely disturbed patients and the predoctoral training of psychologists. In a recent article in the *Journal of Consulting and Clinical Psychology,* he explores the impact of supervision on the development of psychotherapists. His current interests focus on the relationship between treatment and the prediction of dangerousness among judicially committed patients.

# SHEENAH HANKIN-WESSLER

Sheenah Hankin-Wessler is a partner in Cognitive Psychotherapy Associates in New York. She has collaborated with Richard L. Wessler in many publications, and has contributed a chapter to *Cognitive-Behavioral Approaches to Psychotherapy* (Harper & Row, 1986).

# MO THERESE HANNAH

Mo Therese Hannah is currently a doctoral student in clinical psychology at the University of Arizona, Tucson. She has publications in the areas of cross-cultural and community psychology. She is now doing research on the identification of and services provision to the chronically mentally ill.

# W. J. JACOBS

W. J. Jacobs is an NSERC University Research Fellow and an assistant professor at the University of Lethbridge, Alberta, Canada. Dr. Jacobs' research interests include classical conditioning, spatial learning, and the application of animal models to human psychology. His current research and theoretical work is focused upon extending the range of a recently published neurodevelopmental model of simple phobias to panic attack and agoraphobia. He has contributed research and theoretical reports to *Psychological Review, Behavioral and Brain Sciences, American Psychologist, Psychobiology, Physiology, and Behavior, Pharmacology, Biochemistry, and Behavior, Pavlovian Journal of Biological Science, Canadian Journal of Psychology, Quarterly Journal of Experimental Psychology, Archives of Sexual Behavior, Society for the Neurosciences,* and *Advances in Consumer Research.*

# F. MATTHEW KRAMER

F. Matthew Kramer is a research psychologist at the U.S. Army Natick Research, Development, and Engineering Center, in Natick, Massachusetts. He received his doctorate in counseling psychology from the Pennsylvania State University before completing postdoctoral studies at the University of Minnesota and University of Pennsylvania. His research interests include obesity and the role of psychological and environmental factors on food choice and intake, and he has written over a dozen papers in these areas.

# RICHARD S. LAZARUS

Richard S. Lazarus has been a professor of psychology at the University of California at Berkeley for over 30 years. He started his career at Johns Hopkins in 1948, where he did research on personality and perception, and on projective techniques, and did psychotherapy in the campus clinic. He became director of Clinical Training at Clark University from 1953 to 1958 before coming to Berkeley and is a diplomate in clinical psychology of the American Board of Professional Psychology. He is well-known and much honored throughout the world for his programmatic research and theoretical efforts in the fields of psychological stress, emotion, coping, and adaptation, having published a classic book on a cognitive approach to psychological stress in 1966, followed by a recent and widely influential book in 1984 on these subjects.

## RUSSELL C. LEAF

Russell C. Leaf has been a professor of psychology at Rutgers University in New Brunswick for 20 years. Before coming to Rutgers in 1969, he served as Senior Research Psychopharmacologist at the Squibb Institute for Medical Research from 1963–1966, and then taught at Wesleyan University in Connecticut. He is the author of over 70 research articles in the areas of psychopharmacology and, more recently, clinical problems, including drug abuse and personality disorders. He is also the co-editor (with Richard C. DeBold) of *LSD, Man & Society* (Wesleyan University Press, 1967). Since 1986, he has served as director of clinical evaluation at the Institute for Rational-Emotive Therapy in New York.

## BARRY MCCARTHY

Barry McCarthy is a professor of psychology at American University. He has published extensively in the area of sexual function and dysfunction. His latest books are *Sexual Awareness: Enhancing Sexual Pleasure* and *Male Sexual Awareness: Increasing Sexual Pleasures*. Dr. McCarthy maintains a professional practice in clinical psychology, marital therapy, and sex therapy at the Washington Psychological Center. He conducts professional workshops in the areas of sexual trauma and psychotherapy with males.

## THOMAS V. MERLUZZI

Thomas V. Merluzzi is an associate professor of psychology at the University of Notre Dame. He has published articles on methods and uses of cognitive assessment with particular emphasis on the cognitive assessment of social anxiety. He co-edited (with Carol R. Glass and Myles Genest) a volume entitled *Cognitive Assessment,* which is a compilation of work in that area. Dr. Merluzzi's recent research examines information processing approaches to social anxiety and the uses of multidimensional scaling in clinical research.

## L. NADEL

L. Nadel is a professor of psychology and research cognitive scientist at the University of Arizona. His publications include *The Hippocampus as a Cognitive Map* (with John O'Keefe), *Neural Connections, Mental Computations* (with Lynn Cooper, Mike Harnish, and Peter Culicover), and *The Psychobiology of Down Syndrome*. He is editor of *Psychobiology,* and a member of the Scientific Advisory Board of the National Down Syndrome Society. His current research focuses on the implications of late maturation in specific brain systems, and the short-term and long-term impact of various experiences upon brain/behavioral development.

# TERRY M. PACE

Terry M. Pace is currently a doctoral student in counseling psychology at the University of Nebraska-Lincoln. Mr. Pace has published several articles on a variety of topics in counseling and clinical psychology. His most recent research has focused on applications of cognitive theory and methods to psychotherapy research and practice. Mr. Pace is completing his doctoral dissertation entitled "The Reconstruction of Depressive Self-Schemata through Cognitive Psychotherapy." Other areas of professional interest and involvement include applications of social influence theory and research to counseling, consultation, and community psychology, behavioral medicine/health psychology, and professional issues in the training and practice of psychologists and other health service providers.

# CHRISTINE PADESKY

Christine Padesky is a practicing psychotherapist and director of the Center for Cognitive Therapy in Newport Beach, California. Since 1982, she has conducted over 40 training workshops on Cognitive Therapy for mental health professionals throughout the United States and Europe, including year-long advanced training programs for established cognitive therapists. She is a consultant to hospital programs wishing to establish inpatient cognitive therapy units. Dr. Padesky is the founding editor of the *International Cognitive Therapy Newsletter,* and the author of articles on depression, stress, anxiety, children, and personality disorders. She and Dr. Davis are currently writing a book on Cognitive Therapy with women which expands their ideas presented in this handbook.

# CARLO PERRIS

Carlo Perris is a professor of psychiatry at the University of Umëa (Sweden) and Director of the WHO Collaborating Centre for Research and Training in Mental Health at the Umëa University, Department of Psychiatry. He is the President of the Swedish Association for Cognitive Psychotherapy. His publications include: "A study of bipolar (manic depressive) and unipolar recurrent depressive psychoses," which marked the beginning of a distinction between bipolar and unipolar affective disorders. He has published a book on Cognitive Therapy in Swedish. Another two books, *Cognitive Psychotherapy and the Schizophrenic Disorders* (Guilford) and *The Theory and Practice of Cognitive Psychotherapy,* with I. M. Backburn and H. Perris (Springer Verlag), are in press. His most recent research program is concerned with the development of small community based treatment units for intensive cognitive-behavioral psychotherapy with patients suffering from schizophrenic disorders.

# MAURICE F. PROUT

Maurice F. Prout is an assistant professor at Widener University, where he teaches at the Institute for Graduate Clinical Psychology. Dr. Prout is a fellow in the Behavior Therapy and Research Society and is a diplomate in clinical psychology of the American Board of Professional Psychology.

# LAURA RICE

Laura Rice is a professor *emeritus* in the Department of Psychology at York University, Ontario. She is the co-editor of *Patterns of Change: Intensive Analysis of Psychotherapeutic*

*Process* (with L. S. Greenberg) and *Innovations in Client-Centered Therapy* (with D. Wexler). She has published numerous research articles on the process of psychotherapy.

## HUGH ROSEN

Hugh Rosen is a professor in the Department of Mental Health Sciences at Hahnemann University, where he is director of the mental health technology associate and baccalaureate degree programs in the School of Allied Health Professions. He is also associate dean for students in that school. Dr. Rosen's books include *The Development of Sociomoral Knowledge* and *Piagetian Dimensions of Clinical Relevance*. He conducts a limited private practice of psychotherapy in Philadelphia.

## JEREMY SAFRAN

Jeremy Safran is director of the Cognitive Therapy Center at the Clarke Institute of Psychiatry, and an associate professor at the University of Toronto. He has published numerous articles in the area of cognitive interpersonal aspects of psychology. He is also the co-author of *Emotion in Psychotherapy* (with L. S. Greenberg).

## G. RANDOLPH SCHRODT, JR.

G. Randolph Schrodt, Jr., is an assistant professor of psychiatry and behavioral sciences at the University of Louisville School of Medicine, and associate clinical director of Norton Psychiatric Clinic. Dr. Schrodt's research and publications have focused on the psychobiology of adolescent affective disorders and the application of Cognitive Therapy with adolescents.

## BRIAN F. SHAW

Brian F. Shaw is the psychologist-in-chief of the Toronto General Hospital and an associate professor of psychiatry and behavioral science at the University of Toronto. His publications include *Anxiety Disorders: Psychological and Biological Perspectives* and *Cognitive Therapy of Depression*. Dr. Shaw's research focuses on risk factors in major depression and social phobia. He also develops cognitive-behavioral therapies for these disorders.

## KAREN M. SIMON

Karen M. Simon is a clinical associate in psychology in the Department of Psychiatry at the University of Pennsylvania School of Medicine. She is also a supervisor of psychotherapy at Beck's Center for Cognitive Therapy. Books by Dr. Simon, beside the current volume, include *Depression in the Family* (co-edited with Freeman and Epstein) and *Clinical Application of Cognitive Therapy* (co-authored with Freeman, Fleming, and Pretzer). Dr. Simon has published numerous chapters and articles on Cognitive Therapy, self-regulation, and psychopathology.

## LAURIE A. STALKER

Laurie A. Stalker received her doctorate in counseling psychology from the Pennsylvania State University. After completing a postdoctoral fellowship in eating disorders at the University of

Pennsylvania she has joined the faculty of the University of Massachusetts Medical Center. She is a practicing clinician specializing in the treatment of anorexia nervosa and bulimia. She is particularly interested in the development and impact of body image on eating disorders.

## D. J. TATARYN

D. J. Tataryn is working on his Ph.D. in clinical psychology at the University of Arizona. His primary interest is in the area of "unconscious influences on behavior," with published and current research in the areas of psychological repression, subliminal perception, nonconscious processing, and the uses of hypnosis for investigating these types of phenomena. He is also doing research on aspects of statistics and experimental methodology.

## JOHN T. WATKINS

John T. Watkins has been a practitioner, researcher, and teacher of cognitive psychotherapy for over 20 years. He is the principal investigator at the University of Oklahoma Health Sciences Center of the NIMH-sponsored treatment of depression collaborative research program, a multi-site study of the efficacy of psychotherapy in comparison with pharmacotherapy. He is a diplomate in clinical psychology of the American Board of Professional Psychology. Recently, he left full-time academic life to establish a private practice in Atlanta, Georgia.

## MARJORIE WEISHAAR

Marjorie Weishaar is a psychologist in private practice. She trained at the Center for Cognitive Therapy, University of Pennsylvania, and later worked at the V.A. Medical Center, Brown University, Providence, Rhode Island. Dr. Weishaar has written several chapters on cognitive therapy and its applications.

## RICHARD L. WESSLER

Richard L. Wessler is a professor and chairman of the Department of Psychology at Pace University in Westchester. He is a former director of the Institute for Rational-Emotive Therapy in New York, and is the co-author of *Six Group Therapies* (with S. Long) and *Cognitive Therapies with Couples and Groups* (with A. Freeman). He is currently publishing in the area of personality disorders.

## DAVID M. WHITE

David M. White received his doctorate in psychology from the University of Illinois at Urbana-Champaign. He currently is completing his postdoctoral clinical psychology respecialization training at the Department of Mental Health Sciences at Hahnemann University. Dr. White was awarded a fellowship at the California College of Medicine, University of California, Irvine, to evaluate the effects of pharmocological and cognitive-behavioral treatments for "hyperactive" or attention-deficit disordered children. His current professional interests include cognitive-behavioral treatments of pediatric populations, and community-living services for adults with mental illness.

Jesse H. Wright is a professor of psychiatry and behavioral sciences at the University of Louisville and medical director of the Norton Psychiatric Clinic. His research has focused on both biological and cognitive features of depression. Currently Dr. Wright is investigating interactions between pharmocotherapy and Cognitive Therapy. He is the author of *Cognitive Therapy of Depression* in the 1988 American Psychiatric Association's Annual Review of Psychiatry.

# Index

ISBN 0-306-43052-5

90000